ANNALS OF THE NEW YORK ACADEMY OF SCIENCES

Volume 1121

LINKING AFFECT TO ACTION

Critical Contributions of the Orbitofrontal Cortex

Edited by Geoffrey Schoenbaum, Jay A. Gottfried, Elisabeth A. Murray, and Seth J. Ramus

Published by Blackwell Publishing on behalf of the New York Academy of Sciences
Boston, Massachusetts
2007

Library of Congress Cataloging-in-Publication Data

Linking affect to action: critical contributions of the orbitofrontal
cortex/editors, Geoffrey Schoenbaum ... [et al.].
      p.; cm. – (Annals of the New York Academy of Sciences, ISSN
0077-8923)
   Includes bibliographical references.
   ISBN-13: 978-1-57331-683-5 (alk. paper)
   ISBN-10: 1-57331-683-0 (alk. paper)
      1. Prefrontal cortex. 2. Cognition–Physiological aspects. 3. Mental
illness–Physiological aspects. 4. Decision making–Physiological
aspects. I. Schoenbaum, Geoffrey. II. New York Academy of
Sciences. III. Series.
      [DNLM: 1. Prefrontal Cortex–physiology.
2. Prefrontal Cortex–physiopathology. 3. Decision
Making–physiology. 4. Mental Disorders–physiopathology. W1
AN626YL 2007/WL 307 L756 2007]

   QP383.17.L56 2007
   612.8'25–dc22

                                                            2007039309

The *Annals of the New York Academy of Sciences* (ISSN: 0077-8923 [print]; ISSN: 1749-
6632 [online]) is published 28 times a year on behalf of the New York Academy of Sciences
by Blackwell Publishing with offices at 350 Main St., Malden, MA 02148 USA; 9600
Garsington Road, Oxford, OX4 2ZG UK; and 600 North Bridge Rd, #05-01 Parkview
Square, 18878 Singapore.

Information for subscribers: For new orders, renewals, sample copy requests, claims,
changes of address and all other subscription correspondence please contact the Journals
Department at your nearest Blackwell office (address details listed above). UK office phone:
+44 (0)1865 778315, fax +44 (0)1865 471775; US office phone: 1-800-835-6770 (toll free
US) or 1-781-388-8599; fax: 1-781-388-8232; Asia office phone: +65 6511 8000, fax; +44
(0)1865 471775, Email: customerservices@blackwellpublishing.com

Subscription rates:
Institutional Premium   The Americas: $4043   Rest of World: £2246
The Premium institutional price also includes online access to full-text articles from 1997 to
present, where available. For other pricing options or more information about online
access to Blackwell Publishing journals, including access information and terms
and conditions, please visit www.blackwellpublishing. com/nyas
*Customers in Canada should add 6% GST or provide evidence of entitlement to exemption.
**Customer in the UK or EU: add the appropriate rate for VAT EC for non-registered
customers in countries where this is applicable. If you are registered for VAT please supply
your registration number.

Mailing: The *Annals of the New York Academy of Sciences* is mailed Standard Rate. Mailing
to rest of world by International Mail Express (IMEX). Canadian mail is sent by Canadian
publications mail agreement number 40573520. **Postmaster:** Send all address changes to
Annals of the New York Academy of Sciences, Blackwell Publishing Inc., Journals Subscription Department, 350 Main St., Malden, MA 02148-5020.

Membership information: Members may order copies of *Annals* volumes directly from
the Academy by visiting www.nyas.org/annals, emailing membership@nyas.org, faxing
212-298-3650, or calling 800-843-6927 (US only), or 212-298-8640 (International). For
more information on becoming a member of the New York Academy of Sciences, please
visit www.nyas.org/membership. Claims and inquiries on member orders should be directed
to the Academy at email: membership@nyas.org or Tel: 212-298-8640 (International) or
800-843-6927 (US only).

Printed in the USA. Printed on acid-free paper.

Disclaimer: The Publisher, the New York Academy of Sciences and the Editors cannot be held responsible for errors or any consequences arising from the use of information contained in this publication; the views and opinions expressed do not necessarily reflect those of the Publisher, the New York Academy of Sciences, or the Editors.

Annals are available to subscribers online at the New York Academy of Sciences and also at Blackwell Synergy. Visit www.blackwell-synergy.com or www.annalsnyas.org to search the articles and register for table of contents e-mail alerts. Access to full text and PDF downloads of *Annals* articles are available to nonmembers and subscribers on a pay-per-view basis at www.blackwell-synergy.com and www.annalsnyas.org.

The paper used in this publication meets the minimum requirements of the National Standard for Information Sciences Permanence of Paper for Printed Library Materials, ANSI Z39.48-1984.

ISSN: 0077-8923 (print); 1749-6632 (online)
ISBN-10: 1-57331-683-0 (paper); ISBN-13: 978-1-57331-683-5 (paper)

A catalogue record for this title is available from the British Library.

ANNALS OF THE NEW YORK ACADEMY OF SCIENCES

Volume 1121
December 2007

LINKING AFFECT TO ACTION

Critical Contributions of the Orbitofrontal Cortex

Editors
GEOFFREY SCHOENBAUM, JAY A. GOTTFRIED,
ELISABETH A. MURRAY, AND SETH J. RAMUS

This volume is the result of a conference sponsored by the New York Academy of Sciences, entitled **Linking Affect to Action: Critical Contributions of the Orbitofrontal Cortex**, held on March 11–14, 2007 in New York City.

CONTENTS

Financial assistance was received from:

- The National Institute on Drug Abuse/NIH
- The National Institute on Aging/NIH
- The National Institute of Mental Health/NIH
- The National Institute of Neurological Diseases and Stroke/NIH
- Astra Zeneca
- Bowdoin College
- Bristol-Myers Squibb
- Coulbourn Instruments
- Plexon
- Sanofi-Aventis, US, Inc.

Preface

The last 20 years have witnessed an explosive increase in research exploring the function of the orbitofrontal cortex. In 1987, when Dr. Goldman-Rakic described the circuitry of the primate prefrontal cortex and its role in regulating behavior, her seminal work encompassed 44 pages and included several hundred references; yet this article contained less than one page of material about the orbitofrontal subdivision of the prefrontal cortex. Only nine papers published that year included the term *orbitofrontal*.[a]

Since then, interest in the orbitofrontal cortex has increased substantially, with much of that growth occurring only in the last few years. For example, in 2000 the Society for Neuroscience published only 13 abstracts from its annual meeting that mentioned the term *orbitofrontal*, but this number had grown to 34 by 2004.[b] Further, in 2004, 187 papers that included this term were published. Since then, interest in the orbitofrontal cortex has continued to increase, reaching a publication rate of 37.4 papers per month thus far in 2007 (FIG. 1). This accelerated growth is partly attributable to the similarities in orbitofrontal function that appear to exist across species. These similarities are remarkable, despite the numerous subregions discernible within the orbitofrontal cortex and the evolutionary specializations of certain groups, such as primates, which have an expanded frontal cortex relative to other mammals. The relatively widespread recognition of these similarities has promoted research and fostered useful collaborations not only between research laboratories working in different animal models, but also between laboratories studying animal models and those investigating humans. Through this work, it is increasingly apparent that the orbitofrontal cortex figures prominently in a variety of behaviors that are disrupted in neurological and neuropsychiatric diseases. As a result, understanding the functions of this formerly obscure prefrontal cortical area has taken on new urgency.

For this reason, we thought the time was ripe for a scientific meeting on the topic of orbitofrontal cortex function, in part simply to provide a forum in which diverse labs studying the orbitofrontal cortex from different perspectives could interact. For example, the orbitofrontal cortex has been variously described as an olfactory association cortex by those interested in olfactory

---

[a]Numbers of published papers including the term *orbitofrontal* were obtained from searches on PubMed in September 2007; note that PubMed adds articles over time. Thus the numbers for past years may change marginally as additional articles are indexed.

[b]Numbers of abstracts mentioning the term *orbitofrontal* were obtained from searches of abstracts on the Society for Neuroscience Web site.

Ann. N.Y. Acad. Sci. 1121: xi–xiii (2007). © 2007 New York Academy of Sciences.
doi: 10.1196/annals.1401.040

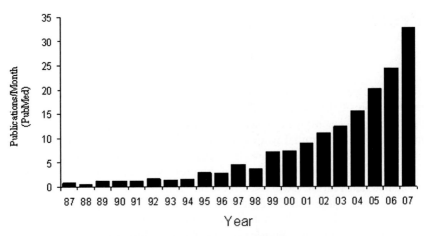

FIGURE 1. "Orbitofrontal" publication rate.

processing, a prefrontal working memory system by those interested in memory function, and a system for controlling emotions by those interested in limbic function. Rarely has the orbitofrontal cortex been considered a critical nexus linking these circuits, with an important general function (or functions) that may inform neural processing within each of these systems.

The chapters in this volume of the *Annals* are a result of this meeting, Linking Affect to Action: Critical Contributions of the Orbitofrontal Cortex, which was held in New York City between March 11–14, 2007 at the conference headquarters of the New York Academy of Sciences in an impressive new building at the World Trade Center. Here, a diverse collection of established investigators and junior researchers with a common interest in understanding the orbitofrontal cortex met to discuss recent work and outstanding issues, and also to consider whether general characteristics of orbitofrontal cortex function could be identified from disparate approaches spanning different species and different methodologies.

Following the organizational scheme of the conference, the present *Annals* volume has been organized into several themes. We start with sections that consider the defining features of the orbitofrontal cortex, including its anatomy in different species, its evolutionary ties to more primitive chemosensory processing systems, and its more recent role in general associative learning. Next, the volume considers how the orbitofrontal cortex interacts with the various circuits that are critical to learning, memory, affect, and decision making, including the hippocampus, amygdala, striatum, and other prefrontal areas. The volume concludes with a focus on orbitofrontal cortex dysfunction as it pertains to aging, addiction, and neuropsychiatric disease, with the hope that ideas generated in earlier chapters might shed light on the importance of pathological changes in the orbitofrontal cortex in these disease states.

It is our sincere hope that the ideas presented in this volume—like those at the meeting—will not only provide a foundation of common ground derived from the last 20 years of work on orbitofrontal cortex function, but also will highlight the critical issues in need of investigation over the next 20 years.

In closing, we would like to thank the speakers who contributed to the success of the meeting and to the content of this volume. We would also like to express our gratitude to all those who made this meeting possible through their generous financial support. Numerous agencies at the National Institutes of Health, including NIDA, NIMH, NINDS, and NIA, provided major support through a scientific grant, without which the meeting and present monograph would not have been possible. We are further grateful to Plexon, Coulbourn, Sanofi-Aventis, AstraZeneca, Bristol-Myers Squibb, and Bowdoin College for their key financial contributions. Finally we would like to thank the New York Academy of Sciences, including Shari Dermer, Kara-Leigh Dockery, and Stacie Bloom, for their excellent job in organizing and hosting such a fruitful meeting; and Kirk Jensen, Linda Mehta, Steven Bohall, and Ralph Brown, for their skillful editorial and production work on this volume.

—GEOFFREY SCHOENBAUM
University of Maryland School of Medicine
Baltimore, Maryland

—JAY A. GOTTFRIED
Northwestern University Feinberg School of Medicine
Chicago, Illinois

—ELISABETH A. MURRAY
National Institute of Mental Health
Bethesda, Maryland

—SETH J. RAMUS
Bowdoin College
Brunswick, Maine

Keynote Address: Revaluing the Orbital Prefrontal Cortex

R. J. DOLAN

Wellcome Trust Centre for Neuroimaging, University College London, London, United Kingdom

ABSTRACT: The importance of orbitofrontal cortex (OFC) in human behavioral regulation is no longer a matter of dispute, though its precise role remains a matter of ongoing investigation. It is ironic that this revaluation of OFC required a major departure from a historical nadir, during which it was viewed as redundant or "silent cortex," a situation that prevailed even up to the latter half of the 20th century. The increasing wealth of data from diverse fields within neuroscience now provides an unambiguous testament to the importance of this cortical region in behavioral regulation and cognition in general.

KEYWORDS: OFC; lobotomy; value

INTRODUCTION

Historically, the lowly status the orbitofrontal cortex (OFC) can be traced back to the 18th century, when the British surgeon Percivall Pott (1713–1788) (who it turns out provided the first account of an environmental basis to cancer, describing scrotal cancer in chimney sweeps), gave expression to what would become a prevailing view. Pott suggested that a brain injury "in or under the frontal bone" was of much less consequence than intracranial damage in any other location. He noted, "I will not assert it to be a general fact, but as far as my own experience and observation go, I think that I have seen more patients get well, whose injuries have been in or under the frontal bone, than any other bones of the cranium. If this should be found to be generally true, may not the reason be worth enquiring into."[1] One hundred years later, John Harlow, who documented the tragic fate of Phineas Gage, may well have been articulating what had become canonical medical lore when he asserted that the sector brain traversed by the tamping iron was "the best fitted of any ... to sustain the injury."[2,3]

Address for correspondence: R. J. Dolan, Wellcome Trust Centre for Neuroimaging, UCL, London WC1N 3BG. Voice: +44 207 833 7453; fax: +44 207 833 1445.
r.dolan@fil.ion.ucl.ac.uk

Ann. N.Y. Acad. Sci. 1121: 1–9 (2007). © 2007 New York Academy of Sciences.
doi: 10.1196/annals.1401.020

1

PSYCHOSURGERY

The lowly status attributed to OFC found an institutional expression with the birth, and widespread tolerance, of psychosurgical lobotomy in the treatment of psychiatric disorders. It is hard to imagine that this practice would have been tolerated had this cortical region been ascribed any reasonably defined function. Cynically, one might conclude that an unchartered sector of brain is as vulnerable as uninhabited patches of earth, ripe for exploitation by the unscrupulous. Apologists for this form of medical intervention have argued that psychosurgery provided relief in an era that preceded the psychopharmacological revolution.[4]

Psychosurgery, a dominant and dramatic form of treatment in psychiatry between the 1940s and the 1960s, was developed by Egas Moniz. Moniz was Professor of Neurology, in Lisbon, Portugal. He became aware of the potential effects of ablation of prefrontal cortex in 1935 when, at a conference in London, he heard a description of the effects on chimpanzees who had ablations to their prefrontal cortex. What grabbed his attention was an observation that one of the animals was apparently "cured" of an "experimental neurosis." The "experimental neurosis" in this case was nothing short of temper tantrums in an animal who was a subject in experiments designed to assess the contribution of the frontal lobes to performance of a delayed-response task. This anecdotal report of the effects of experimental training on a single animal was enough to spur Moniz who, in collaboration with his neurosurgical colleague, Almeida Lima, introduced the technique known as pre-frontal leukotomy just 1 year later. Moniz was not unaware of widespread skepticism in relation to the procedure. Quoting a colleague, he liked to assert that "the indignation of those who oppose lobotomy tests rests in the subconscious conviction that the removal of a part of the brain robs a man of part of his soul."[5]

The procedure preferred by Moniz's surgeon Almeida Lima (1903–1985) involved using an instrument called a leukotome, which was passed into the frontal white matter via burr holes drilled into the vertex of the skull above each frontal lobe. The tip of the leukotome contained a wire loop, which when extended and rotated resulted in a core of tissue being disconnected from the surrounding white matter. Moniz and Lima (1936) published on 20 patients submitted to this new technique, that conformed to the rule of thirds: 7 were considered cured, 7 improved significantly, and 6 were unchanged.[6] The immediate impact of leukotomy can be gauged from the fact that Moniz was awarded the Nobel Prize in Medicine in 1949 for pioneering the development of the technique.

PSYCHOSURGERY AND PSYCHIATRY

Psychosurgery might have been confined to the dustbin of heroic psychiatric practices were it not for the Pauline proselytizing zeal of Walter Freeman, an

American neurologist. In collaboration with his neurosurgical colleague James Watts, he introduced a technique that involved making a cut to the entire white matter of the frontal lobes, his so-called standard lobotomy. At a time where empirical evidence had a low premium, it was often the character of a practitioner that determined the acceptance of a medical treatment. Freeman might reasonably be inferred to have expressed a low risk aversion and indeed, prior to embarking on leukotomy, he had developed a rapid procedure for obtaining a spinal fluid which he referred to as "my jiffy spinal tap," which involved inserting a needle through the foramen magnum into the cisterna magna.[7]

Nor surprisingly, Freeman was interested in a rapid lobotomy technique, and this led him to develop what came to be known as the trans-orbital lobotomy, a procedure that involved gaining access to the frontal lobes by driving an instrument that was akin to an ice-pick behind the eyeballs, passing through the orbital roof, and then cutting the white matter. Here the procedure primarily targeted the connections between the OFC and the rest of the brain. What is now shocking to learn is that Freeman carried out his early operations not in an operating theater, but in his office and was not averse to operating on the those unwilling, or indeed incapable, to give consent. A single operating session might involve performing lobotomies on up to 20 patients, which in practice meant taking no more than 10 min per patient. His most famous patient (operated upon by James Watts) was Rosemary Kennedy, the sister of the future President. During the procedure, performed following administration of a mild tranquillizer he asked her to recite "God Bless America."[7]

Freeman performed his last lobotomy in Berkeley, California, in February 1967 at the age of 72. Throughout his career he continued to advocate lobotomy in the face of all evidence against its effectiveness. Any scientific justification for the procedure remained opaque, though Freeman subscribed to a view that consciousness is mediated by the frontal lobes but added that "we believe there can be too much of a good thing." He suggested its contribution to consciousness is its ability to project an image of the individual into the future coupled with a recognition of this image as the self. A second contribution of the frontal lobes, he asserted, was in providing an "affective facet, the emotional charge connected with that image." At his most articulate, he ascribed to a view that the prefrontal lobotomy acts specifically by reducing the affective component of the image as self as constructed by the frontal lobes, a justification succinctly summed up in his comment, one assumes drawn from anecdotal observation, that "prefrontal lobotomy bleaches the affective component connected with the consciousness of the self."[8]

The shame of the tolerance of lobotomy extends beyond the undoubted harm done to the vulnerable and ill and their undoubtedly disappointed families and loved ones. It indicts, in particular, regulatory authorities who tolerated an extreme procedure for which there was a clear lack of scientific justification, let alone evidence of therapeutic efficacy. Needless to say, there has never been much in the way of systematic evaluation of the effects on cognition of lobotomy, though a notable exception are studies by Stuss *et al*.[9–13]

The era of psychosurgery raises important questions in relation to current interest in the functions of the OFC. Why, if we now assume the OFC is pivotal for human behavioral regulation, were seriously damaging consequences not evident in the thousands of patients subjected to this procedure? One obvious argument might be that its negative effects were masked by virtue of the procedure being inflicted on the mentally ill. I would suggest there was a deeper reason, and this relates to what we now recognize as one of the core functions of OFC, namely in value representation. Historically, psychiatry and neurology, and to a lesser degree psychology, all have had a conceptual difficulty in accepting that subtle aspects of human behavioral regulation and character, including that encompassing the domain of moral behavior, might have a major physiological basis.[14]

REASSESSING THE ROLE OF OFC

Harlow's detailed account of Phineas Gage is widely viewed as the first detailed description of brain injury resulting in a change of character. However, it is almost certainly the case that the problem of acquired character change consequent upon brain damage was already recognized as a source of burden to society. For example, take a 16th century account, from William Shakespeare's Stratford-upon-Avon, of a petition raised requesting that the town be "eased of the charge of one Lewis Gilbert, a maimed soldier in Ireland." Before serving in an Elizabethan military expedition to quell unrest in Ireland, Gilbert was an upstanding member of society who worked as a butcher.[15] On his return he became a public burden being accused of forcible entry, failure to pay debts, and finally stabbing a neighbor to death in a quarrel. Although we have no detail of his actual injury, it is striking that the petition focuses entirely on behavioral changes rather than any physical deformity and implicitly endorses a lack of culpability on his behalf in relation to his misdemeanors and indeed a murder attributed to him.

The highly documented and famous case of Phineas Gage has now been the subject of countless descriptions. It is worth pointing out one class of problem that seems especially relevant to our contemporary understanding of the role of OFC. This is seen in Harlow's observation that his patient "does not estimate size or money accurately, although he has memory as perfect as ever. He would not take $1000 for a few pebbles which he took from an ancient river bed where he was at work." He goes on to describe that he "purchased some articles at the store, enquired to the price, and paid the money with his habitual accuracy; did not appear to be particular as to the price, provided he had money to meet."[16] This description seems particularly pertinent to views that the OFC contributes to valuation, including abstract valuation.

THE REDISCOVERY OF THE OFC

The first half of the 20th century was not without figureheads who recognized the importance of the orbital prefrontal cortex. Alexander Luria, in his book *Higher Cortical Functions in Man* (1980), noted that clinical observation pointed to the fact that no sensory or motor effects arise consequent upon electrical stimulation in the frontal lobes. He noted also that massive lesions of the frontal lobes are unaccompanied by obvious disturbances of visual, auditory, or tactile sensations, or indeed any disturbance of movement. He strongly refuted any conclusion that might seem to logically ensue from such observation, namely that the frontal lobes have no clearly defined function and must, in keeping with prevailing views, be regarded as "silent zones" of cortex. Instead, he noted that "careful observation of complex forms of animal behavior and, in particular, complex forms of human conscious activity lead to completely different conclusions regarding the function of the frontal lobes."[17]

Luria noted that almost all patients with lesions of the frontal lobe loose a "critical faculty" by which he meant an ability to evaluate behavior and the adequacy of actions. He characterized different variants of frontal lobe syndrome based upon an anatomical differentiation. For example, he observed that damage or pathology to the frontal lobes that involves the basal division results in a tendency toward impulsive action, trivial jokes, and euphoria without significant change in intelligence. Furthermore, with lesions to this sector he observed that the syndrome profile shifts towards affective disturbance leading to disturbance of character and personality.[17]

It is important to mention two other key figures who recognized the importance of the OFC, Karl Pribram and William Nauta. Pribram reported that with ablation of prefrontal cortex, reinforcement of motor reactions in a choice situation did not bring about the predicted change in an animal's behavior. In seminal observations, which anticipated reinforcement learning accounts of action learning, he concluded that disregard for the effect of one's own movement, which he referred to as a success signal or mistake signal, is an essential sign of disturbed of behavior consequent upon resection of the frontal lobes.[18] In simple terms Pribram appears to have here captured the idea that a discrepancy between an intention and an outcome, that might be thought of as a prediction error, was no longer expressed in the context of OFC damage.

Nauta highlighted a putative role of OFC in affective guidance of decision making.[19] He suggested that when an individual embarks on a course of action that involves a choice between alternatives, the choice is likely to be strongly determined by a comparison of the affective responses evoked by each of the alternatives. He commented that "if this were indeed the case, it would be readily understandable that loss of frontal cortex as a major mediator of information exchange between cerebral cortex and the limbic system is followed not only by an impairment of strategic choice making, but also by a tendency of projected or current action systems to 'fade out' or become over-ridden by interfering influences."

A landmark account of the role of OFC in behavioral regulation is the clinical paper of Eslinger and Damasio.[20] Their patient, EVR, following resection of an orbitofrontal meningioma, acquired a profound impairment in his ability to make advantageous choices, both in his personal and social life. EVR was described as "not spontaneously motivated for action. He seemed not to have available, automatically, programs of actions capable of driving him to motion." The authors noted that while damage to OFC may not impact on intellectual function, as ascertained in classical tests of intelligence, it does impact on subtle components of behavioral regulation. Thus, the most striking observation was the dissociation between intact cognitive abilities measured in standardized tests and poor utilization of these abilities in real-world environments. The core observation in this single case study has been widely replicated. In a detailed analysis of a large cohort of patients with brain injury, including a large cohort with frontal injuries, it was noted that with ventro-medial prefrontal cortex (VMPFC) damage the most common symptoms include blunted emotional experience, poorly modulated emotional responses, defective social decision making, impaired goal directed behavior, and lack of insight.[21]

THE SOMATIC MARKER HYPOTHESIS

An important theory to emerge out of renewed interest in the behavioral effects of damage to OFC, particularly the VMPFC sector, is the somatic marker hypothesis. A basic premise of this hypothesis is that visceral sensory signals are mapped in OFC. As a consequence, patients with damage to VMPFC make poor decisions partly because they do not elicit somatic responses that index the consequences of their actions as positive or negative. In simple terms the theory proposes that VMPFC elicits visceral responses that reflect the anticipated value of future choices, a process that is enhanced under decision making under uncertainty. Decision making under uncertainty is thus seen as eliciting gut feelings or hunches that inform or bias decision making based upon a forward model.

The idea of guidance of behavior on the basis of future likelihood of reward or punishment, as suggested in the somatic marker hypothesis, is an idea captured within the formalism of reinforcement learning theory of the likely consequences of decision options.[22] Reinforcement learning in its simplest form encapsulates the problem faced by an agent who learns, not by instruction, but through trial-and-error interactions within an environment. The key idea is that under conditions of uncertainty, as in unsupervised settings, learning is driven by a prediction error signal. There is now good evidence that encoding of a prediction error signal for reward is expressed within the OFC, among other regions.[23]

The other key clinical area that has transformed our understanding of OFC is the demarcation of a group of conditions often known as fronto-temporal dementias. These conditions represent a spectrum of disorders in which the brunt of the pathology is expressed in ventral prefrontal cortex and anterior temporal lobes.[24] Descriptions of patients with these conditions indicate that disturbance of emotion and behavior dominate the clinical picture, particularly in early stages, and overshadow any deficits in intellectual function. Among the most frequently noted deficits are disturbances of eating habits often associated with increased acquisition of preferences for sweet foods and lack of satiety, again reflecting problems in value representation in the broad sense.

CONTEMPORARY PERSPECTIVES ON THE ROLE OF OFC

The shift in view regarding the role of the OFC, initially brought about by clinical observation, has led to an ever-increasing interest in defining the behavioral affiliations of this cortical region. Consequently, the OFC is now a prime focus for investigators whose approaches subsume electrophysiology, classical lesion deficit models, neuropsychology, behavioral economics, and functional neuroimaging, to mention a few. One common theme to emerge from these diverse approaches is that this structure is critical to an ability to flexibly represent and update the value of stimuli or states that contribute to long-term behavioral guidance. In this frame of reference, value representation guides behavior by indexing whether options for action are likely to be associated with reward or punishment, not only in the short term but also in the long term. This is nicely encapsulated in the suggestion that OFC is critical for integrating the incentive value of outcomes with predictive cues in the service of behavioral guidance.[25]

Many issues remain regarding the role of OFC, including a key issue of functional specialization, its relative contribution to affect as opposed to cognition, the specification of its precise role in behavioral guidance, the control influences it exerts over more remote structures in emotional regulation, and how neuromodulatory systems bias key functions implemented in this region. At a more clinical level, it seems likely that OFC has a key role in expression of a range of psychopathologies where, as indeed we know to be the case for OFC, there is no primary deficit in intellectual function but major deficits in motivation and behavioral control. Examples here include clinical depression, but also conditions such as psychopathy, obsessive compulsive disorder, addictive behavior, and attention deficit disorders. What no longer seems preposterous, to reprise Moniz, is the idea that that damage to the OFC might indeed rob a person of their very soul.

REFERENCES

1. DOBSON, J. 1972. Percivall Pott. Ann. R. Coll. Surg. Engl. **50:** 54–65.
2. HARLOW, J.M. 1848. Passage of an iron rod through the head. Boston Medical and Surgical Journal **39:** 389–393.
3. HARLOW, J.M. 1868. Recovery from the passage of an iron rod through the head. Massachusetts Medical Society **2:** 327–346.
4. EL-HAI, J. 2007. The Lobotomist: a Maverick Medical Genius and His Tragic Guest to Rid the World of Mental Illness. John Wiley & Sons. Hoboken, New Jersey.
5. MONIZ, E. 1948. How I came to perform prefrontal leucotomy. *In* Proceedings of the First International Congress of Psychosurgery. Lisbon.
6. MONIZ, E. 1936. Essai d'un traitement surgical de certaines psychoses. Bulletin de l'Academie de Medicine **115:** 385–392.
7. VALENSTEIN, E.S. 1986. Great and Desperate Cures: the Rise and Decline of Psychosurgery and Other Radical Treatments for Mental Illness. Harper Collins. New York.
8. FREEMAN, W. & J.W. WATTS. 1941. The frontal lobes and consciousness of self. Psychosom. Med. **3:** 111–119.
9. STUSS, D.T. *et al.* 1984. The effects of prefrontal leucotomy on visuoperceptive and visuoconstructive tests. Bull. Clin. Neurosci. **49:** 43–51.
10. STUSS, D.T. & D.F. BENSON. 1984. Neuropsychological studies of the frontal lobes. Psychol. Bull. **95:** 3–28.
11. STUSS, D.T. *et al.* 1981. Leucotomized and nonleucotomized schizophrenics: comparison on tests of attention. Biol. Psychiatry **16:** 1085–1100.
12. STUSS, D.T. *et al.* 1981. Long-term effects of prefrontal leucotomy–an overview of neuropsychologic residuals. J. Clin. Neuropsychol. **3:** 13–32.
13. BENSON, D.F. *et al.* 1981. The long-term effects of prefrontal leukotomy. Arch. Neurol. **38:** 165–169.
14. DOLAN, R.J. 1999. On the neurology of morals. Nat. Neurosci. **2:** 927–929.
15. SHAPIRO, J. 2005. A Year in the Life of William Shakespeare: 1599. Harper Collins. New York.
16. MACMILLAN, M. 2000. An Odd Kind of Fame. MIT Press. Cambridge, Massachusetts.
17. LURIA, A.R. 1980. The Higher Cortical Functions in Man. Basic Books. New York.
18. PRIBRAM, K.H. 1959. The Intrinsic Systems of the Forebrain. McGraw-Hill. New York.
19. NAUTA, W.J.H. 1971. The problem of the frontal lobe: a reinterpretation. J. Psychiatr. Res. **8:** 167–187.
20. ESLINGER, P.J. & A.R. DAMASIO. 1985. Severe disturbance of higher cognition after bilateral frontal lobe ablation: patient EVR. Neurology **35:** 1731–1741.
21. BARRASH, J., D. TRANEL & S.W. ANDERSON. 2000. Acquired personality disturbances associated with bilateral damage to the ventromedial prefrontal region. Dev. Neuropsychol. **18:** 355–381.
22. SUTTON, R. & A. BARTO. 1998. Reinforcement Learning; An Introduction (Adaptive Computation & Machine Learning). MIT Press. Cambridge, MA.

23. O'DOHERTY, J.P. *et al.* 2003. Temporal difference models and reward-related learning in the human brain. Neuron **38:** 329–337.
24. NEARY, D. *et al.* 1988. Dementia of frontal lobe type. J. Neurol. Neurosurg. Psychiatry **51:** 353–361.
25. SCHOENBAUM, G., M.R. ROESCH & T.A. STALNAKER. 2006. Orbitofrontal cortex, decision-making and drug addiction. Trends Neurosci. **29:** 116–124.

Specialized Elements of Orbitofrontal Cortex in Primates

HELEN BARBAS

Department of Health Sciences, Boston University, Program in Neuroscience, Boston University, Boston, Massachusetts, USA

ABSTRACT: The orbitofrontal cortex is associated with encoding the significance of stimuli within an emotional context, and its connections can be understood in this light. This large cortical region is architectonically heterogeneous, but its connections and functions can be summarized by a broad grouping of areas by cortical type into posterior and anterior sectors. The posterior (limbic) orbitofrontal region is composed of agranular and dysgranular-type cortices and has unique connections with primary olfactory areas and rich connections with high-order sensory association cortices. Posterior orbitofrontal areas are further distinguished by dense and distinct patterns of connections with the amygdala and memory-related anterior temporal lobe structures that may convey signals about emotional import and their memory. The special sets of connections suggest that the posterior orbitofrontal cortex is the primary region for the perception of emotions. In contrast to orbitofrontal areas, posterior medial prefrontal areas in the anterior cingulate are not multi-modal, but have strong connections with auditory association cortices, brain stem vocalization, and autonomic structures, in pathways that may mediate emotional communication and autonomic activation in emotional arousal. Posterior orbitofrontal areas communicate with anterior orbitofrontal areas and, through feedback projections, with lateral prefrontal and other cortices, suggesting a sequence of information processing for emotions. Pathology in orbitofrontal cortex may remove feedback input to sensory cortices, dissociating emotional context from sensory content and impairing the ability to interpret events.

KEYWORDS: orbitofrontal connections; laminar patterns of connections; emotions; inhibitory systems; sequential pathways; emotional memory; temporal structures; intercalated amygdalar neurons; anxiety disorders

Address for correspondence: Helen Barbas, Department of Health Sciences, Program in Neuroscience, Boston University, 635 Commonwealth Ave., Room 431, Boston, MA 02215. Fax: 617-353-7567.
barbas@bu.edu
http://www.bu.edu/neural

Ann. N.Y. Acad. Sci. 1121: 10–32 (2007). © 2007 New York Academy of Sciences.
doi: 10.1196/annals.1401.015

OVERVIEW

The orbitofrontal cortex has been associated with emotional processing in general and specifically with encoding the significance and value of stimuli. As such, stimuli gain or lose relevance based on their association with reward, and the responses of neurons in orbitofrontal cortex reflect this flexibility and paramount regard for context. The anatomic features of the orbitofrontal cortex are best understood within the framework of its salient functional features, and the detailed circuitry, in turn, can inform behavioral and functional studies. A holistic view of the structure and function of the orbitofrontal cortex is necessary to understand its complex organization. This short review focuses on the essential structure and principal connections that underlie the functions that distinguish the orbitofrontal cortices, and which are frequently disrupted in psychiatric diseases.

EXTENT OF ORBITOFRONTAL CORTEX

The orbitofrontal cortex in primates is a large and heterogeneous region, and both its extent and architectonic areas have been variously described. In rhesus monkeys, the basal surface of the prefrontal cortex includes area 13, the orbital part of area 12, the rostrally situated area 11, and the basal part of area 10, which are shown in nearly all maps of the region in macaque monkeys and humans.[1–6] One map distinguishes two other regions in the posterior part of the basal surface of the rhesus monkey (areas OPAll and OPro),[2] and in another map area 13 has been subdivided into several sectors.[3] In a previous study,[2] all these areas have been considered to be the basal part of the basoventral series of prefrontal areas (FIG. 1B). The ventral extension of this series includes the ventrolateral prefrontal cortices[2] (FIG. 1C). References to orbitofrontal cortex here pertain to the basal areas (FIG. 1B).

The orbitofrontal areas are distinct from the series of areas on the medial wall of the prefrontal cortex, which are considered part of a mediodorsal series of cortices.[2] The medial component of this region includes all medial prefrontal areas (FIG. 1A), which are anatomically continuous with dorsolateral prefrontal cortices.[2] The medial prefrontal region can be subdivided into an anterior sector, which includes areas 10, 9, and 14. The posterior part includes the anterior cingulate areas 32, 24, 25, and MPAll. In rhesus monkeys, areas 14 and 25 have a small basal component[2] whose connections are similar to the areas in the anterior cingulate and are part of the mediodorsal series of prefrontal areas. The basal part of area 25 is called caudal area 14 in some maps (e.g., Ref. 3). There is general agreement that the medial areas (including the basal components of areas 14 and 25) have sets of connections that distinguish them from the areas found on the basal surface, as will be described briefly later.

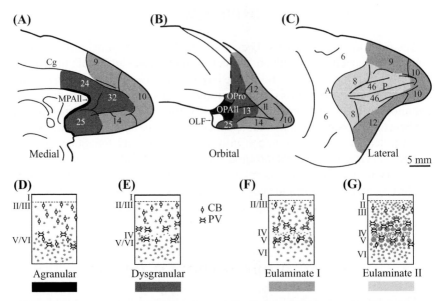

FIGURE 1. The three surfaces of the prefrontal cortex in the rhesus monkey: **(A)** the medial surface; **(B)** the basal surface showing the orbitofrontal cortex; **(C)** the lateral surface. **(D-G)** Cartoon showing differences in the type of cortex: D, agranular; E, dysgranular; F, G, eulaminate. There is an increase in the density of neurons (grey dots) in the direction from agranular (D) to eulaminate II (G) areas, and a concomitant decrease in the density of the neurochemical class of inhibitory neurons labeled with calbindin (CB), and an increase in the density of parvalbumin (PV) inhibitory neurons. Type is depicted in different shades of gray. Numbers designate architectonic areas; Abbreviations: A, arcuate sulcus; Cg, cingulate sulcus; MPAll, medial periallocortical area; OLF, olfactory area; OPAll, orbital periallocortical area; OPro, orbital proisocorticortical area; P, principal sulcus.

ARCHITECTURE OF ORBITOFRONTAL CORTICES

To Lump or to Split?

Situated on the basal surface of the frontal lobe, the orbitofrontal cortex has several architectonic areas that have been variously subdivided (reviewed in Ref. 7). Since the classic map of Walker,[1] some investigators have parcellated this region into relatively broad areas,[2,5,8] while others have proposed finer architectonic subdivisions based on novel markers beyond the classical tools of cytoarchitecture and myeloarchitecture.[3]

Disagreements in placing architectonic borders seem to be based on the tendency of some investigators to split areas at points of subtle differences in architecture, which others consider to be parts of one area. One way to increase agreement among investigators is to use unbiased quantitative approaches to determine the density of specific markers that are sensitive in showing architectonic borders. Quantitative data then can be used for different analyses. For example, the density of neural markers that are differentially expressed across areas, and are thus sensitive in showing architectonic borders, can be used to construct "fingerprints" of areas. If adjacent areas look different using quantitative measures, then the border is justified; if they appear to be similar, then they can be considered to be one area.

FIGURE 2 shows examples of the use of unbiased quantitative methods to construct fingerprints of some key orbitofrontal areas, using the density of all neurons, as well as specific neurochemical classes of inhibitory neurons that express the calcium-binding proteins parvalbumin (PV) or calbindin (CB), which are useful architectonic markers,[3,9–12] as shown in the cartoon in FIGURE 1D–G. Differences in the shape of the triangular plots reflect differences in architecture among the areas. Quantitative data can also be used to carry out multi-dimensional analyses by taking into consideration many architectonic features simultaneously, a task that cannot be easily accomplished by serial observations. Multiple independent analyses can be employed to determine whether they yield the same results. FIGURE 3A shows the results of multi-dimensional analysis of architectonic data in the prefrontal cortex of rhesus monkeys using 17 parameter dimensions.[9] The closer the areas are in the two-dimensional space, the more similar they are in their architectonic features. An independent cluster analysis shows a similar ordering of areas (FIG. 3B).

Architecture and Function

Structure frequently provides important insights on function. The primary visual cortex (area V1) in gyrencephalic primates, for example, has the most recognizable cortical architecture and a readily identified architectonic border with area V2. In early-processing visual cortices, the architecture coincides with detailed maps of the entire sensory periphery in each area. In progressively rostral higher-order visual association areas, however, the borders of areas are more difficult to define and so are the physiological properties of neurons.

Do the functions of the orbitofrontal cortex coincide with architectonic borders? Neurons in the orbitofrontal cortex that show responses to particular stimuli, or fire in distinct aspects of a behavioral task, are not restricted within architectonic areas (reviewed in Ref. 13). Additionally, functional imaging studies in behaving humans have recorded activation within relatively broad areas that encompass several architectonic areas or subareas.[14] This is hardly surprising in view of findings that the responses of orbitofrontal neurons to sensory stimuli depend on behavioral context. For example, in a behavioral task, neurons that respond to a triangle serving as a positive stimulus associated with reward, but not to a square not associated with reward, switch their responses when the association of the stimuli with reward is reversed.[15,16]

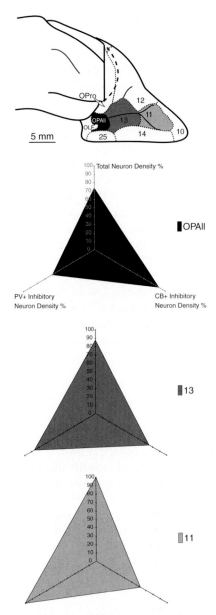

FIGURE 2. Fingerprints of some architectonic areas of the orbitofrontal cortex. The fingerprints were constructed from normalized quantitative data showing the density of all neurons and the density of PV and CB inhibitory neurons, which aid in parcellating architectonic areas. Differences in the shape of the triangles reflect differences in the architecture of these areas along the three parameter dimensions. The depicted orbitofrontal areas are shown on the basal surface (top), and include (from top to bottom), areas OPAll (agranular, type 1), area 13 (dysgranular, type 2) and area 11 (eulaminate, type 3). Scale gradations and labels in central and bottom triangles are as in the top triangle.

(A)   (B)

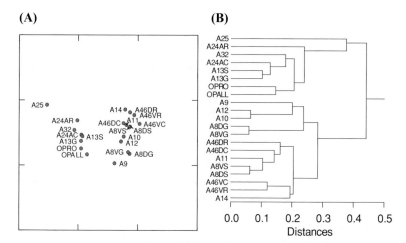

FIGURE 3. Sorting prefrontal architectonic areas by multiple architectonic features. **(A)** Multi-dimensional analysis using 17 parameter dimensions shows that limbic areas (agranular and dysgranular areas) segregate on the left. Orbitofrontal areas are seen at the bottom left (areas 13, OPRO, and OPALL), and anterior cingulate areas are seen at the top left (areas 25, 24, and 32). Eulaminate areas sort to the right. **(B)** An independent cluster analysis shows similar relationship of prefrontal areas to each other as in the multi-dimensional analysis. Reprinted from Ref. 9, with permission.

Architecture and Connections

In some cases architectonic areas coincide with specific connections. The well-defined V1 area in primates, for example, is linked in a highly specific pattern with the thalamic dorsal lateral geniculate nucleus, with cortical area V2, and with area MT. In many cases, however, the connections of cortical areas do not respect architectonic borders. The connections of the orbitofrontal cortex, in particular, are highly distributed. For example, the thalamic connections of orbitofrontal cortex include over 25 nuclei and their subdivisions, even though about half of all thalamic projection neurons are found in the mediodorsal nucleus (for discussion and references see 17, 18). Abrupt disappearance of connection fields close to major anatomic landmarks, such as the depths of sulci, reflect the mechanics of folding of the cortex rather than changes in architecture.[19]

It's clear that neither the function nor the connections coincide with architectonic borders in the orbitofrontal cortex. These findings are consistent with the flexible responses of orbitofrontal neurons within a behavioral context. Below follows a discussion of special aspects of the architecture and connections of orbitofrontal cortex, demonstrating that broader subdivisions of this region are a better match of its anatomic and functional organization.

Global versus Local Architecture and Connections

A different approach to architecture is to group areas by cortical type.[2,8,20] The methods of parcellating by architecture and by type share some features but also have key differences. Architectonic areas are mapped on the basis of local features, such as the shape or size of neurons in different layers, which vary among areas and give each area its unique architectonic signature. Architectonic differences can be seen in Nissl-stained sections, which show all neurons, or in tissue stained for markers that label distinct groups of pyramidal neurons or inhibitory interneurons (e.g., Ref. 3). The fingerprints in FIGURE 2 were constructed using three markers for different architectonic areas of the orbitofrontal cortex.

Grouping architectonic areas by type, on the other hand, relies on global structural features that are common among several areas, such as the number of identifiable layers, the presence or absence of layer IV, neuronal density, and others. For example, areas that have fewer than six layers are different in type than areas that have six layers. To use an analogy, grouping by cortical type is like grouping people by similar height or weight. The people in each group have in common height or weight, though individuals within the group differ in facial features. Grouping areas by type is possible because large cortical systems, such as the prefrontal, visual, auditory, somatosensory, etc., vary gradually and systematically in cortical structure (reviewed in Ref. 21). Limbic areas fall into two major types (agranular and dysgranular), and eulaminate areas can be grouped into two or more types, depending on the structure of the region and by how fine the divisions one wishes to make.

The orbitofrontal cortex can be classified into three types of cortex, as shown in FIGURE 1. The area depicted in black in the posterior orbitofrontal cortex is agranular in type, with only three identifiable layers and a lower neuronal density than the other areas. This area is situated close to the olfactory areas. The adjacent orbitofrontal areas (depicted in dark grey), are dysgranular in type, differing from the agranular by the presence of a poorly developed layer IV. These two types of cortices describe limbic cortices. The anterior part of the orbitofrontal cortex consists of eulaminate cortex (depicted in FIG. 1B in light grey), meaning that it has six layers, including an identifiable granular layer IV. These three types of cortices have also been described for the human orbitofrontal cortex.[22]

Cortical Type and Patterns of Connections in Orbitofrontal Cortex

The significance of type in understanding cortical organization emerged from observations that areas with similar structure are interconnected. Most cortical connections occur between neighboring regions, coinciding with similarity in structure. In the prefrontal cortex, areas are robustly connected with

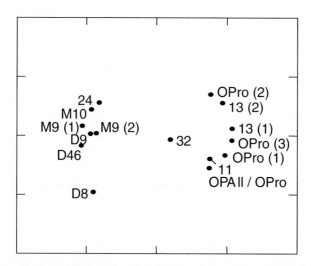

FIGURE 4. Sorting of prefrontal cortices by the entire complement of their connections with other prefrontal cortices. Cases with injection of tracers in orbitofrontal areas sort to the right and cases with injections in medial and lateral prefrontal areas sort to the left. The closer the areas, the greater the similarity in their sets of connections. Numbers in parentheses show results from injection of retrograde tracers in different experiments. Adapted from Ref. 23, with permission.

their immediate neighbors and a neighbor plus one.[2] Connections beyond that are sparser, except for areas that belong to the same structural type.[23] Dysgranular area 32 on the medial surface, for example, is robustly connected with dysgranular posterior orbitofrontal areas, even though they are not close neighbors and differ in their local architecture. FIGURE 4 shows the relatedness of several prefrontal areas by the pattern of their connections with other prefrontal cortices seen after a multi-dimensional analysis.[23] Orbitofrontal cortices cluster to the right by virtue of their similar connections.

Moreover, cortical type underlies the laminar pattern of corticocortical connections.[24] The structural model for connections emerged with the observation that certain areas of the cortex have similar laminar patterns of connections. Limbic areas, for example, which are either agranular or dysgranular in type, project to the six-layered eulaminate areas mostly through their deep layers regardless of their position in the cortex.[20] In contrast, eulaminate areas project to limbic areas mostly through their upper layers. The principal determinant of the laminar pattern of connections is the relative difference in structure between linked areas, as seen in various systems and species.[10,11,25,26] In this model, each area is categorized by cortical type and given a numerical rating based on its structure (1–4 for cortical types D–G in FIG. 1). According to the structural model, feedforward projections, which originate in the upper layers and innervate the middle layers, describe those that link areas with either more layers or higher neuronal density than the area of termination. Feedback connections, which originate in the deep layers and terminate in the superficial layers, link areas with fewer layers or lower neuronal density than the site of termination. Lateral connections, which originate in layers II-III and V-VI and terminate in all layers, link areas with similar structure. Moreover, since the structure of areas within a cortical region, such as the prefrontal, is graded,[2] the relative difference in the structure of areas is also graded, and so is the relative distribution of connections within cortical layers.[24]

Accordingly, the connections of neighboring orbitofrontal areas with similar structure show a columnar pattern of efferent connections. Further predictions can be made on the basis of the relative differences in the type of linked orbitofrontal areas. Broad grouping of areas into structural types of cortex, therefore, can be used to distill complex connections into a few patterns. Further, this approach makes it possible to predict the laminar pattern of connections in humans on the basis of cortical structure.

We have seen that unique connections do not describe specific architectonic areas on the orbitofrontal cortex, but sets and patterns of connections are seen for groups of areas. Below we explore how antero-posterior division of the orbitofrontal cortex based on cortical type provides useful insights on the connectivity and function of the region.

DISTINCTIVE FEATURES OF ORBITOFRONTAL CORTEX

Antero-posterior Orbitofrontal Divisions by Cortical Type

Connections that differentiate orbitofrontal cortices occur along an antero-posterior division, consistent with changes in cortical type (FIG. 1B). The posterior orbitofrontal areas (black and dark gray in FIG. 1B) differ in their connections not only with cortical but also with subcortical structures[8,27,28] (reviewed in Refs. 7, 29, 30). The posterior orbitofrontal cortex is strikingly multi-modal, perhaps the most so among all cortices. It receives projections from primary olfactory areas, the gustatory cortex, and high-order visual, somatosensory, gustatory, and auditory association areas. The latter originate in the superior temporal gyrus and in the lower bank of the lateral fissure,[10,27] which are connected with earlier-processing auditory cortices (reviewed in Ref. 21) and respond to auditory stimuli in macaque monkeys.[31]

The most distinctive feature of posterior orbitofrontal cortex is its prominent connection with the olfactory areas,[27,32] which lie adjacent to posterior orbitofrontal cortex (FIG. 1B, OLF, white area). Olfactory input to posterior orbitofrontal cortex originates from the piriform cortex and the anterior olfactory nucleus,[27] which are primary olfactory areas (reviewed in Ref. 33), a feature it does not share with its rostral neighbors. Interestingly, the primary olfactory areas are thought to represent high levels of processing (for discussion see

Shepherd, this volume[34]), perhaps comparable to the highly processed inputs originating from high-order sensory association and polymodal cortices that also project to orbitofrontal cortex.

Connections of Orbitofrontal Cortex with the Amygdala

The posterior orbitofrontal cortex is further distinguished by its connections with the amygdala. The amygdala has widespread connections with the entire prefrontal cortex (e.g., Refs. 8, 35–44), but its connections with posterior orbitofrontal cortex and the anterior cingulate are considerably denser.[45] Axons from the amygdala terminate densely in bands within layers I-II of many prefrontal cortices.[35,39] However, only the limbic prefrontal areas in the posterior orbitofrontal and anterior cingulate areas receive amygdalar projections in their middle layers as well, or in columns that span the entire cortical thickness.[45] Moreover, unlike other areas, the prefrontal limbic areas issue significant projections to the amygdala from layers II and III, in addition to the predominant projections from layer V.[45]

Specificity of the Connections of Posterior Orbitofrontal Cortex with the Amygdala

The posterior orbitofrontal cortex has a unique pattern of connections with the amygdala, sending projections that terminate in a U-shaped pattern around the borders of the magnocellular basolateral nucleus (FIG. 5). The heaviest terminations in this projection target the intercalated masses of the amygdala,[46] which are entirely inhibitory in primates,[47] as well as in several other species. These small inhibitory neurons project to the central nucleus of the amygdala,[47–52] which sends inhibitory projections to hypothalamic and brain stem autonomic structures.[46,53,54]

The heavy and unique projection to the intercalated masses is unidirectional and originates exclusively from posterior orbitofrontal cortex. The dynamics of this pathway have yet to be investigated at the physiological level. Nevertheless, as shown in FIGURE 6, this pathway has specific functional implications, namely, a net effect of suppressing activity in the central nucleus and removing its inhibitory influence on hypothalamic and brain stem autonomic centers, and may thus increase autonomic drive in emotional arousal.[55] In addition, there is a lighter direct pathway from the posterior orbitofrontal cortex to the central nucleus of the amygdala,[40,46] whose activation would be expected to have the opposite effect, inhibition of autonomic centers (FIG. 6). This pathway potentially can suppress central autonomic drive and help return the system to autonomic homeostasis as circumstances change.

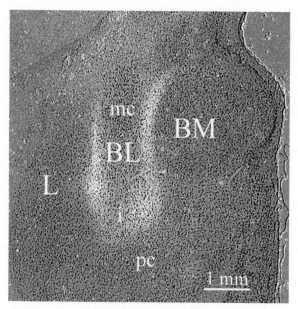

FIGURE 5. The unique innervation of the amygdala by posterior orbitofrontal cortex. Darkfield and brightfield (double exposure) photomicrograph of a coronal section through the amygdala, showing the termination of axons from posterior orbitofrontal cortex in the amygdala. Axons from posterior orbitofrontal cortex terminate heavily (white grain) onto the inhibitory intercalated masses of the amygdala, which are interposed between nuclei of the amygdala, separating the lateral (L) from the basolateral (BL) and basomedial (BM, also known as accessory basal) nuclei. mc and pc refer, respectively, to the magnocellular and parvicellular sectors of the basolateral nucleus. Adapted from Ref. 46.

The Dialogue between the Amygdala and Orbitofrontal Cortex

The amygdala receives projections from the same sensory association cortices as the orbitofrontal cortex (reviewed in Ref. 56). Moreover, projections from auditory and visual association cortices innervate heavily the posterior half of the amygdala, the same parts that are connected with the orbitofrontal cortex.[46] This evidence indicates that the orbitofrontal cortex receives direct projections from sensory association cortices[27,57] and potentially indirect sensory input through the amygdala.[56] Interestingly, projections from the amygdala target each layer of orbitofrontal cortex to a different extent, including significant projections to the middle layers.[45] By analogy with sensory systems, these unusual pathways to the middle layers may convey feedforward information from the amygdala to orbitofrontal cortex pertaining to the emotional significance of events. The strong interactions of the orbitofrontal cortex with the amygdala may help explain why neurons in the orbitofrontal cortex respond within the framework of behavioral context, encoding the value of

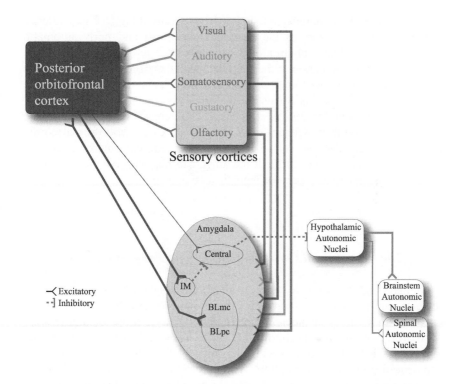

FIGURE 6. Summary of the connections of posterior orbitofrontal cortex. Bidirectional connections of cortices from every sensory modality give the orbitofrontal cortex its multi-modal features. The same sensory association areas project to the amygdala (most of these pathways are likely bidirectional, not shown). The posterior orbitofrontal cortex has robust bidirectional connections with the basal complex of the amygdala (only the basolateral, BL, nucleus is shown). The posterior orbitofrontal cortex also targets robustly the intercalated masses of the amygdala (IM), which project and inhibit the central nucleus of the amygdala, which inhibits hypothalamic autonomic centers; the latter innervate brain stem and spinal autonomic nuclei, which innervate peripheral organs. Activation of this pathway is expected to disinhibit the hypothalamus, allowing its activation in emotional arousal. A lighter pathway from the posterior orbitofrontal cortex innervates the central nucleus of the amygdala. Activation of this pathway is expected to inhibit hypothalamic autonomic centers, perhaps for return of the system to autonomic homeostasis.

stimuli, forming reward associations in cognitive tasks, and responding to stimuli when they are significant for the task at hand, but cease to respond when the reward contingencies change[58–69] (reviewed in Refs. 70–72).

Feedforward projections from the amygdala to orbitofrontal cortex may have additional functions. Activity in the amygdala increases in response to faces showing emotional expressions even when they are presented quickly and below the level of awareness.[73] In rats, a short subcortical loop connecting the amygdala with the thalamus can support fear conditioning.[74] This evidence suggests that the circuits of the amygdala allow fast and fairly automatic processing for vigilance in emotional situations. It is possible that the robust and bidirectional interaction of the amygdala with the orbitofrontal cortex may be necessary for the conscious appreciation of the emotional significance of the environment. This view is consistent with the classic findings of Kennard,[75] who suggested that the cortex is necessary for conscious perception. The direct projections from sensory association cortices to orbitofrontal cortex may provide an overview of the content of the external environment, and the indirect sensory input through the amygdala may provide the emotional context necessary to interpret the significance of events.[56]

The Orbitofrontal Cortex and Memory for Emotional Events

Animals learn to associate stimuli with reward in a large variety of tasks (for reviews see Refs. 76, 77). Neurons in orbitofrontal cortex reflect this ability by encoding in memory changes in reward contingencies in behavioral tasks.[69] Moreover, neurons in the orbitofrontal cortex respond to stimuli that predict reward.[64] What are the pathways that may mediate the process of remembering behaviorally relevant information? The connections of orbitofrontal cortex include a host of cortical and subcortical structures with a demonstrated role in long-term memory. At the cortical level, they include the entorhinal (area 28) and perirhinal (areas 35, 36) cortices.[8,27,40,78] The projections from the orbitofrontal cortex to the entorhinal cortex may underlie the process through which information about the emotional significance of stimuli is remembered, since the entorhinal cortex innervates the hippocampus[79-82] (reviewed in Refs. 83, 84).

Moreover, projections from the dysgranular orbitofrontal cortex terminate in the middle layers of the agranular entorhinal cortex,[57] consistent with the prediction of the structural model for laminar connections, which is based on the structural relationship of linked cortices.[24] Innervation of the middle layers is analogous to feedforward (or bottom-up) projections in sensory cortices. The question then arises, what type of information does the orbitofrontal cortex issue in a feedforward manner to the entorhinal cortex? The orbitofrontal cortex may synthesize its multi-modal input and the robust signals from the amygdala and send the information to the entorhinal cortex, possibly to store motivationally relevant information in long-term memory.[57] The impairment seen in associating objects with rewards after lesions of orbitofrontal cortex[85,86] may be due to disruption of a feedforward pathway to the entorhinal cortex and a return projection from the hippocampal formation, including CA1 and the subiculum to orbitofrontal cortex.[87-89]

Attention for Emotional Events

A striking feature of the innervation of orbitofrontal cortex by the amygdala is the dense projection to the superficial layers I and II of prefrontal cortices, where terminations intermingle with local inhibitory neurons labeled with calbindin.[45] Activity in these inhibitory neurons in prefrontal cortex, and other areas, is associated with focusing attention on relevant features for a task and suppressing distractors.[90] The pathway from the amygdala to orbitofrontal cortex may be engaged to focus attention on stimuli with emotional import,[45] consistent with the role of the amygdala in vigilance (reviewed in Refs. 91–94).

Further, the prefrontal cortex, in general, has a specialized interaction with the inhibitory thalamic reticular nucleus (TRN), which has a role in gating the bidirectional connections of cortical areas with the thalamus. Unlike sensory and motor cortices, which project topographically onto one sector of TRN, some prefrontal areas send widespread projections to the TRN.[95] These projections extend beyond the anterior (prefrontal sector) into the sensory sectors of TRN. In addition, the mediodorsal thalamic nucleus, which is the principal thalamic nucleus for the prefrontal cortex, has widespread bidirectional connections with TRN, including the parts connected with sensory thalamic nuclei. This circuitry suggests a mechanism through which behaviorally relevant stimuli may be selected and distractors filtered out early in information processing through the thalamus.[95] Orbitofrontal area 13 is one of the prefrontal areas with widespread projections to TRN, providing yet another pathway that may facilitate focusing attention on motivationally relevant stimuli.

SIMILARITIES AND DIFFERENCES IN THE CONNECTIONS OF MEDIAL AND ORBITAL AREAS

The discussion thus far has centered on the posterior orbitofrontal cortex (areas OPAll, OPro and 13 in FIG. 1B), which make up the orbital part of the prefrontal limbic region. These posterior orbitofrontal cortices overlap approximately with the posterior half of the "orbital network" of Price and colleagues (this volume).[6] The discussion thus far did not include posterior medial areas in the anterior cingulate (areas MPAll, 25, 32, and 24 in FIG. 1A), which belong to the agranular or dysgranular types of cortices, like the adjacent orbitofrontal. These posterior medial prefrontal areas in the anterior cingulate are part of the prefrontal limbic system,[96,97] and the first to be considered part of the great limbic lobe.[98,99] These anterior cingulate areas correspond to areas 24, 32, 25, and 14c of the "medial network" of Price and colleagues,[6] who do not differentiate between anterior and posterior sectors of medial or orbital networks. As discussed in this review, the division of orbitofrontal and medial prefrontal regions into anterior and posterior sectors is based on cortical type, which, in turn, can help explain their overall topography and pattern of connections. The densest connections with the amygdala, for example, are found in posterior orbitofrontal and posterior medial (anterior cingulate) areas.[45]

There is general agreement that the two components of the prefrontal limbic system share robust connections with cortical and subcortical limbic structures, widespread connections with many thalamic nuclei, the amygdala, the hypothalamus, and memory-related medial temporal cortices. The limbic prefrontal cortices also show a similar laminar pattern of connections with other cortices, as discussed above. Further similarities include bidirectional connections with the basal forebrain and perhaps other neurotransmitter-specific brain stem structures. Other prefrontal areas, including the anterior orbitofrontal and anterior medial areas, receive, but do not send, projections to neurotransmitter-specific structures in primates.[100]

The orbitofrontal and anterior cingulate components of the prefrontal limbic cortex have connectional specializations as well, which were reviewed previously[101] and will be mentioned only briefly here. The two prefrontal limbic components diverge in their connections with sensory association cortices. In sharp contrast to the orbitofrontal cortex, medial prefrontal areas do not have significant connections with sensory association cortices, with the exception of robust connections with auditory association areas.[10,25,102] In addition, although both posterior orbitofrontal cortices and anterior cingulate areas have dense connections with the amygdala (e.g., Refs. 38, 40), their patterns differ markedly,[45,46] as discussed above. Medial and orbitofrontal cortices have some similar connections within the prefrontal cortex, but their entire complement of connections differs.[2,103] These differences are exemplified in the multidimensional analysis of prefrontal interconnections (FIG. 4), which shows that cases with orbitofrontal injections of tracers cluster to the right and cases with medial and dorsolateral injections cluster to the left in the two-dimensional space.

Medial prefrontal cortices differ from the orbitofrontal by their stronger projections to hypothalamic autonomic centers and the spinal cord[104] and brain stem autonomic centers[105] (reviewed in Ref. 106). A pathway from area 32, for example, issues robust projections to hypothalamic autonomic centers, where they synapse through large boutons, suggesting efficient transmission of information.[55] In fact, the anterior cingulate areas have been called the emotional motor system.[107–109]

Based on the above differences in connections, there appears to be a division of labor within the prefrontal limbic system.[101] The posterior orbitofrontal cortices (areas OPAll, OPro and 13 in FIG. 1B), which have robust connections with high-order sensory association cortices and specialized connections with the amygdala, may be the sensors of information pertaining to emotions. On the other hand, posterior medial prefrontal cortices in the anterior cingulate (areas MPAll, 32, 25, and 24), with their extensive connections with hypothalamic, brain stem, and spinal autonomic structures, may be the effectors for emotional arousal. The anterior cingulate areas are connected with brain stem vocalization structures (for reviews see Refs. 7, 110) and have a role in emotional communication, which may help explain their robust connections with auditory association areas.

THE ORBITOFRONTAL CORTEX IN HEALTH AND DISEASE

The connections of the orbitofrontal cortex equip it with information that makes it possible to navigate in a complex social environment, pursuing rewarding goals and avoiding dangers. The posterior orbitofrontal cortex, in particular, appears to be key in these complex functions by its diverse and specialized connections. The posterior orbitofrontal cortex may be viewed as the primary cortical area for emotional processing by its specialized connections with primary olfactory areas, rich connections with high-order sensory association and polymodal cortices, and highly specialized connections with the amygdala and memory-related temporal cortices.

The posterior orbitofrontal cortex, however, must collaborate with the rest of the prefrontal cortex, including areas on the lateral surface that have been implicated in cognitive and executive functions, and can be engaged for action. The posterior orbitofrontal cortex has robust and bidirectional connections with anterior orbitofrontal cortices,[2,103] which are, in turn, linked with lateral prefrontal cortices[2,103] in a pattern that suggests sequential processing of information. The posterior orbitofrontal cortex is also robustly linked with anterior cingulate areas, which innervate autonomic centers and may have a key role in the expression of emotions.

Based on the differences in their sets and pattern of connections, orbitofrontal and medial prefrontal areas may be affected in distinct psychiatric diseases. The anterior cingulate region, for example, has been implicated in schizophrenia, consistent with pathology in specific classes of neurons[111] and hypoactivation in anterior cingulate areas that are connected with auditory association cortices (reviewed in Ref. 7).

The orbitofrontal cortex has been implicated in a wide variety of psychiatric diseases, including anxiety, phobias, obsessive-compulsive disorder, depression, and psychopathic personality disorder (e.g., Refs. 112–114 reviewed in Ref. 115). These diverse diseases likely affect different nodes in the complex pathways that link the orbitofrontal cortex with other cortical and subcortical structures. The pathway from the orbitofrontal cortex to the intercalated masses of the amygdala, which has the potential to allow increase in autonomic gain, may be abnormally active in diseases marked by anxiety.

Projections from structures associated with sensory, mnemonic, and emotional processing to orbitofrontal cortex provide a rich content of information. By virtue of their structure, posterior orbitofrontal areas send robust feedback projections to sensory and other association cortices. In several systems, feedback projections are thought to influence task-related activity.[116–119] Pathology in orbitofrontal cortex may remove feedback input to association areas, dissociating emotional context from sensory, cognitive, and mnemonic content and degrading the ability to interpret events.

AKNOWLEDGEMENTS

I thank my collaborators who participated in the original reports that contributed information for this review and Basilis Zikopoulos and Maya Medalla for help with the figures. Supported by NIH grants from NIMH and NINDS.

REFERENCES

1. WALKER, A.E. 1940. A cytoarchitectural study of the prefrontal area of the macaque monkey. J. Comp. Neurol. **73:** 59–86.
2. BARBAS, H. & D.N. PANDYA. 1989. Architecture and intrinsic connections of the prefrontal cortex in the rhesus monkey. J. Comp. Neurol. **286:** 353–375.
3. CARMICHAEL, S.T. & J.L. PRICE. 1994. Architectonic subdivision of the orbital and medial prefrontal cortex in the macaque monkey. J. Comp. Neurol. **346:** 366–402.
4. PREUSS, T.M. & P.S. GOLDMAN-RAKIC. 1991. Myelo- and cytoarchitecture of the granular frontal cortex and surrounding regions in the strepsirhine primate Galago and the anthropoid primate Macaca. J. Comp. Neurol. **310:** 429–474.
5. PETRIDES, M. & S. MACKEY. 2006. The orbitofrontal cortex: sulcal and gyral morphology and architecture. In The Orbitofrontal Cortex. D.H. Zald & S.L. Rauch, Eds.: 19–37. Oxford University Press. Oxford, UK.
6. PRICE, J. 2007. Definition of the orbital cortex in relation to specific connections with limbic and visceral structures, and other cortical regions. Ann. N.Y. Acad. Sci.
7. BARBAS, H., H. GHASHGHAEI, N. REMPEL-CLOWER & D. XIAO. 2002. Anatomic basis of functional specialization in prefrontal cortices in primates. In Handbook of Neuropsychology. J. Grafman, Ed.: 1–27. Elsevier Science B.V. Amsterdam.
8. MORECRAFT, R.J., C. GEULA & M.-M. MESULAM. 1992. Cytoarchitecture and neural afferents of orbitofrontal cortex in the brain of the monkey. J. Comp. Neurol. **323:** 341–358.
9. DOMBROWSKI, S.M., C.C. HILGETAG & H. BARBAS. 2001. Quantitative architecture distinguishes prefrontal cortical systems in the rhesus monkey. Cereb. Cortex **11:** 975–988.
10. BARBAS, H. et al. 2005. Relationship of prefrontal connections to inhibitory systems in superior temporal areas in the rhesus monkey. Cereb. Cortex **15:** 1356–1370.
11. MEDALLA, M. & H. BARBAS. 2006. Diversity of laminar connections linking periarcuate and lateral intraparietal areas depends on cortical structure. Eur. J. Neurosci. **23:** 161–179.

12. Hof, P.R. *et al.* 1999. Cellular distribution of the calcium-binding proteins parvalbumin, calbindin, and calretinin in the neocortex of mammals: phylogenetic and developmental patterns. J. Chem. Neur. **16:** 77–116.
13. Kringelbach, M.L. & E.T. Rolls. 2004. The functional neuroanatomy of the human orbitofrontal cortex: evidence from neuroimaging and neuropsychology. Prog. Neurobiol. **72:** 341–372.
14. Petrides, M., B. Alivisatos & S. Frey. 2002. Differential activation of the human orbital, mid-ventrolateral, and mid-dorsolateral prefrontal cortex during the processing of visual stimuli. Proc. Natl. Acad. Sci. USA **99:** 5649–5654.
15. Thorpe, S.J., E.T. Rolls & S. Maddison. 1983. The orbitofrontal cortex: neuronal activity in the behaving monkey. Exp. Brain Res. **49:** 93–115.
16. Rolls, E.T. 2004. The functions of the orbitofrontal cortex. Brain Cogn. **55:** 11–29.
17. Barbas, H., T.H. Henion & C.R. Dermon. 1991. Diverse thalamic projections to the prefrontal cortex in the rhesus monkey. J. Comp. Neurol. **313:** 65–94.
18. Dermon, C.R. & H. Barbas. 1994. Contralateral thalamic projections predominantly reach transitional cortices in the rhesus monkey. J. Comp. Neurol. **344:** 508–531.
19. Hilgetag, C.C. & H. Barbas. 2006. Role of mechanical factors in the morphology of the primate cerebral cortex. PLoS Comput. Biol. **2:** e22.
20. Barbas, H. 1986. Pattern in the laminar origin of corticocortical connections. J. Comp. Neurol. **252:** 415–422.
21. Pandya, D.N., B. Seltzer & H. Barbas. 1988. Input-output organization of the primate cerebral cortex. *In* Comparative Primate Biology, Vol. 4: Neurosciences. H.D. Steklis & J. Erwin, Eds.: 39–80. Alan R.Liss. New York.
22. Hof, P.R., E.J. Mufson & J.H. Morrison. 1995. Human orbitofrontal cortex: cytoarchitecture and quantitative immunohistochemical parcellation. J. Comp. Neurol. **359:** 48–68.
23. Barbas, H. *et al.* 2005. Parallel organization of contralateral and ipsilateral prefrontal cortical projections in the rhesus monkey. BMC Neurosci. **6:**32.
24. Barbas, H. & N. Rempel-Clower. 1997. Cortical structure predicts the pattern of corticocortical connections. Cereb. Cortex **7:** 635–646.
25. Barbas, H. *et al.* 1999. Medial prefrontal cortices are unified by common connections with superior temporal cortices and distinguished by input from memory-related areas in the rhesus monkey. J. Comp. Neurol. **410:** 343–367.
26. Grant, S. & C.C. Hilgetag. 2005. Graded classes of cortical connections: quantitative analyses of laminar projections to motion areas of cat extrastriate cortex. Eur. J. Neurosci. **22:** 681–696.
27. Barbas, H. 1993. Organization of cortical afferent input to orbitofrontal areas in the rhesus monkey. Neuroscience **56:** 841–864.
28. Carmichael, S.T. & J.L. Price. 1995. Sensory and premotor connections of the orbital and medial prefrontal cortex of macaque monkeys. J. Comp. Neurol. **363:** 642–664.
29. Cavada, C. *et al.* 2000. The anatomical connections of the macaque monkey orbitofrontal cortex. A review. Cereb. Cortex **10:** 220–242.
30. Barbas, H. & B. Zikopoulos. 2006. Sequential and parallel circuits for emotional processing in primate orbitofrontal cortex. *In* The Orbitofrontal Cortex. D. Zald & S. Rauch, Eds.: 57–91. Oxford University Press. Oxford, UK.
31. Poremba, A. *et al.* 2003. Functional mapping of the primate auditory system. Science **299:** 568–572.

32. CARMICHAEL, S.T., M.-C. CLUGNET & J.L. PRICE. 1994. Central olfactory connections in the macaque monkey. J. Comp. Neurol. **346:** 403–434.
33. PRICE, J.L. 1990. Olfactory system. *In* The Human Nervous System. G. Paxinos, Ed.: 979–998. Academic Press. San Diego.
34. SHEPHERD, G.M. 2007. Perspectives on olfactory processing, conscious perception, and orbitofrontal cortex. Ann. N.Y. Acad. Sci.
35. AMARAL, D.G. & J.L. PRICE. 1984. Amygdalo-cortical projections in the monkey (*Macaca fascicularis*). J. Comp. Neurol. **230:** 465–496.
36. NAUTA, W.J.H. 1961. Fibre degeneration following lesions of the amygdaloid complex in the monkey. J. Anat. **95:** 515–531.
37. JACOBSON, S. & J.Q. TROJANOWSKI. 1975. Amygdaloid projections to prefrontal granular cortex in rhesus monkey demonstrated with horseradish peroxidase. Brain Research **100:** 132–139.
38. BARBAS, H. & J. DE OLMOS. 1990. Projections from the amygdala to basoventral and mediodorsal prefrontal regions in the rhesus monkey. J. Comp. Neurol. **301:** 1–23.
39. PORRINO, L.J., A.M. CRANE & P.S. GOLDMAN-RAKIC. 1981. Direct and indirect pathways from the amygdala to the frontal lobe in rhesus monkeys. J. Comp. Neurol. **198:** 121–136.
40. CARMICHAEL, S.T. & J.L. PRICE. 1995. Limbic connections of the orbital and medial prefrontal cortex in macaque monkeys. J. Comp. Neurol. **363:** 615–641.
41. AGGLETON, J.P., M.J. BURTON & R.E. PASSINGHAM. 1980. Cortical and subcortical afferents to the amygdala of the rhesus monkey (*Macaca mulatta*). Brain Research **190:** 347–368.
42. VAN HOESEN, G.W. 1981. The differential distribution, diversity and sprouting of cortical projections to the amygdala of the rhesus monkey. *In* The Amygdaloid complex. Y. Ben-Ari, Ed.: 77–90. Elsevier/North Holland Biomedical Press. Amsterdam.
43. PANDYA, D.N., G.W. VAN HOESEN & V.B. DOMESICK. 1973. A cingulo-amygdaloid projection in the rhesus monkey. Brain Res. **61:** 369–373.
44. CHIBA, T., T. KAYAHARA & K. NAKANO. 2001. Efferent projections of infralimbic and prelimbic areas of the medial prefrontal cortex in the Japanese monkey, *Macaca fuscata*. Brain Res. **888:** 83–101.
45. GHASHGHAEI, H.T., C.C. HILGETAG & H. BARBAS. 2007. Sequence of information processing for emotions based on the anatomic dialogue between prefrontal cortex and amygdala. Neuroimage **34:** 905–923.
46. GHASHGHAEI, H.T. & H. BARBAS. 2002. Pathways for emotions: interactions of prefrontal and anterior temporal pathways in the amygdala of the rhesus monkey. Neuroscience **115:** 1261–1279.
47. PITKÄNEN, A. & D.G. AMARAL. 1994. The distribution of GABAergic cells, fibers, and terminals in the monkey amygdaloid complex: an immunohistochemical and in situ hybridization study. J. Neurosci. **14:** 2200–2224.
48. NITECKA, L. & Y. BEN ARI. 1987. Distribution of GABA-like immunoreactivity in the rat amygdaloid complex. J. Comp. Neurol. **266:** 45–55.
49. PARÉ, D. & Y. SMITH. 1993. Distribution of GABA immunoreactivity in the amygdaloid complex of the cat. Neuroscience **57:** 1061–1076.
50. PARÉ, D. & Y. SMITH. 1993. The intercalated cell masses project to the central and medial nuclei of the amygdala in cats. Neuroscience **57:** 1077–1090.

51. PARÉ, D. & Y. SMITH. 1994. GABAergic projection from the intercalated cell masses of the amygdala to the basal forebrain in cats. J. Comp. Neurol. **344:** 33–49.

52. MOGA, M.M. & T.S. GRAY. 1985. Peptidergic efferents from the intercalated nuclei of the amygdala to the parabrachial nucleus in the rat. Neurosci. Lett. **61:** 13–18.

53. JONGEN-RELO, A.L. & D.G. AMARAL. 1998. Evidence for a GABAergic projection from the central nucleus of the amygdala to the brainstem of the macaque monkey: a combined retrograde tracing and in situ hybridization study. Eur. J. Neurosci. **10:** 2924–2933.

54. SAHA, S., T.F. BATTEN & Z. HENDERSON. 2000. A GABAergic projection from the central nucleus of the amygdala to the nucleus of the solitary tract: a combined anterograde tracing and electron microscopic immunohistochemical study. Neuroscience **99:** 613–626.

55. BARBAS, H. *et al.* 2003. Serial pathways from primate prefrontal cortex to autonomic areas may influence emotional expression. BMC Neurosci. **4:**25.

56. BARBAS, H. 1995. Anatomic basis of cognitive-emotional interactions in the primate prefrontal cortex. Neurosci. Biobehav. Rev. **19:** 499–510.

57. REMPEL-CLOWER, N.L. & H. BARBAS. 2000. The laminar pattern of connections between prefrontal and anterior temporal cortices in the rhesus monkey is related to cortical structure and function. Cereb. Cortex **10:** 851–865.

58. MALKOVA, L., D. GAFFAN & E.A. MURRAY. 1997. Excitotoxic lesions of the amygdala fail to produce impairment in visual learning for auditory secondary reinforcement but interfere with reinforcer devaluation effects in rhesus monkeys. J. Neurosci. **17:** 6011–6020.

59. HIKOSAKA, K. & M. WATANABE. 2000. Delay activity of orbital and lateral prefrontal neurons of the monkey varying with different rewards. Cereb. Cortex **10:** 263–271.

60. BAXTER, M.G. *et al.* 2000. Control of response selection by reinforcer value requires interaction of amygdala and orbital prefrontal cortex. J. Neurosci. **20:** 4311–4319.

61. SCHOENBAUM, G., A.A. CHIBA & M. GALLAGHER. 1999. Neural encoding in orbitofrontal cortex and basolateral amygdala during olfactory discrimination learning. J. Neurosci. **19:** 1876–1884.

62. WALLIS, J.D. & E.K. MILLER. 2003. Neuronal activity in primate dorsolateral and orbital prefrontal cortex during performance of a reward preference task. Eur. J. Neurosci. **18:** 2069–2081.

63. LIPTON, P.A., P. ALVAREZ & H. EICHENBAUM. 1999. Crossmodal associative memory representations in rodent orbitofrontal cortex. Neuron **2:** 349–359.

64. TREMBLAY, L. & W. SCHULTZ. 1999. Relative reward preference in primate orbitofrontal cortex. Nature **398:** 704–708.

65. SCHOENBAUM, G., A.A. CHIBA & M. GALLAGHER. 2000. Changes in functional connectivity in orbitofrontal cortex and basolateral amygdala during learning and reversal training. J. Neurosci. **20:** 5179–5189.

66. SCHOENBAUM, G. & H. EICHENBAUM. 1995. Information coding in the rodent prefrontal cortex. I. Single-neuron activity in orbitofrontal cortex compared with that in pyriform cortex. J. Neurophysiol. **74:** 733–750.

67. SCHOENBAUM, G. *et al.* 2003. Encoding predicted outcome and acquired value in orbitofrontal cortex during cue sampling depends upon input from basolateral amygdala. Neuron **39:** 855–867.

68. SADDORIS, M.P., M. GALLAGHER & G. SCHOENBAUM. 2005. Rapid associative encoding in basolateral amygdala depends on connections with orbitofrontal cortex. Neuron **46**: 321–331.
69. TREMBLAY, E. & W. SCHULTZ. 2000. Reward-related neuronal activity during go-nogo task performance in primate orbitofrontal cortex. J. Neurophysiol. **83**: 1864–1876.
70. ROLLS, E.T. 2000. The orbitofrontal cortex and reward. Cereb. Cortex **10**: 284–294.
71. SCHULTZ, W., L. TREMBLAY & J.R. HOLLERMAN. 2000. Reward processing in primate orbitofrontal cortex and basal ganglia. Cereb. Cortex **10**: 272–284.
72. BAXTER, M.G. & E.A. MURRAY. 2002. The amygdala and reward. Nat. Rev. Neurosci. **3**: 563–573.
73. WHALEN, P.J. et al. 1998. Masked presentations of emotional facial expressions modulate amygdala activity without explicit knowledge. J. Neurosci. **18**: 411–418.
74. ROMANSKI, L.M. & J.E. LEDOUX. 1992. Equipotentiality of thalamo-amygdala and thalamo-cortico- amygdala circuits in auditory fear conditioning. J. Neurosci. **12**: 4501–4509.
75. KENNARD, M.A. 1945. Focal autonomic representation in the cortex and its relation to sham rage. J. Neuropathol. Exp. Neurol. **4**: 295–304.
76. ROLLS, E.T. 1996. The orbitofrontal cortex. Philos. Trans. R. Soc. Lond. B Biol. Sci. **351**: 1433–143.
77. WATANABE, M. 1998. Cognitive and motivational operations in primate prefrontal neurons. Rev. Neurosci. **9**: 225–241.
78. VAN HOESEN, G.W., D.N. PANDYA & N. BUTTERS. 1975. Some connections of the entorhinal (area 28) and perirhinal (area 35) cortices of the rhesus monkey. II. Frontal lobe afferents. Brain Res. **95**: 25–38.
79. WITTER, M.P., G.W. VAN HOESEN & D.G. AMARAL. 1989. Topographical organization of the entorhinal projection to the dentate gyrus of the monkey. J. Neurosci. **9**: 216–228.
80. LEONARD, B.W. et al. 1995. Transient memory impairment in monkeys with bilateral lesions of the entorhinal cortex. J. Neurosci. **15**: 5637–5659.
81. NAKAMURA, K. & K. KUBOTA. 1995. Mnemonic firing of neurons in the monkey temporal pole during a visual recognition memory task. J. Neurophysiol. **74**: 162–178.
82. SUZUKI, W.A., E.K. MILLER & R. DESIMONE. 1997. Object and place memory in the macaque entorhinal cortex. J. Neurophysiol. **78**: 1062–1081.
83. ROSENE, D.L. & G.W. VAN HOESEN. 1987. The hippocampal formation of the primate brain. A review of some comparative aspects of cytoarchitecture and connections. In Cerebral Cortex, Vol. 6. E.G. Jones & A. Peters, Eds.: 345–455. Plenum Publishing Corporation. New York.
84. SQUIRE, L.R. & S.M. ZOLA. 1996. Structure and function of declarative and nondeclarative memory systems. Proc. Natl. Acad. Sci. USA **93**: 13515–13522.
85. PEARS, A. et al. 2003. Lesions of the orbitofrontal but not medial prefrontal cortex disrupt conditioned reinforcement in primates. J. Neurosci. **23**: 11189–11201.
86. IZQUIERDO, A., R.K. SUDA & E.A. MURRAY. 2004. Bilateral orbital prefrontal cortex lesions in rhesus monkeys disrupt choices guided by both reward value and reward contingency. J. Neurosci. **24**: 7540–7548.

87. ROSENE, D.L. & G.W. VAN HOESEN. 1977. Hippocampal efferents reach widespread areas of cerebral cortex and amygdala in the rhesus monkey. Science **198:** 315–317.
88. BARBAS, H. & G.J. BLATT. 1995. Topographically specific hippocampal projections target functionally distinct prefrontal areas in the rhesus monkey. Hippocampus **5:** 511–533.
89. INSAUSTI, R. & M. MUÑOZ. 2001. Cortical projections of the non-entorhinal hippocampal formation in the cynomolgus monkey (Macaca fascicularis). Eur. J. Neurosci. **14:** 435–451.
90. WANG, X.J. et al. 2004. Division of labor among distinct subtypes of inhibitory neurons in a cortical microcircuit of working memory. Proc. Natl. Acad. Sci. USA **101:** 1368–1373.
91. GALLAGHER, M. & P.C. HOLLAND. 1994. The amygdala complex: multiple roles in associative learning and attention. Proc. Natl. Acad. Sci. USA **91:** 11771–11776.
92. LEDOUX, J.E. 2000. Emotion circuits in the brain. Ann. Rev. Neurosci. **23:** 155–184.
93. DAVIS, M. & P.J. WHALEN. 2001. The amygdala: vigilance and emotion. Mol. Psychiatry **6:** 13–34.
94. ZALD, D.H. 2003. The human amygdala and the emotional evaluation of sensory stimuli. Brain Res. Brain Res. Rev. **41:** 88–123.
95. ZIKOPOULOS, B. & H. BARBAS. 2006. Prefrontal projections to the thalamic reticular nucleus form a unique circuit for attentional mechanisms. J. Neurosci. **26:** 7348–7361.
96. YAKOVLEV, P.I. 1948. Motility, behavior and the brain: Stereodynamic organization and neurocoordinates of behavior. J. Nerv. Ment. Dis. **107:** 313–335.
97. NAUTA, W.J.H. 1979. Expanding borders of the limbic system concept. In Functional Neurosurgery. T. Rasmussen & R. Marino, Eds.: 7–23. Raven Press. New York.
98. BROCA, P. 1878. Anatomie compareé des enconvolutions cérébrales: le grand lobe limbique et la scissure limbique dans la serie des mammifères. Rev. Anthropol. **1:** 385–498.
99. PAPEZ, J.W. 1937. A proposed mechanism of emotion AMA. Arch. Neurol. Psychiat. **38:** 725–743.
100. GHASHGHAEI, H.T. & H. BARBAS. 2001. Neural interaction between the basal forebrain and functionally distinct prefrontal cortices in the rhesus monkey. Neuroscience **103:** 593–614.
101. BARBAS, H. 1997. Two prefrontal limbic systems: their common and unique features. In The Association Cortex: structure and Function. H. Sakata, A. Mikami & J.M. Fuster, Eds.: 99–115. Harwood Academic Publ. Amsterdam.
102. GERMUSKA, M. et al. 2006. Synaptic distinction of laminar specific prefrontal-temporal pathways in primates. Cereb. Cortex **16:** 865–875.
103. CARMICHAEL, S.T. & J.L. PRICE. 1996. Connectional networks within the orbital and medial prefrontal cortex of macaque monkeys. J. Comp. Neurol. **371:** 179–207.
104. REMPEL-CLOWER, N.L. & H. BARBAS. 1998. Topographic organization of connections between the hypothalamus and prefrontal cortex in the rhesus monkey. J. Comp. Neurol. **398:** 393–419.
105. ÖNGUR, D., X. AN & J.L. PRICE. 1998. Prefrontal cortical projections to the hypothalamus in macaque monkeys. J. Comp. Neurol. **401:** 480–505.

106. PETROVICH, G.D., N.S. CANTERAS & L.W. SWANSON. 2001. Combinatorial amygdalar inputs to hippocampal domains and hypothalamic behavior systems. Brain Res. Brain Res. Rev. **38:** 247–289.
107. HOLSTEGE, G. 1991. Descending motor pathways and the spinal motor system: limbic and non-limbic components. Prog. Brain Res. **87:** 307–421.
108. ALHEID, G.F. & L. HEIMER. 1996. Theories of basal forebrain organization and the "emotional motor system". Prog. Brain Res. **107:** 461–484.
109. HOLSTEGE, G., R. BANDLER & C.B. SAPER. 1996. The emotional motor system. Prog. Brain Res. **107:** 3–6.
110. VOGT, B.A. & H. BARBAS. 1988. Structure and connections of the cingulate vocalization region in the rhesus monkey. *In* The Physiological Control of Mammalian Vocalization. J.D. Newman, Ed.: 203–225. Plenum Publ. Corp. New York.
111. BENES, F.M. *et al.* 1991. Deficits in small interneurons in prefrontal and cingulate cortices of schizophrenic and schizoaffective patients. Arch. Gen. Psychiatry **48:** 996–1001.
112. ZALD, D.H. & S.W. KIM. 1996. Anatomy and function of the orbital frontal cortex, I: anatomy, neurocircuitry; and obsessive-compulsive disorder. J. Neuropsychiatry Clin. Neurosci. **8:** 125–138.
113. SIMPSON, J.R. *et al.* 2001. Emotion-induced changes in human medial prefrontal cortex: I. During cognitive task performance. Proc. Natl. Acad. Sci. USA **98:** 683–687.
114. MAYBERG, H.S. 2003. Modulating dysfunctional limbic-cortical circuits in depression: towards development of brain-based algorithms for diagnosis and optimised treatment. Br. Med. Bull. **65:** 193–207.
115. DAVIDSON, R.J. 2002. Anxiety and affective style: role of prefrontal cortex and amygdala. Biol. Psychiatry **51:** 68–80.
116. ULLMAN, S. 1995. Sequence seeking and counter streams: a computational model for bidirectional information in the visual cortex. Cereb. Cortex **5:** 1–11.
117. LAMME, V.A., H. SUPÈR & H. SPEKREIJSE. 1998. Feedforward, horizontal, and feedback processing in the visual cortex. Curr. Opin. Neurobiol. **8:** 529–535.
118. BAR, M. 2003. A cortical mechanism for triggering top-down facilitation in visual object recognition. J. Cogn. Neurosci. **15:** 600–609.
119. RAIZADA, R.D. & S. GROSSBERG. 2003. Towards a theory of the laminar architecture of cerebral cortex: computational clues from the visual system. Cereb. Cortex **13:** 100–113.

The Orbitofrontal Cortex: Novelty, Deviation from Expectation, and Memory

MICHAEL PETRIDES

Montreal Neurological Institute, McGill University, Montreal, Québec, Canada H3A 2B4

ABSTRACT: The orbitofrontal cortex is strongly connected with limbic areas of the medial temporal lobe that are critically involved in the establishment of declarative memories (entorhinal and perirhinal cortex and the hippocampal region) as well as the amygdala and the hypothalamus that are involved in emotional and motivational states. The present article reviews evidence regarding the role of the orbitofrontal cortex in the processing of novel information, breaches of expectation, and memory. Functional neuroimaging evidence is provided that there is a difference between the anterior and posterior orbitofrontal cortex in such processing. Exposure to novel information gives rise to a selective increase of activity in the granular anterior part of the orbitofrontal cortex (area 11) and this activity increases when subjects attempt to encode this information in memory. If the stimuli violate expectations (e.g., inspection of graffiti-like stimuli in the context of other regular stimuli) or are unpleasant (i.e., exposure to the sounds of car crashes), there is increased response in the posteromedial agranular/dysgranular area 13 of the orbitofrontal region. The anatomic data provide a framework within which to understand these functional neuroimaging findings.

KEYWORDS: orbital frontal cortex; macaque monkey; area 11; area 13; memory

The lateral, orbital, and medial surfaces of the human and nonhuman primate frontal cortex consists of several architectonic areas that differ not only in terms of their cellular architecture, [1–6] but also in terms of their connections with other cortical and subcortical areas of the brain.[6–20] Elucidating the contribution of the frontal cortex to any aspect of cognitive processing, including the processing of novel information and memory, will ultimately depend on understanding the nature of the specific neural computations occurring within

Address for correspondence: Michael Petrides, Montreal Neurological Institute, McGill University, 3801 University Street, Montreal, Québec, Canada H3A 2B4. Voice: 1-514-98-8375; fax: 1-514-398-1338.
petrides@ego.psych.mcgill.ca

Ann. N.Y. Acad. Sci. 1121: 33–53 (2007). © 2007 New York Academy of Sciences.
doi: 10.1196/annals.1401.035

particular frontal areas and their functional interactions with the other cortical and subcortical brain areas with which they are connected.[21] It is now clear that the different parts of the lateral prefrontal cortex make distinct contributions to memory performance and that these contributions involve primarily the application of specific control processes to mnemonic information. For instance, the mid-dorsolateral prefrontal cortex plays an important role in the monitoring of information in working memory, while the mid-ventrolateral prefrontal cortex is involved in the active controlled retrieval of information from memory.[21] It can thus be said that the contribution of the lateral prefrontal cortex to memory is rather indirect in that it reflects control processing applied to information in memory. The caudal orbital and medial frontal regions are likely to make more direct contributions to one aspect of memory, namely declarative memory, because these regions maintain the most direct connections (see below) with the limbic medial temporal lobe region which has been repeatedly shown to be the critical part of the brain for the establishment of new declarative memories.[22–27] However, even in the case of the orbital frontal cortex, involvement in memory may not be as central as that of the medial temporal region and may primarily concern the evaluation of novelty and information that radically breaches expectations about sensory input in order to regulate the organism's response to such new information. Such a response to novel and deviant information, which is clearly related to the involvement of the orbitofrontal cortex in the control of emotional and motivational states, will inevitably influence the degree of encoding of novel information in memory and some aspects of the retrieval of memories.

The orbital surface of the frontal lobe extends from the anterior perforated substance, caudally, to the frontal pole, rostrally. At the medial edge of the orbital surface of the frontal lobe there is a straight gyrus, the gyrus rectus, which is delimited by the olfactory sulcus. Typically, the posterior end of the olfactory sulcus lies lateral to its anterior end, making the gyrus rectus wider posteriorly.[28] The largest part of the cortex of the gyrus rectus is occupied by area 14, but area 25 (which occupies mostly the subcallosal gyrus on the medial frontal lobe) extends onto its most caudal part in some cases. The ventromedial margin of the cerebral hemisphere forms the morphologic border of the orbitofrontal cortex but, in terms of architecture, the cortex that lines the medial wall of the gyrus rectus is similar to the cortex that lines the orbital surface of the same gyrus. Lateral to the olfactory sulcus, two longitudinally running sulci can be identified: the medial and lateral orbital sulci, which are joined half-way by the transverse orbital sulcus to form the impression of an H or a K pattern. The anterior orbital gyrus that lies rostral to the transverse orbital sulcus between the anterior branches of the medial and lateral orbital sulci is occupied by area 11. The gyrus that lies caudal to the transverse orbital sulcus between the posterior branches of the medial and lateral orbital sulci is occupied, partly, by area 13, and further caudally by the proisocortical orbitofrontal cortex (FIG. 1).

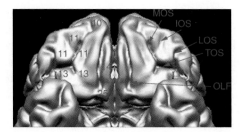

FIGURE 1. Three-dimensional reconstruction of the orbital surface of the human brain from a magnetic resonance image shows the approximate location of the orbital frontal architectonic areas. *Abbreviations:* IOS, intermediate orbital sulcus; LOS, lateral orbital sulcus; MOS, medial orbital sulcus; OLF, olfactory sulcus; TOS, transverse orbital sulcus.

The caudal region of the orbitofrontal cortex has architectonic characteristics similar to those of the limbic areas of the medial temporal lobe (which is critically involved in declarative memory) and constitutes, in terms of architecture and connectivity (see below), an intrinsic component of the same limbic system.[2,5–12,16] On the medial surface of the brain, the caudal limbic frontal region extends from the orbital surface to the subcallosal gyrus (area 25), surrounds the corpus callosum, and includes the anterior cingulate gyrus (area 24). This region on the medial frontal cortex is surrounded by the transitional paralimbic cortex of area 32. On the lateral extent of the orbital frontal surface, the orbital frontal cortex blends with the ventrolateral prefrontal cortex. Indeed, the cortex that lies lateral to the lateral orbital sulcus can be considered, anatomically and functionally, to be the orbital extension of the ventrolateral prefrontal cortical area 47/12.[21]

The limbic region of the medial temporal lobe, which includes the entorhinal and perirhinal cortex, the parahippocampal cortex, the hippocampus and the amygdala, has been shown to play a critical role in declarative memory processing.[22–27] Bilateral damage to this region of the brain gives rise to severe anterograde amnesia (i.e., a failure to acquire new declarative memories), but it leaves the acquisition of procedural memory (e.g., skill learning) intact.[22–25] Recent work has shown that the entorhinal and perirhinal cortex of the limbic medial temporal region are critical for recognition memory.[26,27] The hippocampus and parahippocampal cortex are involved in spatial memory and perhaps other contextual aspects of memory.[29–33] It is therefore of considerable interest that there are major bi-directional connections via the uncinate fasciculus linking the orbitofrontal cortex with the entorhinal and perirhinal cortex, as well as the hippocampal and parahippocampal region.[6–9,11,34–36] The orbital frontal lobe is also closely connected with the amygdaloid system, which plays a critical role in emotional processing and the affective component of mnemonic experience.[37–39] The orbital frontal cortex has both direct connections with the amygdala [10,11,16,40–45] and indirect connections via the temporopolar cortex.[46]

The amygdalo-hippocampal region can also interact with the orbital and medial prefrontal region via connections with the medial thalamus. The anterior nucleus of the thalamus, which receives input from the hippocampal complex directly and through connections with the mammillary bodies,[36,47] projects to the anterior cingulate and subcallosal gyri.[48] In addition, the magnocellular part of the medial dorsal thalamic nucleus, which is linked with the amygdala,[43,47,49] is connected with the orbital frontal region.[18,20,49]

The above brief review of the anatomic evidence demonstrates that the caudal orbital frontal region, as well as the caudal medial frontal cortex that surrounds the rostral part of the corpus callosum, namely the subcallosal gyrus (area 25) and the anterior part of the cingulate gyrus (area 24), have a massive direct interaction with areas of the limbic medial temporal lobe that have been shown to be critical to the establishment of new declarative memories. The following question therefore arises: Can an amnesic syndrome result from damage restricted to the orbito-medial frontal region? This issue has been addressed in lesion studies in the macaque monkey by Bachevalier and Mishkin.[50] These investigators removed, bilaterally, the orbitofrontal cortex from the gyrus rectus to the lateral orbital sulcus, including areas 14, 13, and 11 but not the frontal pole (area 10), as well as the cortex of the subcallosal gyrus (area 25) and the anterior cingulate cortex (areas 24 and 32) on the medial surface of the brain (FIG. 2). In other words, the lesions removed the limbic parts of both the orbital and medial frontal surfaces of the macaque monkey brain. The monkeys were tested on the recognition memory task, the delayed non-matching-to-sample task, which has been successfully used to assess the memory impairment of monkeys with extensive medial temporal lobe lesions.[24,25] In this task, on every trial, the monkey is presented with a novel object (e.g., object A) and, after a short delay, the animal is shown the now-familiar object (object A) together with a novel object (e.g., object B). On the choice phase of the trial, the animal has to choose the novel object (object B), thus displaying knowledge of the fact that object A is familiar and object B is novel. On all subsequent trials, new objects are used. Monkeys with bilateral lesions of both the orbital and medial limbic regions of the frontal lobe were severely impaired in recognition memory. This important study demonstrated the functional involvement of the orbital and caudomedial frontal cortical regions (which are anatomically closely related and linked with the medial temporal limbic region) in recognition memory. In another study, these investigators explored the effects of lesions restricted to either the orbital frontal cortex or the anterior cingulate region.[51] The orbital frontal lesion yielded a severe impairment on visual recognition memory, although not as severe as the combined lesion. In conclusion, these investigations showed that monkeys with lesions restricted to the orbitofrontal cortex exhibit impairments on the same visual recognition memory task (i.e., the delayed non-matching-to-sample task) that was previously used to demonstrate the severe recognition memory loss that follows bilateral medial temporal lobe lesions [24,25] or lesions restricted to the entorhinal

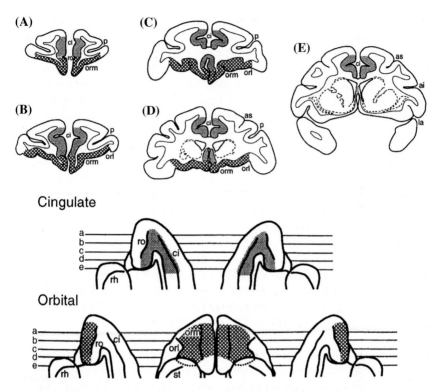

FIGURE 2. Schematic diagrams illustrating the medial (i.e., cingulate and subcallosal) and orbital frontal lesions that were studied by Meunier et al.[51] The combined lesion that includes both the medial and orbital frontal areas yields a severe recognition memory disorder.[50] The orbital lesion alone also yields severe recognition memory impairment, although not as severe as that observed after the combined lesion. **A–E:** Coronal sections through the frontal cortex. *Abbreviations:* ai, inferior branch of the arcuate sulcus; as, superior branch of the arcuate sulcus; ci, cingulate sulcus; la, lateral sulcus; orl, lateral orbital sulcus; orm, medial orbital sulcus; p, principal sulcus; rh, rhinal sulcus; ro, rostral sulcus; st, superior temporal sulcus. From Meunier et al. with permission.

and perirhinal cortex of the limbic medial temporal region.[26,27] Interestingly, the entorhinal and perirhinal cortex are the parts of the medial temporal lobe most heavily linked with the orbitofrontal cortex both directly via the uncinate fasciculus[34,35] and indirectly via the magnocellular part of the dorsomedial thalamic nucleus.[6,8,49,52] Thus, the evidence from the monkey indicates that the orbital region does play a direct role in memory processing. The human evidence, however, remains controversial (see below).

In evaluating the human evidence with regard to the role of the orbitofrontal cortex in memory, it must be borne in mind that just caudal to the orbitomedial margin of the frontal cortex lie certain basal forebrain areas that play a direct role in memory function. For instance, the septal region lies just behind the subcallosal medial frontal cortex. The septal region comprises several nuclei, such as the medial septal nucleus and the nucleus of the diagonal band of Broca,[53] which are massively connected with the hippocampal complex and are an inherent component of that system.[54] Indeed, the anatomic and functional relation between the hippocampus and the septal nuclei is so close that reference is often made to the septo-hippocampal system. Lesions of the septal region deprive the hippocampus of major cholinergic inputs and give rise to memory deficits similar to those observed after damage to the hippocampal region.[55] Furthermore, damage to this basal forebrain region in patients[56-60] gives rise to a severe amnesic syndrome. Thus, lesions of the frontal cortex that include damage to nearby basal forebrain areas do not provide evidence relevant to the issue of whether a basic memory disorder can follow damage *restricted* to the orbital and medial frontal cortex.

EVIDENCE FROM CASES OF TUMOR
OF THE FRONTAL LOBE, RUPTURED ANEURYSMS
OF THE ANTERIOR COMMUNICATING ARTERY,
AND PSYCHOSURGERY

Disturbances of memory have been reported in patients with large tumors affecting the frontal lobes.[61-65] However, conclusions concerning the functions of the frontal cortex from such cases are of questionable validity. Tumors of the frontal lobe, by compressing or infiltrating areas neighboring on the frontal cortex (e.g., the basal forebrain region) or by raising intracranial pressure, can give rise to a variety of symptoms that reflect pathologic changes in widespread regions of the brain. Similar problems of interpretation exist for the amnesic syndrome that often follows ruptured aneurysms of the anterior communicating artery.[56,57,65-70] Although damage to the posterior orbital and adjacent medial frontal cortex can often be demonstrated or presumed in these cases, the extent of damage is not restricted to the frontal cortex, but critically also includes various basal forebrain structures, such as the septal region, nucleus accumbens, and the nucleus basalis of Meynert. It has been suggested that damage to the latter structures may be responsible for the amnesia in cases of ruptured aneurysms of the anterior communicating artery.[68,71,72] More recently, impairment in episodic memory has been reported in a patient with severe traumatic brain injury that involved the ventrolateral prefrontal cortex (area 47/12) and also the uncinate fasciculus, which would certainly disrupt in a major fashion fronto-temporal interactions.[73]

Since the end of World War II, the widespread use of frontal-lobe surgery for the symptomatic relief of psychiatric disorders has furnished the opportunity for a further examination of the effects of damage to the frontal cortex on cognitive functions. Unfortunately the observations made on these patients have often proven more confusing than enlightening because of the difficulties in drawing conclusions from the study of patients with psychotic symptoms and because, in many cases, appropriate control groups were not examined. In addition, formal evaluation of memory function with appropriate tests can only rarely be found in the many publications on the effects of psychosurgical procedures. More recently, Kartsounis et al.[74] studied the cognitive effects, including memory, of bilateral subcaudate (frontal) tractotomy carried out for the treatment of resistant affective disorder (i.e., major depressive disorder, bipolar disorder, etc) in 23 patients. This operation involves the insertion of radioactive yttrium rods which destroy bilaterally pathways located in the caudal orbital region, just below and in front of the head of the caudate nucleus. During the immediate postoperative period (2 weeks) after this operation, massive edema occurs in most of the frontal lobe, but subsides later. The patients were tested 6–9 days before operation, 2 weeks after the operation, and approximately 6 months after the operation. Significant impairments on recognition memory were observed during the immediate postoperative period (2 weeks), but not during the follow-up testing 6 months later. No impairments on the recall of short stories or paired-associate learning were observed at either the immediate or the follow-up testing period. Thus, the impairment in recognition memory was detected only during the immediate postoperative period when massive edema was present in the frontal lobe.

The reported absence of major memory impairment in many investigations of the effects of psychosurgery must be interpreted with caution. A careful consideration of the operative procedures, in those studies in which sufficient information has been provided, raises the possibility that the absence of a severe and general memory loss may have been due to the fact that the lesions did not encroach extensively upon the posterior orbital and adjacent limbic caudal medial frontal cortex. In this context it is interesting to note that Scoville, who introduced the psychosurgical procedure known as "orbital undercutting" (i.e., sectioning of the white matter just above the orbital frontal cortex), reported no clinically evident memory loss in these patients, except for a few cases in which the operation extended too far posteriorly.[75] It is possible that the posterior extension of the undercutting in these operations had brought about a more complete isolation of the orbitomedial frontal lobe from the rest of the brain than might have been the case in more limited psychosurgical procedures confined to either the orbitofrontal or the anterior cingulate regions.

The data presented above indicate that when the caudal orbitomedial region of the frontal cortex is not damaged and the lesions do not include damage to basal forebrain areas (e.g., the septal region), lesions of the orbital frontal cortex do not cause a generalized declarative memory disorder such as that observed after bilateral lesions of the medial temporal region or diencephalic lesions.

EVIDENCE FROM FUNCTIONAL NEUROIMAGING STUDIES

Several studies with modern functional neuroimaging methods have reported changes in activity within the prefrontal cortex during the performance of tasks that required memory processing. The foci within the frontal cortex in such studies have ranged widely within the prefrontal cortex. Activity foci within the mid-dorsolateral prefrontal cortex (areas 46 and 9/46) have been shown to be related to the monitoring of information in working memory, while activity in the mid-ventrolateral prefrontal cortex is related to the active controlled retrieval of information both from short-term and long-term memory (see Petrides[21] for a discussion of these issues). Can activity related to the processing of novel information be selectively demonstrated in the orbital frontal region and how is it related to memory? As pointed out above, research on macaque monkeys showed that bilateral lesions of the orbital frontal cortex can yield impairment on a recognition memory task in which the animals are required to select between a novel and a familiar object.[50] There is also another important piece of information with regard to the orbital frontal cortex that is relevant here: monkeys with lesions to the orbitofrontal cortex do not habituate easily to the presentation of novel stimuli.[76] Given the strong anatomic connections of the caudal orbital frontal cortex with the amygdala[10,11,16,40–45] and hypothalamus,[14,15] as well as many other limbic neural structures, the orbitofrontal cortex may be in a position to regulate the motivational and emotional aspects of novel stimuli. Significant deviations from expectation must be evaluated with regard to their potential positive or negative implications for the organism and the orbitofrontal cortex with its strong and preferential connections with several limbic neural structures is in an ideal position to regulate further information processing in these structures. The greater attention accorded to these novel stimuli/events will inevitably lead to their being better remembered. Thus, there might be an influence of orbital frontal cortical activity to the degree of encoding of information in explicit declarative memory that stems from its primary role in the regulation of the appropriate behavioral and autonomic response to novel environmental stimuli.

On the basis of the above considerations, we designed a series of positron emission tomography studies to address the question of whether the orbitofrontal cortex responds selectively to the presentation of novel stimuli and whether this response is related to memory performance. In one positron emission tomography study,[77] we measured changes in cerebral blood flow in normal human subjects while they viewed novel faces. These faces were presented one at a time on the computer screen and the subjects were told to try to memorize them, but not to attempt to use any verbal tags to remember them. To reduce the chance of any verbal strategies being employed to remember the material, the face stimuli were all of male students of similar ethnic background with standard facial expressions. A black oval mask was placed

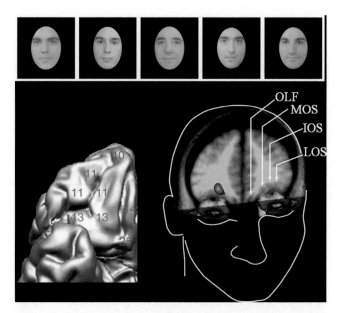

FIGURE 3. Examples of the face stimuli displayed in the center of the screen one at a time during the novel faces viewing condition. The coronal section shows increased activity in the rostral part of the orbitofrontal cortex (area 11) which is related to the viewing of novel faces. There was a positive correlation between face recognition memory performance and activity in this region of the orbital frontal cortex. The activity focus was in the right hemisphere. Note that the activity focus is shown here on the left side of the coronal section (i.e., according to radiologic convention) so that it will be consistent with the three-dimensional rendering of the orbitofrontal surface (*bottom left*) which illustrates the approximate location of the various architectonic areas of the orbital frontal lobe according to Petrides and Pandya.[3] *Abbreviations:* IOS, intermediate orbital sulcus; LOS, lateral orbital sulcus; MOS, medial orbital sulcus; OLF, olfactory sulcus.

around the head to hide the hair and neck region. In the control condition, the subjects viewed the same type of face stimuli, but these were familiar. Comparison of activity recorded during the viewing of novel faces with activity during the viewing of familiar novel faces showed increased activity within the rostral orbitofrontal region specifically related to the viewing of the novel faces (FIG. 3). The focus of activity was close to the rostral branch of the medial orbital sulcus where architectonic area 11 is located according to our architectonic analyses. Importantly, activity in this region correlated positively with memory performance across subjects.

In another positron emission tomography study,[78] we measured changes in cerebral blood flow in normal human subjects during the presentation of sequences of abstract visual designs (FIG. 4). There were four conditions, all of which involved presentation of sequences of colored abstract designs. In the minimal encoding condition (condition 1) that served as the control, the

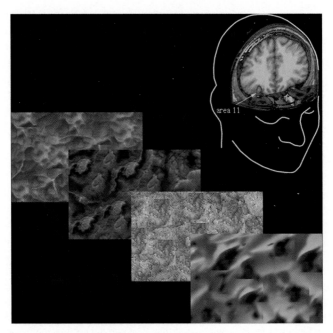

FIGURE 4. Examples of the abstract visual stimuli presented one at time during the various conditions of the memory encoding experiment. In the *inset at top right*, a coronal section of a magnetic resonance image illustrates the increase in activation within the orbitofrontal area 11 in the right hemisphere. Note that the activity focus is shown here on the *left side* of the coronal section (i.e., according to radiologic convention) so that it will be consistent with the orientation used in Figure 3.

subjects viewed three abstract designs presented one at a time in a random order. These three abstract designs were very familiar to the subjects who had seen them many times before scanning (17 times) and, therefore, there was very little new information to be encoded during the presentation of these three familiar stimuli. In condition 2, the subjects viewed 20 moderately familiar stimuli presented one at a time. Although these stimuli were familiar in that the subjects had seen them six times before scanning, there was still information to be encoded as a result of the presentation of these 20 stimuli. In the viewing novel stimuli condition (condition 3), the participants were simply asked to view 20 novel stimuli presented sequentially. In this condition, since the stimuli were all novel, a lot of new information had to be encoded by the participants during viewing. Finally, in condition 4, which required the maximum encoding, again 20 novel stimuli were presented sequentially, but now the subjects were specifically instructed to attempt to memorize these stimuli. After each scanning condition, recognition tests were administered, although the subjects were not informed of this before scanning. All conditions were presented in a random order, with the only restriction that condition 3 should occur before condition 4. Since condition 3 involved the incidental encoding of 20 novel stimuli while condition 4 involved the explicit instructed encoding of 20 novel stimuli, condition 3 had to be presented before condition 4.

The results of this study demonstrated activation in orbitofrontal area 11 (FIG. 4) that increased across the four conditions, that is, from condition 1 (minimal encoding requirements) to condition 4 (maximal encoding require-ments).[78] In addition, there was increased activity within the right parahip-pocampal region. Thus, the right orbitofrontal cortex and the right parahip-pocampal region modulate their activity in relation to the degree to which nonverbal visual information is being encoded in memory. There is consider-able evidence that the right parahippocampal region is critical for the learning of new nonverbal visual information.[22,23] The importance of area 11 in the right hemisphere in the encoding of novel visual stimuli was also demon-strated in two other positron emission tomography studies, one using abstract visual stimuli[79] and the other using auditory stimuli.[80]

In a recent single neuron recording study, Rolls *et al.*[81] reported a population of neurons in area 11 of the macaque monkey that responded selectively to novel but not familiar visual stimuli. Some of these neurons responded to novel faces. The neuronal response to novel stimuli was independent of reward since, in this study, the monkey was rewarded both when the familiar and the novel stimuli were presented. In other words, these neurons coded novelty and not the reward value of the stimuli. Furthermore, the neuronal response habituated very quickly (within 5 or so presentations) and, interestingly, the habituation effect was long lasting (at least 24 hours). For instance, none of these novelty neurons in area 11 responded to a stimulus that had been shown as a novel stimulus on the previous day. Thus, the response of these neurons is affected by long-term encoding of stimuli that are initially novel, suggesting that they may contribute to learning about novel stimuli. These neurons differ from neurons in the amygdala in the sense that neuronal response in the amygdala is closely linked to the reward value of stimuli.

In another positron emission study, we examined the role of the orbitofrontal cortex in the neural response to deviant stimuli.[82] In the control baseline con-dition, the subjects viewed pairs of colored abstract images appearing on the screen. The subjects were instructed to view the pair of images on the screen and then to touch the screen in the space between the two images to advance to the next pair of images. As soon as the subject touched the screen, the previous pair disappeared and a new pair of images appeared. In the deviant stimulation condition, the subjects were presented with pairs of abstract colored images that were deviant in relation to those seen in the control condition and all the other scanning conditions. The deviant stimuli were produced by selecting randomly abstract colored images from a large set and introducing some no-ticeable distortion in them, such as a graffiti-like thick black line, scratches, etc. (FIG. 5). The purpose of these graffiti-like distortions was to make the stimuli noticeable so that the subjects would not fail to notice the distortions when

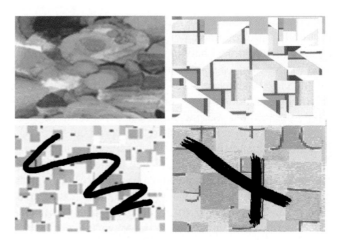

FIGURE 5. Examples of the pairs of abstract nonverbal colored images used in the positron emission tomography study that examined orbitofrontal response to the presentation of deviant graffiti-like stimuli. *Upper panel:* standard stimuli; *lower panel:* stimuli modified by the addition of graffiti-like elements (e.g., black lines) to render them deviant from the standard stimuli.

presented with these stimuli. These changes would not evoke any obvious emotion in subjects, but they would certainly attract attention because they were clearly perceived as elements incongruent with the normal features of the designs. Apart from this change in the type of stimulation presented, all other aspects of the testing in the deviant stimulation condition were the same as those in the control condition, that is, the subjects were required to inspect the pair of visual abstract images presented and to touch the screen in the space between the two stimuli in order to view the next pair of stimuli.

The question whether there would be increased and selective modulation of activity within the human orbital frontal cortex related to the mere inspection of stimuli that deviated from expectation was addressed by comparing activity in the deviant stimulation condition with that in the control condition (FIG. 6). This comparison revealed increased activity within the right orbitofrontal cortex in area 11 and also in area 13. Note that there were no activity differences in any other part of the frontal cortex resulting from this comparison. Note also that no decision was required of the subjects during the inspection of the stimuli and, therefore, the modulation of activity within the orbitofrontal cortex reflects the brain's response to the mere inspection of graffiti-like stimuli, that is, stimuli that deviate from expectation. These focal changes were observed in areas 11 and 13 of the orbitofrontal cortex and both these areas are strongly linked to the anterior inferotemporal cortex,[7,11] which plays a critical role in the processing of visual stimuli. The activity in area 13 was positively correlated with activity in the anterior inferotemporal cortex during inspection of these deviant stimuli.

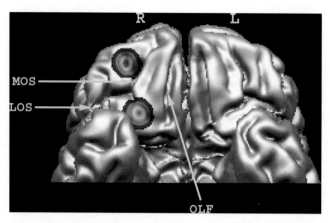

FIGURE 6. Three-dimensional reconstruction of the human orbital frontal surface to illustrate the location of the two peaks of increased activity in the right orbitofrontal region resulting from the exposure of the subjects to deviant stimuli in comparison to standard stimuli. The rostral peak of activity lies between the rostral parts of the medial and lateral orbital sulci and is therefore located in area 11. The caudal peak of activity lies along the caudal end of the medial orbital sulcus and is therefore located in area 13. *Abbreviations:* L, left hemisphere; LOS, lateral orbital sulcus; MOS, medial orbital sulcus; OLF, olfactory sulcus; R, right hemisphere.

In the study described above,[82] the degree of familiarity of the stimuli to the subject, in terms of overall previous exposure, was perfectly matched between the deviant stimulation and control conditions. The increased activity in orbitofrontal areas 11 and 13 was therefore due to changes in the graffiti-like stimuli that made them look inconsistent with the expected type of stimuli (i.e., the activity was related to violations of expectation). Thus, areas 11 and 13 of the orbitofrontal cortex are also engaged when there is a noticeable change in the stimulation to which the organism is exposed. Significant deviations from expectation must be evaluated with regard to their potential positive or negative implications for the organism and the orbitofrontal cortex with its strong and preferential connections with several limbic neural structures is in an ideal position to regulate further information processing in these structures. This argument is consistent with research on human subjects with brain damage,[83] suggesting that the orbital frontal cortex is involved in the regulation of the emotional/motivational states of the organism. There is also evidence at the single neuron level in the rat[84] and monkey[85] that neural activity in the orbitofrontal cortex reflects changes in expectations of the significance of stimuli.

There is considerable evidence that the orbitofrontal cortex is in a position to regulate the central arousal pathways.[86] Furthermore, the posterior orbital and adjacent medial prefrontal cortex projects strongly to the hypothalamus and the periaqueductal gray region,[13–15] regions of the brain that are known to be involved in the regulation of endocrine and visceral control. The caudal region of the orbitofrontal cortex is also closely linked with the amygdala,[10,11,40] which in turn exercises control over the endocrine and visceral systems. Thus, the caudal orbital and medial frontal region is in a position to regulate autonomic responses, such as changes in blood pressure, respiration, and gastric motility, and there is considerable evidence that this is the case. When stimulated, the caudal orbital and medial frontal region in both human subjects[87] and monkeys[88–91] affects heart rate, breathing, and gastric mobility. Similarly, lesions of the orbitomedial frontal cortex in human subjects have been shown to affect visceral responses.[92]

Further evidence that the caudal orbitofrontal cortex is involved in the brain response that is set in motion when stimulation deviates in a major way from what the organism expects comes from a positron emission tomography study in which we examined changes in blood flow in normal human subjects during exposure to unpleasant auditory stimuli.[93] In this study, the subjects were instructed to listen passively to sounds presented during the scanning period. The stimuli used in the control condition were abstract sounds that were generated from an electronic keyboard. These sounds were rather pleasant and familiar to the subjects because they had heard them 24 hours before the scanning session. In the unpleasant sound condition, the subjects listened to the sounds of violent car crashes, such as screeching tires, breaking glass, and sudden impacts, all of which were originally created for use in films. Comparison of brain activity evoked by the pleasant control condition with the unpleasant sound condition revealed increased activity in the caudal orbitofrontal cortex, bilaterally, in area 13 during exposure to the sounds of disturbing events.

The functional neuroimaging data presented above provided evidence with regard to the selective roles of orbitofrontal areas 11 and 13 in the processing of novel, deviant, and disturbing information. The mere exposure to novel information gives rise to a selective increase of activity in area 11 of the orbitofrontal cortex. It is therefore of considerable interest that neurons in area 11 of the macaque monkey exhibit an exaggerated response to novelty and this response habituates very quickly and is long lasting.[81] Furthermore, it should be noted that lesions of the orbitofrontal cortex in the monkey yield a significant impairment in the habituation response to novelty.[76] If the activity violates expectations (e.g., the mere inspection of graffiti-like stimuli) or is unpleasant (e.g., exposure to the sounds of car crashes), there is also increased response in a more caudal and more medial orbitofrontal region, namely area 13. There is evidence that lesions of the orbitofrontal cortex lead to disturbances in the regulation of emotional responses to various environmental stimuli in both the monkey[94] and human subjects.[83]

The anatomic data provide a framework within which to understand the above functional neuroimaging findings. The caudomedial area 13 is part of the agranular/dysgranular caudal orbital frontal cortex that is strongly linked with the amygdala and the hypothalamus. The caudal orbital frontal region, which includes area 13, receives sensory input, directly, from many cortical regions involved with the processing of visual, auditory, somatosensory, gustatory, and olfactory information and, indirectly, from the amygdala and the entorhinal and perirhinal cortex, as well as information about the internal environment from the hypothalamus. Thus, this region of the orbitofrontal cortex has information about the external and the internal environment. This region in turn projects directly to the hypothalamus and the periaqueductal gray, as well as the caudal medial prefrontal cortex and the amygdala, which are also in a position to regulate the hypothalamus and the periaqueductal gray region. Area 13 can thus influence directly and indirectly the autonomic nervous system and is therefore in an ideal position to orchestrate a response when an individual encounters stimuli that breach expectation, regardless of whether these are relatively mild deviations of expectation (e.g., graffiti-like stimuli) or potentially disturbing stimuli (e.g., car crashes). This response, which will involve not only parts of the brain involved with emotion and arousal but also memory, will inevitably lead to greater processing of these stimuli and will contribute to their better encoding. By contrast, the more rostral cortical area 11 is a granular prefrontal area that is linked with area 13, but only moderately with the amygdala and only in a minor way with the hypothalamic region and the caudomedial prefrontal region that regulates the autonomic nervous system. Area 11, however, is strongly linked with the lateral prefrontal areas that are critical in the monitoring of information in working memory and in the controlled retrieval of information from memory. Thus, area 11 is in a position to act as an interface between the cognitive processing of the lateral prefrontal cortex and processing regarding the emotional/motivational life of the individual occurring in the caudal orbitofrontal region. It may thus be one of the key orbitofrontal areas involved in capturing information that is novel relative to current exteroceptive and interoceptive experience and expectations and linking it to the higher cognitive processing occurring in the lateral prefrontal cortex. It can thus mediate between lateral prefrontal areas involved in the monitoring and manipulation of information in working memory and active controlled retrieval and information that is currently perceived as novel and requiring attention. Again, the inevitable directing of attention to novel information would contribute to its deeper processing and thus better encoding of it.

In conclusion, although the orbitofrontal areas clearly contribute to the processing of novel, deviant, and disturbing information, their role may be primarily a modulatory one and any memory impairment that might follow lesions restricted to the orbital frontal cortex may not be as severe as the deficit that follows the limbic medial temporal lobe region, which is essential to the entry of novel information in memory. This argument is consistent with certain findings from investigations that attempted to dissociate the contribution of the orbitofrontal cortex from that of the amygdala in the rat. These investigations provide some evidence that, in contrast to the amygdala, which plays a primary role in the establishment of stimulus–reward associations, the orbitofrontal cortex is not necessary to establish such stimulus–reward associations, but is necessary to integrate information regarding the current internal state of the organism with knowledge of the already established associations in order to regulate choice behavior.[95] Given the anatomic connections of the orbitofrontal cortex, one would expect the orbitofrontal cortex to be involved in the emotional aspects of explicit declarative memories. Most research on emotional memory has focused on the role of the amygdala,[37–39] but in functional neuroimaging research activation of the orbitofrontal cortex is often reported during the retrieval of mnemonic information linked to emotion.[37,96–98] Although there is functional neuroimaging evidence that activity in the orbitofrontal cortex is modulated during emotional memory processing, the precise contribution of the various orbitofrontal areas to emotional memory processing remain to be established.

REFERENCES

1. BRODMANN, K. 1909. Vergleichende Localisationslehre der Grosshirnrinde in ihren Prinzipien dargestellt auf Grund des Zellenbaues. Barth. Leipzig, Germany.
2. ECONOMO, C. & G.N. KOSKINAS. 1925. Die Cytoarchitektonik der Hirnrinde des erwachsenen Menschen. Springer. Wien, Austria.
3. PETRIDES, M. & D.N. PANDYA. 1994. Comparative architectonic analysis of the human and the macaque frontal cortex. In Handbook of Neuropsychology. Vol. 9. F. Boller & J. Grafman, Eds.: 17–58. Elsevier. Amsterdam.
4. BARBAS, H. & D.N. PANDYA. 1989. Architecture and intrinsic connections of the prefrontal cortex in the rhesus monkey. J. Comp. Neurol. **286:** 353–375.
5. CARMICHAEL, S.T. & J.L. PRICE. 1994. Architectonic subdivision of the orbital and medial prefrontal cortex in the macaque monkey. J. Comp. Neurol. **346:** 366–402.
6. MORECRAFT, R.J., C. GEULA & M.-M. MESULAM. 1992. Cytoarchitecture and neural afferents of orbitofrontal cortex in the brain of the monkey. J. Comp. Neurol. **323:** 341–358.
7. BARBAS, H. 1988. Anatomic organization of basoventral and mediodorsal visual recipient prefrontal regions in the rhesus monkey. J. Comp. Neurol. **276:** 313–342.
8. BARBAS, H. 1993. Organization of cortical afferent input to orbitofrontal areas in the rhesus monkey. Neuroscience **56:** 841–864.
9. BARBAS, H. & G.J. BLATT. 1995. Topographically specific hippocampal projections target functionally distinct prefrontal areas in the rhesus monkey. Hippocampus **5:** 511–533.
10. BARBAS, H. & J. DE OLMOS. 1990. Projections from the amygdala to basoventral and mediodorsal prefrontal regions in the rhesus monkey. J. Comp. Neurol. **301:** 1–23.
11. CARMICHAEL, S.T. & J.L. PRICE. 1995. Limbic connections of the orbital and the medial prefrontal cortex in macaque monkeys. J. Comp. Neurol. **363:** 615–641.

12. PETRIDES, M. & D.N. PANDYA. 2002. Association pathways of the prefrontal cortex and functional observations. *In* Principles of Frontal Lobe Function, Chapter 3. D.T. Stuss & R.T. Knight, Eds.: 31–50. Oxford University Press. New York, NY.

13. AN, X., R. BANDLER, D. ÖNGÜR & J.L. PRICE. 1998. Prefrontal cortical projections to longitudinal columns in the midbrain periaqueductal gray in macaque monkeys. J. Comp. Neurol. **401:** 455–479.

14. ÖNGÜR, D., X. AN & J.L. PRICE. 1998. Prefrontal cortical projections to the hypothalamus in macaque monkeys. J. Comp. Neurol. **401:** 480–505.

15. REMPEL-CLOWER, N.L. & H. BARBAS. 1998. Topographic organization of connections between the hypothalamus and prefrontal cortex in the rhesus monkey. J. Comp. Neurol. **398:** 393–419.

16. CAVADA, C., T. COMPANY, J. TEJEDOR, R.J. CRUZ-RIZZOLO & F. REINOSO-SUAREZ. 2000. The anatomical connections of the macaque monkey orbitofrontal cortex: a review. Cereb. Cortex **10:** 220–242.

17. PETRIDES, M. & D.N. PANDYA. 2002. Comparative architectonic analysis of the human and the macaque ventrolateral prefrontal cortex and corticocortical connection patterns in the monkey. Eur. J. Neurosci. **16:** 291–310.

18. GOLDMAN-RAKIC, P.S. & L.J. PORRINO. 1985. The primate medio-dorsal (MD) nucleus and its projections to the frontal lobe. J. Comp. Neurol. **242:** 535–560.

19. CAVADA, C. & P.S. GOLDMAN-RAKIC. 1989. Posterior parietal cortex in rhesus monkey: II. Evidence for segregated corticocortical networks linking sensory and limbic areas with the frontal lobe. J. Comp. Neurol. **287:** 422–445.

20. TOBIAS, T.J. 1975. Afferents to prefrontal cortex from the thalamic mediodorsal nucleus in the rhesus monkey. Brain Res. **83:** 191–212.

21. PETRIDES, M. 2005. Lateral prefrontal cortex: architectonic and functional organization. Phil. Trans. R. Soc. B **360:** 781–795.

22. MILNER, B. 1968. Visual recognition and recall after right temporal-lobe excisions in man. Neuropsychologia **6:** 191–209.

23. MILNER, B. 1972. Disorders of learning and memory after temporal lobe lesions in man. Clin. Neurosurg. **19:** 421–446.

24. MISHKIN, M. 1982. A memory system in the monkey. Phil. Trans. R. Soc. Lond. B. **298:** 85–95.

25. SQUIRE, L.R. & S. ZOLA-MORGAN. 1991. The medial temporal lobe memory system. Science **253:** 1380–1386.

26. MEUNIER, M., J. BACHEVALIER, M. MISHKIN & E.A. MURRAY. 1993. Effects on visual recognition of combined and separate ablations of the entorhinal and perirhinal cortex in rhesus monkeys. J. Neurosci. **13:** 5418–5432.

27. SUZUKI, W., S. ZOLA-MORGAN, L.R. SQUIRE & D.G. AMARAL. 1993. Lesions of the perirhinal and parahippocampal cortices in the monkey produce long lasting memory impairments in the visual and tactual modalities. J. Neurosci. **13:** 2430–2451.

28. CHIAVARAS, M.M. & M. PETRIDES. 2000. Orbitofrontal sulci of the human and macaque monkey brain. J. Comp. Neurol. **422:** 35–54.

29. SMITH, M.L. & B. MILNER. 1989. Right hippocampal impairment in the recall of spatial location: encoding deficit or rapid forgetting? Neuropsychologia **27:** 71–81.

30. PARKINSON, J.K., E.A. MURRAY & M. MISHKIN. 1988. A selective mnemonic role for the hippocampus in monkeys: memory for the location of objects. J. Neurosci. **8:** 4159–4167.

31. BOHBOT, V.D., M. KALINA, K. STEPANKOVA, *et al.* 1998. Spatial memory deficits in patients with lesions to the right hippocampus and to the right parahippocampal cortex. Neuropsychologia **36:** 1217–1238.
32. EICHENBAUM, H., C. STEWART & R.G. MORRIS. 1990. Hippocampal representation in place learning. J. Neurosci. **10:** 3531–3542.
33. IARIA, G., M. PETRIDES, A. DAGHER, *et al.* 2003. Cognitive strategies dependent on the hippocampus and caudate nucleus in human navigation: variability and change with practice. J. Neurosci. **23:** 5945–5952.
34. VAN HOESEN, G.W., D.N. PANDYA & N. BUTTERS. 1972. Cortical afferents to the entorhinal cortex of the rhesus monkey. Science **175:** 1471–1473.
35. VAN HOESEN, G.W., D.N. PANDYA & N. BUTTERS. 1975. Some connections of the entorhinal (area 28) and perirhinal (area 35) cortices of the rhesus monkey. II. Frontal lobe afferents. Brain Res. **95:** 25–38.
36. ROSENE, D.L. & G.W. VAN HOESEN. 1977. Hippocampal efferents reach widespread areas of cerebral cortex and amygdala in the rhesus monkey. Science **198:** 315–317.
37. LABAR, K.S. & CABEZA R. 2006. Cognitive neuroscience of emotional memory. Nature Rev. Neurosci. **7:** 54–64.
38. ROLLS, E.T. 1999. The Brain and Emotion. Oxford University Press. Oxford, UK.
39. LEDOUX, J. 1996. The Emotional Brain. Simon & Shuster. New York.
40. AGGLETON, J.P., M.J. BURTON & R.E. PASSINGHAM. 1980. Cortical and subcortical afferents to the amygdala of the rhesus monkey (*Macaca mulatta*). Brain Res. **190:** 347–368.
41. VAN HOESEN, G.W. 1981. The differential distribution, diversity and sprouting of cortical projections to the amygdala in the rhesus monkey. *In* The Amygdaloid Complex. Y. Ben-Ari, Ed.: 77–90. Elsevier/North-Holland Biomedical Press. New York.
42. AMARAL, D.G. & J.L. PRICE. 1984. Amygdalo-cortical projections in the monkey (*Macaca fascicularis*). J. Comp. Neurol. **230:** 465–496.
43. NAUTA, W.J.H. 1961. Fibre degeneration following lesions of the amygdaloid complex in the monkey. J. Anat. **95:** 515–531.
44. NAUTA, W.J.H. 1962. Neural associations of the amygdaloid complex in the monkey. Brain **85:** 505–520.
45. PORRINO, L.J., A.M. CRANE & P.S. GOLDMAN-RAKIC. 1981. Direct and indirect pathways from the amygdala to the frontal lobe in rhesus monkeys. J. Comp. Neurol. **198:** 121–136.
46. MORAN, M.A., E.J. MUFSON & M.-M. MESULAM. 1987. Neural inputs into the temporopolar cortex of the rhesus monkey. J. Comp. Neurol. **256:** 88–103.
47. AGGLETON, J.P. & M. MISHKIN. 1984. Projections of the amygdala to the thalamus in the cynomologus monkey. J. Comp. Neurol. **222:** 56–68.
48. BALEYDIER, C. & F. MAUGUIERE. 1980. The duality of the cingulate gyrus in the monkey: neuroanatomical study and functional hypothesis. Brain **103:** 525–554.
49. RUSSCHEN, F.T., D.G. AMARAL & J.L. PRICE. 1987. The afferent input to the magnocellular division of the mediodorsal thalamic nucleus in the monkey, *Macaca fascicularis*. J. Comp. Neurol. **256:** 175–210.
50. BACHEVALIER, J. & M. MISHKIN. 1986. Visual recognition impairment follows ventromedial but not dorsolateral prefrontal lesions in monkeys. Behav. Brain Res. **20:** 249–261.

51. MEUNIER, M., J. BACHEVALIER & M. MISHKIN. 1997. Effects of orbital frontal and anterior cingulate lesions on object and spatial memory in rhesus monkeys. Neuropsychologia **35:** 999–1015.

52. AGGLETON, J.P., R. DESIMONE & M. MISHKIN. 1986. The origin, course, and termination of the hippocampo-thalamic projections in the macaque. J. Comp. Neurol. **243:** 409–421.

53. ANDY, O.J. & H. STEPHAN. 1968. The septum in the human brain. J. Comp. Neurol. **133:** 383–410.

54. MESULAM, M.-M., E.J. MULSON, A.I. LEVEY & B.H. WAINER. 1983. Cholinergic innervation of cortex by the basal forebrain: cytochemistry and cortical connections of the septal area, diagonal band nuclei, nucleus basalis (substantia innominata), and the hypothalamus in the rhesus monkey. J. Comp. Neurol. **214:** 170–197.

55. OLTON, D.S., B.S. GIVENS, A.L. MARKOWSKA, et al. 1991. Mnemonic functions of the cholinergic septohippocampal sytem. *In* Memory: Organization and Locus of Change. L.R. Squire, G. Weinberger, G. Lynch & J.L. Mcgaugh, Eds.: 250–269. Oxford University Press. New York.

56. DAMASIO, A.R., N.R. GRAFF-RADFORD, P.J. ESLINGER, et al. 1985. Amnesia following basal forebrain lesions. Arch. Neurol. **42:** 263–271.

57. PHILLIPS, S., V. SANGALANG & G. STERNS. 1987. Basal forebrain infarction: a clinico-pathologic correlation. Arch. Neurol. **44:** 1134–1138.

58. BERTI, A., C. ARIENTA & C. PAPAGNO. 1990. A case of amnesia after excision of the septum pellucidum. J. Neurol. Neurosurg. Psych. **53:** 922–924.

59. MORRIS, M.K., D. BOWEES, A. CHATTERJEE & K.M. HEILMAN. 1992. Amnesia following a discrete basal forebrain lesion. Brain **115:** 1827–1847.

60. CRAMON, D.Y. von, H.J. MARKOWITSCH & U. SCHURI. 1993. The possible contribution of the septal region to memory. Neuropsychologia **31:** 1159–1180.

61. STRAUSS, I. & M. KESCHNER. 1935. Mental symptoms in cases of tumor of the frontal lobe. Arch. Neurol. Psychiatry **33:** 986–1007.

62. PAILLAS, J.E., J. BOURDOURESQUE, J. BONNAL & J. PROVANSAL. 1950. Tumeurs frontales: considerations anatomo-cliniques á propos de 72 tumeurs operées. Rev. Neurol. **83:** 470–473.

63. HECAEN, H. 1964. Mental symptoms associated with tumors of the frontal lobe. *In* The Frontal Granular Cortex and Behavior, Chapter 16. J.M. Warren & K. Akert, Eds.: 335–352. McGraw-Hill. New York.

64. AVERY, T.L. 1971. Seven cases of frontal tumour with psychiatric presentation. Br. J. Psychiatry **119:** 19–23.

65. LURIA, A.R. 1976. The Neuropsychology of Memory. Wiley. New York.

66. LINDQVIST, G. & G. NORLEN. 1966. Korsakoff's syndrome after operation on ruptured aneurysm of the anterior communicating artery. Acta Psych. Scand. **42:** 24–34.

67. TALLAND, G.A., W.H. SWEET & H.T. BALANTINE. 1967. Amnesic syndrome with anterior communicating artery aneurysms. J. Nerv. Ment. Dis. **145:** 179–192.

68. GADE, A. 1982. Amnesia after operations on aneurysms of the anterior communicating artery. Surg. Neurol. **18:** 46–49.

69. VOLPE, B.T. & W. HIRST. 1983. Amnesia following the rupture and repair of an anterior communicating artery aneurysm. J. Neurol. Neurosurg. Psychiatry **46:** 704–709.

70. CORKIN, S, N.J. COHEN, E.V. SULLIVAN, et al. 1985. Analyses of global memory impairments of different etiologies. Ann. N. Y. Acad. Sci. **444:** 10–40.

71. ALEXANDER, M.P. & M. FREEDMAN. 1984. Amnesia after anterior communicating artery aneurysm rupture. Neurol. **34:** 752–757.
72. ESLINGER, P.J. & A.R. DAMASIO. 1985. Severe disturbance of higher cognition after bilateral frontal lobe ablation: patient EVR. Neurology **35:** 1731–1741.
73. LEVINE, B., S.E. BLACK, R. CABEZA, et al. 1998. Episodic memory and the self in a case of isolated retrograde amnesia. Brain **121:** 1951–1973.
74. KARTSOUNIS, L.D., A. POYNTON, P.K. BRIDGES & J.R. BARTLETT. 1991. Neuropsychological correlates of stereotactic subcaudate tractotomy. Brain **114:** 2657–2673.
75. SCOVILLE, W.B. & D.B. BETTIS. 1977. Results of orbital undercutting today: a personal series. *In* Neurosurgical Treatment in Psychiatry, Pain, and Epilepsy. W.H. Sweet, S. Obrador & J.G. Martin-Rodriguez, Eds.: 189–202. University Park Press. Baltimore, MD.
76. BUTTER, C.M. 1964. Habituation of responses to novel stimuli in monkeys with selective frontal lesions. Science **144:** 313–315.
77. FREY, S. & M. PETRIDES. 2003. Greater orbitofrontal activity predicts better memory for faces. Eur. J. Neurosci. **17:** 2755–2758.
78. FREY, S. & M. PETRIDES. 2002. Orbitofrontal cortex and memory formation. Neuron **36:** 171–176.
79. FREY, S. & M. PETRIDES. 2000. Orbitofrontal cortex: a key prefrontal region for encoding information. Proc. Natl. Acad. Sci. USA **97:** 8723–8727.
80. FREY, S., P. KOSTOPOULOS & M. PETRIDES. 2004. Orbitofrontal contribution to auditory encoding. Neuroimage **22:** 1384–1389.
81. ROLLS, E.T., A.S. BROWNING, K. INOUE & S. HERNADI. 2005. Novel visual stimuli activate a population of neurons in the primate orbitofrontal cortex. Neurobiol. Learn. Mem. **84:** 111–123.
82. PETRIDES, M., B. ALIVISATOS & S. FREY. 2002. Differential activation of the human orbital, mid-ventrolateral and mid-dorsolateral prefrontal cortex during the processing of visual stimuli. Proc. Natl. Acad. Sci. USA **99:** 5649–5654.
83. BECHARA, A., D. TRANEL & H. DAMASIO. 2000. Characterization of the decision-making deficit of patients with ventromedial prefrontal cortex lesions. Brain **123:** 1189–2202.
84. SCHOENBAUM, G., A.A. CHIBA & M. GALLAGHER. 1998. Orbitofrontal cortex and basolateral amygdala encode expected outcomes during learning. Nat. Neurosci. **1:** 155–159.
85. TREMBLAY, L. & W. SCHULTZ. 2000. Modifications of reward expectation-related neuronal activity during learning in primate orbitofrontal cortex. J. Neurophysiology **83:** 1877–1885.
86. ROBBINS, T.W., L. CLARK, L.H. CLARKE & A.C. ROBERTS. 2006. Neurochemical modulation of orbitofrontal cortex function. *In* The Orbitofrontal Cortex. D.H. Zald & S.L. Rauch, Eds.: 393–422. Oxford University Press. Oxford, UK.
87. LIVINGSTON, R.B., W.P. CHAPMAN, K.E. LIVINGSTON & L. KRAINTZ. 1948. Stimulation of orbital surface of man prior to frontal lobotomy. Res. Publ. Assoc. Nerv. Ment. Dis. **27:** 421–432.
88. BAILEY, P. & W.H. SWEET. 1940. Effects on respiration, blood pressure and gastric mobility of stimulation of orbital surface of frontal lobe. J. Neurophysiol. **3:** 276–281.
89. DELGADO, J.M.R. & R.B. LIVINGSTON. 1947. Some respiratory, vascular and thermal responses to stimulation of orbital surface of frontal lobe. J. Neurophysiol. **11:** 39–55.

90. HALL, R.E. & K. CORNISH. 1977. Role of the orbital cortex in cardiac dysfunction in unanesthetized rhesus monkey. Exp. Neurol. **56:** 289–297.
91. HALL, R.E., R.B. LIVINGSTON & C.M. BLOOR. 1977. Orbital cortical influences on cardiovascular dynamics and myocardial structure in conscious monkeys. J. Neurosurg. **46:** 638–647.
92. TRANEL, D. & H. DAMASIO. 1994. Neuroanatomical correlates of electrodermal skin conductance responses. Psychophysiology **31:** 427–438.
93. FREY, S., P. KOSTOPOULOS & M. PETRIDES. 2000. Orbitofrontal involvement in the processing of unpleasant auditory information. Eur. J. Neurosci. **12:** 3709–3712.
94. BUTTER, C.M., D.R. SNYDER & J.A. MCDONALD. 1970. Effects of orbital frontal lesions on aversive and aggressive behaviors in rhesus monkeys. J. Comp. Physiol. Psychol. **72:** 132–144.
95. PICKENS, C.L., B. SETLOW, M.P. SADDORIS, *et al.* 2003. Different roles for OFC and basolateral amygdala in a reinforcer devaluation task. J. Neurosci. **23:** 11078–11084.
96. MARKOWITSCH, H.J., M.M. VANDEKERCKHOVE, H. LANFERMANN & M.O. RUSS. 2003. Engagement of lateral and medial prefrontal areas in the ecphory of sad and happy autobiographical memories. Cortex **39:** 643–665.
97. PIEFKE, M., P.H. WEISS, K. ZILLES, *et al.* 2003. Differential remoteness and emotional tone modulate the neural correlates of autobiographical memory. Brain **126:** 650–668.
98. MARATOS, E.J., R.J. DOLAN, J.S. MORRIS, *et al.* 2001. Neural activity associated with episodic memory for emotional context. Neuropsychologia **39:** 910–920.

Definition of the Orbital Cortex in Relation to Specific Connections with Limbic and Visceral Structures and Other Cortical Regions

JOSEPH L. PRICE

Department of Anatomy & Neurobiology, Washington University School of Medicine, St. Louis, Missouri 63110, USA

ABSTRACT: The orbitofrontal cortex is often defined topographically as the cortex on the ventral surface of the frontal lobe. Unfortunately, this definition is not consistently used, and it obscures distinct connectional and functional systems within the orbital cortex. It is difficult to interpret data on the orbital cortex that do not take these different systems into account. Analysis of cortico-cortical connections between areas in the orbital and medial prefrontal cortex indicate two distinct networks in this region. One system, called the orbital network, involves most of the areas in the central orbital cortex. The other system, has been called the medial prefrontal network, though it is actually more complex, since it includes areas on the medial wall, in the medial orbital cortex, and in the posterolateral orbital cortex. Some areas in the medial orbital cortex are involved in both networks. Connections to other brain areas support the distinction between the networks. The orbital network receives several sensory inputs, from olfactory cortex, taste cortex, somatic sensory association cortex, and visual association cortex, and is connected with multisensory areas in the ventrolateral prefrontal cortex and perirhinal cortex. The medial network has outputs to the hypothalamus and brain stem and connects to a cortical circuit that includes the rostral part of the superior temporal gyrus and dorsal bank of the superior temporal sulcus, the cingulate and retrosplenial cortex, the entorhinal and posterior parahippocampal cortex, and the dorsomedial prefrontal cortex.

KEYWORDS: architectonic areas; medial prefrontal cortex; cortico-cortical connections; mediodorsal thalamus; ventral striatum; periaqueductal gray; medial prefrontal network; orbital prefrontal network

Address for correspondence: Joseph L. Price, Ph.D., Department of Anatomy & Neurobiology, Washington University School of Medicine, 660 S. Euclid Avenue, St. Louis, MO 63110. Voice: 314-362-3587; fax: 314-747-1150.
pricej@wustl.edu

Ann. N.Y. Acad. Sci. 1121: 54–71 (2007). © 2007 New York Academy of Sciences.
doi: 10.1196/annals.1401.008

The orbitofrontal or orbital cortex in primates can be defined topographically as the cortex on the ventral surface of the frontal lobe, from the gyrus rectus on the medial side to the ventrolateral convexity laterally, and from the limen insula caudally to the frontal pole. This definition is not used consistently, however, and often the term orbitofrontal cortex is variably extended to include parts of the medial prefrontal cortex. More importantly, a purely topographical definition obscures the fact that there are many distinct areas within the orbitofrontal region. As discussed below, these areas are linked into two, distinct systems that differ in connections and function. Because these two systems have markedly different connections with other parts of the brain, and presumably have different functions, experiments that do not distinguish between them, or do not take their boundaries into account, are difficult to interpret. In order to consider these systems fully, this description will include both the orbital and the medial prefrontal cortex (OMPFC).

The OMPFC is a large and heterogeneous region, which makes up a substantial fraction of the cortex in non-human primates and even more in humans. It is much smaller in rodents, but by comparing the structure and connections of specific areas, a relatively secure correlation can be made between rodents and primates. Only the agranular areas are represented in rodents; these make up approximately the caudal third of the OMPFC in non-human primates, and relatively less in humans.

In primates, including humans, the cortex on both the orbital and medial frontal surfaces varies from the agranular region caudally, at the junction with the insular cortex and the septal nuclei, to a dysgranular zone in the central region, and then a granular region near the frontal pole.[1,2] These broad cortical zones are not homogeneous, however, and each of them can be divided into several architectonic areas that have distinct connections and presumably distinct functions. Although there is considerable variation in the prefrontal cortex across species, especially in the amount of granular versus agranular cortex, similarities in the position and connections of caudal OMPFC indicates that this part of the prefrontal cortex, at least, is relatively comparable across species.[3–5]

ARCHITECTONIC AREAS OF MONKEY, HUMAN, AND RAT

Monkey

Brodmann[6,7] delineated three agranular areas on the medial wall of monkeys, area 24 just dorsal to the genu of the corpus callosum, area 25 in the subgenual region, and area 32 rostral to area 25. His granular area 10 occupies the frontal pole. Brodmann[6,7] did not carry out a detailed study of the orbital cortex, but appeared to include all or most of it in his area 11. A later map by Walker[8] has formed the basis for most recent maps of this region in monkeys.

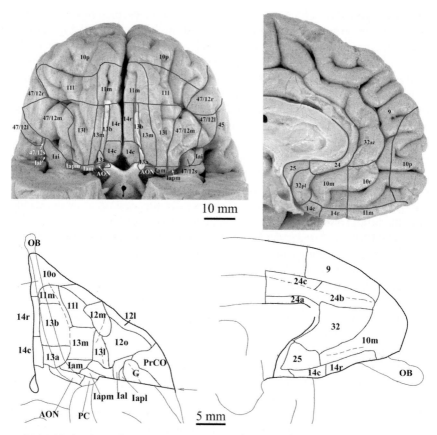

FIGURE 1. Maps of architectonic areas in the OMPFC of humans (above) and monkeys (below). Reproduced from Öngür and Price[5] and Carmichael and Price.[2]

Walker[8] recognized area 10 on the frontal pole and area 11 on the rostral orbital surface. More caudally, his areas 12, 13, and 14 occupy the lateral, central, and medial orbital surface, respectively. Walker[8] also described the medial prefrontal cortex, but his areas with the same number do not have corresponding locations as in Brodmann's maps. Brodmann's maps have formed the basis for most recent analyses of the medial prefrontal cortex.

The description in this chapter will be based primarily on the architectonic analysis by Carmichael and Price,[2] which identified over 20 areas in the OMPFC, many of which are subdivisions of previously recognized areas (FIG. 1). For example, Walker's rostral granular areas 10 and 11 were subdivided into areas 10m, 10o, 11m, and 11l. Of these, areas 10o, 11m, and 11l are in the rostral orbital surface, while area 10m is situated primarily on the medial surface of the hemisphere. In the central part of the orbital surface, Walker's areas 12, 13, and 14 were subdivided into areas 12r, 12l, 12m, 12o,

13a, 13b, 13m, 13l, 14r, and 14c. Finally, five areas (Iam, Iai, Ial, Iapm, and Iapl) were recognized in the posterior orbital cortex that represent a rostral extension of the agranular insular cortex onto the orbital surface.

Human

Brodmann's human map generally resembles his monkey map, although it is clear that they are not identical.[6,7] Thus, in the human map the medial prefrontal cortex consists of areas 10, 11, 24, 25, and 32, while in his monkey (guenon) map there is no area 10 or 25 and area 12 occupies the ventral frontal pole. Further, Brodmann specifically stated that area 32 in the human map is not homologous to area 32 in the monkey map.[6,7] Another terminological problem is related to area 12. In one version of his human map that has been republished in several textbooks and reviews (see Ref. 4 for example). Brodmann included an area 12 on the medial wall anterior to the corpus callosum, but this is not found in the map published in his monograph.[6] Where illustrated, this medial area 12 is clearly different from the area 12 in the lateral orbital cortex in Walker's[8] and subsequent maps of monkeys (see above). The lateral orbital area that is usually denoted as area 12 in monkeys appears to correspond to area 47 in Brodmann's human map. Petrides and Pandya[4] have made an attempt to resolve this by using the term area 47/12 to refer to the lateral orbital areas in both humans and monkeys. Brodmann[6] did not illustrate the rest of the orbital surface, but most of it appears to have been denoted as area 11 in the map of the human brain. Several other investigators have proposed delineations that are in relatively close accord with the map made by Walker[8] in monkeys, with area 14 on the gyrus rectus, area 13 in medial part of the orbital cortex, area 47/12 in the lateral orbital cortex, and area 11 rostrally.[4,9–11]

Öngür *et al.*[12] did a more detailed analysis based on five different histological and immunohistochemical stains, that attempted to translate the monkey map of the OMPFC by Carmichael and Price[2] onto the human brain (FIG. 1). Twenty-three distinct areas were recognized in humans, all of which are correlated with a specific area in monkeys. As in monkeys, many of these areas are subdivisions of previously recognized zones from Walker's map.[4,8,9,11] To a remarkably high degree, the human cortical areas were defined by similar staining characteristics as the corresponding areas in monkeys and were located in similar locations.

Rat

The most prominent cytoarchitectonic feature of the rat prefrontal cortex is that it is composed exclusively of agranular cortical areas. Because of this, there has been concern since the work of Brodmann[6,7] whether rodents have any cortex that can be compared to the granular prefrontal cortex in primates. In an effort to address this question, Rose and Woolsey[13] proposed that equivalent areas could be recognized in different species on the basis of similar connections; specifically they proposed that the "orbitofrontal cortex" of rabbits and cats was similar to the primate prefrontal cortex due to its connections with the mediodorsal thalamic nucleus (MD). Based on this criterion, the "prefrontal cortex" in rats includes the medial frontal cortex (around and rostral to the genu of the corpus callosum), the cortex at the dorsomedial corner of the hemisphere, and the "orbital" cortex in the dorsal bank of the rhinal sulcus.[3,14–16] Unfortunately, this definition does not address the problem of which if any areas in the rat are homologous to the rostral or dorsolateral granular prefrontal cortex in primates. That is, the cortical region that is connected to the mediodorsal thalamic nucleus (by this definition the prefrontal cortex) may include cortical areas in primates (e.g., the rostral and dorsolateral granular areas) that are not present in rodents (see also Refs. 17,18).

The caudal and ventromedial areas of the prefrontal cortex (i.e. all but the rostral parts of the OMPFC) can be recognized in rats, however, based on architectonic and connectional similarities. On topological grounds, it would be expected that the orbital cortex in rats would be situated in the dorsal bank of the rostral end of the rhinal sulcus. Krettek and Price[14] subdivided this region into medial, ventrolateral, and lateral orbital areas (MO, VLO, LO) (FIG. 2). These may be comparable to areas 14, 13a, and 13m/l, respectively, in monkeys. Caudal to the junction of the frontal cortex and the olfactory peduncle, area VLO continues in the depth of the rhinal sulcus, but the dorsal bank and lip of the rhinal sulcus is occupied by the ventral and dorsal agranular insular areas (AIv, AId)[14,16] (FIG. 2). In the initial description, area AId extended rostrally, lateral to the orbital areas,[14] but subsequently the part of area AId rostral to the claustrum was recognized as the dorsolateral orbital area (DLO).[16] AIv may be comparable to areas Iam and Iapm in monkeys, while areas AId and DLO resemble the monkey areas Iai and 12o, respectively. On the medial wall, the infralimbic (IL) and prelimbic (PL) areas presumably correspond to areas 25 and 32, while the anterior cingulate area (AC) corresponds to area 24. More rostrally, Ray and Price[16] also delineated lateral and medial frontal pole areas (FPl and FPm); although these areas still lack a granular layer IV, they may represent the primordium of the granular prefrontal cortex, if anything does in rats.

INTRINSIC CORTICO-CORTICAL CONNECTIONS

Experiments in monkeys in which anterograde or retrograde axonal tracers are injected into the agranular insular areas (Iam, Iapm, Ial, Iapl) at the caudal edge of the orbital surface label substantial connections to areas 12l, 12m, 13l, and 13m in the central orbital cortex (FIG. 3).[19] Those areas, in turn, are

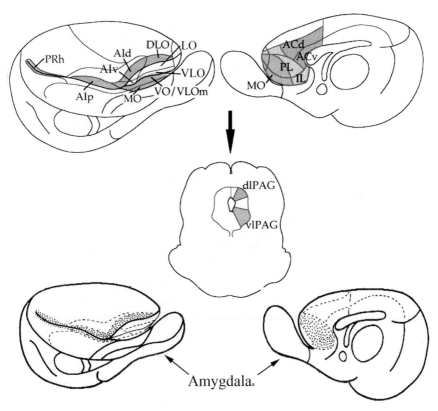

FIGURE 2. Surface drawings of a rat brain, with architectonic areas as analyzed by Krettek and Price[14] and Ray and Price.[16] Above: the areas that project to the PAG are shown by shading.[46] These probably correspond to the medial prefrontal network in monkeys. The intervening areas LO, VLO, and AIv may correspond to the orbital prefrontal network. Below: the dotted regions indicate the areas that receive input from the basal nucleus of the amygdala. Modified from Krettek and Price[51] and Floyd *et al.*[53]

substantially connected with more rostral and lateral areas 11l and 12r. Some of the connections, especially from the lateral orbital areas, extend around the ventrolateral convexity of the frontal lobe and also involve area 45 and the ventral part of area 46. The labeled axons or cells are often arranged in patches or columns; in general, these extend across all layers of the cortex.

The areas in the medial prefrontal cortex (areas 24, 25, 32, and 10m) have a largely complementary pattern of interconnections (FIG. 3).[19] These areas are substantially connected with other medial prefrontal areas, but have few connections with most of the orbital cortex, especially the areas in the central orbital cortex. The exceptions to this rule are areas along the medial edge of the orbital cortex (areas 11m, 13a, 13b, 14c, 14r) and two areas in the caudolateral part of the orbital cortex (areas 12o and Iai). Many of these areas

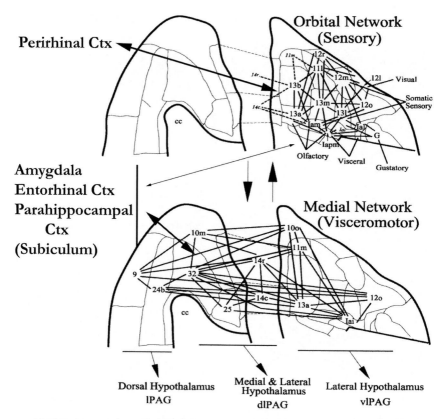

FIGURE 3. Diagrammatic illustration of the intrinsic connections within the OMPFC of monkeys, which define the orbital and medial prefrontal networks.[19] Note that the orbital network includes most of the areas on the orbital surface, while the medial network includes areas on the medial wall plus two areas in the posterolateral orbital cortex. Areas on the gyrus rectus at the medial edge of the orbital cortex tend to be involved in both networks. The orbital network also receives inputs from several sensory modalities, while the medial network has specific outputs to the hypothalamus and PAG. Limbic structures are reciprocally connected primarily to the medial network, with the exception of the perirhinal cortex which is connected mostly to the orbital network. The projection from the subiculum to the medial network is not reciprocated. Modified from Carmichael and Price.[19]

are connected to both the orbital and the medial network areas, but three of them, areas 11m, 14r, and Iai, are primarily connected to the medial areas.

Based on these observations, the areas of the medial and orbital prefrontal cortex of monkeys have been divided into "medial" and "orbital" prefrontal networks (FIG. 3).[19] The areas on the caudal and central part of the orbital surface are included in the orbital network, but areas 11m, 14r, and Iai are part of the "medial" network. The most medial orbital areas, 13a, 13b, 14c, and lateral area 12o, have prominent connections with the medial network, but they also have connections to the orbital network and can be considered intermediate areas that may serve as interfaces between the two networks.

It is critical to stress that the "medial" and "orbital" prefrontal networks are connectional systems and are not synonymous with the topographically defined medial prefrontal cortex or orbital cortex. The medial network includes areas on the medial wall of the prefrontal cortex, *and* areas along the medial edge of the orbital cortex, *and* areas in the caudolateral part of the orbital cortex. The orbital network includes areas in the caudal and central part of the orbital cortex but does *not* include all areas in the orbital cortex.

It is also important to emphasize that, while the medial and orbital networks are distinct, based on differences in both intrinsic connections and extrinsic connections (below), they are not fully separate. There are some interconnections between them, especially through areas along the gyrus rectus at the ventromedial corner of the hemisphere. Further, while the distinction between the two networks has held up through several investigational studies, the boundary between the networks is not always sharp. This subtlety is difficult to express in a short review chapter, and the reader should examine the original research papers referenced below for more nuanced descriptions.

EXTRINSIC CONNECTIONS

Sensory Inputs to Orbital Network

Connections to other brain areas also support the distinction of the orbital and medial networks. The orbital network receives sensory inputs from other cortical areas, including olfactory cortex, taste cortex, parts of SI, SII, and other somatic sensory areas in the insula and parietal cortex, and visual association areas in the inferior temporal cortex. It also is connected with multisensory areas in the ventrolateral prefrontal cortex and the perirhinal cortex.[20]

A chief characteristic of the orbital network is that it receives inputs from cortical areas associated with most of the sensory systems, including olfaction, taste/visceral afferents, vision, and somatic sensation (FIG. 3). The olfactory inputs arise in the piriform cortex and other primary olfactory cortical areas, while the taste/visceral inputs come from the primary taste cortex and from agranular insular areas, both of which receive projections from the taste/visceral thalamic relay nucleus. The inferior temporal cortex (area TE) provides the visual inputs, primarily but not exclusively to ventrolateral prefrontal areas, and parts of SI and SII project somatic sensory information to area 13 m/l in the orbital network.

Taken together, the constellation of sensory inputs suggests that the orbital network is particularly involved in assessment of food. This suggestion is supported by physiological recording studies, which have shown that orbital neurons respond to multisensory, food-related stimuli in a way that appears to

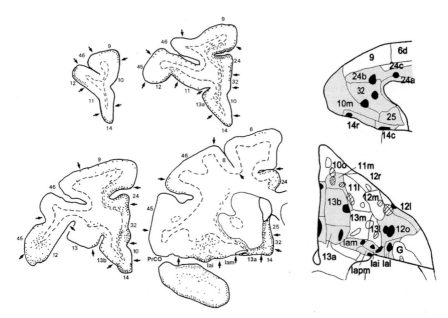

FIGURE 4. Illustrations of the amygdalo-cortical projection to the OMPFC. On the left is a drawing of the distribution of autoradiographically labeled fibers following an injection of 3 H-leucine into the amygdala. Modified from Amaral and Price.[25] Note that there are very few labeled axons in the central part of the orbital cortex, with the exception of area Iai. On the right is a drawing of the position of retrograde tracer injections that either did (*filled outlines*) or did not (*open outlines*) label neurons in the amygdala; the cross-hatched outlines indicate injections that labeled only a few neurons. Areas that had injections that labeled amygdala cells are shaded. Modified from Carmichael and Price.[29] Note that injections in the central and rostral part of the orbital cortex did not label amygdaloid connections.

code for flavor, appearance and texture of food.[21] In addition, the studies also indicate that the orbital neurons respond to affective characteristics (reward versus aversion) as well as sensory characteristics of the stimuli.[22-24] It may be noted that the orbital network is connected with the ventrolateral prefrontal cortex, which also receives multiple sensory inputs, and also may be involved in sensory object assessment.[25]

Limbic Connections

In addition to the sensory inputs, the OMPFC is also reciprocally connected with a number of limbic structures.[26-31] The strongest limbic connections are with the amygdala (especially the basal and accessory basal nuclei), but there are also substantial connections with the entorhinal cortex, the perirhinal cortex, and the posterior parahippocampal cortex (FIGS. 3 and 4). In addition, the subiculum provides a unidirectional projection to the medial prefrontal cortex.

Most of these connections are distributed to the areas of the medial prefrontal network (including the intermediate areas) that are located in the medial wall and along the medial edge and in the caudolateral part of the orbital cortex (FIG. 4). The agranular insular areas in the caudal part of the orbital network also have limbic connections, but even here, the projection from the amygdala is stronger to the medial network area Iai than to adjacent areas such as Iam or Iapm. Further, there are few limbic connections to the central areas in the orbital network (e.g., areas 13m, 13l, and 11l). The only exceptions to this are the connections with the perirhinal cortex (areas 35 and 36), which primarily involve areas of the orbital network.[31]

Visceral Outputs from Medial Network

The medial network receives few direct sensory inputs but has outputs to visceral control structures in the hypothalamus and midbrain, including the periaqueductal gray (PAG)[24,25,32–35](FIG. 3). Both of these brain regions serve to coordinate several aspects of visceral function, and it is likely that the cortical projections are a major pathway for forebrain modulation of bodily reactions.

The strongest projections to the hypothalamus are from areas 25 and 32 in the medial prefrontal cortex, but there are also projections from all of the areas of the medial network, including the ventromedial and caudolateral orbital areas (13a/b and 14c, and Iai/12o)[33](FIG. 3). The fibers from the medial prefrontal cortex are distributed to both medial and lateral hypothalamic nuclei and areas, suggesting that the cortex influences both autonomic and endocrine functions. Fibers from areas 13a, Iai, and 12o, on the other hand, are restricted to the lateral hypothalamus. There are relatively few projections to the hypothalamus from areas of the orbital network, although the agranular insular areas Iam, Iapm, and Ial have light projections to the caudal part of the lateral hypothalamus.[33]

Many of medial network fibers that run through the hypothalamus extend caudally into the ventral midbrain and tegmentum, reaching at least to the PAG[32] (FIG. 3). As in the hypothalamus, the projections to the midbrain arise almost exclusively from the medial prefrontal network and from adjacent related areas such as the dorsomedial prefrontal area 9 and the dorsal temporal pole. There are very few if any fibers from the orbital network to the midbrain.

Thalamic and Striatal Connections

The orbital and medial prefrontal networks also have distinct connections with the thalamus and striatum (FIG. 5). The principal thalamic nucleus related to the orbital cortex is the medial, magnocellular part of the mediodorsal nucleus, but the totality of the connections is complex. Large injections of retrograde axonal tracers in the orbital cortex label cells in many nuclei in

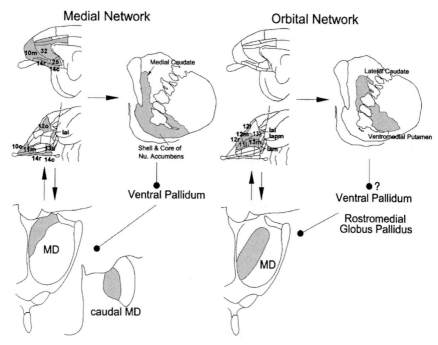

FIGURE 5. Diagram of cortico-striatal-pallidal-thalamic connections of the medial and orbital prefrontal networks. Note that the two networks are related to adjacent but distinct parts of the striatum and mediodorsal thalamic nucleus. Modified from Öngür and Price.[5]

the medial thalamus, including components of the anterior thalamic group, several midline and intralaminar nuclei, and the medial pulvinar, as well as the mediodorsal nucleus.[36] Many of these, including the anteromedial nucleus and many of the midline nuclei, target the areas of the medial network.[29,37] The anteromedial nucleus connects with approximately the same zone along the medial edge of the orbital cortex that is related to the subiculum and posterior parahippocampal cortex.[29,31] The midline nuclei, especially the paraventricular and parataenial nuclei, also project very strongly to the ventromedial striatum, which receives inputs from the medial network (see below). They have few or no connections to orbital network areas.[38]

Within the medial part of the mediodorsal nucleus, different zones are connected to the orbital and medial networks[38] (FIG. 5). The medial network is connected to the dorsomedial and dorsocaudal region of the nucleus, while the orbital network is connected to the ventromedial region of the nucleus. Several limbic areas, including the olfactory cortex, amygdala, entorhinal cortex, and subiculum also provide excitatory inputs to the medial mediodorsal nucleus.[38]

There is a comparable separation in the projections of the orbital and medial networks to the striatum (FIG. 5). The areas of the medial network project

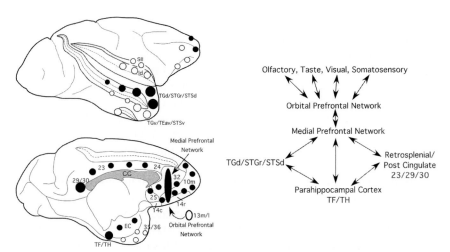

FIGURE 6. Diagram of extrinsic cortical connections of the medial and orbital prefrontal networks, as demonstrated by an experiment with retrograde axonal tracers in the medial prefrontal cortex, and the orbital cortex. (Modified from Saleem et al.[50])

into the classic ventromedial or "limbic" striatum, including the accumbens nucleus, rostromedial caudate nucleus, and ventral putamen.[39] This striatal region is the same that receives input from the amygdala.[40] In comparison, the orbital network areas project to a more central part of striatum, including adjacent portions of the lateral caudate nucleus and medial putamen on either side of the internal capsule.[39]

These striatal regions project to the ventral pallidum and rostral globus pallidus, which in turn projects to the medial part of the mediodorsal thalamic nucleus[16,41] (Fig. 5). Although the details of the pathway have not been fully worked out, there are likely two distinct and separate cortico-striato-pallido-thalamic loops, one for the medial network and one for the orbital network.[5] As in other striato-pallido-thalamic systems, the stiato-pallidal and pallido-thalamic synapses are GABAergic and inhibitory.[42]

Cortical Connections of Medial Network

The medial prefrontal network, including the areas in the ventromedial and caudolateral parts of the orbital cortex, connects to a well-defined cortical circuit that is very different than the constellation of sensory areas that connect to the orbital network (Fig. 6). This circuit related to the medial network includes the dorsal temporal pole, rostral part of the superior temporal gyrus and dorsal bank of the superior temporal sulcus (TGd/STGr/STSd), the cingulate and retrosplenial cortex, the entorhinal and posterior parahippocampal cortex, and the dorsomedial prefrontal cortex (area 9). Except for the TGd/STGr/STSd region, these areas are not specifically sensory or motor in function.

The TGd/STGr/STSd region is usually assumed to have an auditory or polymodal role, but there are several uncertainties about its function. It is adjacent to the auditory belt/parabelt region, but there is little if any overlap with those areas. Rostrally, where the region connected to the medial network occupies the STGr, the auditory areas are restricted to a small region within the lateral sulcus. More caudally, where the auditory areas occupy the STG, the region related to the medial network is displaced into the STSd. Physiological studies have indicated that neurons in the STSd, and possibly in STGr, respond to polymodal signals, including visual, auditory, and somatosensory stimuli.[43-46] Most of the recordings have been made caudal to the TGd/STGr/STSd region, however, and the status of the cortex that is connected with the medial network is not clear. A more recent study that used 2-deoxyglucose in conjunction with complex auditory and visual stimuli has indicated that the region activated by auditory stimuli extends into at least the dorsal aspect of the TGd/STGr/STSd area, although the level of activation does not appear to be as great as in the auditory belt and parabelt areas.[47] The STSd was reported to be activated by both auditory and visual stimuli. Interestingly, areas in the orbital network are also activated by auditory and visual stimuli, but most of the medial network is not activated by either modality stimuli. This is in keeping with the generally sensory nature of the orbital network, and the non-sensory nature of the medial network suggested above.

CORRELATION OF CONNECTIONS IN RAT AND MONKEY

In rats, it appears that the medial and orbital prefrontal networks can be distinguished based on similar cortico-cortical connections, although these have not been studied as thoroughly as in monkeys. Thus, the medial prefrontal prelimbic and infralimbic areas have strong connections to other areas on the medial wall. They also have connections to the agranular insular areas, with relatively fewer connections to the orbital areas in the more rostral part of the rhinal sulcus.[48,49] The connections are especially strong with the dorsal agranular insular area (AId). All of these areas are quite small in rats, however, and a detailed analysis of their cortico-cortical connections has not been published.

Perhaps better indications of the medial and orbital networks in rats come from connections with the amygdala, the hypothalamus, and the periaqueductal gray. As noted above, in monkeys all of these structures are primarily connected to the medial network, including the medial network areas in the medial edge and the caudolateral part of the orbital cortex.[50] Although there are also relatively light connections between these structures and some areas in the orbital network, these are relatively slight compared to the connections with the medial network.

In rats, the major prefrontal connections of the amygdala (especially the basal or basolateral nucleus) are with the prelimbic (PL) and infralimbic (IL) areas on the medial wall of the frontal cortex and the dorsal agranular insular area (AId) laterally.[51] Many of the amygdalo-cortical fibers run through the deep layers of orbital areas just medial to AId, such as the lateral orbital (LO) and ventral agranular insular (AIv) areas, but the termination in these areas appears to be relatively light. It should be noted that lesions of areas LO and AIv, or injections of axonal tracers into these areas, will probably involve the amygdaloid fibers that run through these areas on their way to areas DLO and AId. This distribution is similar to that of the amygdalo-cortical fibers in monkeys, which are concentrated in areas Iai and 12o and are relatively light in other orbital areas, especially 13m and 13l.[25,29]

The cortical output to the PAG in rats also arises primarily from the areas on the medial edge of the frontal cortex, including PL, IL; from the dorsal and ventral anterior cingulate areas and the medial and ventral orbital areas (MO and VO); and from the dorsolateral orbital area (DLO) and AId.[52] There is little projection to the PAG from areas AIv, LO, and the ventrolateral orbital area (VLO) in the dorsal bank of the rhinal sulcus. The origin of outputs to the hypothalamus is less well defined in rats, but the major projection again appears to arise from the medial prefrontal areas and areas AIv and DLO, with less substantial projections from orbital areas such as AIv, VLO, and LO.[53]

Experiments such as this suggest that in rats the medial prefrontal network includes the medial areas PL, IL, and ACv/d, plus the lateral areas AId and DLO. All of these have strong amygdaloid and other limbic inputs and provide substantial output to the hypothalamus and PAG. The orbital network is represented by areas AIv, VLO, and LO. These are strongly related to the olfactory system[54] and probably also receive inputs from other sensory modalities. Areas VO and MO may be similar to the areas on the gyrus rectus of monkeys that are intermediate between the two networks.

CONCLUDING SUMMARY

As discussed in this brief review, the OMPFC is a complex region that in monkeys and humans can be divided into more than 20 areas based on architectonic and connectional distinctions. In rats similar areas can be recognized that appear to correspond to the caudal, agranular parts of the OMPFC, but it is not clear whether rodents have areas equivalent to the more rostral, granular areas seen in primates. In all three species, the areas can be grouped into two systems or networks, based on interconnections within each network and on differential connections with other parts of the brain. Although these have been termed the *medial* and *orbital* prefrontal networks, they are not coextensive with the cortex on the medial or orbital surfaces of the frontal lobe. The medial network includes the medial prefrontal cortex, the cortex along the medial edge of the orbital cortex, and two areas in the caudolateral part of the orbital cortex, while the orbital network consists of areas in the posterior, central, and lateral part of the orbital cortex. The two networks are distinct on several anatomical and functional grounds, but they are not completely separate; in particular, several areas along the ventromedial corner of the frontal lobe have connections with both networks and may provide an interface between them. Functionally, the orbital network has connections with several sensory systems and probably serves as a polymodal integration system for the analysis and assessment of sensory objects, especially food. The medial network does not receive direct sensory inputs, but has strong interconnections with several limbic structures and has outputs to visceral control centers such as the hypothalamus and periaqueductal gray. It is related to emotional regulation and is involved in mood disorders.

ACKNOWLEDGMENT

Supported by USPHS grant R01 MH070941.

REFERENCES

1. BARBAS, H. & D.N. PANDYA. 1989. Architecture and intrinsic connections of the prefrontal cortex in the Rhesus monkey. J. Comp. Neurol. **286:** 353–375.
2. CARMICHAEL, S.T. & J.L. PRICE. 1994. Architectonic subdivision of the orbital and medial prefrontal cortex in the macaque monkey. J. Comp. Neurol. **346:** 366–402.
3. UYLINGS, H.B.M. & C.G. VAN EDEN. 1990. Qualitative and quantitative comparison of the prefrontal cortex in rat and in primates, including humans. Prog. Brain Res. **85:** 31–62.
4. PETRIDES, M. & D.N. PANDYA. 1994. Comparative cytoarchitectonic analysis of the human and the macaque frontal cortex. *In* Handbook of Neuropsychology, Vol. 9. F. Boller & J. Grafman, Eds.: 17–58. Elsevier Science B.V. Amsterdam.
5. ÖNGÜR, D. & J.L. PRICE. 2000. The organization of networks within the orbital and medial prefrontal cortex of rats, monkeys and humans. Cereb. Cortex **10:** 206–219.
6. BRODMANN, K. 1909. Vergleichende Lokalisationslehre der Grosshirnrinde in ihren Prinzipien dargestellt auf Grund des Zellenbaues. JA Barth. Leipzig.
7. GAREY, L.J. 1994. Brodmann's 'Localisation in the Cerebral Cortex'. Smith-Gordon & Co. London.
8. WALKER, A.E. 1940. A cytoarchitectural study of the prefrontal area of the macaque monkey. J. Comp. Neurol. **73:** 59–86.
9. BECK, E. 1949. A cytoarchitectural investigation into the boundaries of cortical areas 13 and 14 in the human brain. J. Anat. **83:** 147–157.
10. SEMENDEFERI, K. *et al.* 1998. Limbic frontal cortex in hominoids: a comparative study of area 13. Am. J. Phys. Anthropol. **106:** 129–155.

11. PETRIDES, M. & D.N. PANDYA. 2002. Comparative cytoarchitectonic analysis of the human and the macaque ventrolateral prefrontal cortex and corticocortical connection patterns in the monkey. Eur. J. Neurosci. **16:** 291–310.

12. ONGUR, D., A.T. FERRY & J.L. PRICE. 2003. Architectonic subdivision of the human orbital and medial prefrontal cortex. J. Comp. Neurol. **460:** 425–449.

13. ROSE, J.E. & C.N. WOOLSEY. 1948a. The orbitofrontal cortex and its connections with the mediodorsal nucleus in rabbit, sheep and cat. Res. Publ. Ass. Nerv. Ment. Dis. **27:** 210–232.

14. KRETTEK, J.E. & J.L. PRICE. 1977. The cortical projections of the mediodorsal nucleus and adjacent thalamic nuclei in the rat. J. Comp. Neurol. **171:** 157–191.

15. GROENEWEGEN, H.J. 1988. Organization of the afferent connections of the mediodorsal thalamic nucleus in the rat, related to mediodorsal-prefrontal topography. Neuroscience **24:** 379–431.

16. RAY, J.P. & J.L. PRICE. 1992. The organization of the thalamocortical connections of the mediodorsal thalamic nucleus in the rat, related to the ventral forebrain-prefrontal cortex topography. J. Comp. Neurol. **323:** 167–197.

17. PREUSS, T.M. 1995. Do rats have prefrontal cortex? The Rose-Woolsey-Akert program reconsidered. J. Cog. Neurosci. **7:** 1–24.

18. UYLINGS, H.B., H.J. GROENEWEGEN & B. KOLB. 2003. Do rats have a prefrontal cortex? Behav. Brain Res. **146:** 3–17.

19. CARMICHAEL, S.T. & J.L. PRICE. 1996. Connectional networks within the orbital and medial prefrontal cortex of macaque monkeys. J. Comp. Neurol. **371:** 179–207.

20. CARMICHAEL, S.T. & J.L. PRICE. 1995. Sensory and premotor connections of the orbital and medial prefrontal cortex. J. Comp. Neurol. **363:** 642–664.

21. ROLLS, E.T. 2005. Taste, olfactory, and food texture processing in the brain, and the control of food intake. Physiol. Behav. **85:** 45–56.

22. ROLLS, E.T. 2000. The orbitofrontal cortex and reward. Cereb. Cortex **10:** 284–294.

23. SCHULTZ, W., L. TREMBLAY & J.R. HOLLERMAN. 2000. Reward processing in primate orbitofrontal cortex and basal ganglia. Cereb. Cortex **10:** 272–284.

24. PADOA-SCHIOPPA, C. & J.A. ASSAD. 2006. Neurons in the orbitofrontal cortex encode economic value. Nature **441:** 223–226.

25. AMARAL, D.G. & J.L. PRICE. 1984. Amygdalo-cortical projections in the monkey. *Macaca fascicularis.* J. Comp. Neurol. **230:** 465–496.

26. PETRIDES, M. 2005. Lateral prefrontal cortex: architectonic and functional organization. Philos. Trans. R. Soc. Lond. B Biol. Sci. **360:** 781–795.

27. BARBAS, H. & J. DE OLMOS. 1990. Projections from the amygdala to basoventral and mediodorsal prefrontal regions in the rhesus monkey. J. Comp. Neurol. **300:** 549–71.

28. BARBAS, H. & G.J. BLATT. 1995. Topographically specific hippocampal projections target functionally distinct prefrontal areas in the rhesus monkey. Hippocampus **5:** 511–33.

29. CARMICHAEL, S.T. & J.L. PRICE. 1995. Limbic connections of the orbital and medial prefrontal cortex in macaque monkeys. J. Comp. Neurol. **363:** 615–641.

30. KONDO, H., K.S. SALEEM & J.L. PRICE. 2003. Differential connections of the temporal pole with the orbital and medial prefrontal networks in macaque monkeys. J. Comp. Neurol. **465:** 499–523.

31. KONDO, H., K.S. SALEEM & J.L. PRICE. 2005. Differential connections of the perirhinal and parahippocampal cortical areas with the orbital and medial prefrontal networks in macaque monkeys. J. Comp. Neurol. **493:** 479–509.

32. AN, X. *et al.* 1998. Prefrontal cortical projections to longitudinal columns in the midbrain periaqueductal gray in macaque monkeys. J. Comp. Neurol. **401:** 455–479.

33. ÖNGÜR, D., X. AN & J.L. PRICE. 1998. Prefrontal cortical projections to the hypothalamus in macaque monkeys. J. Comp. Neurol. **401:** 480–505.

34. REMPEL-CLOWER, N.L. & H. BARBAS. 1998. Topographic organization of connections between the hypothalamus and prefrontal cortex in the rhesus monkey. Comp. Neurol. **398:** 393–419.

35. J. FREEDMAN, L.J., T.R. INSEL & Y. SMITH. 2000. Subcortical projections of area 25 (subgenual cortex) of the macaque monkey. J. Comp. Neurol. **421:** 172–188.

36. CAVADA, C. *et al.* 2000. The anatomical connections of the macaque monkey orbitofrontal cortex. A review. Cereb. Cortex. **10:** 220–42.

37. HSU, D.T. & J.L. PRICE. 2007. Midline and intralaminar thalamic connections with the orbital and medial prefrontal networks in macaque monkeys. J. Comp. Neurol. **504:** 89–111.

38. RAY, J.P. & J.L. PRICE. 1993. The organization of projections from the mediodorsal nucleus of the thalamus to orbital and medial prefrontal cortex in macaque monkeys. J. Comp. Neurol. **337:** 1–31.

39. FERRY, A.T. *et al.* 2000. Prefrontal cortical projections to the striatum in macaque monkeys: evidence for an organization related to prefrontal networks. J. Comp. Neurol. **425:** 447–470.

40. RUSSCHEN, F.T. *et al.* 1985. The amygdalostriatal projections in the monkey. An anterograde tracing study. Brain Res. **329:** 241–257.

41. RUSSCHEN, F.T., D.G. AMARAL & J.L. PRICE. 1987. The afferent input to the magnocellular division of the mediodorsal thalamic nucleus in the monkey, Macaca fascicularis. J. Comp. Neurol. **256:** 175–210.

42. KURODA, M. & J.L. PRICE. 1991. Synaptic organization of projections from basal forebrain structures to the mediodorsal thalamic nucleus of the rat. J. Comp. Neurol. **303:** 513–533.

43. DESIMONE, R. & C.G. GROSS. 1979. Visual areas in the temporal cortex of the macaque. Brain Res. **178:** 363–380.

44. BRUCE, C., R. DESIMONE & C.G. GROSS. 1981. Visual properties of neurons in a polysensory area in superior temporal sulcus of the macaque. J. Neurophysiol. **46:** 369–382.

45. BRUCE, C., R. DESIMONE & C.G. GROSS. 1986. Both striate cortex and superior colliculus contribute to visual properties of neurons in superior temporal polysensory area of macaque monkey. J. Neurophysiol. **55:** 1057–1075.

46. BAYLIS, G.C., E.T. ROLLS & C.M. LEONARD. 1987. Functional subdivisions of the temporal lobe neocortex. J. Neurosci. **7:** 330–342.

47. POREMBA, A., R.M. SAUNDERS & A.M. CRANE. 2003. Functional mapping of the primate auditory system. Science **299:** 568–672.

48. CONDE, F. *et al.* 1995. Afferent connections of the medial frontal cortex of the rat. II. Cortical and subcortical afferents. J. Comp. Neurol. **352:** 567–593.

49. VERTES, R.P. 2004. Differential projections of the infralimbic and prelimbic cortex in the rat. Synapse **51:** 32–58.

50. SALEEM, K.S., H. KONDO & J.L. PRICE. 2007. Complimentary circuits connecting the orbital and medial prefrontal networks with the temporal, insular, and opercular cortex in the macaque monkey. J. Comp. Neurol. In Press.

51. KRETTEK, J.E. & J.L. PRICE. 1977. An autoradiographic study of projections from the amygdaloid complex to the thalamus and cerebral cortex. J. Comp. Neurol. **172:** 723–752.
52. FLOYD, N.S. *et al.* 2001. Orbitomedial prefrontal cortical projections to hypothalamus in the rat. J. Comp. Neurol. **432:** 307–328.
53. FLOYD, N.S. *et al.* 2000. Orbitofrontal prefrontal cortical projections to distinct longitudinal columns of the periaqueductal gray in the rat. J. Comp. Neurol. **422:** 556–578.
54. PRICE, J.L. 1985. Beyond the primary olfactory cortex: olfactory-related areas in the neocortex, thalamus, and hypothalamus. Chem. Senses **10:** 235–258.

Role of Orbitofrontal Cortex Connections in Emotion

NANCY L. REMPEL-CLOWER

Department of Psychology, Grinnell College, Grinnell, Iowa, USA

ABSTRACT: The orbitofrontal cortex is extensively connected with diverse neural areas that underlie its participation in emotional function. It receives extensive sensory input and sends output to areas important for emotional processing and expression, including medial temporal cortical areas, hypothalamic and brain stem autonomic areas, and the amygdala. In the rat, the functional relationship between the orbitofrontal cortex and amygdala has been investigated in numerous recent studies. Clearer understanding of the complex connections between the rat orbitofrontal cortex and the amygdala is fundamental to elucidating the functional contributions of these pathways. Recent work shows that, as in the primate, the subdivisions of the rat orbitofrontal cortex issue different patterns of projections to the amygdala, with intriguing variations in the relative distribution of projections to the sensory-related basal areas compared with output areas, such as the central nucleus. Notably, as has been observed in the monkey, the rat orbitofrontal cortex targets the intercalated nuclei, which contain GABAergic interneurons and provide local inhibitory influences within the amygdala. The complex connections between the orbitofrontal cortex and the amygdala, as well as other areas involved in emotion, suggest important implications for the role of the orbitofrontal cortex in anxiety disorders, in which emotional expression is not appropriate to the situation.

KEYWORDS: amygdala; autonomic; inhibitory influence; intercalated nuclei; hypothalamus

The orbitofrontal cortex is important for flexible responses, allowing an organism to adapt its behavior as situations change.[1–4] In particular, this cortical area is ideally positioned to play a role in regulation of emotion-related responses in the context of a changing environment. The aim of this review is to describe the orbitofrontal cortex in terms of its connections with other neural areas implicated in emotion, paying particular attention to connections that may support a role for orbitofrontal cortex in adaptive responses to emotionally relevant cues or situations. First, connections between the orbitofrontal cortex and areas with emotion-related functions in the primate will be described. Then the

Address for correspondence: Nancy L. Rempel-Clower, Department of Psychology, Grinnell College, Grinnell, IA 50112. Voice: 641-269-3034; fax: 641-269-4285.
   rempelcl@grinnell.edu

Ann. N.Y. Acad. Sci. 1121: 72–86 (2007). © 2007 New York Academy of Sciences.
doi: 10.1196/annals.1401.026

rat orbitofrontal cortex connections with the amygdala will be summarized, describing how the projections of orbitofrontal cortex subregions to the amygdala show both common patterns and interesting differences. Understanding the details of the connections of the orbitofrontal cortex is important for guiding future efforts to better understand its function in normal emotion and in clinical disorders, such as anxiety disorders including post-traumatic stress disorder, phobias, and obsessive compulsive disorder, which are characterized by inappropriate emotional responses to environmental stimuli.[5]

DISTINCT ORBITOFRONTAL CORTEX REGIONS IN THE PRIMATE ARE LIKELY TO PLAY DIFFERENT ROLES IN LINKING AFFECT TO ACTION

In the primate orbitofrontal cortex, the specific regions can be characterized by their cortical structure according to the method of Sanides, as designated by Barbas and Pandya[6] (FIG. 1A). Rostral areas, such as area 11 and the orbital surface of area 12, have six layers, including a granular layer 4. In contrast, caudal areas have fewer than six layers and either lack a layer 4, as in orbital periallocortex (OPAll; comparable to areas delineated as 13a, Iam, and Iapm by Carmichael and Price),[7] or have a poorly defined layer 4, as in areas 13 and orbital proisocortex (OPro; area 13 is comparable to areas 13b, 13m, and 13l, and OPro is comparable to areas Iai, Ial, and Iapl of Carmichael and Price).[7] These structural differences are associated with differences in their connections,[8,9] including those connections with areas that may underlie the role of the orbitofrontal cortex in particular aspects of emotion-related processing. Rostral and caudal regions of the orbitofrontal cortex have some important differences in their specific connections to areas involved in emotion, as described below.

Primate Orbitofrontal Cortex Connections Support a Role in Sensory Processing of Emotionally Salient Stimuli

The primate orbitofrontal cortex is privy to an integrated sensory perspective of the environment, placing it in an ideal position to provide information to other neural regions about the external environment. The orbitofrontal cortex receives sensory input from all modalities.[10,11] Visual, auditory, somatosensory, and gustatory input reach the rostral orbitofrontal cortex, and caudal orbitofrontal cortex receives olfactory input in addition to the other modalities.[12]

Input from the orbitofrontal to the medial temporal lobe may be important for encoding emotionally salient stimuli. The orbitofrontal cortex has bidirectional connections with medial temporal areas, including entorhinal and perirhinal cortex, which form the primary conduit of cortical input to the hippocampus.[7,13–15] For the most part, cortical input flows from the perirhinal

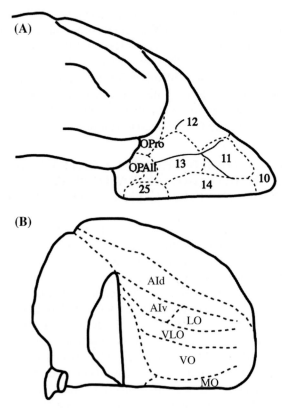

FIGURE 1. **(A)** Ventral view of the rhesus monkey brain indicating orbitofrontal regions according to Barbas and Pandya.[6] **(B)** Ventral view of the rat brain indicating orbitofrontal regions, with the tip of the temporal pole removed. Abbreviations: AId, dorsal agranular insula; AIv, ventral agranular insula; LO, lateral orbital; MO, medial orbital; VLO, ventrolateral orbital; VO, ventral orbital. (Rat brain drawing is adapted with permission from Uylings *et al.*[71])

cortex to entorhinal cortex to reach the hippocampus, a structure important for the encoding of long-term memory.[16–20] The rostral and caudal orbitofrontal cortices communicate with medial temporal areas in different ways. For example, caudal orbitofrontal cortex areas issue robust projections to entorhinal cortex and perirhinal cortex.[8, 13] In contrast, the more rostral areas, such as area 11 and O12, issue weaker projections to perirhinal cortex, but none to entorhinal cortex.[8] This observation suggests that the caudal orbitofrontal cortex has a greater influence over the processing in this area than does the rostral orbitofrontal cortex, and may be particularly important for enhanced encoding of memories about emotionally salient stimuli.

The laminar pattern of connections to medial temporal cortices provides further support for this function of the orbitofrontal cortex. Axons from caudal

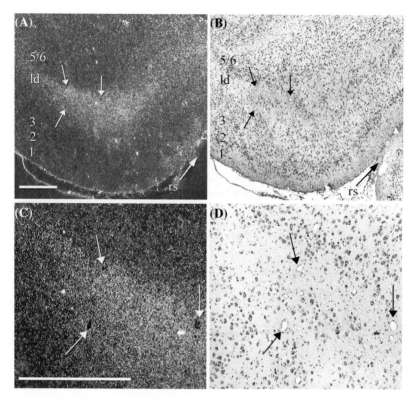

FIGURE 2. Pattern of termination in primate entorhinal cortex from caudal orbitofrontal area OPro. **(A)** Axonal termination in the middle layers of the entorhinal cortex is visible in darkfield illumination. **(B)** In the same view in brightfield illumination, the cell-sparse middle layers (lamina dessicans, ld) of the entorhinal cortex are visible. **(C, D)** Higher magnification of the same section in darkfield and brightfield illumination. Numbers indicate cortical layers. *Arrows* indicate matching blood vessels in all images. Scale bars, 500 μm. (From Rempel-Clower and Barbas.[8] Reproduced by permission.)

orbitofrontal cortex terminate in the middle layers of the entorhinal cortex (FIG. 2), which may be described as a feedforward pattern of communication (analogous to bottom-up), in which earlier processing areas issue projections to later processing areas.[8] Similarly, the more rostral orbital area 11 issues projections in a feedforward pattern of termination to perirhinal cortex.[8] This termination pattern would suggest that the integrated sensory information processed in the orbitofrontal cortex is relayed to the perirhinal and entorhinal cortex, and finally to the hippocampus to encode emotionally relevant information about environmental cues into long-term memories. de Curtis and Paré[21] proposed that the perirhinal and entorhinal cortices function as a gate, selectively allowing only relevant information to the hippocampus. The feedforward input from the orbitofrontal cortex makes this area a likely candidate for one that might "open" the rhinal cortex gate to facilitate the encoding of emotionally relevant stimuli. In support of this idea, a recent PET study revealed increased activity in orbital areas 13 and 11 when black marks (Xs or scribbles drawn across the design) were added to familiar abstract designs, creating a deviation from expectation that might suggest the presence of a threat.[22] This increased activity in the orbitofrontal cortex is consistent with a role in facilitating memory for emotionally salient stimuli.

Orbitofrontal Cortex Connections Support a Role in Emotional Expression

The orbitofrontal cortex also has connections to areas involved in emotional expression, including autonomic activation that accompanies emotional arousal, such as increases in heart rate and blood pressure. For example, the primate orbitofrontal cortex is bidirectionally connected with the hypothalamus.[23–25] Neurons in the hypothalamus, mostly posterior regions of the hypothalamus, issue projections to all parts of orbitofrontal cortex as well as to other prefrontal areas and other cortical areas.[25] However, caudal orbitofrontal cortex sends stronger descending inputs to hypothalamus than do the more rostral areas of the orbitofrontal cortex. In contrast, the lateral prefrontal cortex does not issue descending projections to the hypothalamus.[25] These findings suggest that the orbitofrontal cortex, along with the posterior parts of the medial prefrontal cortex, has a particularly important relationship with the hypothalamus, sending and receiving projections in an overlapping distribution in its autonomic centers. The ascending projections to orbitofrontal cortex areas may provide feedback from autonomic areas that can modulate the descending input to the hypothalamic autonomic areas. Given its denser descending projections, it is likely that the caudal orbitofrontal cortex plays a more direct role than the more rostral orbital areas in the resulting modulation of autonomic responses.

Autonomic responses can be regulated further by direct connections from orbitofrontal cortex to brain stem and spinal cord autonomic areas.[26–28] Moreover, the hypothalamic targets of orbitofrontal cortex neurons issue projections that continue to brain stem and spinal cord autonomic areas.[29] Neurons from caudal orbitofrontal area 13, for example, issue projections into the lateral hypothalamic area, which in turn issues projections to brain stem and spinal cord autonomic areas. Thus, there exist very direct pathways from the orbitofrontal cortex, privy to integrated sensory information about the environment, to the autonomic centers associated with the expression of emotions.

Robust connections between the amygdala and the orbitofrontal cortex are likely to be important for emotion-related processing. The functions of these two areas are complementary. In the amygdala, information about the emotional value of cues is processed, and associated emotional expression is generated through its interaction with the autonomic motor system.[30,31] The

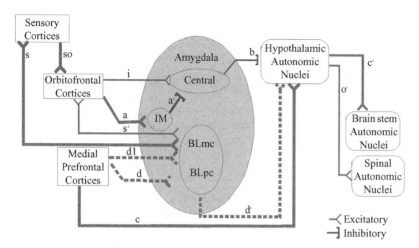

FIGURE 3. Summary of pathways linking primate prefrontal cortex with structures associated with perception and expression of emotions. *Line thickness* indicates the density of projections. The orbitofrontal cortex receives input from every sensory modality (pathway so), as does the magnocellular sector of the basolateral nucleus of the amygdala (BLmc; pathway s). Both of these recipients of sensory information are connected to each other (pathway s′), thus providing indirect sensory information to the amygdala via the orbitofrontal cortex. The orbitofrontal cortex also influences autonomic centers through a pathway to the intercalated nuclei of the amygdala (or intercalated masses, IM; pathway a), which in torn project to the central nucleus (a′), which in turn projects to hypothalamic autonomic centers (pathway b). Activation of pathways (a, a′) leads to disinhibition of hypothalamic autonomic centers, which innervate brain stem and spinal autonomic centers (pathways c′, o′). Activation of a direct pathway from the caudal orbitofrontal cortex to the central nucleus (i) increases the firing of the inhibitory output neurons, thereby suppressing hypothalamic autonomic activity (via pathway b). A direct pathway from medial prefrontal cortex innervates hypothalamic autonomic centers (c), and an indirect pathway from medial prefrontal cortex synapses in the parvicellular sector of the basolateral nucleus (BLpc; pathway d), which issues a presumed excitatory projection to hypothalamic autonomic centers. (From Barbas et al.[29] Reproduced by permission.)

orbitofrontal cortex is important for adapting behavior as an organism learns about the emotional value of cues.[1–4] Like the orbitofrontal cortex, the amygdala receives diverse sensory input and shares bidirectional connections with the hypothalamus. The specific pattern of connections from the primate orbitofrontal cortex to the amygdala provides further support for the role of this prefrontal area in emotion. Of particular interest, caudal orbitofrontal cortex areas issue a dense projection to the posterior part of the amygdala, targeting the border of the basolateral nucleus, the location of the intercalated nuclei, which are clusters of GABAergic inhibitory neurons.[32] Orbitofrontal cortex neurons also target the central, basolateral, and basomedial nuclei and anterior amygdaloid area.[32]

Orbitofrontal Cortex Has Both Direct and Indirect Connections with Areas
Important in the Perception of Emotionally Significant Cues
and the Expression of Emotion

As described above, the orbitofrontal cortex, with its view of the sensory environment, exchanges information with the medial temporal cortex, hypothalamic and brain stem autonomic areas, and the amygdala. Moreover, rather than having independent relationships with each of these areas, the caudal orbitofrontal cortex, in particular, appears to participate in networks through which it interacts with these areas both directly and indirectly. The model represented in FIGURE 3 summarizes the pathways connecting primate prefrontal cortex with other areas important in the perception and expression of emotions.[29] The caudal orbitofrontal cortex has bidirectional connections with the basolateral nucleus, which, like the orbitofrontal cortex, receives widespread sensory input. The circuitry among sensory cortices, the amygdala, and the orbitofrontal cortex is likely to be important in encoding the emotional value of environmental stimuli.

Connections among the orbitofrontal cortex, amygdala, hypothalamus, brain stem, and spinal cord provide multiple avenues through which the orbitofrontal cortex can influence autonomic aspects of emotional expression (FIG. 3). For example, the orbitofrontal cortex provides input to the central nucleus of the amygdala, which, in turn, has an inhibitory effect on autonomic centers in the hypothalamus, brain stem, and spinal cord,[33,34] possibly allowing the orbitofrontal cortex to dampen autonomic activation. Moreover, orbitofrontal cortex projects to the intercalated nuclei surrounding the basolateral nucleus.[32] These inhibitory neurons have been shown to gate information exchanged between the sensory-related basolateral amygdala and the autonomic output of central nucleus.[35] Through these pathways, the caudal orbitofrontal cortex can decrease the inhibitory influence of the central nucleus on autonomic centers, while at the same time providing direct input to these autonomic centers. In addition, both the caudal orbitofrontal cortex and the amygdala issue projections to autonomic centers in the hypothalamus, and the caudal orbitofrontal cortex also sends input to the very areas of the amygdala that issue the hypothalamic projections.[29] In general, the pattern of connections from caudal orbitofrontal cortex suggests it has a more direct and influential role in regulating the activity of these downstream targets than has the rostral orbitofrontal cortex. Thus, the caudal orbitofrontal cortex is positioned prominently in networks that might allow it to regulate emotional processes in particularly comprehensive ways, providing the kind of complex control that would be important for responding to a multifaceted and changing environment. These sorts of connections could permit the enhancement of memory for emotionally salient stimuli and moment-to-moment regulation of appropriate autonomic activation.

DISTINCT ORBITOFRONTAL CORTEX REGIONS
IN THE RAT SEND INPUT TO SENSORY AND AUTONOMIC
REGIONS IN THE AMGYDALA

Over the past decade, there has been increasing interest in the function of the orbital region of the rat prefrontal cortex. Using the nomenclature of Krettek and Price,[36] with later modifications of Groenewegen[37] and Ray and Price,[38] the rat orbitofrontal cortex includes the medial orbital area (MO), ventral orbital area (VO), ventrolateral orbital area (VLO), lateral orbital area (LO), and agranular insular area (AI, which includes ventral and dorsal subdivisions; FIG. 1B). The subdivisions of the rat orbitofrontal cortex largely have been defined, as suggested by Rose and Woolsey,[39] through their connections with the thalamus.[36,38,40,41] The orbital portion of the rat prefrontal cortex shares many of the connectional characteristics of the monkey orbitofrontal cortex, including input from diverse sensory cortices and connections with autonomic areas.[42,43]

Many theories of the role of rat orbitofrontal cortex in emotional processes emphasize its connections with the amygdala.[3,44,45] All parts of the orbitofrontal cortex of the rat receive input from the amygdala, primarily originating from the basolateral, basomedial, and lateral nuclei.[36,40,46] Although studies have shown robust connections from AI to the amygdala,[47,48] there is much less information about how other orbitofrontal areas issue projections to the amygdala.

Recent work to characterize inputs to the amygdala from the various areas of the rat orbitofrontal cortex enhances our understanding of the complex relationship between these areas. Areas across the orbitofrontal cortex of the rat, as in the monkey, differ somewhat in their pattern of projections to the amygdala.[49] The more medially situated VO and VLO issue projections to the anterior portion of the amygdala, with sparse termination distributed across many areas, including the anterior amygdaloid area, basomedial nucleus, medial nucleus, central nucleus, superficial cortical amygdaloid nucleus, and intercalated nuclei. Notably, the VO and VLO provide input to autonomic output areas, including the medial and central nuclei of the amygdala, and issue only weak projections to the basolateral amygdala. Lesions of the VLO impair spatial behavior,[50] and anatomic studies have shown connections between the VLO and medial agranular and posterior parietal areas that would support a role in spatial processing and attention.[40] These more medially situated areas may be particularly important for increasing autonomic activation to orient spatial attention to relevant stimuli, a broad activating function consistent with the observation that the VO projections to the hypothalamus are widely distributed across multiple autonomic areas.[51]

Like those from the VO and VLO, projection neurons from the LO terminate in the anterior portion of the amygdala in a widely distributed fashion, but have particularly strong connections with the basolateral nucleus that suggest a more important role for this area in enhanced processing for emotionally relevant cues.[49] In comparison to the medially located orbitofrontal areas VO and VLO, neurons from the LO terminate more densely in the sensory-related basolateral and lateral nuclei, and less densely in the central nucleus. In addition, neurons in the LO, like those from the VO and VLO, terminate in the intercalated nuclei.[49] The intercalated nuclei contain small, densely packed clusters of GABAergic neurons that provide an inhibitory influence over adjacent areas within the amygdala.[52–54] As described above for the primate, the caudal orbitofrontal cortex issues a strong projection to the intercalated nuclei that surround the basolateral nucleus.[32] A comparable pathway in the rat has not been reported previously, although figures in McDonald et al.[47] show a case with an injection into the LO and the ventral part of AI that contains labeled fibers in the intercalated nuclei. The LO particularly targets the anterior portions of the intercalated nuclei,[49] which are continuous with the more posterior lateral and medial clusters that form a shell around the basolateral nucleus.[55] The LO also provides input to the lateral cluster of this shell, along the lateral edge of the anterior basolateral nucleus.[49] Excitation of the clusters of intercalated nuclei between the basolateral nucleus and the external capsule mediates an inhibitory influence on the basolateral nucleus originating in the cortex.[55] Thus, input from the LO may specifically inhibit incoming cortical signals to the basolateral nucleus.

With both an excitatory and an inhibitory influence over the basolateral amygdala, the LO is ideally positioned to play a role in selection of incoming sensory signals to the amygdala, while its minimal connections to the amygdala's primary output centers, the medial and central nuclei, indicate that it may be involved less directly in regulation of emotional expression. Lesion and electrophysiological studies have indicated that the orbitofrontal cortex and basolateral amygdala together participate in directing behavior according to predicted outcomes.[3] The orbitofrontal cortex appears to facilitate associative learning in the amygdala, and the robust reciprocal connections between the LO and basolateral amygdala support the conclusions of functional studies.[40,49,56–58]

In comparison to the LO, the AI issues a robust projection to the central nucleus as well as to the basolateral and lateral nucleus.[47–49] The AI also targets the intercalated nuclei, including a dense termination zone in the location of its GABAergic neurons between the basolateral and central nucleus.[49] Excitation of these clusters of intercalated nuclei has been shown to have an inhibitory influence on the central nucleus.[59] Royer et al.[35] proposed that the intercalated nuclei act as a gate within the internal circuitry of the amygdala that can influence the resulting expression of emotion in response to the sensory environment. Taken together, these findings suggest that the AI has a direct pathway to the central nucleus as well as an indirect one through the intercalated nucleus.

In sum, the orbitofrontal cortex of the rat, like that of the primate, issues projections to both sensory and autonomic areas of the amygdala. Although the divisions of the rat orbitofrontal cortex all issue projections distributed across multiple areas in the anterior amygdala, the distinct patterns of termination from these areas suggest subtle differences in their influence on amygdala processing. The AI has a complex connectional relationship with the amygdala, issuing projections that may influence both the sensory input zone of the basolateral and lateral nucleus and the autonomic output of the central nucleus, including direct and indirect pathways that can excite and inhibit, respectively, the activity of neurons in the central nucleus. These connections suggest that the AI plays a role in specific regulation of autonomic emotional expression in relation to sensory cues. In comparison, the LO seems to have a more concentrated influence over the sensory-related areas of the amygdala, whereas the influence of the VO and VLO appears to extend broadly to primarily autonomic areas.

Notably, in both the rat and the primate, there are pathways to the amygdala from a discrete region of orbitofrontal cortex that can both excite and inhibit a single target. In particular, subregions of the rat and primate orbitofrontal cortex can provide direct excitation of the central nucleus as well as inhibition of the central nucleus by way of the intercalated nuclei. Medial prefrontal areas in the rat (prelimbic and infralimbic areas) also issue projections to the intercalated nuclei and these connections have been suggested to underlie the role of this area in extinction of fear conditioning.[60,61] The observation of orbitofrontal cortex projections to the intercalated nuclei raises questions about how the medial and orbital prefrontal cortex, which are strongly interconnected,[62–64] together influence the circuitry of the amygdala.

Understanding the Organization of the Rat Orbitofrontal Cortex

The pattern of connections to the amygdala varies across the medial-lateral axis of the rat orbitofrontal cortex. How does this observation in rat orbitofrontal cortex relate to the medial-orbital divisions of the monkey prefrontal cortex? Functionally, the rat orbitofrontal cortex appears to be distinct from medial prefrontal areas. Lesion studies in rats have revealed dissociations between the effects of orbitofrontal and medial prefrontal (specifically infralimbic cortex) lesions.[65–67] Within each of these regions, medial prefrontal and orbitofrontal, there are similarities in connectivity between the rat and monkey. Medial infralimbic and prelimbic cortices in the rat may be comparable to medial areas 25 and 32 in the monkey,[68] and patterns of connections from these areas to the amygdala are similar across species. For example, prelimbic and infralimbic cortex in the rat, like medial areas 24, 25, and 32 in the monkey, issue robust projections to the amygdala.[32,47,69]

Comparison of the pattern of amygdala projections from rat and monkey orbital areas suggests similarity across species for this region as well. The strongest orbitofrontal projections to the amgydala originate in the caudal areas OPro and OPAll in the monkey[32, 69] and in lateral areas AI and LO in the rat.[49] Sparse, widespread projections to the amygdala originate in more rostral orbitofrontal areas in the monkey and more medial orbitofrontal areas in the rat. Thus, the different patterns across the orbital surface of connections with the amygdala suggest a medial-lateral organization in the rat orbitofrontal cortex that may correspond to a rostral–caudal organization in the monkey. More information about the rat orbitofrontal cortex is needed before definitive conclusions can be drawn about homologies between monkey and rat orbitofrontal cortex.

CONCLUSIONS

The complex connections of the orbitofrontal cortex support a role in emotional and behavioral flexibility, the ability to adjust emotional responses according to the characteristics of a situation. These connections are consistent, for example, with the observed role of the orbitofrontal cortex in reversal learning, changing a response to a stimulus when the reinforcement for that response is changed, and choice situations, such as deciding between a smaller, sooner or larger, later reward.[3, 45, 70] Intriguingly, in humans, neuropsychiatric disorders associated with the orbitofrontal cortex include anxiety disorders (such as obsessive–compulsive disorder, panic disorder, and post-traumatic stress disorder) that feature an emotional response, including autonomic activation, that is not appropriate to the environmental context.[5] The complex relationship between the orbitofrontal cortex and other neural regions involved in emotion invites further investigation of the role of this cortical area in cognitive evaluation of a complex and changing environment and the expression of appropriate emotion-related responses.

ACKNOWLEDGMENTS

I thank my collaborators who participated in the original reports that were described in this review. I also thank Martin Cassell and Khristofer Agassanian for their generous advice and assistance in my analysis of the rat amygdala. This work is supported by grants from Grinnell College, the NSF, and the NIH.

REFERENCES

1. ROBERTS, A.C. 2006. Primate orbitofrontal cortex and adaptive behaviour. Trends Cogn. Sci. **10:** 83–90.

2. SCHULTZ, W. & L. TREMBLAY. 2006. Involvement of primate orbitofrontal neurons in reward, uncertainty, and learning. *In* The Orbitofrontal Cortex. D.H. Zald & S.L. Rauch, Eds.: 173–198. Oxford University Press. New York.

3. SCHOENBAUM, G. & M. ROESCH. 2005. Orbitofrontal cortex, associative learning, and expectancies. Neuron **47:** 633–636.

4. FUSTER, J.M. 1997. The Prefrontal Cortex: Anatomy, Physiology, and Neuropsychology of the Frontal Lobe. Lippincott–Raven. Philadelphia, PA.

5. MILAD, M.R. & S.L. RAUCH. 2006. The orbitofrontal cortex and anxiety disorders. *In* The Orbitofrontal Cortex. D.H. Zald & S.L. Rauch, Eds.: 523–543. Oxford University Press. New York.

6. BARBAS, H. & D.N. PANDYA. 1989. Architecture and intrinsic connections of the prefrontal cortex in the rhesus monkey. J. Comp. Neurol. **286:** 353–375.

7. CARMICHAEL, S.T. & J.L. PRICE. 1994. Architectonic subdivision of the orbital and medial prefrontal cortex in the macaque monkey. J. Comp. Neurol. **346:** 366–402.

8. REMPEL-CLOWER, N.L. & H. BARBAS. 2000. The laminar pattern of connections between prefrontal and anterior temporal cortices in the Rhesus monkey is related to cortical structure and function. Cereb. Cortex **10:** 851–865.

9. BARBAS, H. & N. REMPEL-CLOWER. 1997. Cortical structure predicts the pattern of corticocortical connections. Cereb. Cortex **7:** 635–646.

10. ROLLS, E.T. 2004. Convergence of sensory systems in the orbitofrontal cortex in primates and brain design for emotion. Anat. Rec. A. Discov. Mol. Cell. Evol. Biol. **281:** 1212–1225.

11. BARBAS, H., H.T. GHASHGHAEI, N.L. REMPEL-CLOWER, *et al.* 2002. Anatomic basis of functional specialization in prefrontal cortices in primates. Handbook Neuropsychol. **7:** 1–21.

12. BARBAS, H. & B. ZIKOPOULOS. 2006. Sequential and parallel circuits for emotional processing in primate orbitofrontal cortex. *In* The Orbitofrontal Cortex. D.H. Zald & S.L. Rauch, Eds.: 57–91. Oxford University Press. New York.

13. SUZUKI, W.A. & D.G. AMARAL. 1994. Topographic organization of the reciprocal connections between the monkey entorhinal cortex and the perirhinal and parahippocampal cortices. J. Neurosci. **14:** 1856–1877.

14. MORECRAFT, R.J., C. GEULA & M.M. MESULAM. 1992. Cytoarchitecture and neural afferents of orbitofrontal cortex in the brain of the monkey. J. Comp. Neurol. **323:** 341–358.

15. WITTER, M.P., G.W. VAN HOESEN & D.G. AMARAL. 1989. Topographical organization of the entorhinal projection to the dentate gyrus of the monkey. J. Neurosci. **9:** 216–228.

16. SQUIRE, L.R., C.E. STARK & R.E. CLARK. 2004. The medial temporal lobe. Annu. Rev. Neurosci. **27:** 279–306.

17. SUZUKI, W.A. & D.G. AMARAL. 2004. Functional neuroanatomy of the medial temporal lobe memory system. Cortex **40:** 220–222.

18. ZOLA, S.M., L.R. SQUIRE, E. TENG, et al. 2000. Impaired recognition memory in monkeys after damage limited to the hippocampal region. J. Neurosci. **20:** 451–463.

19. REMPEL-CLOWER, N.L., S.M. ZOLA, L.R. SQUIRE, *et al.* 1996. Three cases of enduring memory impairment after bilateral damage limited to the hippocampal formation. J. Neurosci. **16:** 5233–5255.

20. ZOLA-MORGAN, S., L.R. SQUIRE & D.G. AMARAL. 1986. Human amnesia and the medial temporal region: enduring memory impairment following a bilateral le-

sion limited to field CA1 of the hippocampus. J. Neurosci. **6**: 2950–2967.

21. DE CURTIS, M. & D. PARÉ. 2004. The rhinal cortices: a wall of inhibition between the neocortex and the hippocampus. Prog. Neurobiol. **74**: 101–110.

22. PETRIDES, M., B. ALIVISATOS & S. FREY. 2002. Differential activation of the human orbital, mid-ventrolateral, and mid-dorsolateral prefrontal cortex during the processing of visual stimuli. Proc. Natl. Acad. Sci. USA **99**: 5649–5654.

23. CAVADA, C., T. COMPANY, J. TEJEDOR, *et al.* 2000. The anatomical connections of the macaque monkey orbitofrontal cortex. A review. Cereb. Cortex. **10**: 220–242.

24. ÖNGÜR, D., X. AN & J.L. PRICE. 1998. Prefrontal cortical projections to the hypothalamus in macaque monkeys. J. Comp. Neurol. **401**: 480–505.

25. REMPEL-CLOWER, N.L. & H. BARBAS. 1998. Topographic organization of connections between the hypothalamus and prefrontal cortex in the rhesus monkey. J. Comp. Neurol. **398**: 393–419.

26. AN, X., R. BANDLER, D. ÖNGÜR, *et al.* 1998. Prefrontal cortical projections to longitudinal columns in the midbrain periaqueductal gray in macaque monkeys. J. Comp. Neurol. **401**: 455–479.

27. NEAFSEY, E.J. 1990. Prefrontal cortical control of the autonomic nervous system: anatomical and physiological observations. Prog. Brain Res. **85**: 147–165.

28. DEVITO, J.L. & O.A. SMITH, JR. 1964. Subcortical projections of the prefrontal lobe of the monkey. J. Comp. Neurol. **123**: 413–423.

29. BARBAS, H., S. SAHA, N. REMPEL-CLOWER, *et al.* 2003. Serial pathways from primate prefrontal cortex to autonomic areas may influence emotional expression. BMC Neurosci. **4**:25.

30. DAVIS, M. & P.J. WHALEN. 2001. The amygdala: vigilance and emotion. Mol. Psychiatry **6**: 13–34.

31. LEDOUX, J.E. 2000. The amygdala and emotion: a view through fear. *In* The Amygdala: a Functional Analysis. J.P. Aggleton, Ed.: 289–310. Oxford University Press. New York.

32. GHASHGHAEI, H.T. & H. BARBAS. 2002. Pathways for emotion: interactions of prefrontal and anterior temporal pathways in the amygdala of the rhesus monkey. Neuroscience **115**: 1261–1279.

33. SAHA, S., T.F. BATTEN & Z. HENDERSON. 2000. A GABAergic projection from the central nucleus of the amygdala to the nucleus of the solitary tract: a combined anterograde tracing and electron microscopic immunohistochemical study. Neuroscience **99**: 613–626.

34. JONGEN-RELO, A.L. & D.G. AMARAL. 1998. Evidence for a GABAergic projection from the central nucleus of the amygdala to the brainstem of the macaque monkey: a combined retrograde tracing and in situ hybridization study. Eur. J. Neurosci. **10**: 2924–2933.

35. ROYER, S., M. MARTINA & D. PARÉ. 1999. An inhibitory interface gates impulse traffic between the input and output stations of the amygdala. J. Neurosci. **19**: 10575–10583.

36. KRETTEK, J.E. & J.L. PRICE. 1977. Projections from the amygdaloid complex to the cerebral cortex and thalamus in the rat and cat. J. Comp. Neurol. **172**: 687–722.

37. GROENEWEGEN, H.J. 1988. Organization of the afferent connections of the mediodorsal thalamic nucleus in the rat, related to the mediodorsal-prefrontal topography. Neuroscience **24**: 379–431.

38. RAY, J.P. & J.L. PRICE. 1992. The organization of the thalamocortical connections of the mediodorsal thalamic nucleus in the rat, related to the ventral forebrain-prefrontal cortex topography. J. Comp. Neurol. **323**: 167–197.

39. ROSE, J.E. & C.N. WOOLSEY. 1948. The orbitofrontal cortex and its connections with the mediodorsal nucleus in rabbit, sheep and cat. Res. Publ. Assoc. Res. Nerv. Ment. Dis. **27:** 210–232.

40. REEP, R.L., J.V. CORWIN & V. KING. 1996. Neuronal connections of orbital cortex in rats: topography of cortical and thalamic afferents. Exp. Brain Res. **111:** 215–232.

41. LEONARD, C.M. 1969. The prefrontal cortex of the rat. I. Cortical projection of the mediodorsal nucleus. II. Efferent connections. Brain Res. **12:** 321–343.

42. GROENEWEGEN, H.J. & H.B. UYLINGS. 2000. The prefrontal cortex and the integration of sensory, limbic and autonomic information. Prog. Brain Res. **126:** 3–28.

43. ÖNGÜR, D. & J.L. PRICE. 2000. The organization of networks within the orbital and medial prefrontal cortex of rats, monkeys and humans. Cereb. Cortex **10:** 206–219.

44. HOLLAND, P.C. & M. GALLAGHER. 2004. Amygdala-frontal interactions and reward expectancy. Curr. Opin. Neurobiol. **14:** 148–155.

45. CARDINAL, R.N., J.A. PARKINSON, J. HALL, *et al.* 2002. Emotion and motivation: the role of the amygdala, ventral striatum, and prefrontal cortex. Neurosci. Biobehav. Rev. **26:** 321–352.

46. MCDONALD, A.J. 1991. Organization of amygdaloid projections to the prefrontal cortex and associated striatum in the rat. Neuroscience. **44:** 1–14.

47. MCDONALD, A.J., F. MASCAGNI & L. GUO. 1996. Projections of the medial and lateral prefrontal cortices to the amygdala: a *Phaseolus vulgaris* leucoagglutinin study in the rat. Neuroscience **71:** 55–75.

48. SHI, C.J. & M.D. CASSELL. 1998. Cortical, thalamic, and amygdaloid connections of the anterior and posterior insular cortices. J. Comp. Neurol. **399:** 440–468.

49. REMPEL-CLOWER, N.L. 2007. Pattern of projections from orbitofrontal cortex to the amygdala in the rat. Soc. Neurosci. Abstr.

50. CORWIN, J.V., M. FUSSINGER, R.C. MEYER, *et al.* 1994. Bilateral destruction of the ventrolateral orbital cortex produces allocentric but not egocentric spatial deficits in rats. Behav. Brain Res. **61:** 79–86.

51. FLOYD, N.S., J.L. PRICE, A.T. FERRY, *et al.* 2001. Orbitomedial prefrontal cortical projections to hypothalamus in the rat. J. Comp. Neurol. **432:** 307–328.

52. ALHEID, G.F., J.S. DE OLMOS & C.A. BELTRAMINO. 1995. Amygdala and extended amygdala. *In* The Rat Nervous System. G. Paxinos, Ed.: 495–578. Academic Press. San Diego, CA.

53. MILLHOUSE, O.E. 1986. The intercalated cells of the amygdala. J. Comp. Neurol. **247:** 246–271.

54. NITECKA, L. & Y. BEN-ARI. 1987. Distribution of GABA-like immunoreactivity in the rat amygdaloid complex. J. Comp. Neurol. **266:** 45–55.

55. MAROWSKY, A., Y. YANAGAWA, K. OBATA, *et al.* 2005. A specialized subclass of interneurons mediates dopaminergic facilitation of amygdala function. Neuron **48:** 1025–1037.

56. SADDORIS, M.P., M. GALLAGHER & G. SCHOENBAUM. 2005. Rapid associative encoding in basolateral amygdala depends on connections with orbitofrontal cortex. Neuron **46:** 321–331.

57. PICKENS, C.L., M.P. SADDORIS, B. SETLOW, *et al.* 2003. Different roles for orbitofrontal cortex and basolateral amygdala in a reinforcer devaluation task. J. Neurosci. **23:** 11078–11084.

58. SCHOENBAUM, G., B. SETLOW, S.L. NUGENT, et al. 2003. Lesions of orbitofrontal cortex and basolateral amygdala complex disrupt acquisition of odor-guided discriminations and reversals. Learn. Mem. **10:** 129–140.
59. QUIRK, G.J., E. LIKHTIK, J.G. PELLETIER, et al. 2003. Stimulation of medial prefrontal cortex decreases the responsiveness of central amygdala output neurons. J. Neurosci. **23:** 8800–8807.
60. PARÉ, D., G.J. QUIRK & J.E. LEDOUX. 2004. New vistas on amygdala networks in conditioned fear. J. Neurophysiol. **92:** 1–9.
61. SOTRES-BAYON, F., D.E. BUSH & J.E. LEDOUX. 2004. Emotional perseveration: an update on prefrontal-amygdala interactions in fear extinction. Learn. Mem. **11:** 525–535.
62. GABBOTT, P.L., T.A. WARNER, P.R. JAYS, et al. 2003. Areal and synaptic interconnectivity of prelimbic (area 32), infralimbic (area 25) and insular cortices in the rat. Brain Res. **993:** 59–71.
63. TAKAGISHI, M. & T. CHIBA. 1991. Efferent projections of the infralimbic (area 25) region of the medial prefrontal cortex in the rat: an anterograde tracer PHA-L study. Brain Res. **566:** 26–39.
64. SAPER, C.B. 1982. Convergence of autonomic and limbic connections in the insular cortex of the rat. J. Comp. Neurol. **210:** 163–173.
65. EAGLE, D.M., C. BAUNEZ, D.M. HUTCHESON, et al. 2007. Stop-signal reaction-time task performance: role of prefrontal cortex and subthalamic nucleus. Cereb. Cortex Advanced access doi:10.1093/cercor/bhm044
66. CHUDASAMA, Y. & T.W. ROBBINS. 2003. Dissociable contributions of the orbitofrontal and infralimbic cortex to pavlovian autoshaping and discrimination reversal learning: further evidence for the functional heterogeneity of the rodent frontal cortex. J. Neurosci. **23:** 8771–8780.
67. CHUDASAMA, Y., F. PASSETTI, S.E. RHODES, et al. 2003. Dissociable aspects of performance on the 5-choice serial reaction time task following lesions of the dorsal anterior cingulate, infralimbic and orbitofrontal cortex in the rat: differential effects on selectivity, impulsivity and compulsivity. Behav. Brain Res. **146:** 105–119.
68. PRICE, J.L. 2006. Architectonic structure of the orbital and medial prefrontal cortex. In The Orbitofrontal Cortex. D.H. Zald & S.L. Rauch, Eds.: 3–17. Oxford University Press. New York.
69. GHASHGHAEI, H.T., C.C. HILGETAG & H. BARBAS. 2007. Sequence of information processing for emotions based on the anatomic dialogue between prefrontal cortex and amygdala. NeuroImage **34:** 905–923.
70. DALLEY, J.W., R.N. CARDINAL & T.W. ROBBINS. 2004. Prefrontal executive and cognitive functions in rodents: neural and neurochemical substrates. Neurosci. Biobehav. Rev. **28:** 771–784.
71. UYLINGS, H.B., H.J. GROENEWEGEN & B. KOLB. 2003. Do rats have a prefrontal cortex? Behav. Brain Res. **146:** 3–17.

Perspectives on Olfactory Processing, Conscious Perception, and Orbitofrontal Cortex

GORDON M. SHEPHERD

Department of Neurobiology, Yale University School of Medicine, New Haven, Connecticut, USA

ABSTRACT: The orbitofrontal cortex receives inputs from all the major sensory pathways, but olfaction is the only pathway that projects directly to it. We discuss several unique properties with which this is associated. Olfactory stimuli are converted into spatial images, varying in time, in the olfactory bulb, which are processed by the olfactory cortex for input to orbitofrontal cortex. The input from olfactory cortex to orbitofrontal cortex is mostly direct, though some fibers project through mediodorsal thalamus in some species. Studies are needed to determine the specific contributions of olfactory cortex and orbitofrontal cortex to conscious smell perception. A major challenge to the field is accounting for how conscious perception of this sense is coordinated with conscious perceptions of the other major senses, which are known to depend on thalamocortical circuits. The fact that the primary olfactory area at the neocortical level is embedded in the multisensory region of the orbitofrontal cortex indicates that at this level smell perception is heavily influenced by other senses, particularly related to food flavors through retronasal smell, which is being documented in experimental studies in rodents, nonhuman primates, and humans. Also requiring clarification is how behavioral modulation at each step of processing of the odor images is coordinated. In sum, the orbitofrontal cortex is emerging as the next frontier in understanding the neural basis of smell.

KEYWORDS: orbitofrontal cortex; olfactory cortex; thalamus

This symposium brings a welcome focus on the orbitofrontal cortex, a part of the brain of special interest because of its increase during pimate evolution. Among its many functions, the orbitofrontal cortex serves as the first neocortical receiving areas for the olfactory pathway. The cortical olfactory areas in turn have multiple complex relations with other chemosensory areas, and with limbic areas involved in learning, memory, motivation, and emotion. Many of

Address for correspondence: Dr. Gordon M. Shepherd, Department of Neurobiology, Yale University School of Medicine, 333 Cedar Street, New Haven, CT 06510. Tel.: 203-785-4336; fax: 203-785-6990. gordon.shepherd@yale.edu

Ann. N.Y. Acad. Sci. 1121: 87–101 (2007). © 2007 New York Academy of Sciences. doi: 10.1196/annals.1401.032

these functions and relations are documented elsewhere in this volume by the leaders in these studies.

In chairing the session on chemosensory inputs, I would like to take a step back to gain a perspective on the entire olfactory pathway, from the sensory receptors in the nose, through the olfactory bulb and olfactory cortex, to the orbitofrontal cortex. This brings out several key points that are not widely recognized or understood: how odor images are processed at successive steps in the pathway; how orbitofrontal cortical microcircuits may function; the special nature of sensory consciousness in this pathway; and a reminder that a combination of bottom-up sensory processing and top-down behavioral modulation occurs at ever step along this pathway.

OVERVIEW OF THE NEURAL BASIS OF OLFACTORY PROCESSING

The odor stimulus begins as information carried in odor molecules and is transduced by a family of many hundreds of receptors to cover the wide range of odor molecules that an animal may encounter in its environment. In the mammal, a given receptor is expressed by a subset of receptor neurons which project to a module in the olfactory bulb called a *glomerulus*. The activity patterns set up by the differential activation of glomeruli are called "odor maps" or "odor images" (FIG. 1). They also have a temporal dimension with the rise and fall of the stimulus, and the temporal patterns may themselves contain information about the stimulating molecules. As a basis for odor perception, these odor images are therefore equivalent to spatial patterns in the visual system that are the basis for visual perception.[1,2]

Experimental studies with many different imaging techniques tell us that each odor molecule gives rise to its unique spatial activity pattern. Examples from fMRI imaging are shown in FIGURE 1. Some 2000 glomeruli form these patterns in a rodent. We hypothesize that a complex odor object, composed of many odor molecules, such as a perfume or a foodstuff, also has its unique pattern. The ability of a species to detect and discriminate the odors that control its behavior depends in the first instance on the granularity of this glomerular array, which is the result of a combination of numbers of olfactory receptors, olfactory receptor cells, and olfactory glomeruli. These numbers are presently the subject of increasing research in different species.

How much information can be carried in a spatial pattern, such as the array of glomerular modules? An interesting perspective comes from the development of commercial barcodes, which indicates the richness of information coding that is possible by simple spatial patterns (FIG. 2). It is an intriguing hypothesis that a glomerular activity pattern functions as a kind of brain barcode for a specific odor molecule or the combined molecules that make up a complex odor object such as a perfume or a foodstuff.

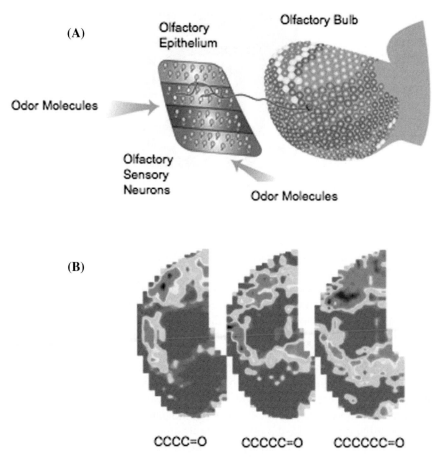

FIGURE 1. (**A**) Representation of the sheet of olfactory receptor cells and their projections to the olfactory bulb in the mouse. (**B**) Odor stimulation with different aldehyde molecule types elicits pattern different patterns of activation of the olfactory glomeruli. (Adapted from Xu *et al.* [2003], in Shepherd.[1])

The activity pattern is only the beginning of the basis of olfactory perception. A critical factor is the degree of processing that takes place through the neural circuits of the olfactory pathway. The odor patterns, laid out in the glomerular layer, are subject to successive steps of processing at the periglomerular and granule cell levels.[3,4] The output is processed in the olfactory cortex before being projected to the olfactory receiving area of the orbitofrontal cortex, the first neocortical level in this pathway. These steps are indicated in FIGURE 3. It has been hypothesized that the increased processing power that has evolved in the human brain, particularly in the orbitofrontal cortex, gives a greatly enhanced ability of the human to carry out complex odor discriminations,

FIGURE 2.   Example of a new generation of two-dimensional barcodes, illustrating the information capacity of spatial activity patterns such as those elicited in the glomerular layer by odor stimulation as in FIGURE 1.

particularly on its retronasal input related to the flavors of food, as we discuss further below.

The nature of the processing through these successive steps is the subject of increasingly intense study. New methods are enabling us to visualize for the first time the organization of cells in the olfactory bulb in terms of cellular columns that appear to form glomerular units, analogous to columns in visual areas of the cerebral cortex.[5] They are also allowing us to visualize ensembles of interconnected columns that appear to provide for an extensive web of lateral interactions independent of distance in processing the odor maps. Both physiological and computational studies are demonstrating the kind of synaptic organization and functional circuits that can mediate these interactions.[6]

In the olfactory cortex, the olfactory bulb input appears to be distributed relatively widely. Within this distribution, there may be clusters of input fiber terminals and output cells. The signature organizational principle appears to be to receive this distributed pattern and add iterative recurrent re-excitatory patterns through long recurrent axon collaterals of the pyramidal neurons. The organization has been likened to that of the face area of higher visual association areas.[7] It has the function of a content-addressable memory in storing the input patterns in a widely distributed manner—in other words, an organization well adapted to process complex spatial patterns, such as those of FIGURES 1 AND 3.

From olfactory cortex, there are two main output streams. One is to subcortical limbic regions for activation of systems involved in control of hypothalamic, motivational, and emotional responses to odors. Presumably this subcortically mediated behavior is "unconscious," a question to which we will return. Some of this information involves pheromones. In some species pheromone information is mediated by both the main and the accessory olfactory system acting in parallel; in the human both ordinary odors and pheromones are processed through the main olfactory pathway. The other output stream is to the

Sequence of
Functional Operations

Odor determinants differentially activate
olfactory receptor binding pockets

Odor image of the determinants is formed
in the glomerular layer

Enhanced odor image is formed
by glomerular layer microcircuits

Contextual odor image is formed by
mitral/tufted and granule cell
microcircuits

Content addressable memory
is formed by olfactory cortex
microcircuits

Perception mediated by
orbitofrontal cortex microcircuits?

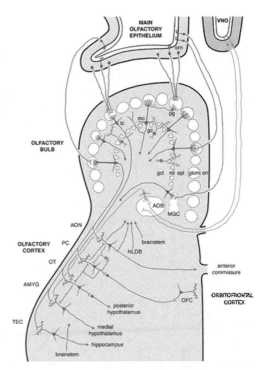

FIGURE 3.   Overview of the mammalian olfactory pathway (*right*) with steps in odor processing (*left*). VNO, vomeronasal organ; mc, mitral cell; tc, tufted cell; pg, periglomerular cell; gc, granule cell; glom, glomerulus; on, olfactory nerve; AOB, accessory olfactory bulb; MGC, modified glomerular complex; OFC, orbitofrontal cortex; NLDB, nucleus of the horizontal limb of the diagonal band; AON, anterior olfactory nucleus; PC, piriform cortex; OT, olfactory tubercle; AMYG, amygdala; TEC, transitional entorhinal cortex.

olfactory area of the orbitofrontal cortex, the level of neocortex at which, classically, conscious perception arises.

How is the olfactory cortex able to sort the incoming information from the olfactory bulb into these two output streams? At present this is not understood. The division of the output cells into smaller tufted cells and larger mitral cells may be a key (FIG. 3). A working hypothesis is that pheromone information is conveyed mainly through the tufted cell pathway, whereas common smells are conveyed mainly through the mitral cell pathway. These pathways would be processed selectively at the olfactory cortical level by differential projections to different olfactory cortical areas, and different parallel microcircuits within the primary olfactory cortex. This would be in addition to the mainly, but not exclusively, pheromonal pathway through the accessory olfactory pathway in some species (FIG. 3). This suggestion at least provides a testable hypothesis for future experiments.

The projection from the olfactory cortex to the orbitofrontal cortex is both direct and indirect (FIG. 3). The direct projection is carried by the output axons of the pyramidal cells, the same axons that give rise to the long re-excitatory association fibers and which also carry centrifugal information back to the olfactory bulb. The indirect projection is through activation by the pyramidal cells of cells in the endopiriform nucleus just deep to the pyriform cortex; their axons project to the mediodorsal thalamus, where they make synapses on cells that project to the olfactory orbitofrontal area.[8]

THE NATURE OF CONSCIOUS SMELL PERCEPTION

A big challenge is to understand the special nature of the direct projection, which does not pass through the thalamus, a feature that makes the olfactory pathway unique among sensory systems. Surprisingly little attention has been given to this remarkable feature.

The implications for conscious sensory perception should be one of the most intriguing challenges in cognitive neuroscience. There are two possibilities. One is that conscious smell perception arises already at the level of olfactory cortex. This idea is supported by the finding, reported by Verrity Brown[9] at this meeting, that rodents with lesions of the olfactory area of orbitofrontal cortex can still perform normally on an odor-identification task. If behaving rodents are regarded as "conscious," this finding is significant for two reasons. First, it means that this is the only sensory pathway that gives rise to conscious sensory perception without reaching the neocortex and without engaging the thalamocortical system. Second, if this is so, we must ask: what are the subcortical mechanisms that replace the thalamus and the neocortex, in terms of thalamic arousal and the attentional "searchlight" that are essential in the other sensory systems for conscious perception? And if these mechanisms can be identified, how are they coordinated with the thalamocortical mechanisms so that our perception appears to be conscious for smell in the same way as it is for the other system?

A recent study of olfactory cortex provides evidence that may bear on this question. Murakami et al. asked: does the olfactory system have neural mechanisms for state-dependent gating of its sensory information flow from olfactory cortex to the neocortex that does not require a thalamic relay?[10] They focused on mechanisms controlling different behavioral states that could relate to different levels of consciousness. They first confirmed that, in anesthetized rats, the neocortical electroencephalogram (EEG) undergoes alternation between a slow-wave state (SWS) and a fast-wave state (FWS), similar to the differences seen during slow-wave and fast-wave sleep. With single-cell recordings in the olfactory cortex, they found that odor stimulation could drive cells strongly during FWS, but only weakly during SWS, similar to the differences in sensory driving in other systems during slow- and fast-wave sleep. Stimulation of the ascending reticular activating system in the brainstem desynchronized the neocortical EEG while enhancing olfactory cortical neuron responses to odors. A small percentage of cells in the olfactory bulb also showed state-dependent sensitivity, which may reflect the coupling between olfactory cortex and olfactory bulb through long association fibers from olfactory cortex (see FIG. 3). The authors conclude (see also Shepherd[11]) that "state-dependent sensory gating in the olfactory system is in synchrony with other sensory systems," through the coordinating actions of the brainstem activating system.

How do these mechanisms account for where the "consciousness" of a smell arises? The neural mechanisms of consciousness have become a growth industry in neuroscience, with most of the focus on the visual system. In a well-known synthesis, Crick and Koch first define "consciousness" in a relatively narrow sense, as "perceiving the specific color, shape, or movement of an object."[12] They outline a framework in which primary sensory cortex at the "back" of the brain contains cells and microcircuits that act as "feature detectors" of the information relayed from the thalamus. Feature detection is believed to be largely "unconscious." According to Crick and Koch, "The conscious mode for vision depends largely on the early visual areas (beyond V1) and especially on the ventral stream [in the temporal lobe]." This response is then relayed forward to the "front" of the brain, followed by complex backward and forward interactions between prefrontal cortex and the visual association areas. One suggestion is that the forward connections are largely "driving" and the backward connections are largely "modulatory." "Consciousness" in this view arises from special (as yet unspecified) firing properties of cortical neurons, in particular those that project from the sensory association areas to integrative (not primarily motor or sensory) prefrontal areas.

No indication is given of how olfactory "conscious" perception would fit into this framework. Toward that end the following considerations may be relevant. In olfactory perception there is no "back" of the brain; the primary neocortical receptive area is in the orbitofrontal cortex, which is at the core of the prefrontal area. Thus, in olfaction, all of the sequences of processing necessary to get from the back to the front of the brain are compressed within the front of the brain itself. This reflects the evolutionary position of smell, with its privileged input to the highest centers of the frontal lobe throughout the evolution of the vertebrate brain. From this perspective, the basic architecture of the neural basis of consciousness in mammals, including primates, should be sought in the olfactory system, with adaptations for the other sensory pathways reflecting their relative importance in the different species.

These two different perspectives may be illustrated by the following considerations. In the visual system, experiments in which lesions have been made in lateral orbitofrontal cortex and visual stimuli have been used to test animals' behavior, it is obvious that the animals are responding "consciously" to a visual perception that is received in the primary visual area (V1), and processed in the intact visual association areas and other areas to which they are connected. By contrast, in the olfactory system, when lesions have been made in the sensory orbitofrontal cortex and smell has been used to test an animal's behavior, the exclusive primary neocortical area for smell perception has been removed. This also precludes further processing in neocortical association areas, together with higher processing in other prefrontal areas, and connections to limbic structures. It therefore should have much more profound effects on smell perception.

A number of questions arise, for which answers are still not available. In this case, does the animal still show normal behavioral responses to smell stimuli? If so, does this show that neocortex is necessary for conscious smell perception?, and if so, does this reflect the mediodorsal thalamic pathway? In addition, are the animals "conscious" of the odor perception in the way that visual stimuli are conscious? If the animals still show "conscious" smell perception despite the orbitofrontal cortex lesions, does this mean that conscious smell perception is mediated "sub-neocortically" by olfactory cortex? This would be a type of perceptual consciousness distinct from that of all other sensory pathways that have an obligatory relay through the thalamus, and which depend on the tight interactions between neocortex and thalamus through thalamo-cortical and cortico-thalamic loops.

The other possibility is that conscious smell perception does depend on the neocortical level, through the projection to the olfactory area of lateral orbitofrontal cortex, particularly for primates, including humans. In favor of this is the finding by Tanabe et al. that in the monkey unit responses to odor show increasingly narrow selectivity for different odor molecules, from olfactory bulb through olfactory cortex to the olfactory orbitofrontal area.[13] These are the molecular features that are encoded in the odor maps of FIGURE 1, and this is precisely the type of feature selectivity on which Crick and Koch focus.[12] This suggests that the orbitofrontal area is not processing an odor image that has been increasingly refined and abstracted, similar to the progression in other sensory systems.

This neocortical level for conscious odor perception also gives a function to the parallel indirect projection through mediodorsal thalamus in analogy with other sensory systems. In a recent study in awake behaving rats, some cells in the mediodorsal thalamic nucleus responded to odor cues, discriminating between cues and changing their responses according to reward contingency.[14] The authors suggested that "these mediodorsal thalamic neurons are the neural substrates for association learning of olfactory stimuli with rewards." If associative learning with rewards implies a consciously responding animal, these findings could be construed as reflecting associative learning already at the level of the olfactory cortex projecting, through the endopiriform nucleus, to the thalamus.

An intriguing insight into this question comes from comparing the equivalent stages of processing in the olfactory pathway with other sensory systems. Here we find an amazing range (see FIG. 4). The olfactory bulb, for example, was

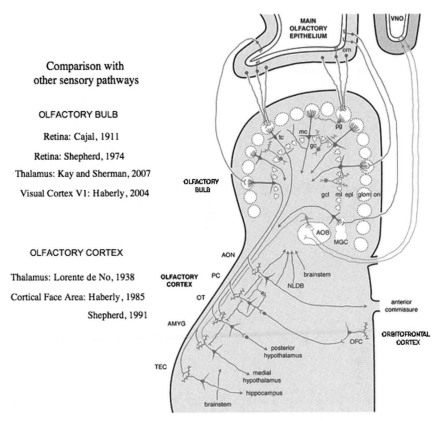

FIGURE 4. Comparisons of different steps of processing in the olfactory pathway with analogies with other sensory pathways that have been suggested.

initially compared by Cajal with the retina,[15] and modern research has provided evidence of similarities in their synaptic organization at the two successive levels of synaptic interactions. The finding of odor images in the glomerular layer, and their processing by the granule cell layer, has supported that idea.

Many years ago Lorente de No suggested that olfactory cortex might function as a kind of thalamus, representing this stage for input to neocortex.[16] The results of Murakami *et al.* cited earlier on state-dependent mechanisms in the olfactory cortex might be construed as supporting that view.[10] In other views, also based on experimental evidence, the olfactory bulb has been compared to V1 in the visual pathway, anterior olfactory cortex to higher visual areas, and posterior olfactory cortex to the face area, as mentioned above. Recently the olfactory bulb itself was compared to thalamus. Olfactory cortex has also been compared with hippocampus in terms of its basic neuronal circuits. Another hypothesis is that olfactory cortex is equivalent to the layer 4 stellate cells of granular cortex in providing a staging center for formatting the input to

Comparison of visual and olfactory pathways

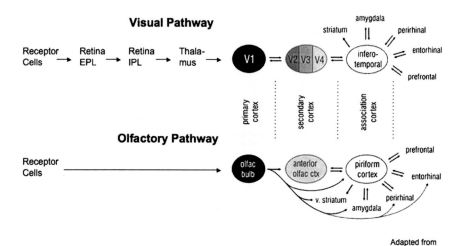

Adapted from
Haberly, 2001

FIGURE 5. Comparison of steps of sensory processing in the olfactory and visual pathways. EPL, external plexiform layer; IPL, internal plexiform layer. (Adapted from Neville and Haberly.[18])

the different cortical laminae. FIGURE 5 summarizes some of these studies and suggestions.[17,18]

The lesson from these comparisons is that the truth likely lies with all of the above. This explanation requires understanding the different sensory modalities. In comparison with vision, the olfactory pathway is relieved of having to keep track of external space and time, which, in the visual system, is known to be extremely expensive of computational power. It can therefore be much more efficient in carrying out successive stages of information processing of its spatial pattern input. These steps presumably include such basic operations as signal-to-noise detection, feature-from-ground abstraction, object recognition, etc. To do this, this pathway can build circuits that overlap within a structure (such as the two levels of the olfactory bulb) as well as between structures (as in the feedback loops between olfactory cortex and olfactory bulb).

This suggestion brings us back to the nature of the sensory information that is processed in this pathway. The glomerulus is the near-universal principle of neuronal organization, and the layer of glomeruli forms the odor images that are the basis for successive processing in the olfactory pathway. It is therefore a reasonable working hypothesis that the odor image, reformatted by the circuits of the olfactory bulb and olfactory cortex, is the input that is processed by the olfactory area of the orbitofrontal cortex. A great deal is known about the processing of visual objects,[19] and there is therefore the opportunity to draw on that knowledge for a deeper insight into the nature of processing of odor objects by orbitofrontal cortex.

IS THERE A BASIC MICROCIRCUIT FOR ORBITOFRONTAL CORTEX?

Comparing smell processing with visual processing brings out the fact that we lack critical knowledge about the synaptic organization of orbitofrontal cortex. In vision, understanding of mechanisms of visual processing is built on a detailed knowledge of the circuits and their operation at each step of the pathway, from the two successive stages in the retina, through thalamus, to V1 and beyond. In olfaction, we are building a similar understanding of mechanisms of olfactory processing at the two successive stages in the olfactory bulb to the olfactory cortex, as summarized above.

In orbitofrontal cortex, we have detailed analyses of connectivity by Price,[8] and detailed recordings of unit responses to smell stimuli by Rolls and colleagues.[20] However, there is not yet the analysis of synaptic organization that has been so essential for understanding other brain regions at the cellular and molecular level. The needed information includes: the types of circuits that perform the essential input–output operations on the sensory inputs, the generation of intrinsic excitability properties, the sequences of dendritic processing; the types of lateral inhibitory mechanisms; the synaptic actions of the specific inputs from other areas; the synaptic modulation by inputs reflecting behavioral states, etc.

A working hypothesis is that, as an area of agranular cortex, orbitofrontal cortex contains a basic type of cortical microcircuit[21] consisting of superficial and deep pyramidal cells; these have recurrent axon collaterals that mediate re-excitation as well as lateral inhibition feedback and lateral inhibition through subclasses of inhibitory interneurons, and apical and basal dendritic trees which have basic integrative properties similar to those of other cortical areas. How these general properties are fine-tuned to produce the special functional operations within the olfactory area and the other orbitofrontal areas constitutes the next frontier of cortical circuit investigation. In view of the evidence that this area reaches its highest development in primates, and especially humans, a high priority should be put on revealing these intrinsic mechanisms.

In addition to its specific olfactory sensory role, a special feature of orbitofrontal cortex is that, during feeding behavior, the information contained in the odor images is immediately combined with inputs from taste, somatosensation, audition, and vision into the multimodal perception of flavor. From these sensory areas in lateral orbitofrontal cortex, the integrated information is transferred to medial visceral orbitofrontal output areas that are interconnected with basolateral amygdala and related areas to provide the motivational and emotional dimensions of the feeding experience, with hypothalamic areas involved in control of feeding behavior[8]; and, in humans, with language areas involved in smell and flavor identification and verbal characterization of these perceptions. Together these form a brain–flavor system that is unique to humans.[1,20,22] It has been hypothesized that flavor is one of the most important sensory experiences in the evolution of human behavior.

TOP-DOWN MODULATION OF OLFACTORY PROCESSING

We have seen that this higher cognitive function, as far as the olfactory pathway is concerned, arises only three synapses from the receptor event in the nose. This compression of processing stages brings us to our last observation, on how the sensory input information is modulated. We need to keep in mind that a property recorded at the level of the orbitofrontal cortex may reflect processing not at that level but at a lower level in the pathway. A simple example is adaptation of a response to repeated stimulation. This occurs already at the level of the receptor cells, where it may involve several properties, such as desensitization of the receptor or one of the steps in the second-messenger cascade, or at the cyclic nucleotide gated channel that generates the receptor potential. Adaptation also occurs in the synaptic responses of mitral cells in the olfactory bulb, and at the level of pyramidal cell responses in the olfactory cortex.[23]

Another property is top-down modulation by the behavioral state of the animal. Modulation by states of hunger and satiety, for example, is a common finding in recordings from the olfactory area of orbitofrontal cortex. However, it has been known for some time that a similar modulation is shown by mitral cells in the olfactory bulb, which show increased responses to food odors in hungry rats compared with subdued responses in rats fed to satiety. A similar modulation in relation to these states has been shown by pyramidal cells in the olfactory cortex. Both the olfactory bulb and olfactory cortex are richly supplied with fibers from brainstem and basal forebrain modulatory systems (cholinergic, noradrenergic, serotonergic). How these modulatory systems act at these successive levels up to and including the orbitofrontal cortex will be a big challenge.

CHALLENGES FOR THE FUTURE

The methods for analyzing the sensory responses to smell and taste and the other modalities contributing to flavor perception are increasingly sophisticated, involving cutting-edge technologies in single-unit recordings from primates and functional imaging in humans. Despite these advances, it is still not possible in the human to obtain the resolution needed to discern the nature of the image processing that we have postulated. Nor is it usually possible to monitor the lower levels in the olfactory pathway to assess modulatory systems that act in a coordinated fashion at the successive stages of processing, but new experiments are making this possible (see monitoring of orbitofrontal cortex and olfactory cortex in the studies of Gottfried[24]). In this respect the animal experiments provide critical information, through higher-resolution methods and closer stimulus control. Together, the two approaches should provide an increasingly revealing understanding of the neural basis of odor image formation and flavor perception mediated by orbitofrontal cortex, and the critical role it plays in human behavior.

To address these problems in this symposium, Jay Gottfried provides an orientation to imaging smell responses in the human.[24] Tom Pritchard reviews the studies of responses in the taste area of human orbitofrontal cortex.[25] Dana Small describes human imaging studies showing how retronasal smell and taste responses combine to give rise to flavor perception.[22] Taken together, this session provides the latest report from leading laboratories on the remarkable progress in revealing the central role of the chemical senses in the higher-level cognitive processing that takes place in the human orbitofrontal cortex.

ACKNOWLEDGMENTS

Our studies have been generously supported by the National Institutes of Health through the NIDCD and the Human Brain Project.

REFERENCES

1. SHEPHERD, G.M. 2006. Smell images and the flavour system in the human brain. Nature **444:** 316–321.
2. XU, F.Q., N. LIU, I. KIDA, et al. 2003. Odor maps of aldehydes and esters revealed by fMRI in the glomerular layer of the mouse olfactory bulb. Proc. Natl. Acad. Sci. USA **100:** 11029–11034.
3. SHEPHERD, G.M., W. R. CHEN & C. A. GREER. 2004. Olfactory bulb. In The Synaptic Organization of the Brain, 5th ed. G.M. Shepherd, Ed., 165–216. Oxford University Press. New York.
4. YAKSI, E., B. JUDKEWITZ & R. W. FRIEDRICH. 2007. Topological reorganization of odor representations in the olfactory bulb. PLoS Biol. **5:** e178.
5. WILLHITE, D.C., K. T. NGUYEN, A. V. MASURKAR, et al. 2006. Viral tracing identifies distributed columnar organization in the olfactory bulb. Proc. Natl. Acad. Sci. USA **103:** 12592–12597.
6. MIGLIORE, M. & G. M. SHEPHERD. 2007. Dendritic action potentials connect distributed dendrodendritic microcircuits. J. Computat. Neurosci. Aug. 3 [Epub ahead of print].
7. HABERLY, L.B. 1985. Neuronal circuitry in olfactory cortex: anatomy and functional implications. Chem. Senses **10:** 219–238.

8. PRICE, J.L. 2007. Definition of the orbital cortex in relation to specific connections with limbic and visceral structures, and other cortical regions. This volume.

9. TAIT, D.S. & V. J. BROWN 2007. Difficulty overcoming learned non-reward during reversal learning in rats with ibotenic acid lesions of orbital prefrontal cortex. This volume.

10. MURAKAMI, M., H. KASHIWADANI, Y. KIRINO & K. MORI. 2005. State-dependent sensory gating in olfactory cortex. Neuron **46:** 285–296.

11. SHEPHERD, G.M. 2005. Perception without a thalamus: How does olfaction do it? Neuron **46:** 166–168.

12. CRICK, F. & C. KOCH. 2003. A framework for consciousness. Nat. Neurosci. **6:** 119–126.

13. TANABE, T., M. IIONO & S. F. TAKAGI. 1975. Discrimination of odors in olfactory bulb, pyriform-amygdaloid areas, and orbitofrontal cortex of the monkey. J. Neurophysiol. **38:** 1284–1296.

14. KAWAGOE, T., R. TAMURA, T. UWANO, et al. 2007. Neural correlates of stimulus-reward association in the rat mediodorsal thalamus. Neuroreport **18:** 683–688.

15. CAJAL, RAMONY, S. 1911. Histologie du Système Nerveux chez l'Homme et des Vertébrés. Maloine. Paris.

16. LORENTE DE NO, R. 1938. The cerebral cortex: architecture, intracortical connections and motor projections. In Physiology of the Nervous System, J.F. Fulton, Ed.: 291–325. Oxford University Press. London.

17. HABERLY, L.B. 2001. Parallel-distributed processing in olfactory cortex: new insights from morphological and physiological analysis of neuronal circuitry. Chem. Senses. **26:** 551–576.

18. NEVILLE, K.R. & L. B. HABERLY. 2004. Olfactory cortex. In The Synaptic Organization of the Brain, 5th ed. G.M. Shepherd, Ed.: 415–454. Oxford University Press. New York.

19. STERLING, P. & J. B. DEMB. 2004. Retina. In The Synaptic Organization of the Brain, 5th ed. G.M. Shepherd, Ed.: 217–270. Oxford University Press. New York.

20. ROLLS, E.T. 2006. Brain mechanisms underlying flavour and appetite. Philos. Trans. R. Soc. Lond. B Biol Sci. **361:** 1123–1136.

21. SHEPHERD, G.M. 2004. Introduction to synaptic circuits. In The Synaptic Organization of the Brain, 5th ed. G.M. Shepherd, Ed.: 1–38. Oxford University Press. New York.

22. SMALL, D.M. et al. 2007. The role of the human orbital frontal cortex in taste and flavor processing. This volume.

23. LINSTER, C., L. HENRY, M. KADOHISA & D. A. WILSON. 2007. Synaptic adaptation and odor-background segmentation. Neurobiol. Learn. Mem. **87:** 352–360.

24. GOTTFRIED, J.A. 2007. What can an orbitofrontal cortex-endowed animal do with smells? This volume.

25. PRITCHARD, T.C. et al. 2007. Taste in the medial orbitofrontal cortex of the macaque. This volume.

OTHER REFERENCE SOURCES

KAY, L.M. & S.M. SHERMAN. 2007. An argument for an olfactory thalamus. Trends Neurosci. **30:** 47–53.

SHEPHERD, G.M. 1974. The Synaptic Organization of the Brain. Oxford University Press. New York.

SHEPHERD, G.M. 1991. Computational structure of the olfactory system. *In* Olfaction: A Model for Computational Neuroscience. H. Eichenbaum & J. Davis, Eds.: 3–42. MIT Press. Cambridge, MA.

What Can an Orbitofrontal Cortex-Endowed Animal Do with Smells?

JAY A. GOTTFRIED

Cognitive Neurology & Alzheimer's Disease Center and the Department of Neurology, Northwestern University Feinberg School of Medicine, Chicago, Illinois, USA

ABSTRACT: It is widely presumed that odor quality is a direct outcome of odorant molecular structure, but increasing evidence suggests that learning, experience, and context play important roles in human olfactory perception. Such data suggest that a given set of olfactory receptors activated by an odorant does not map directly onto a given odor percept. Rather, odor perception may rely on more synthetic, or integrative, mechanisms subserved by higher-order brain regions. Results presented here explore the specific role of human orbitofrontal cortex (OFC) in the formation and modulation of odor quality coding. Combining olfactory psychophysical techniques and functional imaging approaches, we have found that sensory-specific information about an odorant is not static or fixed within human olfactory OFC, but is highly malleable and can be rapidly updated by perceptual experience. Critically, the magnitude of OFC activation predicts subsequent behavioral improvement in olfactory perception. Our findings highlight the pivotal role of OFC in linking olfactory sensation, perception, and experience. It is worth considering that many of the current proposed functions attributed to the (distinctively mammalian) OFC are an extension of mechanisms that originally evolved to mediate response flexibility between chemosensory signals and appropriate behavioral actions.

KEYWORDS: orbitofrontal cortex; limbic system; olfactory cortex; olfaction; smell; sensory processing; perceptual learning; aversive conditioning

INTRODUCTION

The original title of this chapter was "Smelling to Learn in Human Orbitofrontal Cortex," and much of what follows will focus on the topics of smelling, learning, and experience. However, after organizing my oral presentation for the New York Academy Sciences conference on orbitofrontal cortex

Address for correspondence: Jay A. Gottfried, M.D., Ph.D., Cognitive Neurology & Alzheimer's Disease Center, Northwestern University Feinberg School of Medicine, 320 E. Superior St., Searle 11-453, Chicago, IL 60611. Voice: (312) 503-1834; fax: (312) 908-8789.
j-gottfried@northwestern.edu

Ann. N.Y. Acad. Sci. 1121: 102–120 (2007). © 2007 New York Academy of Sciences.
doi: 10.1196/annals.1401.018

(OFC), I was inclined toward a different title that more faithfully captures the broad themes raised in the Keynote talks: "What Can an Orbitofrontal Cortex-Endowed Animal Do with Smells?" This somewhat non-traditional approach to the topic of chemosensory processing and the OFC is motivated by a simple fact (which was admittedly difficult for an olfactory neuroscientist, such as myself to accept). The fact is, the sense of smell does not require an OFC.

A casual glance at the animal kingdom makes this abundantly clear. There are thousands of vertebrate and invertebrate species using their sense of smell quite efficiently without the least remnant of prefrontal cortex (PFC) or OFC. Maternal bonding, kinship identification, mating choice, hunting and feeding, defining home and territory, evading predators—all of these behaviors are frequently under the spell of odor stimuli, but for many of the animals engaged in these activities, there is no OFC to which olfactory information can even be projected. So while it may be true that the smells are processed in the OFC, or that odor inputs gain access to OFC in as few as three synapses, these statements are not especially enlightening or informative, because the real question is to understand the *unique* features that an OFC contributes to odor processing.

A brief evolutionary interlude may shed some light on these issues. Phylogenetic analyses (FIG. 1) indicate that PFC first emerged in vertebrate evolution about 175 million years ago,[1] traced back to a mammalian ancestor that gave rise to one line of now-extinct mammals and to one line of modern mammals (including egg-laying monotremes, pouch-bearing marsupials, and placentals). Of the remaining living vertebrates, this leaves roughly 30,000 species of bony fish, 6,000 species of amphibians, 8,000 species of reptiles, and 10,000 species of birds, all surviving quite well without prefrontal neocortical brain structures. Thus it is clear that smelling, tasting, hunting, scavenging, eating, and copulating can all be accomplished in the absence of a PFC.

An interesting corollary follows from these considerations: what are the behavioral limitations of an animal *without* a PFC? The green lizard *Lacerta* provides a good example of PFC-less behavior. Wagner showed 75 years ago that *Lacerta* is compelled to approach the color green[2] (discussed in Schneirla[3]), an innate response that no doubt has social and nutritional importance for a green species living in a green environment. When Wagner allowed the lizard to choose between a tasty mealworm placed in front of a red panel, and a noxious (salt-saturated) mealworm placed in front of a green panel, it consistently selected the salty worm, and only learned to switch its response pattern after hundreds of trials, if at all.

The great difficulty of this reptile to use experience to modify its behavior adaptively illustrates the advantages of a PFC. The ability to suppress natural response tendencies, to form new predictions about old stimuli, and to update information about sensory inputs, particularly for "emotionally" (biologically) important events, are some of the unique features that PFC and OFC contribute

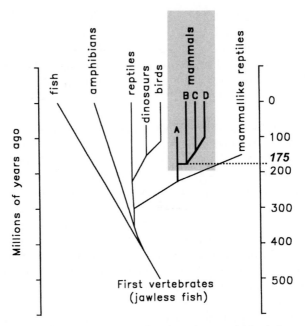

FIGURE 1. Evolutionary appearance of prefrontal cortex. This phylogenetic diagram of vertebrate evolution illustrates that prefrontal cortex arose approximately 175 million years ago in an ancestral species common to the line of modern-day mammals (*grey box*), including monotremes **(B)**, marsupials **(C)**, and placentals **(D)**. The group of now-extinct mammals, such as trichonodonts and multituberculates, is indicated at **A**. It is important to emphasize that thousands of non-mammalian vertebrate species, spanning fish, amphibians, reptiles, and birds, have an acute sense of smell despite the absence of a prefrontal cortex. [Figure modified from Fig. 1.3 of: H.J. Jerison, Evolution of prefrontal cortex. 1997. *In* N.A. Krasnegor, G.R. Lyon & P.S. Goldman-Rakic, Eds., Development of the prefrontal cortex: evolution, neurobiology, and behavior, Baltimore, MD: Paul H. Brookes Publishing Co., Inc. Copyright (1997), reprinted and adapted by permission of Brookes Publishing and the author.[1]]

to olfactory processing. It is intriguing to speculate that further neocortical differentiation over the last 175 million years has enabled an appropriation of neural machinery originally tuned to handle the interface of odor, behavior, and experience. The OFC of modern-day mammals ensures that a wide variety of experiences, including non-olfactory sensations and interoceptive states, can guide behavior adaptively, with maximal flexibility.

Defining the OFC of modern-day mammals presents its own challenges. The rat is endowed with a tremendous sense of smell but with very little recognizable OFC, at least on cytoarchitectonic grounds, given the absence of granular cortex. Its frontal agranular neocortex has been loosely divided into a medial wall (including medial orbital [MO], infralimbic [IL], and prelimbic [PL] areas) and a ventral/lateral segment (including ventral and posterior agranular insula [AIv and AIp], ventrolateral orbital [VLO], and lateral orbital [LO] areas).[4] This latter group of structures (AIv, AIp, VLO, LO) receives direct projections from rodent piriform cortex and responds with short-latency action potentials to electrical stimulation of the olfactory bulb.[5] From electrophysiological recordings in rodents, it is evident that these same structures are involved in olfactory discrimination learning,[6,7] lending support to the idea that the OFC of "sub-primate" mammals was chiefly dedicated to the handling of behaviorally salient odor information.

The olfactory OFC in monkeys is broadly comparable to the rodent, though evidence for a definitive homology is still lacking.[5] Physiological[8,9] and anatomical[5,10] studies suggest that primary olfactory cortex (including piriform cortex, olfactory tubercle, and cortical amygdaloid nuclei) projects most densely to posterior orbital cortex in areas Iam, Iapm, and 13a, corresponding to the rodent areas AIv, AIp, and VLO, respectively. Research by Tanabe and colleagues in the 1970's on monkeys suggested that an odor has access to neocortical structures by either of two routes: a direct path from piriform cortex to OFC or an indirect path from piriform cortex to OFC via an intermediary in mediodorsal thalamus.[8,9] Thus an odorous sensation at the nasal periphery is no more than two synapses removed from olfactory neocortex.

By comparison, the putative human olfactory OFC appears to be strikingly more anterior than one would predict on the basis of the animal data. A recent meta-analysis of 13 human olfactory imaging studies[11] demonstrates that odor stimulation consistently activates a bilateral area close to the transverse orbital sulcus (the horizontal limb of the "H"-shaped sulcus), roughly corresponding to the posterior part of granular OFC area 11l in human OFC.[12] Methodological issues notwithstanding, it is interesting to speculate that these cross-species anatomical differences might reflect behavioral differences in the role that the sense of smell plays in these two species. For example, the amygdala provides strong input to agranular OFC, but very scant projections to central anterior OFC (such as area 11l), implying that limbic (amygdala) influences on odor processing in OFC may be limited in the human brain.

This brief survey is meant to illustrate the considerable anatomical variation in the organization of olfactory OFC across mammalian species, suggesting important potential constraints upon extrapolating human OFC function from animal data (for detailed discussion see Gottfried and Zald[11]). These differences are likely to be even more exaggerated in rostral areas of OFC, where increasing cellular granularity leads to further interspecies divergence. Now with these provisos impartially aired, the remainder of this chapter will focus on OFC and olfaction in the human brain. Specifically, as an epitome of the neuro-behavioral interface between sensation, learning, and experience, the following section describes two recent functional magnetic resonance imaging (fMRI) experiments from our laboratory demonstrating the role of human OFC in olfactory perceptual learning and associative (Pavlovian) conditioning. Together these studies reveal how experience-dependent modification of odor representations in OFC underlies the capacity for sensory refinement of human olfactory perception.

METHODS AND RESULTS

Olfactory Perceptual Learning

The idea that sensory exposure and experience can induce long-term changes in behavior and brain function, even in the absence of direct behavioral reinforcement, is referred to as perceptual learning.[13,14] This form of plasticity has been documented in numerous non-olfactory systems including visual,[15,16] auditory,[17,18] and somatosensory[19] cortices.

In the olfactory domain, perceptual learning is well documented at the behavioral level. For example, repeated presentations of an odor reduce olfactory detection thresholds[20,21] and can boost olfactory sensitivity in anosmic subjects.[22,23] Exposure to wine[24] or beer[25] is sufficient to improve sensitivity toward stimuli whose chief sensory property is olfactory. Experience and familiarity significantly enhance odor quality discrimination,[26,27] while exposure to odor mixtures alters the perceived quality of the individual components.[28] Notably, despite growing behavioral evidence for olfactory perceptual learning, how this form of learning updates odor quality codes in the human brain is unknown.

In the present study,[29] Dr. Wen Li and I combined fMRI techniques with an olfactory habituation paradigm[30–32] to test whether prolonged olfactory exposure (as a simple form of perceptual learning) leads to sensory plasticity within the human brain. Our main hypothesis was that prolonged sensory experience would modulate neural representations of odor quality in areas previously implicated in coding of this perceptual feature, including piriform cortex[33,34] and OFC.[6,33,35–37] Moreover, in parallel to the neural effects, we hypothesized that odor experience would facilitate perceptual differentiation between odorants sharing critical qualitative or structural attributes. Note, as used throughout the rest of this chapter, the term "odor quality" is meant to refer to the specific character or identity of a smell emanating from an odorous object (such as its mintiness or floweriness), in contrast to other features, such as intensity, pleasantness, or pungency.

During event-related fMRI scanning, 16 human volunteers (mean age, 24 years) smelled a target odorant (TG) destined for habituation; a quality-related odorant (QR, either "floral" or "mint"); a functional group-related odorant (GR, either ketone or alcohol); and a control odorant (CT) unrelated to TG either in quality or group, both before and after 3.5-min continuous exposure to the TG stimulus (FIG. 2). As orthogonal factors in the study design, the GR odorants systematically differed in perceptual quality, and the QR odorants systematically differed in functional group. Thus, inclusion of the

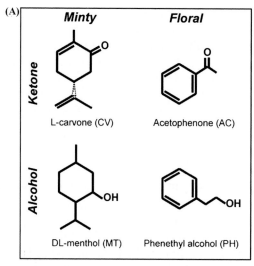

FIGURE 2. Experimental paradigm of olfactory perceptual learning. (**A**) Subjects smelled four different odorants that systematically differed in perceptual quality (minty or floral) and in molecular functional group (ketone or alcohol). (**B**) Odorants were assigned to four conditions: a target odorant (TG) destined for habituation, an odorant related in perceptual quality (QR) to TG, an odorant related in molecular functional group (GR) to TG, and a control odorant (CT) unrelated in either quality or functional group to TG. Across subjects, the assignment of a given odorant as the TG stimulus was evenly counterbalanced (N, number of subjects), thereby minimizing perceptual differences between TG, QR, GR, and CT conditions. (**C**) fMRI scanning was divided into three sequential sessions. During pre-habituation and post-habituation, there were 14 2-sec presentations of each of the four odorants. During habituation, the TG odorant was presented continuously for 3.5 min. [Reprinted and modified from Figs. 1 and 2 in: W. Li, E. Luxenberg, T. Parrish & J.A. Gottfried, Learning to smell the roses: experience-dependent neural plasticity in human piriform and orbitofrontal cortices, Neuron, Vol. 52, Pages 1097–1108, Copyright (2006), with permission from Elsevier.[29]]

QR and GR conditions enabled us to probe the specificity of learning-induced changes across the dimensions of odor quality and odorant group independently, while the CT condition provided a base line to adjust for non-specific effects. Importantly, the selection of odorants (L-carvone, menthol, acetophenone, and phenethyl alcohol) made it possible to assign the stimuli to each of the four conditions (TG, QR, GR, CT), counterbalanced across subjects, to minimize odorant-specific confounds. Pairwise similarity ratings of odor quality,[28] collected 30 min before and 30 min. after prolonged TG exposure, provided a behavioral index of perceptual learning.

Using an integrated parallel acquisition technique known as GRAPPA, we obtained T2*-weighted echoplanar images on a Siemens Trio 3-T MRI scanner (Siemens Medical Solutions, Erlangen, Germany) equipped with an 8-channel head array coil. In combination with a matrix size of 128 mm, a slice thickness of 2 mm, an echo time (TE) of 20 ms, and a tilted acquisition angle (30° to the intercommissural line), this imaging protocol exhibits excellent sensitivity for detecting BOLD (blood-oxygen-level dependent) contrast changes in olfactory regions of the brain that are highly susceptible to signal dropout and distortion.

Behaviorally, from pre-exposure to post-exposure, quality similarity ratings decreased (indicating more *dissimilarity*) for the TG:QR pair and the TG:GR pair, compared to control pairs (FIG. 3). The implication is that sensory experience with the TG odorant successfully enhanced the discriminative capacity (or expertise) for odorants similar in perceptual quality or chemical structure. For example, subjects exposed to L-carvone (the minty ketone) became mint "experts," and they simultaneously became experts at distinguishing among ketone-bearing odorants. Importantly, the four odorants did not differ in intensity at the time of pre-testing or post-testing, making it unlikely that subjects relied on intensity factors to make their similarity judgments. Moreover, by the end of the post-habituation session, there were no significant behavioral differences in valence or pungency among the four odorant conditions, ruling out the likelihood that the impact of TG exposure on odor quality differentiation was due to mere perceptual variations in these other perceptual features. Finally, a complementary behavioral study on an independent group of 16 subjects revealed that these perceptual effects persisted for up to 24 hours after initial exposure and even generalized to novel odorants within the same odor category.[29]

Analysis of the fMRI data set was performed using the software package SPM2 (www.fil.ion.ucl.ac.uk/spm/). Subject-specific comparisons (contrasts) between the different odor conditions, at pre-habituation versus, post-habituation, were entered into a series of one-sample *t*-tests or ANOVAs, each constituting a group-level (random-effects) analysis, permitting population-based inference testing. These results demonstrated experience-dependent response enhancement in both piriform and orbitofrontal cortices, in parallel to (and preceding) the behavioral effects. In posterior piriform cortex, neural activity elicited by the QR odorant increased from pre-habituation to

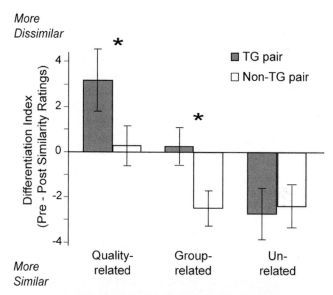

FIGURE 3. Odor exposure enhances perceptual expertise. Similarity ratings of odor quality between pairs of odorants indicate that from pre-exposure to post-exposure, subjects were better able to differentiate odorant pairs related in perceptual quality (TG:QR), in comparison to unrelated pairs (TG:CT) and in comparison to quality-related pairs (GR:CT) whose qualitative features differed from the TG category (for example, if TG and QR were both minty smells, then GR and CT were both floral smells). Discrimination was also improved between odorants sharing functional groups (TG:GR). These effects persisted for 24 hours (data not shown). *Significant compared with non-TG pairs; $P < 0.05$. [Reprinted and modified from Fig. 4 in: W. Li, E. Luxenberg, T. Parrish & J.A. Gottfried, Learning to smell the roses: experience-dependent neural plasticity in human piriform and orbitofrontal cortices, Neuron, Vol. 52, Pages 1097–1108, Copyright (2006), with permission from Elsevier.[29]]

post-habituation; in olfactory OFC, increased activation was seen in response to both the QR and GR odorants.

The above findings provide solid evidence for behavioral and neural plasticity in response to sensory experience, but are unable to demonstrate whether there is a predictive relationship between the magnitude of response change in OFC (or piriform cortex) and the behavioral improvement in perceptual learning. To address this question, we conducted a correlation analysis by regressing subject-specific changes in neural activity (post-habituation minus pre-habituation) against changes in odor quality similarity (post minus pre). In olfactory OFC, there was a significant correlation ($R = 0.75$; $P < 0.05$ corrected for small volume) between neural and behavioral indices of learning (FIG. 4). No such effect was observed in piriform cortex. These additional results suggest that OFC is a critical locus for guiding experience-dependent behavioral improvements in perceptual expertise.

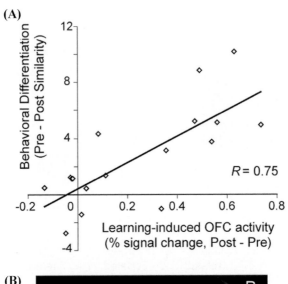

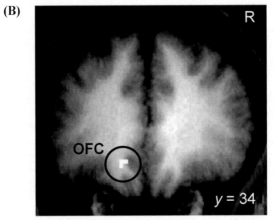

FIGURE 4. Neural activity in OFC predicts subsequent enhancement in perceptual differentiation. (**A**) Regression analysis demonstrates that the magnitude of learning-induced change in OFC (abscissa) directly correlates with the degree of perceptual enhancement (ordinate), on a subject-by-subject basis. Each *diamond* represents a different subject. (**B**) The mean effect of the behavioral correlation in OFC ($N = 16$ subjects) is shown superimposed on a coronal section of the group-averaged T1-weighted anatomical scan (threshold, $P < 0.005$ uncorrected). [Reprinted and modified from Fig. 5 in: W. Li, E. Luxenberg, T. Parrish & J.A. Gottfried, Learning to smell the roses: experience-dependent neural plasticity in human piriform and orbitofrontal cortices, Neuron, Vol. 52, Pages 1097–1108, Copyright (2006), with permission from Elsevier[29].]

Together these findings demonstrate that mere odor exposure is sufficient to enhance odor differentiation and elicit perceptual expertise for both odor perceptual quality and odorant functional group. These behavioral effects are paralleled (and preceded) by experience-induced neural plasticity in OFC and piriform cortex. Our data suggest that experience specifically updates sensory-specific representations in olfactory OFC, guiding subsequent improvements in odor perception.

Olfactory Aversive Conditioning

As a model of associative learning, classical (Pavlovian) conditioning has been used to investigate how neutral sensory cues in the environment become endowed with behavioral salience. Non-olfactory studies of aversive conditioning in animals[38-40] and humans[41-44] indicate that this form of learning elicits robust neural changes in sensory-specific brain regions. For example, in an aversive conditioning task that used a tone as the conditioned stimulus, fMRI responses were robustly enhanced in auditory regions of the brain for a conditioned (but not for a non-conditioned) tone, reflecting experience-dependent plasticity in sensory-specific cortex.[43,44] Findings such as these indicate that the pairing of a sensory stimulus (the conditioned stimulus, or CS+) with an emotionally charged event (the unconditioned stimulus, or UCS) is sufficient to modulate neural representations of the original sensory input. In turn these learning-dependent changes in sensory coding may underlie subsequent modifications in sensory perception. In preliminary studies we have devised an aversive conditioning fMRI paradigm between an odor (CS+) and an electric shock (UCS) to test the following questions: What is the effect of emotional learning on human odor perception? Does associative pairing between an odor and shock alter cortical representations of smell? Is the magnitude of experience-dependent neural change predictive of behavioral perceptual enhancement?

To address these questions, Dr. Wen Li and colleagues in my laboratory presented healthy human subjects with four odorants: two pairs of odor enantiomers (mirror-image "chiral" molecules) that were perceptually indistinguishable, based on Laska et al.[45] After a baseline (pre-conditioning) session, subjects underwent aversive conditioning between one of the four odorants and an electric shock. The level of electrical stimulation was titrated individually for each subject, to a point which was uncomfortable but still tolerable. The other three odorants (including the chiral twin of the conditioned odorant, and the other enantiomer pair) were never paired with shock. This conditioning session was followed by a final post-conditioning phase, identical to pre-conditioning, which permitted a direct examination of conditioning-specific neural plasticity by comparing post-conditioning and pre-conditioning sessions. To assess the impact of conditioning on behavioral discrimination, subjects also took part in a triangle test both at the start and at end of the scanning study, in which they were given sets of three bottles (two containing the same odorant, a third containing its chiral opposite) and asked to identify the "odd" bottle.

Our preliminary results[46] suggest that prior to conditioning, subjects were unable to discriminate between the enantiomer pairs, as expected. However, as a result of aversive conditioning, behavioral discrimination was selectively enhanced for the conditioned odorant and its chiral opposite, but discrimination remained at chance for the other pair of enantiomers that had not been involved in the conditioning procedure. In parallel to these behavioral effects, the amplitude of OFC activity evoked by the odor CS+ increased in response to conditioning. Interestingly, OFC response enhancement was also observed for the chiral-related odorant (which itself had never been associated with electric shock), suggesting that associative learning partially generalizes to odorants similar in perceptual quality. Finally, on a subject-by-subject basis, the magnitude of learning-induced OFC activity closely correlated with the level of behavioral odor discrimination. Although further work remains to be done, these initial findings suggest that olfactory aversive learning can enhance sensory discrimination, such that odorants initially smelling the same become perceptually distinct. These perceptual changes are accompanied by conditioning-specific neural plasticity in OFC, with generalization to odorants sharing qualitative attributes. Together our data suggest that OFC plays a critical role in the modulation of odor perception via emotional experience.

DISCUSSION

The data presented here indicate that sensory-specific neural representations of odor quality are not static or fixed in OFC, but are modifiable and can be updated by sensory, emotional, and associative experience. The idea that context, learning, and experience can modulate odor perception receives support from a variety of recent fMRI studies. For example, O'Doherty and colleagues[47] were among the first to show that appetite and motivational state could influence sensory-specific odor representations in human OFC. On alternating fMRI blocks, subjects were presented with banana or vanilla odor, both before and after a lunch of bananas until they became sated for this item. As a result of this manipulation, the neural activity evoked by the banana odor (but not the vanilla odor) was selectively diminished in OFC, indicating that this brain region was sensitive to the current rewarding properties of an olfactory stimulus. Using a different paradigm, Gottfried and Dolan[48] showed that visual semantic context also modulates odor coding in OFC. Neural activation in this area was increased when an odor (e.g., smell of a rose) was presented in combination with a congruent image (e.g., picture of a flower), as opposed to an incongruent image (e.g., picture of a bus). Thus, the same sensory input evoked different responses depending on whether it was experienced in a semantically appropriate context. Similar effects of sensory context on odor processing in OFC have been demonstrated with combinations of odors and tastes[49] and odors and verbal labels.[50] That OFC activity is common to

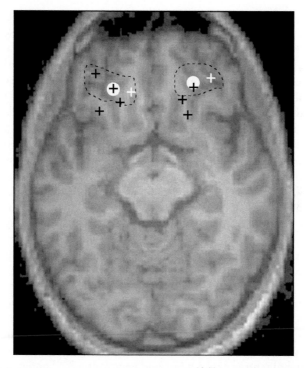

FIGURE 5. Neural representations of odor quality[29,33] in OFC (*white crosses*) overlap the putative human olfactory OFC[11] (*white circles*) and are adjacent to regions that code the reward value of food smells[47] and flavors[51,52] and the predictive reward value of olfactory reinforcers[53] (*black crosses*). Area 111 in human OFC is roughly approximated by the dashed black lines, following Fig. 2 of Ongur and Price.[12] For presentation, activations are presented on a normalized axial T1-weighted image and collapsed across the *z*-axis (superior-inferior) in order to display all activations on a single slice. The right side of the image corresponds to the right side of space. See text for further details.

all of these studies highlights its pivotal role in linking olfactory sensation, perception, and experience.

Interestingly the region of OFC shown here to participate in the modulation of odor quality coding[29] overlaps fairly closely with the human orbitofrontal areas involved in sensory-specific satiation of food odors[47] and flavors[51,52] and in reinforcer devaluation of pleasant food odor,[53] as well as with neural representations of odor quality itself.[33] In the majority of these fMRI studies, the activations fall within human anterior OFC area 111 (with reference to the human cytoarchitectonic map of Ongur *et al.*[12]), clustering near the putative human olfactory OFC.[11] This anatomical correspondence (FIG. 5) raises the intriguing idea that experimental manipulations designed to devalue odor reward might actually elicit qualitative changes in the odor itself. For example, the same odor experienced in a state of hunger may take on a different perceptual quality when later experienced in a state of satiety, over and above changes in reward value. The possibility that satiety induces sensory-specific changes in odor quality has a certain ecological plausibility (if for instance one considers the sensory reaction to a grilled 40-oz dry-aged porterhouse steak before and after its consumption), and also raises general questions about the use of devaluation procedures to assess reward-related processing in the brain.

It is worth considering that experience-dependent fMRI plasticity in OFC (as well as in posterior piriform cortex) might actually reflect inputs from lower-level regions. For example, as a result of tight feedback loops between piriform cortex and olfactory bulb,[54-56] any changes in response plasticity seen in piriform cortex may simply mirror equivalent changes in olfactory bulb. Indeed, centrifugal feedback from learning-modified regions in piriform cortex might be highly instrumental in sculpting sensory response profiles in olfactory bulb, streamlining bottom-up information processing for behaviorally salient odorants. Alternatively, it is possible that the response plasticity in orbitofrontal and piriform cortices is related to a common input from the amygdala, which in rats[54,57] and monkeys[5,58] projects to both of these areas. However, it is not clear whether amygdala projections to piriform cortex arise from the same amygdala nuclei that project to OFC,[54,59] and in any event we have not observed fMRI evidence for experience-dependent updating of odor quality information in the amygdala. Rather, our own prior studies are more compatible with the role of amygdala in the learning of novel associations between emotionally provocative odors and neutral cues[60,61] and in the signaling of motivationally salient odors.[53,62]

Notably, our studies have not identified learning-induced neural plasticity in *anterior* piriform cortex. We speculate that the absence of changes in this region would ensure stimulus constancy of the original sensory input, in keeping with the purported role of anterior piriform in encoding odorant structure.[33] It is plausible that the observed differences in neural plasticity between anterior and posterior piriform cortex[63] accentuate the underlying anatomical connectivity of these regions: anterior piriform is the principal target of olfactory bulb[55] and therefore contains a labeled line for odorant structure, whereas posterior piriform receives the bulk of its inputs from associational fiber systems and would be a better candidate for experience-dependent modulation.[55,63]

The ability of experience to sculpt sensory processing at both the behavioral and neural levels has important implications for contemporary models of olfaction. In particular, the findings described here indicate that the perceptual quality of an odor does *not* necessarily follow from its underlying molecular chemical composition. Ever since the first multigene family of olfactory receptors was identified in rodents,[64] the dominant view of odor perception is that molecular chemical knowledge of an odorant is sufficient to predict its perceptual attributes. Behavioral studies in rodents demonstrate that odorants evoking similar electrophysiological patterns in the olfactory bulb are perceived as being more similar,[65-68] leading to the idea that odor-specific spatial maps in the olfactory bulb may underpin odor perception and that neural representations of odor quality are reflected in ensemble olfactory bulb activity encoding complex configurations of molecular features.[69]

On the other hand, these "bottom-up" models of odor perception conflict with a growing number of studies suggesting that even elementary aspects of olfactory processing are highly contingent on learning and experience. Odor detection thresholds, adaptation rates, and intensity judgments are all strongly modulated by visual, perceptual, and cognitive factors.[70-73] Olfactory discrimination in general is highly plastic and can be modified by contextual cues.[26,27,74-76] It is often noted that the perception of an odor is a synthetic process—the smell of chocolate may contain dozens, if not hundreds, of volatile organic compounds,[77] yet the olfactory system synthesizes this complex mixture seamlessly into one odor. Recent psychophysical studies have demonstrated the integrative nature of odor perception.[28,78,79] In this manner, the smell of a rose is as much defined by a myriad of molecular determinants as by previously stored odor representations and ongoing sensory context.[79]

In all likelihood there are multiple personifications of an odor map or code, with progressive transformations occurring at each level of the olfactory neuraxis. However, the critical issue is to understand the form these maps take that ultimately determines sensory perception and to understand how learning and experience refine these maps in the service of behavior. These questions are not unique to the olfactory system, but apply generally to all of the sensory channels—even for a widely studied sense like vision, it is by no means clear how a behaviorally relevant percept is assembled out of visual maps in the brain. Some of the data presented here suggest that olfactory OFC is a primary target of odor experience, but in comparison to the olfactory bulb and piriform cortex, virtually nothing is known about its finer details. As discussed in the chapter by Shepherd (this volume), a challenge of future work will be to delineate the intrinsic neuronal properties, synaptic organization, and connectivity of olfactory OFC.

Prior fMRI data from our laboratory indicate that neural representations of odor quality and odorant structure (molecular functional group) are encoded in separable olfactory areas of the human brain.[33] Importantly, the identification of odor quality codes across a network of olfactory regions, including posterior piriform cortex, OFC, and hippocampus,[36,37] was independent of any simple molecular configuration.[33] Our recent data on perceptual learning and aversive conditioning extend these findings by implying that neural codes of odor quality rely on experience and learning for their formation, rather than simply existing as a product of structure-based ensembles. We suspect that neural representations of odor quality are a dynamic product of lower-level coding from olfactory bulb and higher-level cortical inputs, under the regulation of learning and experience,[79] attention,[80] sensory context,[48,73] and language.[50,75,81] The results presented here indicate that the OFC (as a distinctively mammalian brain region) is a critical neurobiological interface that flexibly links affect and action, providing advantages for adaptation and survival that exceed the everyday reach of our OFC-impoverished vertebrate (piscine, amphibian, reptilian, avian) kin.

REFERENCES

1. JERISON, H.J. 1997. Evolution of prefrontal cortex. *In* Development of the Prefrontal Cortex: Evolution, Neurobiology, and Behavior. N.A. Krasnegor, G.R. Lyon & P.S. Goldman-Rakic, Eds.: 27–47. Paul H. Brookes Publ. Baltimore, MD.

2. WAGNER, H. 1932. Uber den Farbensinn der Eidechsen. J. Comp. Physiol.[A]: Neuroethology **18:** 378–392.

3. SCHNEIRLA, T.C. 1959. An evolutionary and developmental theory of biphasic processes underlying approach and withdrawal. *In* Nebraska Symposium on Motivation. M.R. Jones, Ed.: 1–43. University of Nebraska Press. Lincoln, NB.

4. KRETTEK, J.E. & J.L. PRICE. 1977. The cortical projections of the mediodorsal nucleus and adjacent thalamic nuclei in the rat. J. Comp. Neurol. **171:** 157–191.

5. CARMICHAEL, S.T., M.C. CLUGNET & J.L. PRICE. 1994. Central olfactory connections in the macaque monkey. J. Comp. Neurol. **346:** 403–434.

6. SCHOENBAUM, G. & H. EICHENBAUM. 1995. Information coding in the rodent prefrontal cortex. I. Single-neuron activity in orbitofrontal cortex compared with that in pyriform cortex. J. Neurophysiol. **74:** 733–750.

7. SCHOENBAUM, G., A.A. CHIBA & M. GALLAGHER. 1999. Neural encoding in orbitofrontal cortex and basolateral amygdala during olfactory discrimination learning. J. Neurosci. **19:** 1876–1884.

8. TANABE, T. *et al.* 1975. An olfactory projection area in orbitofrontal cortex of the monkey. J. Neurophysiol. **38:** 1269–1283.

9. YARITA, H. *et al.* 1980. A transthalamic olfactory pathway to orbitofrontal cortex in the monkey. J. Neurophysiol. **43:** 69–85.

10. MORECRAFT, R.J., C. GEULA & M.M. MESULAM. 1992. Cytoarchitecture and neural afferents of orbitofrontal cortex in the brain of the monkey. J. Comp. Neurol. **323:** 341–358.

11. GOTTFRIED, J.A. & D.H. ZALD. 2005. On the scent of human olfactory orbitofrontal cortex: meta-analysis and comparison to non-human primates. Brain Res. Brain Res. Rev. **50:** 287–304.

12. ONGUR, D., A.T. FERRY & J.L. PRICE. 2003. Architectonic subdivision of the human orbital and medial prefrontal cortex. J. Comp. Neurol. **460:** 425–449.

13. GIBSON, E.J. 1991. An Odyssey in Learning and Perception. MIT Press. Cambridge, MA.

14. GOLDSTONE, R.L. 1998. Perceptual learning. Ann. Rev. Psychol. **49:** 585–612.

15. CRIST, R.E., W. LI & C.D. GILBERT. 2001. Learning to see: experience and attention in primary visual cortex. Nat. Neurosci. **4:** 519–525.

16. YANG, T. & J.H. MAUNSELL. 2004. The effect of perceptual learning on neuronal responses in monkey visual area V4. J. Neurosci. **24:** 1617–1626.

17. CONDON, C.D. & N.M. WEINBERGER. 1991. Habituation produces frequency-specific plasticity of receptive fields in the auditory cortex. Behav. Neurosci. **105:** 416–430.

18. JENKINS, W.M. *et al.* 1990. Functional reorganization of primary somatosensory cortex in adult owl monkeys after behaviorally controlled tactile stimulation. J. Neurophysiol. **63:** 82–104.

19. KOSSUT, M. *et al.* 1988. Single vibrissal cortical column in SI cortex of rat and its alterations in neonatal and adult vibrissa-deafferented animals: a quantitative 2DG study. J. Neurophysiol. **60:** 829–852.

20. DALTON, P., N. DOOLITTLE & P.A. BRESLIN. 2002. Gender-specific induction of enhanced sensitivity to odors. Nat. Neurosci. **5:** 199–200.

21. STEVENS, D.A. & R.J. O'CONNELL. 1995. Enhanced sensitivity to androstenone following regular exposure to pemenone. Chem. Senses **20:** 413–419.

22. MAINLAND, J.D. *et al.* 2002. Olfactory plasticity: one nostril knows what the other learns. Nature **419:**802.

23. WYSOCKI, C.J., K.M. DORRIES & G.K. BEAUCHAMP. 1989. Ability to perceive androstenone can be acquired by ostensibly anosmic people. Proc. Natl. Acad. Sci. U.S.A. **86:** 7976–7978.

24. OWEN, D.H. & P.K. MACHAMER. 1979. Bias-free improvement in wine discrimination. Perception **8:** 199–209.

25. PERON, R.M. & G.L. ALLEN. 1988. Attempts to train novices for beer flavor discrimination: a matter of taste. J. Gen. Psychol. **115:** 403–418.

26. JEHL, C., J.P. ROYET & A. HOLLEY. 1995. Odor discrimination and recognition memory as a function of familiarization. Percept. Psychophys. **57:** 1002–1011.

27. RABIN, M.D. 1988. Experience facilitates olfactory quality discrimination. Percept. Psychophys. **44:** 532–540.

28. STEVENSON, R.J. 2001. The acquisition of odour qualities. Q. J. Exp. Psychol. **54:** 561–577.

29. LI, W. *et al.* 2006. Learning to smell the roses: experience-dependent neural plasticity in human piriform and orbitofrontal cortices. Neuron **52:** 1097–1108.

30. WILSON, D.A. 2000. Comparison of odor receptive field plasticity in the rat olfactory bulb and anterior piriform cortex. J. Neurophysiol. **84:** 3036–3042.

31. WILSON, D.A. 2000. Odor specificity of habituation in the rat anterior piriform cortex. J. Neurophysiol. **83:** 139–145.

32. WILSON, D.A. 2003. Rapid, experience-induced enhancement in odorant discrimination by anterior piriform cortex neurons. J. Neurophysiol. **90:** 65–72.

33. GOTTFRIED, J.A., J.S. WINSTON & R.J. DOLAN. 2006. Dissociable codes of odor quality and odorant structure in human piriform cortex. Neuron **49:** 467–479.

34. KADOHISA, M. & D.A. WILSON. 2006. Separate encoding of identity and similarity of complex familiar odors in piriform cortex. Proc. Natl. Acad. Sci. USA **103:** 15206–15211.

35. DADE, L.A., R.J. ZATORRE & M. JONES-GOTMAN. 2002. Olfactory learning: convergent findings from lesion and brain imaging studies in humans. Brain **125:** 86–101.

36. ROYET, J.P. *et al.* 2001. Functional neuroanatomy of different olfactory judgments. Neuroimage **13:** 506–519.

37. SAVIC, I. *et al.* 2000. Olfactory functions are mediated by parallel and hierarchical processing. Neuron **26:** 735–745.

38. DIAMOND, D.M. & N.M. WEINBERGER. 1986. Classical conditioning rapidly induces specific changes in frequency receptive fields of single neurons in secondary and ventral ectosylvian auditory cortical fields. Brain Res. **372:** 357–360.

39. GONZALEZ-LIMA, F. & H. SCHEICH. 1986. Neural substrates for tone-conditioned bradycardia demonstrated with 2-deoxyglucose. II. Auditory cortex plasticity. Behav. Brain Res. **20:** 281–293.
40. SIUCINSKA, E. & M. KOSSUT. 1996. Short-lasting classical conditioning induces reversible changes of representational maps of vibrissae in mouse SI cortex–a 2DG study. Cereb. Cortex **6:** 506–513.
41. MOLCHAN, S.E., T. SUNDERLAND, A.R. MCINTOSH, *et al.* 1994. A functional anatomical study of associative learning in humans. Proc. Natl. Acad. Sci. USA **91:** 8122–8126.
42. MORRIS, J.S., A. OHMAN & R.J. DOLAN. 1998. Conscious and unconscious emotional learning in the human amygdala. Nature **393:** 467–470.
43. THIEL, C.M., P. BENTLEY & R.J. DOLAN. 2002. Effects of cholinergic enhancement on conditioning-related responses in human auditory cortex. Eur. J. Neurosci. **16:** 2199–2206.
44. THIEL, C.M., K.J. FRISTON & R.J. DOLAN. 2002. Cholinergic modulation of experience-dependent plasticity in human auditory cortex. Neuron **35:** 567–574.
45. LASKA, M., A. LIESEN & P. TEUBNER. 1999. Enantioselectivity of odor perception in squirrel monkeys and humans. Am. J. Physiol. **277:** R1098–R1103.
46. LI, W., J. HOWARD & J.A. GOTTFRIED. 2007. NYAS Conference Abstract: a shock to the senses. *In* From Affect to Action: Linking. G. Schoenbaum, *et al.*, Eds.: New York Academy of Sciences. New York.
47. O'DOHERTY, J. *et al.* 2000. Sensory-specific satiety-related olfactory activation of the human orbitofrontal cortex. Neuroreport **11:** 893–897.
48. GOTTFRIED, J.A. & R.J. DOLAN. 2003. The nose smells what the eye sees: cross-modal visual facilitation of human olfactory perception. Neuron **39:** 375–386.
49. SMALL, D.M. *et al.* 2004. Experience-dependent neural integration of taste and smell in the human brain. J. Neurophysiol. **92:** 1892–1903.
50. DE ARAUJO, I.E. *et al.* 2005. Cognitive modulation of olfactory processing. Neuron **46:** 671–679.
51. SMALL, D.M. *et al.* 2001. Changes in brain activity related to eating chocolate: from pleasure to aversion. Brain **124:** 1720–1733.
52. KRINGELBACH, M.L. *et al.* 2003. Activation of the human orbitofrontal cortex to a liquid food stimulus is correlated with subjective pleasantness. Cereb. Cortex **13:** 1064–1071.
53. GOTTFRIED, J.A., J. O'DOHERTY & R.J. DOLAN. 2003. Encoding predictive reward value in human amygdala and orbitofrontal cortex. Science **301:** 1104–1107.
54. LUSKIN, M.B. & J.L. PRICE. 1983. The topographic organization of associational fibers of the olfactory system in the rat, including centrifugal fibers to the olfactory bulb. J. Comp. Neurol. **216:** 264–291.
55. HABERLY, L.B. 1998. Olfactory cortex. *In* The Synaptic Organization of the Brain. G.M. Shepherd, Ed.: 377–416. Oxford University Press. New York.
56. WILLHITE, D.C. *et al.* 2006. Viral tracing identifies distributed columnar organization in the olfactory bulb. Proc. Natl. Acad. Sci. USA **103:** 12592–12597.
57. HABERLY, L.B. & J.L. PRICE. 1978. Association and commissural fiber systems of the olfactory cortex of the rat. J. Comp. Neurol. **178:** 711–740.

58. CARMICHAEL, S.T. & J.L. PRICE. 1995. Limbic connections of the orbital and medial prefrontal cortex in macaque monkeys. J. Comp. Neurol. **363:** 615–641.

59. KRETTEK, J.E. & J.L. PRICE. 1977. Projections from the amygdaloid complex to the cerebral cortex and thalamus in the rat and cat. J. Comp. Neurol. **172:** 225–254.

60. GOTTFRIED, J.A., J. O'DOHERTY & R.J. DOLAN. 2002. Appetitive and aversive olfactory learning in humans studied using event-related functional magnetic resonance imaging. J. Neurosci. **22:** 10829–10837.

61. GOTTFRIED, J.A. & R.J. DOLAN. 2004. Human orbitofrontal cortex mediates extinction learning while accessing conditioned representations of value. Nat. Neurosci. **7:** 1144–1152.

62. WINSTON, J.S. *et al.* 2005. Integrated neural representations of odor intensity and affective valence in human amygdala. J. Neurosci. **25:** 8903–8907.

63. WILSON, D.A. & R.M. SULLIVAN. 2003. Sensory physiology of central olfactory pathways. *In* Handbook of Olfaction and Gustation. R.L. Doty, Ed.: 181–201. Marcel Dekker. New York.

64. BUCK, L. & R. AXEL. 1991. A novel multigene family may encode odorant receptors: a molecular basis for odor recognition. Cell **65:** 175–187.

65. CLELAND, T.A. *et al.* 2002. Behavioral models of odor similarity. Behav. Neurosci. **116:** 222–231.

66. LINSTER, C. & M.E. HASSELMO. 1999. Behavioral responses to aliphatic aldehydes can be predicted from known electrophysiological responses of mitral cells in the olfactory bulb. Physiol. Behav. **66:** 497–502.

67. LINSTER, C. *et al.* 2002. Spontaneous versus reinforced olfactory discriminations. J. Neurosci. **22:** 6842–6845.

68. LINSTER, C. *et al.* 2001. Perceptual correlates of neural representations evoked by odorant enantiomers. J. Neurosci. **21:** 9837–9843.

69. FIRESTEIN, S. 2001. How the olfactory system makes sense of scents. Nature **413:** 211–218.

70. DALTON, P. 1996. Odor perception and beliefs about risk. Chem. Senses **21:** 447–458.

71. DALTON, P. *et al.* 2000. The merging of the senses: integration of subthreshold taste and smell. Nat. Neurosci. **3:** 431–432.

72. DISTEL, H. *et al.* 1999. Perception of everyday odors–correlation between intensity, familiarity and strength of hedonic judgement. Chem. Senses **24:** 191–199.

73. ZELLNER, D.A. & M.A. KAUTZ. 1990. Color affects perceived odor intensity. J. Exp. Psychol. Hum. Percept. Perform. **16:** 391–397.

74. CAIN, W.S. 1979. To know with the nose: keys to odor identification. Science **203:** 467–470.

75. HERZ, R.S. & J. VON CLEF. 2001. The influence of verbal labeling on the perception of odors: evidence for olfactory illusions? Perception **30:** 381–391.

76. MORROT, G., F. BROCHET & D. DUBOURDIEU. 2001. The color of odors. Brain Lang. **79:** 309–320.

77. COUNET, C. *et al.* 2002. Use of gas chromatography-olfactometry to identify key odorant compounds in dark chocolate. Comparison of samples before and after conching. J. Agric. Food Chem. **50:** 2385–2391.

78. STEVENSON, R.J. 2001. Associative learning and odor quality perception: how sniffing an odor mixture can alter the smell of its parts. Learning Motiv. **32:** 154–177.

79. WILSON, D.A. & R.J. STEVENSON. 2003. The fundamental role of memory in olfactory perception. Trends Neurosci. **26:** 243–247.
80. ZELANO, C. *et al.* 2005. Attentional modulation in human primary olfactory cortex. Nat. Neurosci. **8:** 114–120.
81. SHEPHERD, G.M. 2004. The human sense of smell: are we better than we think? PLoS Biol **2:** E146.

Taste in the Medial Orbitofrontal Cortex of the Macaque

THOMAS C. PRITCHARD,[a] GARY J. SCHWARTZ,[b]
AND THOMAS R. SCOTT[c]

[a]Department of Neural and Behavioral Science, The Pennsylvania State University College of Medicine, Hershey, Pennsylvania 17033, USA

[b]Departments of Medicine & Neuroscience, Albert Einstein College of Medicine, Bronx, New York 10461, USA

[c]Office of Graduate and Research Affairs, San Diego State University, San Diego, California 92182, USA

ABSTRACT: Taste activates about 6% of the neurons in the anterior insula (primary taste cortex) of the macaque. The anterior insula has many direct and indirect projections to the orbitofrontal cortex (OFC), including the caudolateral OFC (clOFC), where only 2% of the neurons respond to taste. We have identified a 12-mm^2 region in the medial OFC (mOFC) where taste represents 7–28% of the population. This rich trove of taste cells has functional characteristics typical of both the insular cortex that projects to it and the clOFC to which it projects. Mean spontaneous rate was 3.1 spikes/s, nearly identical to that in the insula, but double that of the clOFC. In the mOFC, 19% of the taste cells also responded to other modalities, most commonly olfaction and touch, slightly less than the 27% in the clOFC. The distribution of best stimulus neurons was almost even across the four prototypical stimuli in the mOFC, as in insula, but discrepant from the clOFC, where sugar responsiveness dominated. The broadly tuned taste neurons in the mOFC were similar to those in the insula and strikingly different from the more specialized cells of the clOFC. Whereas the responsiveness to the taste of a satiating stimulus declines among the narrowly tuned clOFC cells, satiety has much less impact on the responsiveness of mOFC neurons. The mOFC is a robust area worthy of exploration for its involvement in gustatory coding, the amalgamation of sensory inputs to create flavor, and the hedonics that guide feeding.

KEYWORDS: taste; orbitofrontal cortex; monkey

INTRODUCTION

The lateral and posterior orbitofrontal cortex (OFC) of Old World monkeys is an elaborate network that receives widespread projections from the

Address for correspondence: Thomas C. Pritchard, Ph.D., The Pennsylvania State University College of Medicine, 500 University Drive, Department of Neural and Behavioral Science, H181, Hershey, PA 17033. Voice: 717-531-6410; fax: 717-531-6916.
tcp1@psu.edu

Ann. N.Y. Acad. Sci. 1121: 121–135 (2007). © 2007 New York Academy of Sciences.
doi: 10.1196/annals.1401.007

visual, somatosensory, olfactory, and gustatory cortical areas.[1-3] Electrophysiological, lesion-behavioral, and imaging experiments, as well as clinical case
studies, have shown that this sensory information supports a variety of goal-
directed and reward-related behaviors.[4-7] For example, OFC neurons are active during discrimination between appetitive and aversive stimuli[8] as well
as during execution of goal-directed responses based on fluctuating reward
contingencies.[9,10] The activity of neurons in the OFC is also affected by the
expectation of reward[11] as well as by the relative value of primary (e.g.,
taste)[12,13] and secondary (learned) reinforcers.[14] Rolls et al. described a small
population of gustatory neurons within the caudolateral OFC (clOFC) whose
responses vary inversely with the animal's level of satiety.[15] For example, the
responses evoked by glucose in a food-deprived macaque gradually wane and
finally disappear as the monkey consumes glucose to satiety at which point
the sugar loses its hedonic appeal.

Given the involvement of the OFC in reward mechanisms, the gustatory
system should be well represented there. In fact, gustatory neurons have been
recorded across a broad swath of the OFC, as far laterally as Brodmann area
(BA) 47/12o, which forms the boundary between the OFC and the lateral
convexity, and as far medially as BA 14, which is adjacent to the midline.[15,16]
These studies have focused on a variety of issues, but surprisingly, all report
that gustatory neurons represent only a small percentage (2–8%) of the cells
within the OFC.[17,18]

Based upon anatomical studies by Carmichael and Price, we hypothesized
that OFC taste neurons would be prevalent within BA 13l and 13m.[19] BA 13l
receives direct projections from the gustatory insula (primary taste cortex) as
well as direct and indirect projections from the ventral agranular insula via BA
13m.[3,20] Rather than receiving direct projections from primary taste cortex, BA
13m receives projections from parts of the dysgranular and agranular insula
that receive efferents from the gustatory insula. (Pritchard et al., unpublished
data)[1,3]

This report describes the distribution and response properties of gustatory
neurons located primarily within BA 13m of the medial OFC (mOFC). The
mOFC, unlike other areas of the orbital cortex, contains a significant population of gustatory-responsive neurons. From both anatomical and functional
standpoints, these taste neurons occupy an intermediate position between the
primary taste cortex and the gustatory area in the clOFC.

MATERIALS AND METHODS

Animals

Data were collected from three male cynomolgus monkeys (*Macaca fascicularis*), weighing 5.0–6.4 kg, under 17 h of water and food deprivation. Prior

to surgery, each monkey was trained with juice and fruit reinforcement to sit in a primate chair specifically designed for neurophysiological recording. This research was approved by the Institutional Animal Care and Use Committee of The Pennsylvania State University College of Medicine. The research conformed to the guidelines of the Society for Neuroscience *(Policies on the Use of Animals and Humans in Neuroscience Research (1995))*.

Anesthesia and Surgery

With the monkey under full anesthesia and using sterile technique, a chronic recording chamber was attached to the skull overlying the OFC in a dedicated primate operating room. Pre-surgical radiographs (anterior/posterior [A-P] and medial/lateral [M-L] planes) and an MRI series were used to guide chamber placement. Stainless steel wires fixed 20 mm into the brain were used as fiduciary marks during recording to confirm or correct electrode placement. Two stainless steel tubes (7 mm i.d.) were mounted transversely behind the recording chamber. These tubes were used during recording to secure the monkey's head to the primate chair. See Pritchard *et al.* for a more detailed description of the anesthetic, surgical, and recording techniques.[21]

Electrophysiological Recording

Two weeks following surgery, the monkey was returned to the primate chair and was trained to sit with its head immobilized. The monkey was otherwise free to move its arms and feet during recording and typically adopted a relaxed position. Neurophysiological recording began after the monkey became accustomed to sitting with its head restrained. Heat sterilized Epoxylite-coated microelectrodes (Frederic Haer & Co., Bowdoinham, ME; $Z = 2$–$4M\Omega$ @ 1 kHz) were used to record extracellular action potentials. The microelectrodes were placed in a sterile 21-ga. stainless steel guide tube secured to an x-y stage mounted on top of the recording chamber. The guide tube penetrated the dura and provided lateral support for the microelectrodes during their descent to the OFC. After the microelectrode was advanced manually to within 5mm of the OFC, a Narishige hydraulic microdrive was used to lower the microelectrode to the recording site. A 1-mm grid search pattern was used to map the OFC.

Conventional electrophysiological recording techniques for differential amplification and display, combined with an analog delay device (2 ms) and a window discriminator, were used to identify action potentials with a consistent time course and amplitude. All neural data and voice commentary were digitized and stored on computer (Spike2, Cambridge Electronic Design, Cambridge, UK) for later off-line analysis. The location of the microelectrode within the OFC was determined by taking an x-ray of the head in the A-P and M-L planes when the electrode was at the bottom of each recording track. We confirmed the location of data collection by comparing the locus of the electrode on the x-ray to the bony landmarks of the skull and the three fiduciary wires.

Sensory Stimulation

Gustatory responsiveness was tested with the four prototypical stimuli: 0.3 M sodium chloride (NaCl), 1.0M glucose, 0.01M hydrochloric acid (HCl), and 0.001M quinine hydrochloride (QHCl). These mid-range concentrations were chosen to permit comparison with previously published studies. The stimuli were administered at room temperature as a 0.5-cc bolus from a plastic 1-cc syringe with its tip cut off. Each fluid application was preceded by one or more applications of distilled water (dH_2O) and followed by at least one dH_2O rinse (1 mL). Gustatory testing was done with an interstimulus interval of at least 45 s. Other stimuli included warm (37°C) and cold (17°C) dH_2O and odors (geraniol, benzaldehyde, iso-amylacetate, limonene, and phenethyl alcohol). Tactile stimulation of the tongue, face, lips, gingivae, and teeth was conducted, but probing of the intraoral cavity typically could not be done with precision.

Histological Procedures and Location of Recording Sites

After data collection was complete, wheat germ agglutinin-horseradish per-oxidase (WGA-HRP; 100–200 nL) was injected into the center of the taste-responsive area. The three monkeys were sacrificed and their brains were processed histologically to determine the precise locations of data collection. The BA boundaries within the posterior OFC were determined from neutral red, cresyl violet, and parvalbumin material using the cytoarchitectonic criteria of Carmichael and Price.[19] Each BA was plotted on a photograph of a coronal section of that monkey's brain. A composite map of the OFC was constructed for each monkey by measuring the distance of each cytoarchitectural boundary (through layer IV of the OFC) from a point 5 mm lateral to the midline. By measuring the BA boundaries from a fixed point close to the recording area, we minimized the local distortion that takes place when a gyrencephalic area of the brain is reconstructed as a two-dimensional map.

Data Analyses

Responses to sapid stimuli that differed from the mean response to dH_2O by 1.96 s.d. (95% confidence interval) were considered excitatory (or inhibitory)

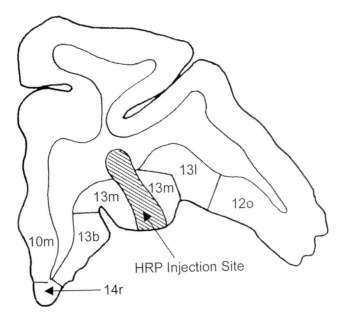

FIGURE 1. Diagram showing a WGA-HRP injection in the taste-responsive region of the mOFC in monkey SAT2.

responses. Comparing taste-evoked to water-evoked responses enabled us to control for possible thermal, visual, somatomotor, and anticipatory activation that might accompany the presentation and consumption of fluids by an alert animal. Responses to dH_2O that exceeded the mean spontaneous rate by 1.96 s.d. were deemed significant. Similarly, responses elicited by the odorants were defined as significant if they exceeded the mean response evoked by a comparable application of clean air by 1.96 s.d.

RESULTS

Location and Extent of the Gustatory Region

Gustatory neurons were collected from a 20-mm^2 area, which was divided into a 12-mm^2 center and a 1-mm wide perimeter. The center of this taste-responsive area was located approximately 8 mm lateral to the midline and approximately 6 mm rostral to the anterior clinoid process of the sphenoid bone (FIG. 1). Taste neurons constituted 19.7% of the cells of the core and 7.8% of the neurons in the perimeter. The high percentage of taste neurons in this part of the OFC enabled us to record multineuron gustatory activity within both the center (11 of 12 coordinates) and the perimeter (3 of 20 coordinates). Although most of the core area was located within BA 13m and the rostral

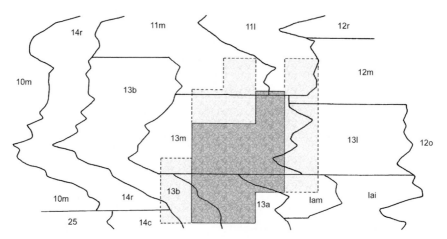

FIGURE 2. An unfolded map of the OFC showing the core (dark shaded) and perimeter (light shaded) taste areas in the mOFC.

half of BA 13a, there was secondary involvement of BA 13b and the medial agranular insula (FIG. 2). The perimeter taste area included adjacent tissue within BAs 13l and 12m laterally, BA 11m rostrally, and BA 13b caudally. The proportion of taste cells declined across the 1-mm perimeter such that further exploration was not warranted (FIG. 3).

Sensory Demographics

There were 242 (12.5%) taste-responsive neurons among the 1943 OFC neurons tested in the three monkeys. As time permitted, many cells were tested with the olfactory stimuli (N = 967 neurons) and with perioral tactile (N = 784 neurons) and thermal (N = 746 neurons) stimulation. Of these 242 taste cells, 196 (81%) responded only to gustatory stimuli. The remaining 46 gustatory neurons also responded to one or more of the other sensory stimuli; 38 of these neurons had bimodal sensitivity. Twenty three (61%) of the bimodal gustatory neurons responded to odors.

Taste was clearly the dominant sensory presence within this part of the OFC. Whereas 10.1% of the responsive neurons were exclusively gustatory, just 2.6% responded exclusively to tactile, 0.9% to thermal, 0.9% to visual, and 0.7% to olfactory stimulation. An additional 0.7% of the sample responded exclusively to dH_2O. Another 1.7% discharged reliably as the syringe approached the monkey's mouth, regardless of whether taste or dH_2O was being delivered. We could not determine the adequate stimulus for these anticipatory responses.

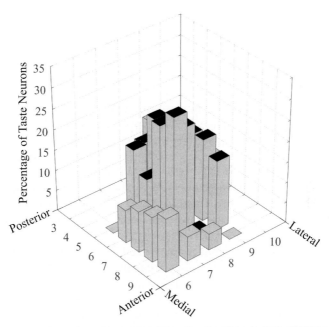

FIGURE 3. A three-dimensional histogram showing the percentage of taste neurons recorded within the mOFC on monkey SAT2. The coordinates (in mm) are relative to the anterior clinoid process of the sphenoid bone. The bars with dark tops were located within the core of the taste-responsive region.

Characteristics of Taste Cells

Spontaneous and Water-Evoked Activity

Neurons for which we had incomplete data ($N = 43$) or that only responded to a tastant in the extended stimulus array ($N = 57$) are not described further in this report. The remaining 142 neurons responded to one of the four basic taste stimuli. These neurons had a mean spontaneous discharge rate of 3.1 ± 5.6 spikes/s (range: 0.0–46.4 spikes/s). The average response evoked by dH_2O was 3.9 ± 6.9 spikes/s (range: 0.0–61.0 spikes/s).

Excitation, Inhibition, and Response Magnitude

Of the 568 stimulus-neuron interactions (4 stimuli $\times$ 142 neurons), 258 (45%) yielded excitatory responses; 10 (2%) were inhibitory, and 300 (53%) failed to satisfy either criterion. Thus, with few exceptions, the responses of taste neurons in the mOFC were excitatory. Even though the mean response to the four prototypical taste stimuli fell in a narrow range

(5.2–5.9 spikes/s), the defining stimulus of each group contributed a majority of the total spikes evoked by all four of the basic taste stimuli (range 51–63%).

Response Breadth

One of the basic characteristics of gustatory neurons is their breadth of sensitivity or breadth of tuning (BOT) across the four basic taste qualities. One measure of response breadth is the percentage of basic taste stimuli to which each neuron responds. In our sample of 142 taste neurons, 62 (44%) responded to only one of the four basic stimuli; 43 (30%) to two, 28 (20%) to three, and 9 (6%) to all four. Because response breadth depends on the criterion established by the investigator, it is sometimes difficult to make comparisons across studies. One way to standardize response breadth is to use the entropy coefficient (H) of each neuron.[22] The entropy coefficient ranges from 0.00, when all of the action potentials are evoked by a single stimulus, to 1.00 when the evoked activity is distributed equally across all four taste stimuli. Because all of our analyses (except spontaneous rate) were based on "net spike activity," an accommodation had to be made for negative numbers, which the entropy formula cannot accept. We used the absolute value of each cell's net response to calculate the entropy coefficients, based upon the assumption that both negative and positive numbers impact the nervous system to the same degree, albeit in opposite directions.[23] For the 142 taste cells tested in this study, the mean BOT was 0.79 ± 0.15 (range $= 0.28$–0.98).

Topographic Distribution of Taste Sensitivity

Even though the search for a topographic organization of taste quality within cortex has met with limited success, we felt obligated to examine this issue in the mOFC, which has not been systematically examined previously. First, we divided the 12-mm^2 core region of one monkey into four quadrants: anteromedial, anterolateral, posteromedial, and posterolateral. A chi-square analysis revealed no significant differences in the proportion of glucose-best, NaCl-best, HCl-best, and QHCl-best neurons among the four quadrants. We calculated the average coordinate within the mOFC for the four best-stimulus classes of cells and, once again, found no evidence of a chemotopic organization. Thus, the mOFC, like the gustatory areas in the medulla, thalamus, and insula, offers no evidence of using a chemotopic organization to code taste quality.[24–26]

Responses to the Basic Taste Stimuli

The mean response to the basic taste stimuli across all 142 cells was 5.9 spikes/s (uncorrected for dH_2O), or 2.0 spikes/s above the response evoked by dH_2O. After correcting for dH_2O, the mean responses for each of the basic taste stimuli were both low and limited in range: in spikes/s, Glucose = 2.0, NaCl = 1.8, HCl = 2.4, and QHCl = 1.7. The narrow range of discharge frequencies within the mOFC is illustrated by the fact that only 24 of the 258 excitatory responses exceeded 10 spikes/s. These 24 responses were distributed almost equally across the four best stimulus classes (Glucose-best = 5; NaCl-best = 6; HCl-best = 8; QHCl-best = 5).

DISCUSSION

Previous studies that have examined the afferent projections of the OFC suggest that the mOFC should contain at least one area with a high percentage of taste neurons.[3] In this electrophysiological investigation of the mOFC, we have found such an area where gustatory neurons were more concentrated than has been reported in either primary taste cortex or the clOFC. Gustatory neurons in the mOFC have response properties typical of both the insula, which projects to this area, and of the clOFC, to which it projects.[20]

Several studies have reported that the posterior OFC contains taste-responsive neurons, but in each instance the percentage was small. Rolls *et al.* sampled 3120 neurons within BA 12o and reported that only 49 (1.6%) responded to taste.[17] More medial explorations near the regions described in this paper revealed 39 taste cells in a sample of 494 neurons (7.9%).[8] In another large electrophysiological survey of the OFC, Rolls *et al.* identified 65 (6.5%) taste-responsive cells in a sample of approximately 1000 neurons.[14] Rolls and Baylis reported that 108 (5.4%) neurons in a sample of about 2000 cells responded to taste.[16] These neurons were recorded from a broad area of the anterior insula and the posterior OFC (BAs 11, 12, 13, and 14), and while the precise number of cells recorded in each area was not disclosed, most were located either in primary taste cortex or further rostrally in BA 12o.

In the 12-mm^2 region of the mOFC that we explored, 19.7% of the cells responded to sapid stimulation of the tongue. In the center of this core region, taste neurons accounted for as many as 28% of the cells tested. This dense concentration of taste-responsive neurons in the mOFC enabled us to record multi-unit responses there, which have never been reported for either primary taste cortex[27] or the clOFC,[17] where the percentage of taste cells is close to 5%. The high percentage of taste-responsive neurons within the mOFC is not due to our having used more concentrated stimuli or a less stringent response criterion than previous investigators. We used the same concentrations of glucose and QHCl that Smith-Swintosky *et al.* used in the insula,[28] and that Rolls *et al.* used in the clOFC.[17] Because NaCl can be an irritant at high concentrations, we used a lower concentration (0.3M versus 1.0M) than used by Rolls *et al.*[17] We elected to use a higher concentration of HCl (0.03M versus 0.01M) than either of the other studies because Old World monkeys are relatively insensitive to HCl.

A higher percentage of taste-responsive neurons would be expected if we used a more liberal criterion for taste responsivity than previous studies. We examined this possibility and found no evidence to support it. The response criterion used by Smith-Swintosky et al. in the insula[28] and Rolls et al. in the clOFC[17] was 2.33 s.d. ($P < 0.01$) above the cell's spontaneous firing rate. In this study, we compensated for possible coincident tactile, thermal, and somatomotor stimulation and non-specific activity caused by our interactions with the monkey during fluid delivery by demanding that taste-elicited activity exceed the dH_2O-evoked response by 1.96 s.d. ($P < 0.05$). We also analyzed the data with the criterion of Smith-Swintosky and Rolls (spontaneous ± 2.33 s.d.) to determine if our criterion had resulted in a spuriously high taste cell count. Using our dH_2O-based criterion and an alpha level of $P < 0.05$, we found that 19.7% of the cells in the core responded to taste; the proportion of taste cells in the core was 19.9% when the criterion was based on the level of spontaneous activity and an alpha level of $P < 0.01$. In the perimeter, the two percentages were 7.8 and 6.7, respectively. Thus, it does not appear that the high percentage of taste cells in the mOFC was caused by use of a more liberal response criterion. The high percentage of taste-responsive neurons in the mOFC reported here may reflect our focus on a relatively circumscribed area, unlike the studies cited above which covered much larger areas of the OFC. Thus, the feature that distinguishes the mOFC from other areas of the OFC is its high concentration of taste-responsive neurons.

Taste Processing in the Human Orbitofrontal Cortex

Numerous positron emission tomography (PET),[29] and functional MRI,[30] studies have identified taste- and food-related areas within the human OFC. In most experiments, these OFC areas were activated by affectively charged stimuli[31,32] or responded to the subject's internal state, such as their level of hunger/satiety[33,34] (although see LaBar et al. and Del Parigi et al.).[34,35] Reports of satiety-modulated taste neurons within the mOFC and the clOFC of macaques provide a neurophysiological basis for the human imaging studies, but they suggest that the OFC hunger/satiety areas are much smaller in the macaque than in humans.[15,36] Using PET, Tataranni et al. have shown that most of the caudal OFC is activated by hunger and that part of the anterior OFC responds to satiation.[37] In macaques, satiety-modulated taste responses have been reported for a limited part of BA 12o and only an 8-mm^2 area in the vicinity of BA 13m.[15,36] In addition, the responses of only a fraction of the neurons in BA 12o (1.6%) and BA 13m ($\sim$10%) of the macaque were modulated by satiety. The more widespread distribution for taste-related behavior in the human imaging literature may reflect activation of neural systems related to reward or reward comparison, rather than taste per se.[5,38]

Response Properties

Spontaneous Rate

The average spontaneous rate of gustatory neurons in the mOFC (3.1 ± 5.6 spikes/s) was nearly identical to the rate reported for taste cells in primary taste cortex (3.2 spikes/s)[27] and nearly twice that of neurons in the clOFC (1.6 spikes/s).[17]

Multimodality

Taste cells in primary taste cortex rarely respond to other sensory modalities.[27] In the clOFC, by comparison, convergence of olfactory, visual, and textural information is relatively common. Rolls and Baylis found that 27% (30/112) of taste cells in the posterior orbital area and the anterior insula also responded significantly to olfactory (13.4%) and visual (13.4%) stimulation.[16] Verhagen *et al.* reported that the textural component of fat activated 31% (13/42) of taste cells in the clOFC.[39] In the present experiment, approximately 2.5% of the taste neurons responded to either olfactory or tactile stimulation. Clearly, taste is the dominant sensory modality in the mOFC, but sideband sensitivity to olfactory, tactile, and visual stimuli may serve as a foundation for perception of flavor, which appears to be more fully expressed in the clOFC.

Breadth of Tuning

Gustatory neurons in the clOFC are more narrowly tuned than those in primary taste cortex. The average BOT coefficient across some 800 neurons in primary taste cortex is 0.70,[27] similar to that reported within the nucleus of the solitary tract (0.87)[24] and the gustatory thalamus (0.73).[26] In the clOFC, however, taste neurons have a mean BOT coefficient of 0.39.[17] Gustatory neurons in the mOFC have a mean BOT coefficient of 0.79, which is close to that reported for the primary taste cortex.[a] The striking difference in the entropy coefficients between the mOFC and the clOFC is reflected in the number of basic taste stimuli that drive neurons in each area. In the mOFC, 44% of the neurons respond to only one of the four basic taste stimuli; the corresponding percentage in the clOFC is 82%. Rolls *et al.* have speculated that specificity of gustatory neurons in the clOFC provides the basis for the mechanism of sensory-specific satiety.[15] Sensory-specific satiety is the decrease in consumption of a particular food that develops over the course of a

---

[a]The entropy coefficient in the mOFC is 0.64 when the calculation is performed with negative values replaced with zeros to accommodate the entropy formula which does not accept negative values.

meal as the subject gradually becomes satiated to that food.[40] At the neuro-physiological level, Rolls and colleagues have reported that the effectiveness of a taste stimulus decreases as monkeys are fed to the point of satiety.[15] This decrease in neural responsiveness is correlated to the loss of hedonic value for that taste, as measured behaviorally.[41] The narrow tuning of gustatory neurons within the clOFC ensures that the hedonic value of other foods remains high, which increases the probability that the animal, still hungry but sated on one food, will switch to a different food.[41]

Evoked Activity Levels

Scott and Plata-Salamán concluded that 73% of the taste neurons in primary taste cortex respond to glucose or NaCl (38% and 35%, respectively), whereas only 27% detect QHCl and HCl (22% and 5%).[27] In the clOFC, glucose was the most effective stimulus for 82% of their sample. In addition, the average glucose response was nearly four times the mean response evoked by the other basic taste stimuli.[17] In the mOFC, neither glucose nor NaCl had such a clear advantage.

Cortical Taste Pathways

Primary taste cortex is located in the rostral, dorsal part of the granular insula that caps the ascending limb of the circular sulcus.[42] Although the details are not known with certainty, the available evidence suggests that neurons in the primary gustatory cortex project to the dysgranular and agranular insulae, which in turn, have widespread projections to the posterior OFC.[1,3,20,43–45] Based on the detailed anatomical reports of Barbas[1] and Carmichael and Price,[3] the two regions of the OFC that are most likely to contain a significant population of gustatory neurons are BAs 13m and 13l. The gustatory area described in this report lies primarily within BA 13m, which we are calling the mOFC taste area. These cells display some of the features of taste neurons in the anterior insula (broad tuning, spontaneous levels of activity) and others more in keeping with neurons of the clOFC (multimodal responses). Some attributes of the mOFC taste neurons do not resemble those of either the primary taste cortex or the clOFC (nearly equal responses to all four basic stimuli, high density of taste cells).

Given the role of the OFC in reward evaluation, it is not surprising that the gustatory system has a representation there. Even though taste neurons may not be the largest functional tenant in the mOFC, and their contributions to taste perception and reward evaluation are currently unknown, it seems appropriate to designate this area as part of higher-order taste cortex. Wearing this mantle does not deny that other nongustatory functions take place in the mOFC, just as they do in the clOFC, where the gustatory system has an even smaller footprint. It is worth noting that taste neurons do not represent a majority within any central nervous system nucleus. Even the anterior insula, which is considered primary taste cortex because it receives direct projections from the gustatory relay in the thalamus, has been implicated in nociception[46] and autonomic function.[47,48]

In summary, the mOFC contains a higher percentage of taste neurons than any other area of the cerebral cortex yet explored. Future studies will be needed to determine the afferent projections of the mOFC and its role in gustatory neural coding, the sensory amalgamation of flavor, the hedonic control of feeding behavior, and reward.

ACKNOWLEDGMENTS

This research was supported by PHS grant DK59549. We would like to thank Erin Nedderman, Erin Edwards, Andrew Petticoffer, Carrie Smith, Thomas Maryniak, Andrew Gavlick, and Kristen Hilgert for their excellent technical assistance.

REFERENCES

1. BARBAS, H. 1993. Organization of cortical afferent input to orbitofrontal areas in the rhesus monkey. Neuroscience **56:** 841–864.
2. BAYLIS, L.L., E.T. ROLLS & G.C. BAYLIS. 1995. Afferent connections of the caudolateral orbitofrontal cortex taste area of the primate. Neuroscience **64:** 801–812.
3. CARMICHAEL, S.T. & J.L. PRICE. 1995. Sensory and premotor connections of the orbital and medial prefrontal cortex of the macaque monkey. J. Comp. Neurol. **363:** 642–664.
4. ROGERS, R.D. *et al.* 1999. Choosing between small, likely rewards and large, unlikely rewards activates inferior and orbital prefrontal cortex. J. Neurosci. **20:** 9029–9038.
5. KRINGELBACH, M.L. & E.T. ROLLS. 2004. The functional neuroanatomy of the human orbitofrontal cortex: evidence from neuroimaging and neuropsychology. Prog. Neurobiol. **72:** 341–372.
6. KRINGELBACH, M.L. 2005. The human orbitofrontal cortex: linking reward to hedonic experience. Nature Rev. Neurosci. **6:** 691–702.
7. SCHULTZ, W. 2006. Behavioral theories and the neurophysiology of reward. Ann. Rev. Psychol. **57:** 87–115.
8. THORPE, S.J., E.T. ROLLS & S. MADDISON. 1983. The orbitofrontal cortex: neuronal activity in the behaving monkey. Exp. Brain Res. **49:** 93–115.
9. TREMBLAY, L. & W. SCHULTZ. 1999. Relative reward preference in primate orbitofrontal cortex. Nature **398:** 704–708.
10. TREMBLAY, L. & W. SCHULTZ. 2000. Modification of reward expectation-related neuronal activity during learning in primate orbitofrontal cortex. J. Neurophysiol. **83:** 1877–1885.

11. SCHOENBAUM, G., A.A. CHIBA & M. GALLAGHER. 1998. Orbitofrontal cortex and basolateral amygdala encode expected outcomes during learning. Nature Neurosci. **1:** 155–159.

12. WALLIS, J.D. & E.K. MILLER. 2003. Neuronal activity in primate dorsolateral and orbital prefrontal cortex during performance of a reward preference task. Eur. J. Neurosci. **18:** 2069–2081.

13. ROESCH, M.R. & C.R. OLSON. 2004. Neuronal activity related to reward value and motivation in primate frontal cortex. Science **304:** 307–310.

14. ROLLS, E.T. *et al.* 1996. Orbitofrontal cortex neurons: role in olfactory and visual association learning. J. Neurophysiol. **75:** 1970–1981.

15. ROLLS, E.T., Z.J. SIENKIEWICZ & S. YAXLEY. 1989. Hunger modulates the responses to gustatory stimuli of single neurons in the caudolateral orbitofrontal cortex of the macaque monkey. Eur. J. Neurosci. **1:** 53–60.

16. ROLLS, E.T. & L.L. BAYLIS. 1994. Gustatory, olfactory, and visual convergence within the primate orbitofrontal cortex. J. Neurosci. **14:** 5437–5452.

17. ROLLS, E.T., S. YAXLEY & Z.J. SIENKIEWICZ. 1990. Gustatory responses of single neurons in the caudolateral orbitofrontal cortex of the macaque monkey. J. Neurophysiol. **64:** 1055–1066.

18. ROLLS, E.T. *et al.* 1999. Responses to the sensory properties of fat of neurons in the primate orbitofrontal cortex. J. Neurosci. **19:** 1532–1540.

19. CARMICHAEL, S.T. & J.L. PRICE. 1994. Architectonic subdivision of the orbital and medial prefrontal cortex in the macaque monkey. J. Comp. Neurol. **346:** 366–402.

20. CARMICHAEL, S.T. & J.L. PRICE. 1996. Connectional networks within the orbital and medial prefrontal cortex of macaque monkeys. J. Comp. Neurol. **371:** 179–207.

21. PRITCHARD, T.C. *et al.* 2005. Gustatory neural responses in the medial orbitofrontal cortex of the Old World monkey. J. Neurosci. **25:** 6047–6056.

22. SMITH, D.V. & J.B. TRAVERS. 1979. A metric for the breadth of tuning of gustatory neurons. Chem. Senses **4:** 215–229.

23. MIYAOKA, Y. & T.C. PRITCHARD. 1996. Responses of primate cortical neurons to unitary and binary taste stimuli. J. Neurophysiol. **75:** 396–411.

24. SCOTT, T.R. *et al.* 1986. Gustatory responses in the nucleus tractus solitarius of the alert cynomolgus money. J. Neurophysiol. **55:** 182–200.

25. SCOTT, T.R. *et al.* 1986. Gustatory responses in the frontal opercular cortex of the alert cynomolgus monkey. J. Neurophysiol. **56:** 876–890.

26. PRITCHARD, T.C., R.B. HAMILTON & R. NORGREN. 1989. Neural coding of gustatory information in the thalamus of *Macaca mulatta.* J. Neurophysiol. **61:** 1–14.

27. SCOTT, T.R. & C.R. PLATA-SALAMÁN. 1999. Taste in the monkey cortex. Physiol. Behav. **67:** 489–511.

28. SMITH-SWINTOSKY, V.L., C.R. PLATA-SALAMÁN & T.R. SCOTT. 1991. Gustatory neural coding in the monkey cortex: stimulus quality. J. Neurophysiol. **66:** 1156–1165.

29. ZALD, D.H. *et al.* 1998. Aversive gustatory stimulation activates limbic circuits in humans. Brain **121:** 1143–1154.

30. FRANK, G.K. *et al.* 2003. The evaluation of brain activity in response to taste stimuli—a pilot study and method for central taste activation as assessed by event-related fMRI. J. Neurosci. Methods **131:** 99–105.

31. DE ARAUJO, I.E.T. *et al.* 2003. Human cortical responses to water in the mouth, and the effects of thirst. J. Neurophysiol. **90:** 1865–1876.

32. SMALL, D.M. *et al.* 2003. Dissociation of neural representation of intensity and affective valuation in human gustation. Neuron **39:** 701–711.
33. GAUTIER, J.-F. *et al.* 2000. Differential brain responses to satiation in obese and lean men. Diabetes **49:** 838–846.
34. DEL PARIGI, A. *et al.* 2002. Neuroimaging and obesity: mapping the brain responses to hunger and satiation in humans using positron emission tomography. Ann. N. Y. Acad. Sci. **967:** 389–397.
35. LABAR, K.S. *et al.* 2001. Hunger selectively modulates corticolimbic activation to food stimuli in humans. Behav. Neurosci. **115:** 493–500.
36. PRITCHARD, T.C. *et al.* 2007. Satiety-responsive neurons in the medial orbitofrontal cortex of the macaque. Behav. Neurosci. In press.
37. TATARANNI, P.A. *et al.* 1999. Neuroanatomical correlates of hunger and satiation in humans using positron emission tomography. Proc. Natl. Acad. Sci. USA **96:** 4569–4574.
38. O'DOHERTY, J.P. *et al.* 2002. Neural responses during anticipation of a primary taste reward. Neuron **33:** 815–826.
39. VERHAGEN, J.V., E.T. ROLLS & M. KADOHISA. 2003. Neurons in primate orbitofrontal cortex respond to fat texture independently of viscosity. J Neurophysiol. **90:** 1514–1525.
40. ROLLS, E.T., B.J. ROLLS & E.A. ROWE. 1983. Sensory-specific and motivation-specific satiety for the sight and taste of food and water in man. Physiol. Behav. **30:** 185–192.
41. ROLLS, B.J. *et al.* 1981. Sensory specific satiety in man. Physiol. Behav. **27:** 137–142.
42. PRITCHARD, T.C. *et al.* 1986. Projections of thalamic gustatory and lingual areas in the monkey, *Macaca fascicularis*. J. Comp. Neurol. **244:** 213–228.
43. MUFSON, E.J. & M-M. MESULAM. 1982. Insula of the Old World monkey. II: afferent cortical input and comments on the claustrum. J. Comp. Neurol. **212:** 23–37.
44. MESULAM, M.-M. & E.J. MUFSON. 1985. The insula of Reil in man and monkey. *In* Cerebral Cortex, Vol. 4. A. Peters & E.G. Jones, Eds.: 179–226. Plenum Press. New York, NY.
45. PRITCHARD, T.C. & R. NORGREN. 2004. Gustatory system. *In* The Human Nervous System. G. Paxinos & J. Mai, Eds.: 1171–1196. Academic Press. New York, NY.
46. BENARROCH, E.E. 2001. Pain-autonomic interactions: a selective review. Clin. Auton. Res. **11:** 343–349.
47. LADABAUM, U., T.P. ROBERTS & D.J. MCGONIGLE. 2007. Gastric fundic distension activates fronto-limbic structures but not primary somatosensory cortex: a functional magnetic resonance imaging study. Neuroimage **34:** 724–732.
48. DERBYSHIRE, S.W. 2003. A systematic review of neuroimaging data during visceral stimulation. Am. J. Gastroenterol. **98:** 12–20.

The Role of the Human Orbitofrontal Cortex in Taste and Flavor Processing

DANA M. SMALL,[a–d] GENEVIEVE BENDER,[a,c]
MARIA G. VELDHUIZEN,[a,b] KRISTIN RUDENGA,[a,c]
DANIELLE NACHTIGAL,[a] AND JENNIFER FELSTED[a]

[a]The John B Pierce Laboratory, New Haven, Connecticut 06519, USA

[b]Department of Psychiatry, Yale University School of Medicine, New Haven, Connecticut 06519, USA

[c]Interdepartmental Neuroscience Program, Yale University School of Medicine, New Haven, Connecticut 06519, USA

[d]Department of Psychology, Yale University, New Haven, Connecticut 06519, USA

ABSTRACT: The human orbitofrontal cortex (OFC) plays an important role in representing taste, flavor, and food reward. The primary role of the OFC in taste is thought to be the encoding of affective value and the computation of perceived pleasantness. The OFC also encodes retronasal olfaction and oral somatosensation. During eating, distinct sensory inputs fuse into a unitary flavor percept, and there is evidence that this percept is encoded in the orbital cortex. Studies examining the effect of internal state on neural representation of food and drink further suggest that processing in the OFC is critical for representing the reward value of foods. Thus, it is likely that, in addition to serving as higher-order gustatory cortex, the OFC integrates multiple sensory inputs and computes reward value to guide feeding behavior.

KEYWORDS: gustation; flavor; multisensory integration; feeding; food reward; motivation; obesity; addiction; human; neuroimaging; functional magnetic resonance imaging (fMRI); positron emission tomography (PET)

INTRODUCTION

Taste refers to the qualities of sweet, sour, salty, bitter, and savory. What we colloquially refer to as taste is actually flavor, the combined sensation of taste, retronasal olfaction, and oral somatosensation. However, because all of these sensations are co-localized to the mouth via the olfactory localization illusion, we perceive a unitary flavor percept arising from the mouth and refer to the

Address for correspondence: Dana M. Small, The John B Pierce Laboratory, 290 Congress Avenue, New Haven, CT 06519. Voice: 203-401-6242; fax: 203-624-4950.
dsmall@jbpierce.org

Ann. N.Y. Acad. Sci. 1121: 136–151 (2007). © 2007 New York Academy of Sciences.
doi: 10.1196/annals.1401.002

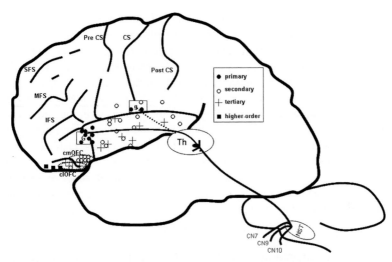

FIGURE 1. Human Gustatory Pathway. A line drawing depicting the presumed human gustatory pathway. NST, nucleus of the solitary; Th, Thalamus; Post CS, postcentral sulcus; CS, central sulcus; Pre CS, precentral sulcus; SFS, superior frontal sulcus; MFS, middle frontal sulcus; IFS, inferior frontal sulcus; cmOFC, caudomedial orbitofrontal cortex; clOFC, caudolateral orbitofrontal cortex.

sensation as taste.[1–3] The human orbitofrontal cortex (OFC) plays a role in encoding taste and flavor. It is also critically involved in encoding food reward. Thus, the OFC receives multiple sensory and affective signals about food and likely plays an important role in integrating these signals in the service of feeding behavior.

THE GUSTATORY PATHWAY AND THE LOCATION OF CORTICAL GUSTATORY AREAS

The gustatory pathway is presumed to be similar in human and nonhuman primates. Gustatory information travels through cranial nerves VII, IX, and X to the nucleus of the solitary tract[4] (FIG. 1). Second-order gustatory fibers leave the nucleus of the solitary tract to join the central tegmental tract and project to the parvocellular division of the ventral posterior medial nucleus (VPM) of the thalamus.[4] Neuroanatomical tract-tracing studies have identified two projections from the gustatory thalamus VPM to the cortex.[5,6] The primary projection terminates in ipsilateral anterior insula/frontal operculum (AIFO) adjacent to the superior limiting sulcus and extends rostrally to the caudal OFC. A secondary ipsilateral projection terminates at areas 3a, 3b, and 1 along the lateral margin of the precentral gyrus at the base of the central sulcus (Pritchard *et al.*[6]), although the extent to which this projection represents taste versus oral somatosensation has been questioned (personal communication with Tom Pritchard, March 2007). However, consistent with dual projection, electrical stimulation of the primate gustatory nerves gives rise to evoked potentials within these two regions.[7] In FIGURE 1 we have represented the dominant projection by a solid line terminating in area "G" and the secondary projection from a dotted line terminating in area "g." The location of the presumed primary representation is depicted by solid black circles. The insula and operculum also contain higher-order gustatory regions adjacent to the primary termination zone(s).[8] Findings from human neuroimaging studies of taste in humans clearly demonstrate that there are multiple taste-responsive regions in the insula and overlying opercula.[9–23] In FIGURE 1 this representation is indicated by empty circles and plusses. Empty circles signify proposed secondary representations, and plusses signify proposed tertiary representation, but this is speculative as it is currently not known what order relay these responses reflect. Interestingly, it is not the case that all neuroimaging studies report activity in all regions. Rather there is considerable variability in the location of taste-elicited activity. Although there are a number of potential reasons that could explain the variability, one likely explanation is that functional specialization exists and the use of different tasks and stimuli results in differential recruitment of specialized regions or networks. Consistent with this possibility, we have reported that different regions of the insula/operculum respond to taste compared to tasteless solutions, depending upon the nature of the task performed.[24] However, despite this functional specialization, AIFO responds to the comparison of taste-tasteless, irrespective of the nature of the task performed. Together, findings suggests that as is the case in olfaction,[25] gustatory functions are mediated by parallel and hierarchical processing.

Three orbital gustatory regions have been identified in nonhuman primates.[26–29] The best characterized region is dysgranular caudolateral OFC (clOFC) (see Ref. 30 for review). This region has been referred to as the secondary gustatory area in the past; however, we refer to it by anatomical reference since there are clearly multiple "secondary" areas. More recently, a caudomedial region (cmOFC) has been identified in which there is the highest density of gustatory neurons in any cortical region.[26] Based on the anatomy and the characteristics of the evoked taste responses in this region, it is suggested to be a relay between AI and clOFC. In FIGURE 1 these regions are labeled and represented by empty circles and plusses depending on whether they are thought to represent secondary (empty circles) or tertiary (plusses) zones. Gustatory neurons have also been identified in a more anterior and medial region of OFC, corresponding to the rostral-most section of area 13.[29] FIGURE 2 displays a cartoon of human OFC based upon anatomical work by Chiavaras and Petrides.[31] The three orbitofrontal gustatory regions identified in monkeys are presented as red dots located in what is presumed to be the anatomically homologous region of human cortex.

The human OFC is frequently activated in response to gustatory stimulation.[32–39] However, the area of activation is often anterior and medial to the

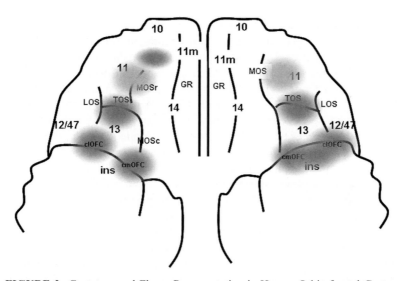

FIGURE 2. Gustatory and Flavor Representation in Human Orbitofrontal Cortex. A line drawing based upon anatomical work of Chiavaras and Petrides.[31] Red blobs represent gustatory regions identified in nonhuman primates projected onto human cortex. Turquoise blobs represent approximate location of the region(s) of anterior OFC that human imaging studies have identified as taste-responsive. Grey blobs represent regions where supra-additive responses to taste and smell stimuli have been observed.

orbital taste regions described in monkeys.[16] Small and colleagues[16] used the anatomical descriptions of the clOFC taste area in the monkey provided by Rolls and colleagues[27] to identify the anatomically homologous region in the human brain. Activation foci generated in response to taste stimulation from all published (and some unpublished) positron emission tomography (PET) studies of human gustation were plotted onto a high-resolution MRI image. Eighteen peaks localized to the OFC. However, of these 18 peaks, only two were located in the region anatomically homologous to the monkey orbital taste area (corresponding to clOFC in FIG. 2), while the remaining peaks were dispersed throughout areas 11, 13, and 14, according to the terminology employed by Petrides and Pandya.[40] This raises the possibility of inter-species differences in the precise location of the orbital gustatory area. Alternatively, it could reflect different methodologies or the anterior activations may represent higher-order processing of taste-related information. In FIG. 2, we have used turquoise blobs to depict the approximate location of the anterior orbital taste response frequently observed in human imaging studies.

CONTRIBUTIONS OF THE OFC TO GUSTATORY PROCESSING

The primary contribution of the OFC to gustatory processing is thought to be the encoding of affective value. In the human brain, stimulus-specific responses to pure tastes have been consistently observed in the OFC.[34,38,41] For example, aversive bitter taste consistently activates a region of left anterior orbital cortex (turquoise blob in FIG. 2), likely corresponding to area 11 (using the terminology of Chiavaras and Petrides),[31] whereas sweet tastes tend to activate right clOFC, as well as the two anterior right hemisphere gustatory zones.[38,41] (See Ref. 42 for a more in depth discussion.) These stimulus-specific responses have been interpreted as reflecting the affective value of the taste stimulus. However, a unique feature of the gustatory sense is that there is a relatively stable, though not immutable,[43-47] relationship between quality, physiological significance, and affective value. There are five major categories of taste quality: sweet, sour, salty, bitter, and savory. Each taste category is tuned to identify a specific nutrient or physiological threat; namely, ensuring energy reserves (sweet), maintaining electrolyte balance (salty), guarding pH (sour, bitter), motivating protein intake (savory), and avoiding toxins (bitter).[48,49] Thus the stimulus-specific responses may reflect valence, physiological significance, quality, or the integration of these factors. Consequently, although the specific responses to sweet versus bitter are generally interpreted as affective in nature, it is important to note that it is not possible to rule out contributions related encoding of quality and/or physiological significance. Additionally, as with all studies of higher-order processing at the neocortical level, there is the possibility that responses reflect mechanisms at lower levels than local processing. Determining if these dimensions are encoded separately and if so, identifying the separate networks that encode the dimensions is the subject of ongoing work in our lab.

Hedonic value may also be influenced by intensity, and the nature of this interaction depends upon quality. For example, pure bitter is perceived as unpleasant at all concentrations, whereas sweet is generally perceived to be increasingly pleasant as its concentration increases, though at very high concentrations its pleasantness plateaus or declines. In an attempt to dissociate neural response to intensity and valence, we asked subjects to rate the perceived pleasantness and intensity of sweet and bitter solutions.[41] We then selected subjects for whom we could identify four stimuli (two sweet and two bitter) for which subjects gave ratings in the target range, such that the weak tastes were equally weak, the strong tastes equally strong, the sweet tastes equally pleasant and the bitter tastes equally unpleasant. Functional magnetic resonance imaging (fMRI) was then used to probe for responses specific to weak and strong sweet compared to base line (a tasteless artificial saliva solution) or weak and strong bitter compared to base line. Sweet-specific intensity-independent responses were observed bilaterally in the clOFC (area 13L) and in a more rostral region (likely area 11) of right OFC (turquoise blob in right hemisphere in FIG. 2). Bitter-specific intensity-independent responses were isolated in left clOFC and left area 11 (turquoise blob in left hemisphere in FIG. 2). These findings demonstrate that stimulus-specific responses can be independent of intensity and that the encoding of intensity is at least partially dissociated from encoding valence/quality. In turn, this suggests that the influence of intensity upon perceived pleasantness might result from orbital integration of inputs from regions that encode intensity, or perhaps the combination of intensity and valence, such as the insula and amygdala.[41,50,51]

It is also noteworthy that the segregation of responses to sweet compared to bitter stimuli accord with earlier imaging work[34,38] and with more recent data from transgenic mice showing segregated encoding of sweet and bitter taste throughout the entire neuroaxis.[52] We therefore coded taste peaks according to whether they represented pleasant or unpleasant taste and plotted all the orbital peaks onto a single axial section of OFC. A consistent pattern emerged in that there was preferential response in the right clOFC to sweet pleasant taste.[42] These data examining differences between sweet and bitter encoding coalesce with many other studies showing profound effects of physiological significance upon the gustatory neural code[53–57] and suggest that physiological significance is the primary organizing principle in neural encoding of taste.

In addition to stimulus-specific responses, which may reflect quality, valence, physiological significance, or some combination of these factors, recent unpublished data from our laboratory suggest that the far lateral caudal OFC (area 47/12) plays a role in evaluation of taste pleasantness (FIG. 3; not depicted in FIG. 1 or 2). In this study subjects received weak taste (sweet, sour, or salty) or tasteless/odorless solutions under four different conditions: 1) detect, in which subjects indicated whether or not a taste was present; 2) randomly press, in which they made a random response (button press); 3) quality judgment, in which they pressed a different button for sweet, salty, sour, or tasteless; and 4) pleasantness judgment, in which they used the buttons to indicate how pleasant or unpleasant they found the solution. The data were analyzed using an analysis of variance with stimulus (taste versus tasteless) and task (detect, random, quality, pleasantness) as within-subject variables. A main effect of task was observed in the caudal far lateral OFC (FIG. 3). This region responded preferentially when subjects evaluated stimulus pleasantness regardless of the nature of the stimulus (i.e., taste versus tasteless). This result is consistent with a role for this region in evaluation of pleasantness of multiple types of sensory information.[58] We therefore questioned whether this lateral area might be preferentially connected to earlier gustatory relays when subjects perceive taste compared to tasteless solutions. A psychophysiological interaction analysis indicated that indeed this was the case; connectivity between the far clOFC and the earlier relays (cmOFC and AI) was greater when a taste was present (FIG. 3). These findings suggest that area 47/12 is important for evaluating perceived pleasantness of stimuli in the mouth and that processing in this region helps to organize retrieval of sensory information from earlier taste relays in the service of computing the perceived pleasantness of taste.

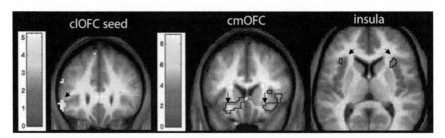

FIGURE 3. Orbitofrontal response during evaluation of stimulus pleasantness. Three images showing the results from an experiment in which subjects were presented with taste and tasteless solutions and asked to perform one of four different tasks: 1) detect, in which subjects indicated whether or not a taste was present; 2) randomly press, in which they made a random response (button press); 3) quality judgment, in which they pressed a different button for sweet, salty, sour, or tasteless; and 4) pleasantness judgment, in which they used the buttons to indicate how pleasant or unpleasant they found the solution. The image on the left shows activation in clOFC indicated by the arrow (-54, 30, -6; z = 3.8; cluster size = 144; $P = 0.001$ whole brain corrected) that was preferentially activated during the pleasantness task irrespective of whether the subject received a taste or tasteless stimulus. To determine if this region was differentially connected with other brain regions depending on the type of stimulus, a psychophysiological interaction (PPI) was performed using the clOFC peak as a seed region. PPI results are shown in the middle and right image and revealed that clOFC was preferentially connected to cmOFC indicated by arrows (33, 18, -9; z = 4.97; $P = 0.001$ and -24, 18, -12; z = 3.70; $P = 0.01$) and insula indicated by arrows (-36, 24, 9; z = 3.26; $P = 0.001$ uncorrected and 45, 18, 3; z = 3.64; $P = 0.0001$ uncorrected) when subjects received taste compared to tasteless solutions. Results were analyzed in SPM 2 using procedures previously described. All t-map thresholds were set to $P < 0.001$ with a minimum cluster threshold of k < 3. The grey-scale bars indicate t-values from group random effects analyses. Activations in the cmOFC and insula have been outlined in black to facilitate identification.

FLAVOR

The sensation of taste always occurs in conjunction with oral somatosensory stimulation and almost always with retronasal olfaction (which occurs when volatiles in foods reach the olfactory epithelium by traversing the nasophyarnx). There are multiple views of how flavor is encoded.[3,59–61] We propose that flavor is an experience-dependent perceptual modality formed over time by experiencing taste, retronasal olfaction, and oral somatosensation as a fused unitary percept (D.M. Small manuscript submitted for publication). It is proposed that this fusion is achieved via the oral capture illusion, which causes all three senses to be localized to a common location; namely, the place where a food contacts the mouth.[62,63] The resulting percept is not analytic, in that perceptions do appear to be blended,[64] nor is it synthetic, in that the parts are still identifiable.[65,66] Rather, the inputs are fused into a unitary flavor percept in which the parts are identifiable but the boundaries between them are ill-defined.[67] Thus one refers to flavors as singular perceptions. For example, we say something tastes wonderful rather than exclaiming that it tastes, smells, and feels wonderful.

The mechanism by which the oral capture illusion is achieved is currently unknown. However we have shown that the oral somato-motor cortex is preferentially engaged during perception of retronasally compared to orthonasally perceived odors and have suggested that this activation reflects the fact that retronasal but not orthonasal odors are localized to the mouth.[68] It is therefore suggested that this region plays a key role in flavor fusion. Once flavor fusion is achieved the unitary percept must then be encoded. Although the OFC may or may not play a primary role in flavor fusion *per se*, it is clear that taste, oral somatosensation, and retronasal olfaction are represented in the OFC and there is good evidence that the OFC encodes flavor percepts.[26,27,36,69-72]

Rolls and Baylis sampled 2000 orbital neurons for their responsiveness to taste, smell, flavor, and visual stimuli.[73] One hundred and fifty-eight neurons responded to stimulation. Forty-five of these responded in more than one modality. Although unimodal cells were concentrated in different areas, considerable overlap occurred, and bimodal and trimodal cells were interspersed throughout. Notably, all multimodal cells were driven by corresponding stimulation across modalities. For example, a cell that responded to sweet taste would respond to fruity but not fishy odors and the sight of a banana but not the sight of pliers. Rolls and colleagues therefore suggested that these neurons represented flavors.

In the human, several neuroimaging studies have been performed where unimodal stimulation with a taste or an odor were compared to bimodal (simultaneous) presentation of the same tastes and odors.[36,70,72] The results converge to highlight a role for two regions of human OFC experience-dependent taste-odor integration. These regions are depicted as grey blobs in FIGURE 2. Small and colleagues showed that a region of anteroventral insula/caudal OFC responded preferentially to a congruent taste-odor mixture (sweet vanilla) compared to the summed response of the components (sweet taste, vanilla retronasal olfaction) and compared to an incongruent mixture (salty vanilla) (FIG. 5 in Small *et al.*[72]). This result was interpreted as reflecting an experience-dependent supra-additive response.[72] In another study, de Araujo and colleagues reported that caudal OFC responded to sweet taste, strawberry odor, and a sweet strawberry mixture, providing additional evidence for the role of this region in representing flavor. They further identified a region of anteromedial OFC (probably corresponding to area 11) in which the response to the mixture correlated positively with subjective consonance ratings.[70] Taken together these findings suggest that learned flavor percepts are encoded in the OFC.

If flavor is an experience-dependent modality formed from the perception of taste, oral somatosensation, and retronasal olfaction as a fused flavor percept, then odors that are experienced retronasally should come to have a separate neural representation from odors that are not experienced as flavors. In essence, such an organization would reflect the existence of category-specific processing akin to the fusiform face area or the parahippocampal place area described in vision.[74–76] To investigate this possibility we collaborated with Dr. Thomas Hummel's laboratory and used fMRI to examine brain response to odors delivered orthonasally and retronasally. The test odors were administered as vapors via tubes inserted under endoscopic guidance so that one tube ended at the external nares (orthonasal olfaction) and the other at the nasopharynx (retronasal olfaction).[68] Four odors were delivered using this technique, one food odor (chocolate) and three nonfood odors (butanol, farnesol, and lavender). Comparison of all odors minus odorless revealed bilateral activity in piriform cortex and medial OFC (i.e., classical olfactory sensory regions). Food-odor specific activations were observed in the insula and the OFC. The mid-dorsal insula responded preferentially to the chocolate odor irrespective of route of administration.[77] This region responds to taste stimulation.[16] Therefore its recruitment may reflect re-activation of the gustatory component of the original neural signature of the unitary flavor percept by the experience of the olfactory component (i.e., food odor) of the flavor percept. In OFC an interaction between odorant type and route of administration was observed. The caudal-most region of OFC (corresponding to the right caudal grey blob in FIG. 2), as well as the amygdala, responded preferentially to orthonasally delivered chocolate odor, whereas an anteromedial region (gyrus rectus and anterior cingulate at the genu of the corpus callosum) responded preferentially to retronasally delivered chocolate odor (not indicated in FIG. 2). This interaction was interpreted as reflecting response specificity to different aspects of food reward since orthonasal perception of food odor is associated with the anticipatory phase of food reward, whereas retronasal perception of food odor is associated with the consummatory phase of food reward. This speculation was based on prior work suggesting that separate regions of the human brain encode the devaluation of anticipation compared to the devaluation of food consumption. For example, amygdala responds to visual cues that predict food aromas, and response in this region decreases selectively to cues predicting the aroma representing a meal eaten to satiety.[78] In contrast, amygdala response during consumption of chocolate does not change as a function of satiety, even though ratings of perceived chocolate pleasantness significantly decrease.[79] Rather, response in medial OFC appears to track changes in comsummatory food reward.[79] Regardless of whether the differential response to orthonasally compared to retronasally sensed chocolate odor observed in the OFC reflects separable networks for anticipatory versus consummatory food reward, the findings support our hypothesis that there is category-specific processing in olfaction by indicating that OFC represents food odors separately from nonfood odors. One caveat is that it is theoretically possible that these responses may be specific to chocolate rather than food in general. A follow-up study has recently been completed to address this possibility.

THE PLEASURE OF FOOD

The perceived pleasure experienced when eating and drinking can be influenced by 1) sensory features, such as taste quality; 2) experience, such as prior exposure to taste-odor mixtures; 3) internal state; and 4) cognitive context, such as information about brand. A remarkable feature of the OFC is that all determinants of perceived pleasure are represented.[69,70,72,79–83]

We have already outlined data supporting a role for the OFC in encoding the affective value and perceived pleasantness of taste. We have also discussed the role of the OFC in experience-dependent encoding of flavor. In both studies of taste-odor integration, congruency was correlated with perceived pleasantness.[70,72] Thus preferential orbital response to congruent stimuli may well reflect perceived pleasantness, which is a function of prior experience with taste-odor mixtures.

The OFC is also critical for encoding alliesthesia, a term coined by Cabanac to refer to the decrease in perceived pleasure of a food as it is eaten to satiety.[84] For example, we used PET to examine neural response to eating chocolate as subjects ate chocolate to beyond satiety.[79] Activity in the medial OFC, extending from area 25 to the medial aspect of the ventral surface (areas 13 and 14), correlated with ratings of the perceived pleasantness of the chocolate, which decreased linearly as a function of satiety. In contrast, activity in lateral OFC (area 47/12) increased with satiety and hence, decreases in perceived pleasantness. It was therefore argued that the medial OFC encoded alliesthesia whereas the lateral OFC played an important role in meal termination. The proposal regarding lateral orbital function is consistent with classic work by Iverson and Mishkin showing that medial orbital lesions give rise to impairments associating stimuli with reward value, whereas lateral orbital lesions result in failure to inhibit responding to previously reward stimuli.[85] More recently, Del Parigi and colleagues reported an inverse relationship between dietary restraint and activation in lateral OFC, again supporting a role for this region in the inhibition of eating and possibly suggesting a role for dysfunction in this region in overeating.[86] The proposal that medial OFC encodes alliesthesia contrasts with work in primates from Izquierdo and colleagues, who showed that bilateral orbital lesions impair reversal learning but not food preference when preference differs as a function of stimulus attributes or satiety.[87] Specifically, their finding suggests that satiety mechanisms and the ability to assign value to familiar foods are intact, and this possibility contrasts with our suggestion that medial OFC encodes alliesthesia. Although the reason for the discrepancy is unclear, one possibility is that; A) conscious perceived pleasantness, the variable we measured, is represented separately from food selection, the variable measured by Izquierdo and colleagues, and B) the experimental lesion in monkeys did not infringe upon the medial region that we propose represents perceived pleasantness of food in humans. Inspection of the photomicrographs from the Izquierdo study supports this possibility as the lesioned area did not appear to extend onto the medial surface. Another possibility is that there are interspecies differences.

Intriguingly, it appears that cognitive factors such as information about brand can override sensory determinants of perceived pleasure represented in medial OFC to change eating behavior. McClure and colleagues found preferential response during consumption of a preferred soft drink in medial OFC.[82] However, when subjects were given information about the brand, behavioral preference changed and response in the medial OFC no longer correlated with preference.

Finally, we note that reward is multifaceted and that we have only discussed one aspect of food reward, perceived pleasure. For further discussion of the role of the human OFC in food reward, the reader is referred to Gottfried, Small, and Zald[42] and Kringelbach.[88] Here we only note that in addition to perceived pleasure, there is very strong evidence to support a role for the OFC in predictive encoding of food reward in humans (e.g., Refs. 78, 89).

GENERAL CONCLUSION

Gustatory information reaches several regions of the OFC. Collectively these regions are thought to be important for encoding the affective value of taste, which may depend upon local integration of physiological significance and quality, as well as integration of intensity signals from earlier taste relays. Interestingly, the right clOFC appears to be preferentially responsive to pleasant sweet taste. This same region shows supra-additive responses to congruent taste-odor mixtures compared to the sum of the activity in response to independent presentation of the components and compared to the response to incongruent mixtures. Taken together, these data suggest that this region is important for integrating sensory signals into flavor percepts and food concepts. Thus sensory information about food and flavor is available locally to support reward learning, which almost invariably includes food and food-related stimuli.

In summary, the OFC should be understood not only as a critical region for reward learning, but also as higher-order chemosensory cortex. As noted by Carmichael and Price:

> At first consideration, there appears to be a discrepancy between the suggestion from the lesion results that the orbital cortex has a behavioral role in stimulus-reward association and the indication from the connectional data that there is a sensory hierarchy related to feeding. On further consideration, however, such apparent discrepancy may be an artifact of experimental methodology. In fact, the hierarchical processing of chemical and visceral sensations and the formation of reward may be the same thing (p. 205).[90]

We concur with this sentiment in that it is clear that chemosensory and affective processing overlap and evolved to serve a common purpose; namely avoiding toxins and incorporating nutrients. However, we also note that it is clear that objects other than food can become the targets of goal-directed behavior and that the variety of such objects multiply in humans. Thus cortex that may have originally represented nutrients and toxins, evolved to encode predictors of such stimuli, provide flexibility in response and goal selection, and then gradually organized to encode such higher order rewards, such as the beauty of a face[91] and the joy of a Brahms symphony.[92,93] At what point in evolution did "reward" and "pleasure" emerge as distinct from chemosensation. Perhaps comparison between neural encoding of different classes of reward will help shed light on this issue and determine whether aesthetic appreciation really is a matter of taste.

ACKNOWLEDGMENTS

This work was supported by NIH/NIDCD R01DC6706-01 and NIH/NIDCD R03DC006169

REFERENCES

1. MURPHY, C., W.S. CAIN & L.M. BARTOSHUK. 1977. Mutual action of taste and olfaction. Sens. Processes **1:** 204–211.
2. ROZIN, P. 1982. "Taste-smell confusions" and the duality of the olfactory sense. Percept. & Psychophys. **31:** 397–401.
3. SMALL, D.M. & J. PRESCOTT. 2005. Odor/taste integration and the perception of flavor. Exp. Brain Res. **166:** 345–357.
4. BECKSTEAD, R.M., J.R. MORSE & R. NORGREN. 1980. The nucleus of the solitary tract in the monkey: Projections to the thalamus and brain stem nuclei. J. Comp. Neurol. **190:** 259–282.
5. MUFSON, E.J. & M.-M. MESULAM. 1984. Thalamic connections of the insula in the rhesus monkey and comments on the paralimbic connectivity of the medial pulvinar nucleus. J. Comp. Neurol. **227:** 109–120.
6. PRITCHARD, T.C. *et al.* 1986. Projections of thalamic gustatory and lingual areas in the monkey, Macaca fascicularis. J. Comp. Neurol. **244:** 213–228.
7. OGAWA, H., S. ITO & T. NOMURA. 1985. Two distinct projection areas from tongue nerves in the frontal operculum of macaque monkeys as revealed with evoked potential mapping. Neurosci. Res. **2:** 447–459.
8. OGAWA, H. 1994. Gustatory cortex of primates: Anatomy and physiology. Neurosci. Res. **20:** 1–13.
9. KINOMURA, S. *et al.* 1994. Functional anatomy of taste perception in the human brain studied with positron emission tomography. Brain Res. **659:** 263–266.
10. SMALL, D.M. *et al.* 1997. A role for the right anterior temporal lobe in taste quality recognition. J. Neurosci. **17:** 5136–5142.
11. CERF, B. *et al.* 1998. Functional lateralization of human gustatory cortex related to handedness disclosed by fMRI study. Ann. N. Y. Acad. Sci. **855:** 575–578.
12. FAURION, A. *et al.* 1998. fMRI study of taste cortical areas in humans. Ann. N. Y. Acad. Sci. **855:** 535–545.

13. FAURION, A. *et al.* 1999. Human taste cortical areas studied with functional magnetic resonance imaging: Evidence of functional lateralization related to handedness. Neurosci. Lett. **277:** 189–192.

14. FREY, S. & M. PETRIDES. 1999. Re-examination of the human taste region: a positron emission tomography study. Eur. J. Neurosci. **11:** 2985–2988.

15. KOBAYAKAWA, T. *et al.* 1999. Spatio-temporal analysis of cortical activity evoked by gustatory stimulation in humans. Chem. Senses **24:** 201–209.

16. SMALL, D.M. *et al.* 1999. Human cortical gustatory areas: A review of functional neuroimaging data. Neuroreport **10:** 7–14.

17. ZALD, D.H. & J.V. PARDO. 2000. Cortical activation induced by intraoral stimulation with water in humans. Chem. Senses **25:** 267–275.

18. CERF-DUCASTEL, B. *et al.* 2001. Interaction of gustatory and lingual somatosensory perceptions at the cortical level in the human: A functional magnetic resonance imaging study. Chem. Senses **26:** 371–383.

19. O'DOHERTY, J. *et al.* 2001. Representation of pleasant and aversive taste in the human brain. J. Neurophysiol. **85:** 1315–1321.

20. O'DOHERTY, J.P. *et al.* 2002. Neural responses during anticipation of a primary taste reward. Neuron **33:** 815–826.

21. ZALD, D.H., M.C. HAGEN & J.V. PARDO. 2002. Neural correlates of tasting concentrated quinine and sugar solutions. J. Neurophysiol. **87:** 1068–1075.

22. FRANK, G.K. *et al.* 2003. The evaluation of brain activity in response to taste stimuli—a pilot study and method for central taste activation as assessed by event-related fMRI. J. Neurosci. Methods **131:** 99–105.

23. OGAWA, H. *et al.* 2005. Functional MRI detection of activation in the primary gustatory cortices in humans. Chem. Senses **30:** 583–592.

24. BENDER, G., Y.E. MAK & D.M. SMALL. 2005. The interaction between evaluative and passive response to taste in the human brain. Chem. Senses **30:** A188.

25. SAVIC, I. *et al.* 2000. Olfactory functions are mediated by parallel and hierarchical processing. Neuron **26:** 735–745.

26. PRITCHARD, T.C. *et al.* 2005. Gustatory neural responses in the medial orbitofrontal cortex of the old world monkey. J. Neurosci. **25:** 6047–6065.

27. ROLLS, E.T., S. YAXLEY & Z.J. SIENKIEWICZ. 1990. Gustatory responses of single neurons in the caudolateral orbitofrontal cortex of the macaque monkey. J. Neurophysiol. **64:** 1055–1066.

28. BAYLIS, L.L., E.T. ROLLS & G.C. BAYLIS. 1995. Afferent connections of the caudolateral orbitofrontal cortex taste area of the primate. Neuroscience **64:** 801–812.

29. THORPE, S.J., E.T. ROLLS & S. MADDISON. 1983. The orbitofrontal cortex: neuronal activity in the behaving monkey. Exp. Brain Res. **49:** 93–115.

30. ROLLS, E.T. 1997. Taste and olfactory processing in the brain and its relation to the control of eating. Crit. Rev. Neurobiol. **11:** 263–287.

31. CHIAVARAS, M.M. & M. PETRIDES. 2000. Orbitofrontal sulci of the human and Macaque monkey brain. J. Comp. Neurol. **422:** 35–54.

32. FRANCIS, S. *et al.* 1999. The representation of pleasant touch in the brain and its relationship with taste and olfactory areas. Neuroreport **10:** 435–459.

33. FREY, S. & M. PETRIDES. 1999. Re-examination of the human taste region: A positron emission tomography study. Eur. J. Neurosci. **11:** 2985–2988.

34. O'DOHERTY, J. *et al.* 2001. Representation of pleasant and aversive taste in the human brain. J. Neurophysiol. **85:** 1315–1321.

35. SMALL, D.M. *et al.* 1997. A role for the right anterior temporal lobe in taste quality recognition. J. Neurosci. **17:** 5136–5142.
36. SMALL, D.M. *et al.* 1997. Flavor processing: More than the sum of its parts. Neuroreport **8:** 3913–3917.
37. ZALD, D.H. *et al.* 1998. Aversive gustatory stimulation activates limbic circuits in humans. Brain **121**(Pt 6): 1143–1154.
38. ZALD, D.H., M.C. HAGEN & J.V. PARDO. 2002. Neural correlates of tasting concentrated quinine and sugar solutions. J. Neurophysiol. **87:** 1068–1075.
39. O'DOHERTY, J.P. *et al.* 2002. Neural responses during anticipation of a primary taste reward. Neuron **33:** 815–826.
40. PETRIDES, M. & D. PANDYA. 1994. Comparative architectonic analysis of the human and macaque frontal cortex. *In* Handbook of Neuropsychology. F. Boller & J. Grafman, Eds.: 17–58. Elsevier. Amsterdam.
41. SMALL, D.M. *et al.* 2003. Dissociation of neural representation of intensity and affective valuation in human gustation. Neuron **39:** 701–711.
42. GOTTFRIED, J.A., D.M. SMALL & D.H. ZALD. 2006. The chemical senses. *In* The Orbitofrontal Cortex. D.H. Zald & S.L. Rauch, Eds.: 125–171. Oxford University Press. New York.
43. PITTMAN, D.W. & R.J. CONTRERAS. 2002. Dietary NaCl influences the organization of chorda tympani neurons projecting to the nucleus of the solitary tract in rats. Chem. Senses **27:** 333–341.
44. SHULER, M.G., R.F. KRIMM & D.L. HILL. 2004. Neuron/target plasticity in the peripheral gustatory system. J. Comp. Neurol. **472:** 183–192.
45. KRIMM, R.F. & D.L. HILL. 1999. Early dietary sodium restriction disrupts the peripheral anatomical development of the gustatory system. J. of Neurobiol. **39:** 218–226.
46. HENDRICKS, S.J., P.C. BRUNJES & D.L. HILL. 2004. Taste bud cell dynamics during normal and sodium-restricted development. J. Comp. Neurol. **472:** 173–182.
47. HILL, D.L. & P.R. PRZEKOP, JR. 1988. Influences of dietary sodium on functional taste receptor development: a sensitive period. Science **241:** 1826–1828.
48. BARTOSHUK, L.M. 1991. Taste, smell & pleasure. *In* The Hedonics of Taste and Smell. R.C. Bolles, Ed.: 15–28. Lawrence Erlbaum Associates. New Jersey.
49. SCOTT, T.R. &. C.R. PLATA-SALAMAN. 1999. Taste in the monkey cortex. Physiol. Behav. **67:** 489–511.
50. WINSTON, J.S. *et al.* 2005. Integrated neural representation of odor intensity and affective valence in human amygdala. J. Neurosci. **25:** 8903–8907.
51. SMALL, D.M., R.J. ZATORRE & M. JONES-GOTMAN. 2001. Increased intensity perception of aversive taste following right anteromedial temporal lobe removal in humans. Brain **124**(Pt 8): 1566–1575.
52. SUGITA, M. & Y. SHIBA. 2005. Genetic tracing shows segregation of taste neuronal circuitries for bitter and sweet. Science **309:** 781–785.
53. ACCOLLA, R. *et al.* 2007. Differential spatial representation of taste modalities in the rat gustatory cortex. J. Neurosci. **27:** 1396–1404.
54. CHANG, F.C. & T.R. SCOTT. 1984. Conditioned taste aversions modify neural responses in the rat nucleus tractus solitarius. J. Neurosci. **4:** 1850–1862.
55. KATZ, D.B., M.A. NICOLELIS & S.A. SIMON. 2000. Nutrient tasting and signaling mechanisms in the gut. IV. There is more to taste than meets the tongue. Am. J. of Physiol. Gastrointest Liver Physiol **278:** G6–G9.

56. SCOTT, T.R. 1992. Taste, feeding, and pleasure. *In* Progress in Psychobiology and Physiological Psychology. A.N. Epstein & A.R. Morrison, Eds.: 231–291. Academic Press. San Diego.

57. SCOTT, T.R. & B.K. GIZA. 1995. Theories of gustatory neural coding. *In* Handbook of olfaction and gustation. R.L. Doty, Ed.: 573–603. Marcel Dekker, Inc. New York.

58. ROYET, J.P. *et al.* 2000. Emotional responses to pleasant and unpleasant olfactory, visual, and auditory stimuli: a positron emission tomography study. J. Neurosci. **20:** 7752–7759.

59. STEVENSON, R.J. & R.A. BOAKES. 2004. Sweet and sour smells: learned synaesthesia between the senses of taste and smell. *In* The Handbook of Multisensory Integration. C.S.G.A. Calvert & B.E. Stein, Eds.: 69–83. MIT Press. Cambridge, MA.

60. VERHAGEN, J.V. & L. ENGELEN. 2006. The neurocognitive bases of human multimodal food perception: Sensory integration. Neurosci. Biobehav. Rev. **30:** 613–650.

61. ROLLS, E.T. 1999. The functions of the orbitofrontal cortex. Neurocase **5:** 301–312.

62. MURPHY, C.A. & W.S. CAIN. 1980. Taste and olfaction: independence vs interaction. Physiol. Behav. **24:** 601–605.

63. GREEN, B.G. 2002. Studying taste as a cutaneous sense. Food Qual. Pref. **14:** 99–109.

64. STEVENSON, R.J., J. PRESCOTT & R.A. BOAKES. 1999. Confusing tastes and smells: how odours can influence the perception of sweet and sour tastes. Chem. Senses **24:** 627–635.

65. FRANK, R.A., N.J. VAN DER KLAAUW & H.N. SCHIFFERSTEIN. 1993. Both perceptual and conceptual factors influence taste-odor and taste-taste interactions. Percept. Psychophys. **54:** 343–354.

66. PRESCOTT, J., V. JOHNSTONE & J. FRANCIS. 2004. Odor-taste interactions: Effects of attentional strategies during exposure. Chem. Senses **29:** 331–340.

67. MCBURNY, D.H. 1986. Taste, smell, and flavor terminology: taking the confusion of of fusion. *In* Clinical Measurement of Taste and Smell. R.S.R.H.L. Meiselman, Ed.: 117–125. Macmillan. New York.

68. SMALL, D.M. *et al.* 2005. Differential neural responses evoked by orthonasal versus retronasal odorant perception in humans. Neuron **47:** 593–605.

69. DE ARAUJO, E. & E.T. ROLLS. 2004. Representation in the human brain of food texture and oral fat. J. Neurosci. **24:** 3086–3093.

70. DE ARAUJO, E. *et al.* 2003. Taste-olfactory conergence, and the representation of the pleasantness of flavour in the human brain. Eur. J. Neurosci. **18:** 2059–2068.

71. ROLLS, E.T., J.V. VERHAGEN & M. KADOHISA. 2003. Representation of the texture of food in the primate orbitofrontal cortex: neurons responding to viscosity, grittiness, and capsaicin. J. Neurophysiol. **90:** 3711–3724.

72. SMALL, D.M. *et al.* 2004. Experience-dependent neural integration of taste and smell in the human brain. J. Neurophysiol. **92:** 1892–1903.

73. ROLLS, E.T. & L.L. BAYLIS. 1994. Gustatory, olfactory, and visual convergence within the primate orbitofrontal cortex. J. Neurosci. **14:** 5437–5452.

74. KANWISHER, N., J. MCDERMOTT & M.M. CHUN. 1997. The fusiform face area: a module in human extrastriate cortex specialized for face perception. J. Neurosci. **17:** 4302–4311.

75. KANWISHER, N. & E. WOJCIULIK. 2000. Visual attention: Insights from brain imaging. Nat. Rev. Neurosci. **1:** 91–100.

76. O'CRAVEN, K.M., P.E. DOWNING & N. KANWISHER. 1999. fMRI evidence for objects as the units of attentional selection. Nature **401:** 584–587.

77. LEGER, G.C. *et al.* 2003. Retronasal presentation of a food odor preferentially activates cortical chemosensory areas compared to orthonasal presentation of the same odor and retronasal presentation of a nonfood odor. Chem. Senses **28:** 554.

78. GOTTFRIED, J.A., J. O'DOHERTY & R.J. DOLAN. 2003. Encoding predictive reward value in human amygdala and orbitofrontal cortex. Science **301:** 1104–1107.

79. SMALL, D.M. *et al.* 2001. Changes in brain activity related to eating chocolate: from pleasure to aversion. Brain **124**(Pt 9): 1720–1733.

80. BERNS, G.S. *et al.* 2001. Predictability modulates human brain response to reward. J. Neurosci. **21:** 2793–2798.

81. KRINGELBACH, M.L. *et al.* 2003. Activation of the human orbitofrontal cortex to a liquid food stimulus is correlated with its subjective pleasantness. Cerebral Cortex **13:** 1064–1071.

82. MCCLURE, S.M. *et al.* 2004. Neural correlates of behavioral preference for culturally familiar drinks. Neuron **44:** 379–387.

83. SMALL, D.M. *et al.* 2005. Neural correlates of the affective processing of oral texture. Chem. Senses **30**(Suppl): A63.

84. CABANAC, M. 1971. Physiological role of pleasure. Science **173:** 1103–1107.

85. IVERSEN, S.D. & M. MISHKIN. 1970. Perseverative interference in monkeys following selective lesions of the inferior prefrontal convexity. Exp. Brain Res. **11:** 376–386.

86. DEL PARIGI, A. *et al.* 2006. Successful dieters have increased neural activity in cortical areas involved in the control of behavior. Int. J. Obes. 1–9.

87. IZQUIERDO, A., R.K. SUDA & E.A. MURRAY. 2004. Bilateral orbital prefrontal cortex lesions in rhesus monkeys disrupt choices guided by both reward value and reward contingency. J. Neurosci. **24:** 7540–7548.

88. KRINGELBACH, M.L. 2004. Food for thought: Hedonic experience beyond homeostasis in the human brain. Neuroscience **126:** 807–819.

89. O'DOHERTY, J.P. *et al.* 2002. Neural responses during anticipation of a primary taste reward [see comment]. Neuron **33:** 815–826.

90. CARMICHAEL, S.T. & J.L. PRICE. 1996. Connectional networks within the orbital and medial prefrontal cortex of Macaque monkeys. J. Comp. Physiol. Psychol. **371:** 179–207.

91. O'DOHERTY, J. *et al.* 2003. Beauty in a smile: The role of medial orbitofrontal cortex in facial attractiveness. Neuropsychologia **41:** 147–155.

92. BLOOD, A.J. & R.J. ZATORRE. 2001. Intensely pleasurable responses to music correlate with activity in brain regions implicated in reward and emotion. Proc. Nat. Acad. Sci. U.S.A. **98:** 11818–11823.

93. BLOOD, A.J. *et al.* 1999. Emotional responses to pleasant and unpleasant music correlate with activity in paralimbic brain regions. Nat. Neurosci. **2:** 382–387.

The Role of the Orbitofrontal Cortex in Sensory-Specific Encoding of Associations in Pavlovian and Instrumental Conditioning

ANDREW R. DELAMATER

Psychology Department, Brooklyn College, City University of New York, Brooklyn, New York 11210, USA

ABSTRACT: A wide variety of associative learning tasks have been employed to assess the functional role of the orbitofrontal cortex (OFC) and related structures in learning. Many of these tasks were designed to assess the learning of highly specific associations between Pavlovian conditioned stimuli (or instrumental responses) and the sensory properties of reinforcement (i.e., sensory-specific associations). Current research suggests that OFC lesions impair behavioral control by these sensory-specific associations in unconditioned stimulus (US) devaluation, differential outcome, and Pavlovian-to-instrumental transfer experiments. In addition, although the OFC has been shown to be important in conditioned reinforcement but not in potentiated feeding tasks, versions of these tasks that assess control by sensory-specific associations have either not been run or they have not examined the effects of OFC lesions. Thus, firm conclusions from conditioned reinforcement and potentiated feeding studies cannot yet be drawn. Furthermore, studies examining the OFC's involvement in reversal learning have also suggested that associations between stimuli and reinforcement importantly depend upon a functioning OFC, possibly because this structure is needed to generate outcome expectancies useful in the computation of prediction errors ultimately used to "update" associations elsewhere (e.g., basolateral amygdala). Other work has shown that both original and reversed sensory-specific associations can control performance after different time delays following reversal learning. This suggests that structures outside of the OFC may be involved in the storage of originally acquired associations. Overall, this review makes clear that the OFC plays an important role in the encoding of sensory-specific associations in a wide variety of learning tasks.

KEYWORDS: orbitofrontal cortex; associative learning; US devaluation; differential outcome effect; cue potentiated feeding; conditioned reinforcement; sensory-specific learning

Address for correspondence: Andrew R. Delamater, Psychology Department, Brooklyn College, CUNY, 2900 Bedford Avenue, Brooklyn, NY 11210. Voice: 718-951-5000; ext.: 6026; fax: (718) 951-4814.

andrewd@brooklyn.cuny.edu

Ann. N.Y. Acad. Sci. 1121: 152–173 (2007). © 2007 New York Academy of Sciences.
doi: 10.1196/annals.1401.030

INTRODUCTION

One of the fundamental problems in associative learning is determining the associative structures that mediate learned behavior. Psychologists studying Pavlovian learning, for instance, have examined what features of the conditioned and unconditioned stimuli (CSs and USs) become associatively connected. The presumption is that CSs and USs can be represented by the brain in multiple ways, and that an "association" means that some new connection has been established between the neural representations of CSs and USs. Determining the nature of the representations involved in this new "associative structure" becomes critical for an adequate understanding of associative learning.

One of the complexities in solving this problem comes with the increasingly recognized fact that different, but superficially similar, learning tasks can sometimes engage quite different associative structures. This fact becomes crucially important when one attempts to identify the functional significance of particular central nervous system (CNS) structures because use of different tasks will frequently have different implications for specifying neural functions. On the other hand, multiple CNS structures are likely to be engaged by a particular behavioral task. Indeed, a particular associative structure that may be prominent in a particular behavioral task may reflect the interaction among multiple CNS structures. Thus, there are a variety of issues faced by neuroscientists interested in understanding the neural mechanisms of associative learning. Chief among these include identifying the associative structures involved in a particular task, understanding which CNS structures are important, and understanding the nature of the interactions among different CNS structures, if any, that occur while subjects perform in the task. A good understanding of these issues should lead to solid information concerning the functional significance of different CNS structures.

Investigations of the role of the orbitofrontal cortex (OFC) in associative learning have been especially illuminating toward this end, although an emerging consensus as to just how the OFC relates to associative learning has remained somewhat elusive. Part of the reason for this has to do with the variety of tasks used to study OFC and learning, as well as the acknowledgement that OFC's functions in associative learning depend in part upon its interactions with other structures, most notably the basolateral amygdala (BLA), and studies directed toward an understanding of how these structures interact in various tasks are only just beginning. The purpose of the present paper is not to provide a comprehensive review of studies examining OFC and associative learning— the aim is much more modest than that. I would like to first provide a very brief overview of some of the ideas on the types of associative structures thought to underlie performance in simple Pavlovian and instrumental conditioning. Next I will describe how several of the tasks used to study OFC functioning may be interpreted in terms of associative structures, and how the results from

Pavlovian   Instrumental

Binary Associations:

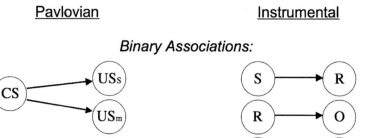

Hierarchical Associations:

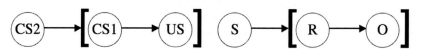

FIGURE 1. Some possible associative structures in Pavlovian and instrumental learning. Various binary and hierarchical structures can be learned in each case. See text for further details.

OFC lesion experiments, primarily, may be interpreted in these terms. Finally, I would like to point to some remaining issues that have not been addressed in the study of OFC functioning, particularly as it relates to possible similarities between reversal learning and processes involved in extinction.

ASSOCIATIVE STRUCTURES IN PAVLOVIAN AND INSTRUMENTAL LEARNING

A comprehensive review of this topic has been provided by Hall.[1] The present comments, therefore, will necessarily be brief. FIGURE 1 illustrates some of the possible associations that may be established in simple Pavlovian conditioning.[2,3] A CS can enter into associations with different features of the US. For example, if an initially neutral olfactory CS is paired with a biologically valuable event such as a liquid sucrose US, then the CS may form independent associations with the general motivational properties of sucrose and with its specific sensory properties. Which of these associations occurs may have important implications for the type of conditioned response that may be observed.[4,5] Traditionally, it has been assumed that "preparatory" responses are more reflective of associations with the motivationally activating effects of the US, whereas highly specific "consummatory" responses are more reflective of associations with the specific sensory properties of the US. In practice, however, it is rarely easy to rely on conditioned responses alone to determine the nature of the learning. Instead, learning theorists have relied on a variety of special tests to establish when learning can best be described as involving associations between the CS and the motivational or sensory properties of the US. Some of these tests will be described in later sections.

Additional types of associations may be learned in Pavlovian conditioning as well. Those mentioned above are essentially binary in form (because they involve an association between two basic elements), but hierarchical associations may also be acquired. In certain tasks, for example, the organism can learn that a CS1-US association is dependent on the presence of CS2. For instance, in a positive occasion-setting task two types of conditioning trials are presented to the organism. On some occasions, CS2 is followed by CS1, which, in turn, is then followed by the US (i.e., a CS2-CS1-US trial), and on other occasions CS1 occurs without the US (a CS1- trial). The organism learns to respond to CS1 when it follows CS2, but not otherwise. In this case, one can say that CS2 "sets the occasion" for the CS1-US association.[6] While there are different ways in which this occasion-setting function has been conceptualized,[6,7] it is worth realizing that more complicated associative structures than the binary ones noted above may also result from many Pavlovian learning tasks. One such hierarchical structure is indicated in FIGURE 1. It shows that a representation of CS2 itself associates with a representation of the binary CS1-US association.

FIGURE 1 also indicates some of the simple associative structures that may arise from instrumental learning situations. Simple binary and hierarchical associations are thought to characterize learning here as well. Indeed, a strong case has been made for the parallels between learning in Pavlovian and instrumental conditioning domains.[8] Evidence for several types of binary associations in simple instrumental learning has been provided. In the most basic task, for example, the hungry rat's lever-press response is reinforced with a food pellet, and the issue concerns what associations govern responding. These include associations between the instrumental response and the reinforcing outcome (R-O, or lever press–pellet association), between the ambient stimulus situation and the instrumental response (S-R, or stimulus context–lever press association), and also between the reinforcing outcome and the instrumental response (O-R, or pellet–lever press association). The issue, important in Pavlovian conditioning as well, as to whether learning about the outcome consists of learning about its specific sensory properties or its more general motivational properties, has also been an important one in the study of instrumental learning. Conceptually similar experimental procedures (to those used in Pavlovian studies) have been used to determine when the instrumental response enters into an association with the specific sensory properties of the reinforcer.

Similarly, studies have also been conducted to show that hierarchical associative structures are learned in some instrumental conditioning tasks especially those involving discriminated operant procedures.[9] The most common task of this sort is one in which an instrumental response (e.g., lever pressing) is reinforced with some outcome (e.g., food pellet), but only in the presence of

Reinforcer Devaluation Test

Training	*Devaluation*	*Extinction Test*
CS1 - US1	Devalue US1	CS1-
CS2 - US2		CS2-

FIGURE 2. Experimental design used to study reinforcer devaluation effects in Pavlovian learning. Decreased CS1 responding during the test indicates that sensory-specific CS-US associations were learned.

a discriminative stimulus (e.g., a tone). In the absence of the discriminative stimulus, then responding is nonreinforced. This task, S:R-O, R-, is formally quite similar to the Pavlovian positive occasion-setting task described above, and as is true there hierarchical associative structures are also thought to be learned in the instrumental version of the task. FIGURE 1 illustrates one possible hierarchical structure. Here it is assumed that the discriminative stimulus, S, enters into an association with the binary R-O association formed during initial instrumental training.

In short, intensive research over the last couple of decades has shown that a number of binary and hierarchical associative structures can be learned in different situations, and that multiple features of the reinforcing outcome in both Pavlovian and instrumental learning situations can enter into these associations. These are important considerations to keep in mind when interpreting the results of various studies directed at the neural systems level of analysis.

DIFFERENT TASKS USED TO STUDY OFC AND ASSOCIATIVE STRUCTURES

The Reinforcer Devaluation Task

One important task that has helped learning theorists understand the structure of the association in learning is the reinforcer (or US) devaluation task. This task was first introduced by Tolman,[10] and was later recognized by Rozeboom[11] as an important procedure in helping solve the problem of what was learned in conditioning experiments. FIGURE 2 illustrates the basic experimental design.

In the Pavlovian version of this experiment, two different CSs are each reinforced with motivationally equivalent USs (such as two different flavored foods) that differ along several sensory dimensions. It is assumed that CS1-US1 and CS2-US2 associations are learned in this part of the experiment, but at issue is whether the two CSs have associated with specific sensory or more general motivational features of the USs. To address this question, one of the USs is devalued in the second part of the experiment (either by allowing the animal to become fully satiated on one of the USs or by associating one of the USs with an emetic that causes a selective aversion to that food item). The effect of this selective US devaluation treatment on conditioned responses supported by CS1 and CS2 is then assessed in a test conducted under extinction conditions (where no US is presented). It is important that no US be presented in the test phase because the opportunity for differential learning involving the two USs in the test could contaminate our assessment of what was learned originally. If devaluation of US1 were to result in selective suppression of responses to CS1, but not CS2, then this would indicate that sensory-specific CS-US associations had been established in training. In other words, it would suggest that the CSs had associated with the sensory features of the USs. This follows from the fact that the sensory features of US1 were devalued. If CS1 had associated with the sensory features of US1, then devaluation of those features should also affect responding to CS1, but not CS2. On the other hand, if both CSs had associated only with the shared motivational characteristics of the two USs, then neither stimulus should be affected by selective devaluation of US1 because the motivational characteristics of the USs, per se, were not devalued.

A variety of studies have provided evidence for the claim that sensory-specific associations are learned in many different Pavlovian procedures.[12] Of additional interest is that several different studies have examined the effects of OFC lesions on sensitivity to US devaluation. Gallagher and colleagues demonstrated with rats performing in a magazine approach conditioning paradigm that OFC lesions occurring prior to Pavlovian conditioning had no effect on the development of conditioned responses to the CS as a result of CS-US pairings, but it did eliminate the US devaluation effect.[13] Subsequent studies demonstrated that OFC lesions made after Pavlovian training and before[14] or after[15] US devaluation similarly abolished the US devaluation effect. Of additional interest was the finding that BLA lesions conducted before Pavlovian training also abolished the US devaluation effect on conditioned responses,[16] but that lesions conducted after Pavlovian training and before US devaluation training left the effect intact,[14] suggesting differential roles for BLA and OFC in maintaining this effect.

One interpretation of these results is that the sensory-specific CS-US association depends upon a functioning OFC and BLA (at least early in training). Exactly why this is the case, however, requires more analysis. For instance, one possibility is that a representation of the sensory features of the US, the so-called US expectancy, itself depends on the OFC and BLA. If this representation does not form in rats with OFC or BLA lesions, then the US devaluation effect should not be seen either.

Another interpretation is that the sensory representation of the US is not itself undermined by OFC or BLA lesions, but the ability to adjust the "value" of that representation after US devaluation is affected by such lesions. Under this view, the CS is still capable of evoking a sensory-specific representation of the US, but one which cannot have its value updated because it lacks the ability to, perhaps, recognize that this representation is related to the actual US that was devalued earlier.

It is not easy to distinguish among these alternative interpretations in the current literature, although it is worth noting that the second alternative is probably unlikely to be true in subjects with BLA lesions. Blundell and colleagues[17] found that while BLA lesions eliminated the US devaluation effect in an appetitive lever-press autoshaping task with rats, these same lesions had no effect on sensory preconditioning with flavor CSs. In this task, two relatively neutral flavor cues are initially mixed together in solution to encourage the development of an association between those cues. Subsequently, one of these flavor cues is paired on its own with a toxin to produce an aversion to this substance. The ability of this aversion to transfer to the other flavor cue is then assessed. Blundell and colleagues found that BLA-lesioned rats displayed normal sensory preconditioning.[17] They asserted that a deficit should have been found in these rats if BLA lesions made it difficult for the value of sensory representations to be adjusted after aversion conditioning, for this is precisely what is required of successful sensory preconditioning. Instead, they argued that the BLA is critical for the development of sensory-specific representations of motivationally significant events. The sensory preconditioning effect was not so affected because this phenomenon depends upon the establishment of sensory-specific associations among neutral events, which presumably depends upon other brain structures.[18] It remains to be seen whether sensory preconditioning is similarly spared in animals with OFC lesions.

Finally, the reinforcer devaluation technique has also been used to assess the effects of OFC lesions[19] and OFC-BLA disconnection[20] in rhesus monkeys performing in a more complex instrumental categorization learning task. Deficits were found in both of these experiments in subjects given OFC lesions or disconnections; however, interpretation is made more difficult in these studies given that the two differentially valued reinforcers were presented during the devaluation test itself. This could have allowed for new learning to occur during the test in normal subjects that was absent in subjects with lesions.

The Stimulus-Potentiated Feeding Test

Another potentially important task used to study OFC functioning in associative learning is the stimulus-potentiated feeding test. FIGURE 3 illustrates the basic procedure. Weingarten demonstrated that animals trained to associate an auditory CS with food while hungry would be more inclined to consume that food when they were later tested satiated if the food was signaled by the auditory CS, than if the food was signaled by a different CS not previously paired with the food US.[21] More recently, Holland and his colleagues have demonstrated that this effect is US specific. In other words, a CS for one food

Potentiated Feeding Tests

Non-specific Potentiated feeding test:

Training	Satiation	Consumption Test
CS1 - US	Sate on	CS1 + US
CS2-	home cage chow	CS2 + US

US-Specific Potentiated feeding test:

Training	Satiation	Consumption Test
CS1 - US1	Sate on	CS1 + US1
CS2 - US2	home cage chow	CS2 + US1

FIGURE 3. Experimental designs used to study CS-potentiated feeding effects. Note that both non-specific and US-specific versions of the experiment differ in terms of the information they convey regarding the underlying associative structure in Pavlovian learning. Non-specific CS-potentiated feeding could occur because of sensory-specific or general motivational associations with the CS, but US-specific potentiated feeding indicates that sensory-specific CS-US associations were learned.

type was shown to potentiate eating in sated rats of that food, but not other foods.[22,23]

The interesting implication of this result is that these US-specific effects reflect the learning of a sensory-specific CS-US association. If the CS had associated with the more general motivationally valued components shared by the two USs, then non-specific potentiation of feeding should have been observed. But this was not the case, and the result more strongly implies that the CS had associated with a more detailed sensory representation of the US. Thus, as was true of the US devaluation test, the stimulus-potentiated feeding test can also be used profitably to assess the effects of OFC and BLA lesions and disconnections.

There are very little data available to examine these issues to date. Holland and colleagues demonstrated that BLA lesions abolished stimulus-potentiated feeding,[24] and that OFC lesions[25] had no effect on cue-potentiated feeding. However, in neither of these cases was a design used that would permit for an examination of US-specific potentiated feeding. Given the results described in the reinforcer devaluation section, it would be surprising if a different pattern of data would emerge here.

Differential Outcome Effect

Gp Differential   *Gp Nondifferential*

S1: R1 - O1, R2-   S1: R1 - O1/O2, R2-
S2: R1-,   R2 - O2   S2: R1-,   R2 - O1/O2

FIGURE 4. One common design used to study differential outcome effects in instrumental discrimination learning. Gp differential acquires this discrimination more rapidly than gp nondifferential, indicating that specific S-O associations are learned in this task.

The Differential Outcome Effect

Another procedure has also been used to imply that subjects must be learning about the sensory-specific properties of the reinforcer. This task has most commonly used an instrumental discriminative conditioning procedure and is illustrated in FIGURE 4. Most typically different groups of subjects are trained to choose one of two instrumental responses (R1 or R2) for reinforcement (O1 or O2) in the presence of one stimulus (S1), but to choose the other action in the presence of a second stimulus (S2). For the "differential outcomes" group, in the presence of S1, R1 is reinforced with O1, and in the presence of S2, R2 is reinforced with O2. For the "nondifferential outcome" group, the two reinforcing outcomes, O1 and O2, are delivered randomly for correct responses made in the presence of both discriminative stimuli (S1 and S2). Thus, both groups are trained to choose different correct responses in the presence of the different stimuli, but reinforcement is given differentially or non-differentially. The usual result is that the group trained with differential reinforcement learns the task more rapidly.[26] This has most commonly been understood in terms of the animals developing associations between the stimuli and the sensory-specific representations of the outcomes, the latter of which serve as additional discriminative stimuli making the task easier to solve in subjects trained with differential outcomes.[27]

It is of interest that this effect is also abolished by OFC lesions,[25] as well as BLA lesions.[28] Again, these results suggest a similarity in functioning of OFC and BLA in representing the sensory-specific properties of the reinforcer. Since this task does not require reinforcer value adjustments to be made at any time during the experiment, the most parsimonious explanation for similar lesion effects in these two tasks is that they have a common basis, namely, interference with the representation of the specific sensory properties of the reinforcer.

Outcome-specific Conditioned Reinforcement

	Pav Train	Instr Train	Conditioned Reinforcement
Gp Consistent	CS1 - O1 CS2 - O2	R1 - O1 R2 - O2	R1 - CS1 R2 - CS2
Gp Inconsistent	CS1 - O1 CS2 - O2	R1 - O1 R2 - O2	R1 - CS2 R2 - CS1

FIGURE 5. An experimental design that could determine whether conditioned reinforcement depends upon sensory-specific CS-US associations. If this were the case, then Gps Consistent and Inconsistent would display unequal levels of instrumental responding during the test. See text for further details.

Conditioned Reinforcement and Pavlovian Second-Order Conditioning Tests

In conditioned reinforcement, a previously established CS for a food US is presented contingent upon some instrumental response. If successful conditioning has occurred to that CS, then the CS should be able to support instrumental responding when the CS is presented contingent upon that response. A related procedure is Pavlovian second-order conditioning where the CS is used to support new Pavlovian learning to a second CS. As Balleine and Killcross have noted, it is sometimes difficult to know exactly why conditioned reinforcement (or by extension second-order conditioning) works.[3] For instance, they suggest that a CS can support instrumental learning through its association with specific (sensory) or general (motivational) properties of the US. These possibilities complicate matters a great deal because a simple demonstration of conditioned reinforcement could be understood in either way. Thus, when it is observed that OFC lesions interfere with conditioned reinforcement in marmosets,[29] or that BLA lesions interfere with Pavlovian second-order conditioning in rats,[16, 30] then the basis of the lesion effects is unclear.

To explore this distinction further, one could use an experimental design like that depicted in FIGURE 5. The question this hypothetical experiment asks is whether a CS will be a more effective conditioned reinforcer when it is asked to reinforce a response with which it shares a reinforcing outcome compared to when it is asked to reinforce a response with which it does not share a reinforcing outcome. Thus, in this experiment CS1-US1 and CS2-US2 associations are trained in one phase, while R1-US1 and R2-US2 associations are trained during a separate instrumental learning phase. Subsequently, one group receives R1-CS1 and R2-CS2 secondary reinforcement training, while another group receives R1-CS2 and R2-CS1 secondary reinforcement training. The groups should differ to the extent that sensory-specific associative processes are important in conditioned reinforcement. For instance, it might be anticipated that Gp Consistent would respond more than Gp Inconsistent during the conditioned reinforcement test. This result would suggest that conditioned reinforcement is more easily accomplished when the CS and the response it is reinforcing have been paired with the same as opposed to different outcomes, and would indicate a role of sensory-specific learning in conditioned reinforcement.

Precisely why this advantage occurs would require additional experimental analysis. One possibility is that secondary reinforcement by a CS paired with the same outcome as the response could retard the rate of extinction of the R-O association. Another possibility is that when the response and CS have been paired with the same outcome this could promote faster learning during the conditioned reinforcement test, for instance, between the response and the CS, the response and the sensory representation evoked by the CS, or between the response and the appetitive motivational state evoked by the CS. Either of these possibilities could make sense of the pattern of results anticipated.

It is also possible that the two groups in this experiment would not differ. If this were observed, then it would suggest that motivational processes are more important for conditioned reinforcement than sensory processes. However, in this case it would additionally have to be shown that these two groups would respond more than a control group (e.g., one that received zero contingency training during the initial Pavlovian training phase). Nevertheless, assuming that a result favoring the importance of sensory-specific processes were to be obtained in this hypothetical experiment (and to the best of my knowledge this experiment has not been performed), then one would expect a similar pattern of lesion results in this procedure compared to the reinforcer devaluation, differential outcome, and US-specific potentiated feeding tasks described above.

While these ideas have yet to be explored, a recent study by Burke *et al.* in this volume is encouraging. These investigators provided evidence that US-specific blocking depends upon the OFC. Rat subjects initially learned two distinct S1-O1 and S2-O2 associations before subsequently being trained with S1S3-O1 and S2S4-O1 associations. The amount of learning occurring to S3 and S4 was then assessed in different ways. First, it was observed that responding to S4 was greater than to S3, presumably because S2 was less successful at blocking conditioning to S4 than S1 was at blocking conditioning to S3. This result is sensible from the perspective that unanticipated USs are more effective at supporting new learning than are anticipated USs. It is important to note that in this study O1 and O2 were different-flavored food pellets. Thus, the sensory differences between these two outcomes must have been responsible for the differences in learning to S3 and S4. In addition, S4 was shown to be a more successful conditioned reinforcer of instrumental responding than S3. Both of these differences between S4 and S3 were absent, however, in subjects

Pavlovian - Instrumental Transfer

Pav Train	Instr Train	Transfer Test
CS1 - O1	R1 - O1	CS1: R1 vs R2
CS2 - O2	R2 - O2	CS2: R1 vs R2

FIGURE 6. An experimental design used commonly to study Pavlovian-to-instrumental transfer of control. More R1 than R2 responding in the presence of CS1 and more R2 than R1 responding in the presence of CS2 during the test indicates that specific CS-US associations were learned. See text for further details.

that received pretraining OFC lesions. These results are therefore consistent with those reported above concerning the importance of OFC in processing sensory-specific CS-US associations.

The Pavlovian-to-Instrumental Transfer Test

Another task that has been helpful at identifying when sensory-specific CS-US associations are learned is the Pavlovian-to-instrumental transfer (PIT) test. The basic experiment consists of separate Pavlovian and instrumental conditioning phases followed by a test phase in which the effects of the CS on instrumental performance is assessed. Early studies exploring these effects were mostly concerned with motivational interactions that might arise in this procedure when, for example, a CS for an aversive shock US is presented to an animal pressing a lever for food reinforcement. Other potential interactions were also studied fairly extensively.[31] One common procedure that has received more attention in recent years is illustrated in FIGURE 6. In this case two different instrumental responses are each reinforced with different reinforcing outcomes, R1-O1 and R2-O2. Separately, Pavlovian conditioning occurs with different CSs each reinforced with one or the other of these outcomes, CS1-O1 and CS2-O2. In a transfer test the effects of the CSs on instrumental responding are assessed, and it is typically found that the CSs selectively control the instrumental response with which they share a reinforcing outcome even though no outcomes are presented during the test. This result indicates that the CSs have associated with sensory-specific aspects of the USs because if this was not the case, then selective transfer of control should not have been obtained.

Another result has also been obtained in studies using this or similar designs. Whereas a given CS is shown to selectively elevate over baseline levels the instrumental response with which it shares an outcome, sometimes the CS also elevates to a lesser degree an instrumental response with which it does not share an outcome.[32,33] Although the selective effect is said to reflect learning of an association between the CS and the sensory properties of the outcome, the general elevation of the other response is said to reflect learning of an association between the CS and the general motivational properties of the outcome.[3]

The importance of the amygdala in supporting these specific and general PIT effects has been clearly established, but the role of the OFC has not yet been extensively studied. In particular, Balleine and his colleague have provided clear evidence to suggest that the sensory-specific form of PIT depends upon the BLA, whereas the general form of PIT depends upon the central nucleus of the amygdala.[32] Given that other tests described above show that sensory-specific CS-US associations seem to be impaired by BLA and by OFC lesions, one might expect OFC lesions to similarly impair selective PIT. There are few data on this question, but Balleine and Ostlund have provided some early data in this volume to confirm that this is the case.[34]

Reversal Learning

It has been known for some time that OFC lesions disrupt the ability of animals to acquire a discrimination reversal. The nature of this deficit has been studied extensively by Schoenbaum and his colleagues using electrophysiological recording and lesion techniques.[35] Schoenbaum's basic discrimination reversal-learning experimental design is depicted in FIGURE 7. It is an instrumental learning task that involves subjects first learning to make an instrumental response in the presence of S1 for a reinforcing outcome O1+ (sucrose), but that this response will be followed by a punishing outcome O2– (quinine) if made in the presence of S2. Both sham- and OFC-lesioned rats learn quite readily to respond in the presence of S1, but not S2. During the reversal phase, these reinforcement contingencies are switched such that responding in the presence of S1 is followed by O2– and responding in the presence of S2 is followed by O1+. Rats with OFC lesions show deficits in learning this reversal.[36]

Data from electrophysiological recording studies suggests that BLA and OFC interact in interesting ways in this task. First, in normal rats, cells in the BLA and OFC develop firing patterns that track the outcomes in each phase. For instance, one cell type increases its firing rate just after S1, but not S2, in the initial learning phase, but respond more to S2 than S1 during the reversal phase. In other words, these cells fire more in response to a stimulus signaling sucrose reinforcement in both phases of the experiment. Another cell type shows exactly the opposite pattern (responding more to S2 than S1 initially and then more to S1 than S2 during reversal). It is tempting to speculate that these cells are coding the specific S-O associations that can be learned in this task. Further, since these cell types are found in both BLA and OFC it would

Reversal Learning

Instrumental Task:

Original Discrimination
S1: R - O1(+)
S2: R - O2(-)

Reversed Discrimination
S1: R - O2(-)
S2: R - O1(+)

FIGURE 7. Schoenbaum's experimental design used to study reversal learning. In this instrumental task, R is reinforced with an appetitive outcome, O1(+), if this response occurs after S1, but it is punished by an aversive outcome, O2(−), if this response occurs after S2. The response contingencies are reversed in a subsequent phase. See text for further details.

appear as though these two structures interact in some fashion to produce these S-O associations as well as their reversals.

More direct evidence for this presumed interaction comes from studies that have lesioned one structure and recorded in the other. Schoenbaum and colleagues recorded in the OFC while BLA-lesioned rats performed in this task and found that such lesions eliminated the occurrence of these outcome-selective cells in the OFC firing in response to the stimuli during the reversal phase.[37] In addition, Saddoris and colleagues observed fewer outcome-selective cells in the BLA firing in response to the stimuli in OFC-lesioned rats both during initial training and during the reversal phase.[38] Thus, it would appear as though S-O associative encoding within these structures depends to some degree on the integrity of both structures.

Stalnaker and colleagues recently examined the hypothesis that outcome expectations are generated in the OFC for the purposes of evaluating the accuracy of outcome predictions.[39] Once prediction errors occur, they suggest, this could signal other structures, like BLA, to alter their coding relations. This idea was suggested by the fact that outcome-selective cells are more in abundance in the BLA during reversal learning, and they reverse more rapidly in the BLA than in the OFC. The idea suggests that the nature of the reversal-learning deficit seen in OFC-lesioned rats has to do with their inability to adjust their S-O encodings in the BLA during the reversal phase. Stalnaker, *et al.* examined this by determining whether BLA lesions might overcome the harmful effects for reversal learning produced by OFC lesions. Thus, subjects with BLA lesions learned the discrimination and reversals normally, while subjects with OFC lesions learned the discrimination normally, but were slow to acquire the reversal. Of most interest, subjects with BLA and OFC lesions learned the discrimination and reversals normally.[39] This result suggests that whereas the BLA might produce "inflexible" S-O associations that disrupt reversal learning in rats with OFC lesions, other structures where S-O associations are presumably not encoded (or at least do not depend upon the OFC) exist outside of the BLA and OFC and are responsible for allowing subjects with BLA and OFC lesions to acquire their reversal more normally. Just what these other structures are and how these subjects are learning this task is a matter for additional research.

The picture that seems to be emerging from this research is that BLA and OFC are intimately involved in coding specific S-O associations and are also involved in the relatively rapid adjustments that help organisms acquire discrimination reversals. There is one problem with these ideas that suggests the analysis is incomplete. A fair amount of behavioral research has suggested that specific S-O associations once they are acquired are not lost, and, indeed, can be called upon to influence performance.[40–43] Thus, if the originally learned associations are preserved and can contribute to performance even after reversal learning has taken place, then where can such coding be occurring?

Reversal Learning and Recovery of the Original Associations

To illustrate this problem, we have recently completed an experiment that involves reversal learning using a flavor preference conditioning procedure. In this task, thirsty rats were given two compound flavor solutions to drink over a series of days. These flavor compounds consisted of different flavor extracts (almond or banana) mixed in solution with different nutrients (sucrose or polycose solutions) to form two stimulus compounds, A+N1 and B+N2. During a series of reversal sessions, subjects were exposed to the reversed flavor compounds, A+N2 and B+N1. At this point, we were interested in understanding whether subsequent intake of the A and B flavors would be determined by the associations learned during phase 1, phase 2, or both. We examined this by conditioning an aversion to one of the nutrients in a subsequent (nutrient devaluation) phase, and then offering the subjects a choice between the A and B flavors alone (FIG. 8). If the original associations controlled performance and N1 was devalued, then subjects should avoid consuming flavor A. However, if during the reversal phase the specific flavor-nutrient associations were "updated" such that their representations were changed to reflect the current contingencies, then subjects should avoid flavor B (the flavor most recently associated with the devalued N1).

Preliminary results from our lab suggest that which of these possibilities is true depends upon how soon after reversal learning the flavors are tested. FIGURE 8 shows the results from one experiment. The left set of bars shows that intake of the flavor that was most recently associated with the devalued nutrient, B, was reduced in subjects devalued and then tested 1 day after reversal training.

Pavlovian Flavor Preference Reversals

Phase 1	Phase 2	Nutrient Devaluation	Preference Test
A + Nutr 1	A + Nutr 2	Nutr 1 - Illness	A vs B
B + Nutr 2	B + Nutr 1	Nutr 2 -	

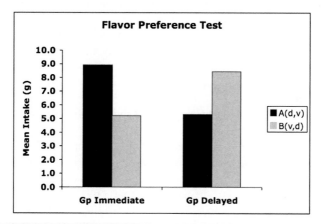

FIGURE 8.   Experimental design and data from a study examining Pavlovian reversal learning. This design can be used to assess the status of the specific flavor-nutrient associations after reversal learning by selectively devaluing one of the nutrients and then testing for a preference between the two flavor cues. The test data show that subjects avoided the flavor most recently paired with the devalued nutrient when this test occurred shortly after reversal learning, but they avoided the flavor that was originally paired with the devalued nutrient when the test occurred several weeks after reversal learning. See text for further details.

The right set of bars, however, shows that intake of the flavor that was originally associated with the devalued nutrient, A, was reduced in subjects devalued and tested 3 weeks after reversal training. It is as though testing subjects soon after reversal learning reveals control by the recently learned associations, but that testing them several weeks later brings back control by the originally learned associations. This result suggests that if the S-O associations are updated, for example, in the BLA because OFC-generated outcome expectancies lead to prediction errors, then this updating is by no means permanent. Perhaps as the updating occurs during the reversal phase, then some record of the original associations is stored elsewhere and ready for subsequent retrieval. Just what CNS structures might be involved in this and what the rules are determining selective retrieval of one or the other association remains a puzzle for future researchers to solve.

It is noteworthy that the sort of recovery effect seen here is reminiscent of a phenomenon extensively studied in the extinction literature—spontaneous recovery. In spontaneous recovery, there is a return of conditioned responses to a CS that has undergone extinction when the CS is tested well after extinction had taken place. Reversal learning may also be regarded as a kind of extinction procedure,[40] since the outcomes in phase 1 fail to occur in the presence of the appropriate stimuli during the reversal phase. If this is the case, then it suggests that there should be some overlap in the neural mechanisms that are involved in reversal learning, on the one hand, and in extinction, on the other. There has not been an extensive amount of work directed at the neural mechanisms of extinction of appetitive conditioning, but that which has been done suggests that the prefrontal cortex may play an important role.[44,45] Future studies examining this parallel may prove to be worthwhile.

SUMMARY AND CONCLUSIONS

Studies of the OFC and associative learning have provided a wealth of information concerning the role of this structure in a variety of tasks. I have chosen a rather limited approach in trying to find commonalities among the various tasks employed in terms of the associative structures that are likely to be engaged and assessed by these different tasks. To the extent that different tasks presumed to assess similar underlying psychological mechanisms (e.g., associative structures) are each affected by OFC manipulations in similar ways, this would give fairly strong support for the OFC's functional role in these tasks. Toward this end I have focused largely on the ability of various tasks to assess the learning of sensory-specific CS-US associations. Some of these tasks were specifically designed to assess such learning, like the US devaluation test, the differential outcomes effect, and the specific form of PIT, whereas other tasks can be adapted to make such assessments. In particular, the potentiated feeding task has been shown to be US specific, and specific CS-US associations can also be assessed using the reversal learning paradigm from our lab described above. In neither of these cases has intensive study begun as to the role of the OFC or other structures, although we are currently conducting a study examining the effects of BLA or OFC lesions on reversal learning. Furthermore, the conditioned reinforcement technique described above has traditionally been thought of as reflecting acquired motivational properties, but as Balleine and Killcross point out,[3] sensory-specific learning processes are also likely to play a role even here. I have described a way in which this can be made more obvious and future studies directed towards this could also be fruitful. Indeed, Burke et al.[46] have already reported data to encourage the view that sensory-specific conditioned reinforcement depends on a functioning OFC. It would surely be impressive if a wide variety of tasks, each of which assess sensory-specific CS-US associations in different ways, could be shown to be similarly affected by OFC lesions.

Some early indications are encouraging. Studies examining the US devaluation effect, the differential outcomes effect, and specific PIT all seem to point to similar deficits produced by OFC lesions. This fact strongly suggests that OFC lesions produce their effect by interfering in some fashion with sensory-specific associative processes. The simplest explanation is that such lesions interfere with the establishment of a sensory representation of the US. Another interpretation (that most readily applies to the US devaluation experiment) is based on the idea that the OFC codes for US value. As noted above, this idea could make sense of the fact that OFC lesions impair US devaluation effects if one were to assume that such lesions make it difficult for animals to attach a new decreased value to the outcome representation that is otherwise intact. However, while this sort of analysis could handle results from the US devaluation experiment, it is difficult to see how a value-based account could also apply to the results from differential outcome and specific PIT experiments since these procedures do not involve any value manipulations. The situation is made even more difficult for such an account when one considers evidence suggesting that equivalent PIT occurs when the basis of that transfer is an association between the CS and a US that is valued or devalued.[33,47] This equivalence suggests that the value of the US is irrelevant for specific PIT. By extension, this suggests that the CNS structure(s) that code sensory-specific CS-US associations can be separable from those structures that code the value of those associations. Future work will be needed to clarify precisely how sensory and value representations of the US might interact in their control of performance, and what CNS structures might be involved, but from the perspective of the several different types of studies reviewed here it seems most parsimonious to regard the OFC as somehow being involved in coding the sensory representation of the US.

Additional work will also be required to make the case more strongly that OFC lesion-induced deficits are produced because such lesions interfere with formation or utilization of specific CS-US associations. It seems clear that if specific CS-US associations are impaired by OFC lesions in a variety of tasks, the most parsimonious way of understanding this is to assume that specific sensory encoding mechanisms are impaired in their formation. It would be more difficult to show that such associations are intact, but cannot be utilized. One strategy has been used in BLA lesion studies and the data do not support this possibility. Blundell and colleagues[17] demonstrated that the US devaluation effect is unimpaired by BLA lesions when the CS has been paired with a motivationally neutral "US" (as in sensory preconditioning). This fact, together with their additional finding that BLA lesions abolish the US devaluation effect when the CS has been paired with a motivationally valuable US implies that the nature of the deficit is not merely a failure to utilize information concerning the devalued event. It appears as though there may be a distinction in the sensory encoding of outcomes with and without motivational significance, with the sensory encoding of valuable outcomes being BLA dependent. Whether or not this same distinction also applies to the OFC represents yet another level of complexity.

There are still other ways of assessing OFC functioning in associative learning tasks, and it seems like this assessment is just beginning. A variety of additional tasks that assess still other types of associative structures have yet to be employed. For instance, some of the hierarchical structures mentioned above may yet prove to be important. To assess these it will be important to devise tasks that are specifically designed to assess particular psychological mechanisms. In addition, one important aspect of associative learning I have not emphasized here is the possibility that Pavlovian and instrumental learning may involve quite different neural processes, and although seemingly parallel associative mechanisms may apply, these may be differentially sensitive to OFC manipulations.[34]

Another area that I have only alluded to concerns possible similarities between reversal learning and extinction learning phenomena. What we have attempted to show is that recovery of originally established associations can occur if subjects are tested after some delay following reversal learning. This phenomenon is in some ways analogous to the recovery shown to occur in spontaneous recovery from extinction experiments. Thus, there may be further links between OFC studies on reversal learning and extinction worth exploring. This problem would seem to present special difficulties for our understanding of OFC functioning. Through the elegant studies of Schoenbaum and his colleagues we can appreciate that OFC and BLA interact in important ways in different tasks.[37–39] One characterization of that interaction is that OFC generates an outcome expectancy that could feed into a prediction error computation (performed by some other structure)[48] that ultimately signals the BLA to change its associative encoding. This flexibility is normally regarded as useful. However, if original associations can recover over time, then would such recovery be occurring elsewhere? If the "updated" associations within the BLA essentially erase traces of the original associations, then it seems hard to understand how OFC-BLA interactions could be involved in this recovery. Clearly, more research is required to adequately understand these effects.

Overall, there is an impressive array of research suggesting that the OFC plays a fundamentally important role in a variety of associative learning tasks, specifically those that assess the integrity of sensory-specific S-O associations. Understanding the precise roles of the OFC and related structures in these tasks will continue to be a challenging endeavor and should for some time continue providing us with a wealth of interesting information.

ACKNOWLEDGEMENTS

This research was supported by grants from the NIMH (065947) and PSC-CUNY (67378) awarded to the author. I would like to thank Janina Scarlet for her role in collecting the data reported here.

REFERENCES

1. HALL, G. 2002. Associative structures in Pavlovian and instrumental conditioning. *In* Steven's Handbook of Experimental Psychology, 3rd ed. Vol 3: Learning, Motivation, and Emotion. H. Pashler & R. Gallistel, Eds.: 1–45. John Wiley. New York.

2. DELAMATER, A.R. & S. OAKESHOTT. 2007. Learning about multiple attributes of reward in Pavlovian conditioning. Ann. N. Y. Acad. Sci. **1104:** 1–20.

3. BALLEINE, B.W. & S. KILLCROSS. 2006. Parallel incentive processing: an integrated view of amygdala function. Trends Neurosci. **29:** 272–279.

4. KONORSKI, J. 1967. Integrative Activity of the Brain. University of Chicago Press. Chicago, IL.

5. WAGNER, A.R. & S.E. BRANDON. 1989. Evolution of a Structured Connectionist Model of Pavlovian Conditioning (AESOP). *In* Contemporary Learning Theories: Pavlovian Conditioning and the Status of Traditional Learning Theory. S.B. Klein & R.R. Mowrer, Eds.: 149–189. Lawrence Erlbaum. Hillsdale, NJ.

6. SCHMAJUK, N.A. & P.C. HOLLAND. 1998. Occasion Setting: Associative Learning and Cognition in Animals. American Psychological Association. Washington, DC.

7. SCHMAJUK, N.A., J.A. LAMOUREUX & P.C. HOLLAND. 1998. Occasion setting: a neural network approach. Psychol. Rev. **105:** 3–32.

8. MACKINTOSH, N.J. 1983. Conditioning and Associative Learning. Oxford University Press. New York.

9. COLWILL, R.M. & R.A. RESCORLA. 1990. Evidence for the hierarchical structure of instrumental learning. Anim. Learn. Behav. **18:** 71–82.

10. TOLMAN, E.C. 1933. Sign-gestalt or conditioned reflex? Psychol. Rev. **40:** 391–411.

11. ROZEBOOM, W.W. 1958. "What is learned?" An empirical enigma. Psychol. Rev. **65:** 22–33.

12. DELAMATER, A.R. & V.M. LoLORDO. 1991. Event Revaluation Procedures and Associative Structures in Pavlovian Conditioning. *In* Current Topics in Animal Learning: Brain, Emotion, and Cognition. L. Dachowski & C.F. Flaherty, Eds.: 55–94. Lawrence Erlbaum. Hillsdale, NJ.

13. GALLAGHER, M., R.W. MCMAHAN & G. SCHOENBAUM. 1999. Orbitofrontal cortex and representation of incentive value in associative learning. J. Neurosci. **19:** 6610–6614.

14. PICKENS, C.L., M.P. SADDORIS, B. SETLOW, *et al.* 2003. Different roles for orbitofrontal cortex and basolateral amygdala in a reinforcer devaluation task. J. Neurosci. **23:** 11078–11084.

15. PICKENS, C.L., M.P. SADDORIS, M. GALLAGHER & P.C. HOLLAND. 2005. Orbitofrontal lesions impair use of cue-outcome associations in a devaluation task. Behav. Neurosci. **119:** 317–322.

16. HATFIELD, T., J.S. HAN, M. CONLEY, *et al.* 1996. Neurotoxic lesions of basolateral, but not central, amygdala interfere with Pavlovian second-order conditioning and reinforcer devaluation effects. J. Neurosci. **16:** 5256–5265.

17. BLUNDELL, P., G. HALL & S. KILLCROSS. 2003. Preserved sensitivity to outcome value after lesions of the basolateral amygdala. J. Neurosci. **23:** 7702–7709.

18. NICHOLSON, D.A. & J.H. FREEMAN JR. 2000. Lesions of the perirhinal cortex impair sensory preconditioning in rats. Behav. Brain Res. **112:** 69–75.

19. IZQUIERDO, A., R.K. SUDA & E.A. MURRAY. 2004. Bilateral orbital prefrontal cortex lesions in rhesus monkeys disrupt choices guided by both reward value and reward contingency. J. Neurosci. **24:** 7540–7548.
20. BAXTER, M.G., A. PARKER, C.C. LINDNER, *et al.* 2000. Control of response selection by reinforcer value requires interaction of amygdala and orbital prefrontal cortex. J. Neurosci. **20:** 4311–4319.
21. WEINGARTEN, H.P. 1983. Conditioned cues elicit feeding in sated rats: a role for learning in meal initiation. Science **220:** 431–433.
22. GALARCE, E.M., H.S. CROMBAG & P.C. HOLLAND. 2007. Reinforcer-specificity of appetitive and consummatory behavior of rats after Pavlovian conditioning with food reinforcers. Physiol. Behav. **91:** 95–105.
23. PETROVICH, G.D., C.A. ROSS, M. GALLAGHER & P.C. HOLLAND. 2007. Learned contextual cue potentiates eating in rats. Physiol. Behav. **90:** 362–367.
24. HOLLAND, P.C., G.D. PETROVICH & M. GALLAGHER. 2002. The effects of amygdala lesions on conditioned stimulus-potentiated eating in rats. Physiol. Behav. **76:** 117–129.
25. MCDANNALD, M.A., M.P. SADDORIS, M. GALLAGHER & P.C. HOLLAND. 2005. Lesions of orbitofrontal cortex impair rats' differential outcome expectancy learning but not conditioned stimulus-potentiated feeding. J. Neurosci. **25:** 4626–4632.
26. TRAPOLD, M.A. 1970. Are expectancies based upon different positive reinforcing events discriminably different? Learn. Motiv. **1:** 129–140.
27. TRAPOLD, M.A. & J.B. OVERMIER. 1972. The Second Learning Process in Instrumental Learning. *In* Classical Conditioning II: Current Research and Theory. A.H.P. Black & W.F. Prokasy, Eds.: 427–452. Appleton-Century-Crofts. New York.
28. BLUNDELL, P., G. HALL & S. KILLCROSS. 2001. Lesions of the basolateral amygdala disrupt selective aspects of reinforcer representation in rats. J. Neurosci. **21:** 9018–9026.
29. PEARS, A., J.A. PARKINSON, L. HOPEWELL, *et al.* 2003. Lesions of the orbitofrontal but not medial prefrontal cortex disrupt conditioned reinforcement in primates. J. Neurosci **23:** 11189–11201.
30. SETLOW, B., M. GALLAGHER & P.C. HOLLAND. 2002. The basolateral complex of the amygdala is necessary for acquisition but not expression of CS motivational value in appetitive Pavlovian second-order conditioning. Eur. J. Neurosci **15:** 1841–1853.
31. RESCORLA, R.A. & R.L. SOLOMON. 1967. Two-process learning theory: relationships between Pavlovian conditioning and instrumental learning. Psychol. Rev. **74:** 151–182.
32. CORBIT, L.H. & B.W. BALLEINE. 2005. Double dissociation of basolateral and central amygdala lesions on the general and outcome-specific forms of Pavlovian-instrumental transfer. J. Neurosci. **25:** 962–970.
33. HOLLAND, P.C. 2004. Relations between Pavlovian-instrumental transfer and reinforcer devaluation. J. Exp. Psychol. Anim. Behav. Process **30:** 104–117.
34. BALLEINE, B. & S. OSTLUND. 2007. This volume.
35. SCHOENBAUM, G. 2007. This volume.
36. SCHOENBAUM, G., B. SETLOW, S.L. NUGENT, *et al.* 2003. Lesions of orbitofrontal cortex and basolateral amygdala complex disrupt acquisition of odor-guided discriminations and reversals. Learn. Mem. **10:** 129–140.

37. SCHOENBAUM, G., B. SETLOW, M.P. SADDORIS & M. GALLAGHER. 2003. Encoding predicted outcome and acquired value in orbitofrontal cortex during cue sampling depends upon input from basolateral amygdala. Neuron **39:** 855–867.
38. SADDORIS, M.P., M. GALLAGHER & G. SCHOENBAUM. 2005. Rapid associative encoding in basolateral amygdala depends on connections with orbitofrontal cortex. Neuron **46:** 321–331.
39. STALNAKER, T.A., T.M. FRANZ, T. SINGH & G. SCHOENBAUM. 2007. Basolateral amygdala lesions abolish orbitofrontal-dependent reversal impairments. Neuron **54:** 51–58.
40. DELAMATER, A.R. 1996. Effects of several extinction treatments upon the integrity of Pavlovian stimulus-outcome associations. Anim. Learn. Behav. **24:** 437–449.
41. RESCORLA, R.A. 1991. Associations of multiple outcomes with an instrumental response. J. Exp. Psychol. Anim. Behav. Processes **17:** 465–474.
42. RESCORLA, R.A. 1992. Associations between an instrumental discriminative stimulus and multiple outcomes. J. Exp. Psychol. Anim. Behav. Processes **18:** 95–104.
43. RESCORLA, R.A. 1996. Preservation of Pavlovian associations through extinction. Q. J. Exp. Psychol. Sect. B Comp. Physiol. Psychol. **49:** 245–258.
44. DELAMATER, A.R. 2004. Experimental extinction in Pavlovian conditioning: behavioural and neuroscience perspectives. Q. J. Exp. Psychol. Sect. B Comp. Physiol. Psychol. **57:** 97–132.
45. RHODES, S.E. & S. KILLCROSS. 2004. Lesions of rat infralimbic cortex enhance recovery and reinstatement of an appetitive Pavlovian response. Learn Mem. **11:** 611–616.
46. BURKE, K.A., D.N. MILLER, T.M. FRANZ & G. SCHOENBAUM. 2007. Orbitofrontal cortex lesions abolish conditioned reinforcement mediated by a representation of the expected outcome. Ann. N. Y. Acad. Sci. In press.
47. RESCORLA, R.A. 1994. Transfer of instrumental control mediated by a devalued outcome. Anim. Learn. Behav. **22:** 27–33.
48. CALU, D.J., M.R. ROESCH & G. SCHOENBAUM. 2007. A comparison of reward-related activity during learning in VTA and OFC. Ann. N. Y. Acad. Sci. In press.

The Contribution of Orbitofrontal Cortex to Action Selection

SEAN B. OSTLUND AND BERNARD W. BALLEINE

Department of Psychology and the Brain Research Institute, University of California at Los Angeles, Los Angeles, California, USA

ABSTRACT: A number of recent findings suggest that the orbitofrontal cortex (OFC) influences action selection by providing information about the incentive value of behavioral goals or outcomes. However, much of this evidence has been derived from experiments using Pavlovian conditioning preparations of one form or another, making it difficult to determine whether the OFC is selectively involved in stimulus–outcome learning or whether it plays a more general role in processing reward value. Although many theorists have argued that these are fundamentally similar processes (i.e., that stimulus-reward learning provides the basis for choosing between actions based on anticipated reward value), several behavioral findings indicate that they are, in fact, dissociable. We have recently investigated the role of the OFC in the control of free operant lever pressing using tests that independently target the effect of stimulus–outcome learning and outcome devaluation on performance. We found that OFC lesions disrupted the tendency of Pavlovian cues to facilitate instrumental performance but left intact the suppressive effects of outcome devaluation. Rather than processing goal value, therefore, we hypothesize that the contribution of the OFC to goal-directed action is limited to encoding predictive stimulus–outcome relationships that can bias instrumental response selection.

KEYWORDS: instrumental conditioning; goal-directed action; Pavlovian conditioning

INTRODUCTION

The orbitofrontal cortex (OFC) is thought by many to be a critical neural substrate of reward learning and action selection.[1-6] How the OFC actually contributes to action selection, however, remains a matter of considerable debate. One possibility is that it is responsible for processing the motivational value of expected rewards. In support for this general account, damage to the OFC has been shown to disrupt the sensitivity of conditioned responses, including

Address for correspondence: Sean Ostlund, Department of Psychology, UCLA, Box 951563, Los Angeles, CA 90095-14563. Voice: 310.825.2998; fax: 310.206.5895.
sostlund@ucla.edu

Ann. N.Y. Acad. Sci. 1121: 174–192 (2007). © 2007 New York Academy of Sciences.
doi: 10.1196/annals.1401.033

anticipatory approach[7-9] and conditioned reaching,[10] to manipulations of expected reward value. Furthermore, a number of functional neuroimaging[11,12] and single-unit recording studies[13,14] have found anticipatory activity in the OFC corresponding to motivational features (e.g., magnitude and valence) of the expected outcome.

However, other evidence suggests that the OFC contributes more to action selection than a simple evaluation of the incentive-motivational status of reward. For instance, some OFC neurons display anticipatory firing patterns related to the timing and location of reward delivery.[15,16] In addition, although it is true that the anticipatory firing of some OFC neurons can be modulated by sensory-specific satiety (i.e., by selectively sating the subject on one of several food outcomes), the activity of a significant proportion of these neurons appears to be unaffected by this treatment.[13] OFC neurons have also been shown to display preferences for sensory features of the anticipated outcome, like texture and taste.[17] Such findings suggest that, rather than merely processing reward value, the OFC is involved in encoding a rich representation of the training outcome.

In this paper we review several recent findings from our lab that call into question the simple reward processing view of OFC function. Much of the evidence implicating the OFC in processing outcome value has been obtained using behavioral tasks that rely predominantly on stimulus–outcome (S-O) learning. As we will see, however, S-O learning tasks are ill suited for studying the processes that underlie truly goal-directed action selection and that involve deciding between different courses of action based on the value of their consequences. Using tasks that are better suited to assess goal-directed action selection, however, we have found that the OFC plays an important but highly selective role in this selection process. Although these experiments suggest that the OFC plays little, if any, direct role in the way that the relative reward value of the instrumental outcome affects action selection and choice, it does appear to be critically involved in the way animals extract information from predictive relations between environmental cues regarding the likelihood of certain consequences and use this information to guide action selection accordingly; that is, the OFC appears to affect choice by influencing reward prediction rather than reward value.

GOAL-DIRECTED ACTIONS IN RATS

When it comes to action selection, not all actions are alike. Some are selected because they produce a desired outcome or goal whereas others are reflexively elicited whenever certain stimulus conditions arise. Of course, most naturally occurring activity can appear "goal directed" to an outside observer and, as a consequence, specific tests have to be conducted to ascertain the nature of the processes controlling any specific action. For example, it is perfectly rational for a woodlouse to seek out shade when it finds itself in direct sunlight, but we would not want to mistake their negative phototaxis for a deliberated, goal-directed action. We therefore need empirically based criteria for distinguishing goal-directed actions from conditioned and unconditioned reflexes in nonhuman subjects.

It has been argued that, in order to be considered goal directed, an action must satisfy two diagnostic criteria: the goal criterion and the contingency criterion.[18,19] In order to satisfy the *goal criterion*, the performance of the action must be shown to depend on the desirability its consequences or outcome. Goal-directed actions should therefore be sensitive to motivational manipulations that render the outcome either more or less valuable to the organism. To satisfy the *contingency criterion*, an action must be shown to be dependent on the specific consequences that it produces; that is, it must be demonstrated that the performance of the action is mediated by the subject's knowledge of the specific contingency, or causal relationship, that exists between the action and its outcome.

Conditioned Approach Responses

To see how these criteria are applied, consider first a typical Pavlovian conditioning study in which a hungry rat is given repeated pairings between a tone and a food outcome (FIG. 1). Aside from an orienting response, initially, the tone will have little impact on the rat's behavior. Over the course of training, however, the rat will come to approach the location of the food delivery whenever the tone is presented. Does this conditioned approach behavior satisfy the criteria for goal-directed action? In order to answer this question, we must know much more than the conditioning procedure that was used. We must determine what the subject actually learned during training.

It turns out that there are at least three forms of learning that could support approach responding in this situation (FIG. 1). One possibility is that this conditioned approach behavior is the natural consequence of encoding the tone–food relationship that was scheduled by the experimenter. According to this S-O view of learning, the tone comes to evoke an expectation of food, which will in turn elicit a set of species-typical foraging behaviors that prepare the rat for the food delivery, including, of course, the approach response. However, it is also true that the rat will tend to experience an incidental relationship between the approach response and food, since it must approach the food cup in order to consume the outcome. Encoding this approach-food, or response–outcome (R-O), relationship would also increase their performance of the approach response. In this case, however, the rat should approach the food cup because it believes that this action *produces* food, not because it *anticipates* food based on the cue presentation. A third possibility is that conditioned approach is supported by stimulus–response (S-R) learning. Indeed, many early

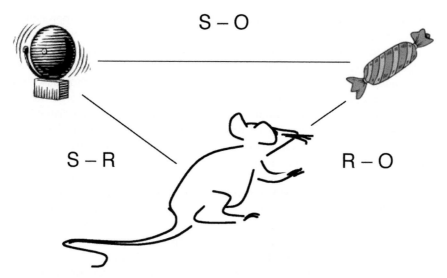

FIGURE 1. Relationships that could support conditioned approach performance. See text for details.

learning theorists posited that this single form of learning provides the basis for all acquired behavior.[20] This view assumes that the outcome itself plays no direct role in controlling performance, but is instead responsible for modulating the strength of S-R associations according to a reinforcement/punishment process; whereas an appetitive outcome, or reinforcer, will tend to strengthen S-R associations, an aversive outcome, or punisher, will tend to weaken them. According to this account, conditioned approach behavior should be supported by a direct association between the tone stimulus and the approach response.

These accounts make different predictions about the sensitivity of approach performance to post-training manipulations of outcome value. Both the R-O and S-O account assume that a representation of the training outcome serves as a critical mediating link in the chain of events that governs response selection. Therefore, both accounts predict that a reduction in outcome value will produce a corresponding response decrement. In contrast, the S-R view assumes that primary function of the outcome is catalytic; it reinforces the S-R association. As the outcome itself is not encoded in this associative structure, this S-R view predicts that post-training manipulations of outcome value should have no effect on performance. In contrast to this prediction, however, it has been repeatedly shown that manipulations of outcome value strongly affect conditioned approach performance.[21,22] For example, Colwill and Motzkin[22] trained rats on two distinct S-O contingencies, such that each stimulus (a tone and light) was paired with a different outcome (sucrose solution and food pellets). One of the outcomes was then devalued through lithium chloride–induced conditioned taste aversion training (i.e., subjects were made nauseous after consuming the outcome). In a subsequent test, the rats displayed less conditioned approach to the food cup during the stimulus that had been paired with the now devalued outcome than during the other stimulus, whose training outcome remained valuable. Several features of this experiment are worth noting. First, the test was conducted in extinction to preclude an alternative interpretation based on the S-R account. Had the devalued outcome actually been delivered during this session, it would have had the opportunity to weaken the supporting S-R association. The observation of a devaluation effect in extinction, therefore, demonstrates that approach performance depends on an associative structure that incorporates a representation of the training outcome. Second, the outcome selectivity of this effect nicely rules out alternative interpretations based on nonspecific motivational or behavioral effects that might have resulted from the devaluation treatment. For instance, had the subjects been generally nauseous or inactive, a response decrement should have been observed for both stimuli regardless of which outcome they signaled during training.

With regard to our criteria of goal-directed action, conditioned approach performance clearly satisfies the goal criterion. However, considerable evidence suggests that it fails the contingency criterion. Assessments of conditioned approach suggest that this response is not controlled by the R-O contingency; that is, its performance is not dependent on its relationship to its consequences. Holland[23] exposed hungry rats to a situation in which a tone was paired with food delivery. Unlike the case in a typical conditioned approach experiment, however, these rats had to refrain from approaching the food source during the tone presentation in order to gain access to the food outcome; that is, the food delivery was cancelled on any trial in which an approach response was performed. On any goal-directed analysis of approach responding, rats should never acquire an approach response in this situation. Nevertheless, relative to a group that received the signal and food in an unpaired relation, Holland found that rats on this schedule acquired and maintained the approach response during the tone even though this resulted in the loss of a significant portion of the food available to them. Indeed, their level of responding was indistinguishable from that of rats exposed to a consistent pairing between the signal and food without the omission contingency. These results suggest that this simple anticipatory approach response is not acquired through R-O learning, but is instead the product of S-O learning.

If the conditioned approach response is indeed acquired through a learning process that encodes the S-O association, then it should be particularly sensitive to manipulations of the *Pavlovian* contingency. In support of this hypothesis it has been shown that conditioned approach depends on how reliably the eliciting stimulus signals its particular outcome. An effective method for reducing the predictive status of a stimulus is to deliver its outcome noncontingently. This treatment ensures that, even though the stimulus continues to be paired with its outcome, it no longer serves as a *reliable* predictor of that outcome. Several studies have shown that this kind of manipulation, known as contingency degradation, weakens the capacity of a stimulus to elicit conditioned approach.[24-26] For example, Delamater[24] trained rats on two Pavlovian contingencies, such that each stimulus terminated with the delivery of a different food outcome. After this initial training phase, one of the S-O relationships was degraded by delivering its corresponding outcome noncontingently during the intertrial interval. The rats were found to adjust their approach behavior accordingly; that is, they approached the food cup less during the stimulus that no longer reliably signaled its outcome than during the other stimulus, even though both stimuli continued to be paired with their respective outcomes. Importantly, by employing an outcome-selective design, Delamater was able to control for nonspecific motivational (e.g., satiation) and behavioral (e.g., response competition) effects that might have complicated an interpretation of the results. This finding, therefore, provides strong evidence that conditioned approach is mediated primarily by the S-O contingency.

Free Operant Performance

The investigation of the learning and motivational processes that support the performance of conditioned approach has provided clear evidence that this response is controlled by predictive learning involving the S-O association and is not controlled by the R-O contingency. In contrast, recent evidence suggests that responses trained in the free operant situation have all the hallmarks of goal-directed actions. In free operant conditioning rats are taught to perform arbitrary actions to gain access to some valued goals or other; in the paradigm case, hungry rats are taught to press a freely available lever to gain access to a food reward. There is, in fact, considerable evidence that free operant lever pressing in rats is sensitive to the causal relation between the action and its consequences; not only will rats stop responding if lever pressing no longer delivers a valued food, but they will also stop responding even faster if their performance cancels otherwise freely available food (i.e., leads to the omission of the outcome).[27,28] Likewise, when the situation is arranged such that access to a particular rewarding outcome is equally probable whether a rat presses the lever that delivers that reward or not, rats quickly stop performing the specific response that gains access to that outcome while maintaining their performance of other actions.[18,29,30]

Likewise, a number of studies have investigated the sensitivity of instrumental performance to post-training outcome devaluation.[31,32] These studies have established that, under most training conditions, instrumental performance satisfies the goal criterion of goal-directed action. In a recent example, we trained hungry rats to press two levers, one for food pellets and another for sucrose solution.[33] A specific-satiety treatment was then used to selectively devalue one of the two training outcomes; that is, rats were allowed to freely consume one outcome for 1 hour before the rats were returned to the experimental chamber for a test in which they were allowed to choose between the two levers in extinction. The rats were found to substantially reduce their performance of the action that had earned the pre-fed (devalued) outcome, but continued to perform the other action at a high rate.

These findings confirm that a dichotomy exists between the processes that control conditioned responses, like the anticipatory approach response, and those that control goal-directed instrumental actions. Importantly, although both categories of behavior display sensitivity to outcome devaluation, indicating that neither is the product of a purely S-R structure, only instrumental performance exhibits sensitivity to manipulations of R-O contingency. The conditioned approach response and free operant lever pressing differ qualitatively; rats approach because they anticipate a valuable outcome, but they lever press because they believe that this action will produce a valuable outcome. This distinction is particularly important for researchers interested in the neural basis of action selection. It seems unlikely that much will be revealed about the neural processes unique to goal-directed action selection by studying the substrates of Pavlovian S-O learning. This distinction also raises a warning: it is possible to devise a behavioral task that uses nominally instrumental procedures but that generates S-O learning. If the behavioral product of the task can be construed as a conditioned approach response directed at the goal location or the signal itself, it is difficult to argue that it represents an arbitrary, instrumental action. In this case, care must be taken to determine what role the scheduled R-O contingency actually plays in controlling performance.

But what about the influence of changes in outcome value on conditioned approach behavior? As with lever pressing, the approach response exhibits sensitivity to outcome devaluation and although lever pressing and conditioned approach seem to be supported by fundamentally different associative structures, it remains a possibility, therefore, that they rely on a common reward process. Indeed, as we will see in the next section, it has been argued that Pavlovian learning provides the motivational support for instrumental performance. However, we will also review a number of recent findings that are incompatible with this view and that suggest, instead, that instrumental action selection is governed by a separate reward-evaluation process.

OUTCOME VALUE AND THE OFC

As mentioned in the introduction, there is considerable evidence that the OFC plays a role in processing outcome value. One of the most convincing pieces of evidence for this claim is the finding that although rats with OFC lesions readily acquire the anticipatory approach response to a stimulus paired with a food reward, their performance of this response is insensitive to the devaluation of the rewarding outcome.[7–9] Similarly, the effect of outcome devaluation on approach performance can also be abolished by lesions of the basolateral amygdala[34] (BLA), a structure that has long been implicated in the processing of the emotional properties of events.[35] The BLA shares reciprocal connections with the OFC,[36–39] and recent evidence suggests that the sensitivity of a conditioned reaching task to changes in outcome value depends on the interaction of the BLA and OFC. For example, Baxter et al.[40] trained monkeys on a task in which the identity of a target object signaled which of two outcomes (e.g., fruit or peanut) could be earned by displacing that object. The performance of unoperated monkeys on this task was found to be sensitive to outcome devaluation; when pre-fed to satiety on one of the two outcomes, the unoperated group tended to select an object that signaled the non–pre-fed (valued) outcome over an object that signaled the pre-fed (devalued) outcome. In contrast, the performance of monkeys with a unilateral lesion of the OFC plus a unilateral lesion of the contralateral BLA was found to be significantly less sensitive to outcome devaluation and, indeed, their impairment was similar to that observed when either of these structures was lesioned bilaterally.[41,42] Furthermore, this deficit did not appear to be due to a simple additive effect of OFC and BLA damage, as monkeys with ipsilateral lesions of the OFC and BLA did not show an equivalent level of impairment.[43] Generally, these results have been interpreted as suggesting that the BLA and OFC work in tandem as parts of a broader circuit that uses anticipated value to guide response selection.

Other studies using a range of species and experimental techniques have implicated the OFC in outcome encoding. Single-unit recording studies have found cue-evoked, anticipatory firing in the OFC during go/no-go performance.[14,44] When it is considered that the object displacement task used in primates, although nominally instrumental, involves a clear S-O learning component, and when taken together with evidence that OFC lesions abolish the sensitivity of conditioned approach to outcome devaluation[7–9] and disrupt the influence of Pavlovian outcome expectations on instrumental response selection,[45] it becomes clear that there is scant evidence directly implicating the OFC in instrumental R-O learning. Although this might seem trivial—as mentioned above, sensitivity to outcome devaluation has been found in both Pavlovian conditioned responses and goal-directed instrumental actions—it is of prime importance. In fact, current evidence suggests that instrumental and Pavlovian "values" are not mediated by a common process, but are in fact determined by distinct evaluative processes mediated by independent neural systems.[18,19,29]

Pavlovian and Instrumental Values

Although they are clearly supported by distinct associative structures, it has long been assumed that Pavlovian conditioned responses and instrumental actions rely on a common incentive or reward process. This view is often expressed in the form of one or other version of two-process theory.[46–48] As mentioned earlier, the fact that instrumental actions are typically performed on some manipulandum or other ensures that there is an embedded Pavlovian relationship between the sensory features of that manipulandum (e.g., the sight of a lever) and the outcome delivery. Many theories of instrumental performance place heavy emphasis on this relationship, proposing that the Pavlovian process that it engages is responsible for modulating the expression of instrumental learning; specifically, environmental cues that signal reward are assumed to facilitate or invigorate instrumental actions.

In line with this account, the influence of Pavlovian learning over instrumental performance can be demonstrated using the Pavlovian-instrumental transfer effect; introducing a stimulus that has been independently paired with food into the instrumental learning situation has long been known to facilitate instrumental performance.[49] The transfer effect has since been well established and, in some cases, shown to be outcome specific.[22,50,51] The top panel of FIGURE 2 depicts the results of a typical transfer experiment from our laboratory.[33] Hungry rats were first given Pavlovian training with two S-O contingencies (e.g., white noise → grain pellets & tone → sucrose solution) before being given instrumental training on two R-O contingencies (e.g., left lever press → grain pellets & right lever press → sucrose solution). After training, the rats were returned to the chamber for a test session in which they were allowed to perform both actions in extinction (i.e., no outcomes were delivered) and, at various points in the session, the two stimuli were presented while the rats were lever pressing. As can be seen in the figure, stimulus presentations selectively facilitated the action with which it shared a common outcome (Same), relative to the action that earned a different outcome (Different).

A number of theorists have argued that this Pavlovian-instrumental interaction is responsible for mediating the influence of manipulations of incentive-motivation on instrumental performance.[48] From this perspective, outcome devaluation is thought to affect performance indirectly by attenuating the facilitatory contribution of the Pavlovian process. Importantly, this account posits that the impact of outcome devaluation on both Pavlovian conditioned approach and instrumental lever pressing is mediated by the same incentive process that underlies the transfer effect. Consequently, all three phenomena should also depend on a common neural circuitry. Given the evidence described above, one might predict that this circuit involves both the OFC and BLA. Alternatively, of course, it is possible that instrumental reward processing does not rely on Pavlovian learning. In this case, we should expect to find both behavioral and neural dissociations between these three phenomena.

Dissociating Transfer and Devaluation

A number of studies have shown that lesions of the BLA made before training disrupt both instrumental outcome devaluation and outcome-selective transfer.[52–54] In addition, a preliminary study from our laboratory found that

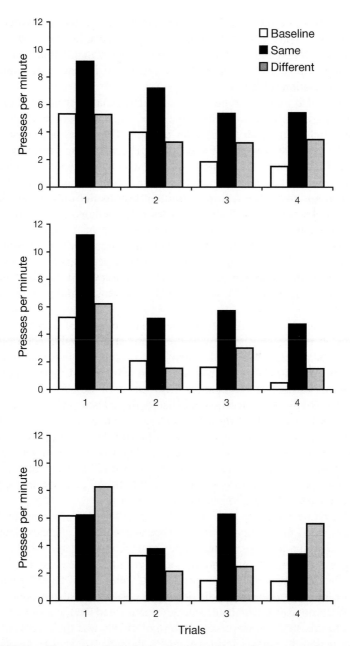

FIGURE 2. The results of a Pavlovian-instrumental transfer test, plotted across successive 2-min trials for the Baseline (pre-stimulus) period and for stimuli Same and Different. The *top panel* presents a typical effect, taken from a sham-lesioned control group. The middle and bottom panels present the results of OFC-lesioned rats that underwent surgery either before (*middle*) or after (*bottom*) training.

excitotoxic BLA lesions made after training were also effective in abolishing these effects.[55] Thus, the BLA seems to be involved in incentive processing for both conditioned approach and instrumental performance and also appears to play a critical role in mediating the influence of Pavlovian learning over instrumental action selection.

The OFC also appears to be involved in Pavlovian-instrumental transfer. For instance, we recently contrasted the effects of OFC lesions made before or after initial training on the transfer effect.[33] These data are presented in the middle (Pre-training group) and bottom (Post-training group) panels of FIGURE 2, directly under the "typical" transfer data which came from the group that served as a sham-lesioned control in this study. Although pre-training lesions had no apparent effect, post-training lesions did impair transfer performance. This pattern of findings suggests that although OFC contributes to transfer performance under normal conditions, it may not play an essential role. In the absence of the OFC, other structures, perhaps including the BLA, may be sufficient to support normal transfer performance. Of course, it is also possible that compensation occurred at the level of the OFC and that more complete damage to this region prior to training would have resulted in impairment.

This finding clearly implicates the OFC in the control of instrumental performance. It is also consistent with the notion that the OFC contributes to a general incentive-motivational system that is responsible for both transfer and reward processing. In order to assess this claim, and thereby provide a more thorough characterization of the involvement of the OFC in instrumental action selection, we also investigated whether these lesions would have an impact on the sensitivity of instrumental performance to outcome devaluation. In contrast to the simple reward processing view of OFC function, however, we found that both pre- and post-training lesioned groups exhibited normal shifts in their choice performance after outcome devaluation. Instrumental outcome devaluation appears, therefore, to be dissociable from Pavlovian-instrumental transfer, at least at the level of the OFC.[33]

These findings indicate that the OFC is particularly important for using S-O learning to guide action selection. They also call into question the notion that reward evaluation in instrumental performance is mediated by a Pavlovian learning process. In fact, this is not the first piece of evidence against this latter view of incentive processing. For instance, Corbit and Balleine[56] found that lesions of the prelimbic area of the prefrontal cortex (PL) also produce dissociable effects on instrumental outcome devaluation and Pavlovian-instrumental transfer. In this study, however, the pattern of effects was the reverse of those observed in the OFC; that is, lesions of the PL abolished the sensitivity of instrumental performance to outcome devaluation but had no effect on transfer. PL lesions have also been shown to impair instrumental contingency degradation learning, indicating that this structure is important for encoding R-O associations.[19,29,56] When taken together, therefore, these studies provide evidence that the respective contributions of S-O and R-O associations to instrumental action selection can be doubly dissociated at the level of the prefrontal cortex, with the OFC supporting the former and the PL supporting the latter.

The incentive-motivational version of two-process theory is also challenged by studies that have investigated the nature of the transfer effect. For instance, the notion that Pavlovian learning provides *motivational* support for action selection is not easily reconciled with the selectivity typically found in transfer studies using outcomes of approximately the same motivational value (e.g., food pellets and sucrose solution). Indeed, Pavlovian cues have been shown to guide response selection based on features of the outcome representation that are motivationally neutral.[57] Of course, such findings are not entirely incompatible with an incentive-motivational interpretation of transfer, they merely argue that this phenomenon is supported, at least in part, by a sensorily rich expectation of the training outcome. More damning still, however, is evidence that transfer stimuli and outcome devaluation can act independently of one another in controlling performance. In order to explain the outcome devaluation effect, the two-process account assumes that the influence of Pavlovian learning over response selection is gated by the current value of the mediating outcome. With standard instrumental lever pressing, the sight of the lever should remind the rat of its associated outcome, but whether this facilitates pressing or not must depend on how desirable that outcome is to the rat. Similarly, in transfer, the potency of a particular cue in facilitating performance should depend on the value of the anticipated outcome. In contrast to this prediction, several studies have found that reducing an outcome's value does not affect its capacity to mediate Pavlovian-instrumental transfer.[58-60]

INFORMATION, CHOICE, AND THE OFC

Thus, there seems to be overwhelming evidence against the claim that the influence of reward value on instrumental response selection is mediated by S-O learning. We do not deny, of course, that Pavlovian cues influence choice. Rather, it is clear that the influences of reward value and of predictive cues on choice performance are mediated by distinct processes that are subserved by distinct neural systems. If, however, Pavlovian learning does not influence instrumental performance though an incentive or motivational mechanism then it remains to be determined how it acts to guide action selection.

Some two-process theories apply a cognitive interpretation to transfer-like phenomena,[60-62] suggesting that Pavlovian cues have the capacity to elicit an expectation of their outcome that, in turn, results in the selection of any action (or actions) associated with that outcome. According to this account, the tendency of an environmental cue to remind the agent of a particular outcome is enough to bias the agent's decision to perform an action associated with that outcome. In line with this interpretation, the influence of Pavlovian cues on action selection has been shown to depend on the predictive status of that cue.[24,63] One piece of evidence comes from the Delamater[24] study we mentioned earlier. After selectively degrading one of two S-O contingencies and observing the effect of this treatment on conditioned approach performance, Delamater conducted a test of Pavlovian-instrumental transfer using these stimuli. He found that the stimulus from the degraded contingency had not only lost its capacity to elicit approach, but it was also ineffective in facilitating instrumental performance. In contrast to the degraded contingency, the stimulus from the other, nondegraded contingency was unaffected and generated clear evidence of transfer.

When carefully considered, this finding suggests a possible hypothesis as to why OFC lesions disrupt the influence of Pavlovian cues on action selection. As mentioned above, Pavlovian conditioned responses are not under the subject's control; these responses are elicited by conditioned stimuli and, in that sense, are not truly *selected* in the same way one selects the best option among alternatives. Although Pavlovian cues are of limited value in selecting a conditioned response, cues with a relatively high predictive validity are of considerable value in selecting between different courses of action. Stimuli that provide information on the likely payoff associated with selecting one as opposed to another course of action reduces uncertainty and, as such, can and should bias action selection. Hence, stimuli that are highly predictive of specific consequences are likely to bias choice toward actions associated with those consequences. This analysis of transfer explains why reducing the predictive validity of a cue reduces its influence on action selection. It also suggests that the reason why OFC lesions abolish transfer is because they too remove the capacity of cues to provide information about their specific outcomes. From this perspective, the contribution of the OFC to goal-directed instrumental performance has little to do with processing reward value and instead involves encoding the predictive status of cues so that they may bias action selection.

If this account is true, then animals with lesions of the OFC should be relatively insensitive to changes in the predictive status of Pavlovian cues. In order to test this hypothesis, we assessed the effect of OFC lesions on Pavlovian contingency degradation learning.[33] Rats were trained to asymptote on two distinct S-O relationships (e.g., noise → grain & tone → sucrose) before being given sham or excitotoxic lesions of the OFC. Training resumed after a brief recovery period. During this phase, however, one of the two S-O relationships was degraded by delivering the corresponding outcome with a fixed probability throughout the session regardless of whether its stimulus was present or absent. The results of this experiment are presented in FIGURE 3. The sham group displayed normal Pavlovian contingency learning, withholding their magazine approach performance during the stimulus that was paired with the noncontingent outcome (Degraded), but maintaining their performance to the control stimulus (Nondegraded). In contrast, the OFC group exhibited a general decrease in responding to both stimuli, regardless of their predictive status.

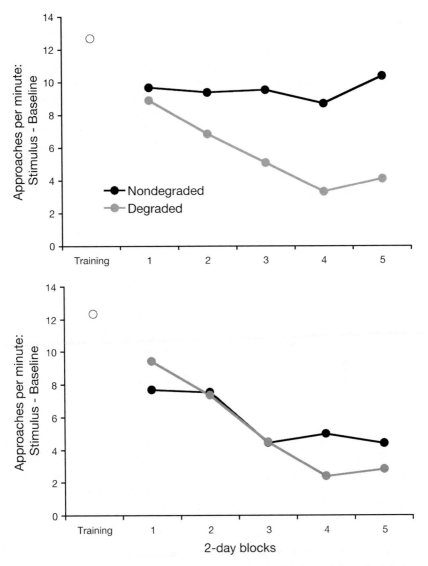

FIGURE 3. The results of Pavlovian contingency degradation training, plotted across successive 2-day blocks for the Degraded stimulus and the Nondegraded stimulus. The *top panel* displays the results of the sham-lesioned group and the *bottom panel* displays the results of the OFC-lesioned group. Open circles represent approach performance on the last day of Pavlovian training.

These data reveal that, although not necessary for conditioned approach performance per se, the OFC is critical for encoding and updating predictive S-O relationships; that is, for establishing the relative validity of predictive cues with respect to their specific consequences. Without this capacity, it seems likely that conditioned approach performance comes under the control of alternative learning processes. For instance, one interpretation of the nonspecific reduction in responding displayed by the OFC group is that their performance is supported by their intact capacity for R-O learning. In this experiment, of course, although no explicit contingency was scheduled between the approach response and food, occasional approach-food pairings could have supported some indiscriminate approach behavior (i.e., approach should have been equally likely during both stimuli and the inter-trial interval). This account also fits nicely with an early finding that OFC lesions render conditioned approach performance abnormally sensitive to the introduction of an instrumental contingency,[64] confirming that this structure is selectively involved in S-O but not R-O learning.

CONCLUSIONS

These findings call into question the simple view that the OFC is generally involved in processing the incentive value of outcomes. As we have seen, the OFC of rodents and the lateral but likely not the differentiated medial part of the OFC of primates[65] (the latter being, perhaps, homologous to the rodent prelimbic cortex[66]) only appears to be necessary for processing outcome value when task performance is likely to be mediated by S-O learning. This analysis also applies to electrophysiological and functional imaging studies reporting evidence of OFC involvement in reward processing. The fact that OFC activity can reflect the motivational value of expected outcomes has been well established.[11–14] These studies, however, tend to involve substantial S-O learning components, raising the possibility that this neural activity reflects a purely Pavlovian incentive process.

Nevertheless, the OFC appears to be involved in more than just processing the incentive value of Pavlovian outcomes; it also appears to encode the predictive relationship between specific cues and their respective outcomes and, hence, is important in mediating the way that this learning influences instrumental performance. Although the OFC does not appear to mediate the influence of goal value over instrumental action selection, the findings reviewed here suggest that it is involved in the way information extracted from the environment is used to decide between alternative courses of action.

ACKNOWLEDGMENT

The preparation of this article and much of the research that it describes was supported by Grant No. 56446 from the National Institute of Mental Health.

REFERENCES

1. HOLLAND, P.C. & M. GALLAGHER. 2004. Amygdala-frontal interactions and reward expectancy. Curr. Opin. Neurobiol. **14:** 148–155.
2. HOLLERMAN, J.R., L. TREMBLAY & W. SCHULTZ. 2000. Involvement of basal ganglia and orbitofrontal cortex in goal-directed behavior. Prog. Brain Res. **126:** 193–215.
3. O'DOHERTY, J.P. 2004. Reward representations and reward-related learning in the human brain: insights from neuroimaging. Curr. Opin. Neurobiol. **14:** 769–776.
4. ROLLS, E.T. 2004. The functions of the orbitofrontal cortex. Brain Cogn. **55:** 11–29.
5. ROBERTS, A.C. 2006. Primate orbitofrontal cortex and adaptive behaviour. Trends Cogn. Sci. **10:** 83–90.
6. SCHOENBAUM, G. & M. ROESCH. 2005. Orbitofrontal cortex, associative learning, and expectancies. Neuron **47:** 633–636.
7. GALLAGHER, M., R.W. MCMAHAN & G. SCHOENBAUM. 1999. Orbitofrontal cortex and representation of incentive value in associative learning. J. Neurosci. **19:** 6610–6614.
8. PICKENS, C.L. et al. 2003. Different roles for orbitofrontal cortex and basolateral amygdala in a reinforcer devaluation task. J. Neurosci. **23:** 11078–11084.
9. PICKENS, C.L. et al. 2005. Orbitofrontal lesions impair use of cue-outcome associations in a devaluation task. Behav. Neurosci. **119:** 317–322.
10. IZQUIERDO, A., R.K. SUDA & E.A. MURRAY. 2004. Bilateral orbital prefrontal cortex lesions in rhesus monkeys disrupt choices guided by both reward value and reward contingency. J. Neurosci. **24:** 7540–7548.
11. GOTTFRIED, J.A., J. O'DOHERTY & R.J. DOLAN. 2003. Encoding predictive reward value in human amygdala and orbitofrontal cortex. Science **301:** 1104–1107.
12. O'DOHERTY, J. et al. 2000. Sensory-specific satiety-related olfactory activation of the human orbitofrontal cortex. Neuroreport **11:** 893–897.
13. CRITCHLEY, H.D. & E.T. ROLLS. 1996. Hunger and satiety modify the responses of olfactory and visual neurons in the primate orbitofrontal cortex. J. Neurophysiol. **75:** 1673–1686.
14. TREMBLAY, L. & W. SCHULTZ. 1999. Relative reward preference in primate orbitofrontal cortex. Nature **398:** 704–708.
15. LIPTON, P.A., P. ALVAREZ & H. EICHENBAUM. 1999. Crossmodal associative memory representations in rodent orbitofrontal cortex. Neuron **22:** 349–359.
16. ROESCH, M.R., A.R. TAYLOR & G. SCHOENBAUM. 2006. Encoding of time-discounted rewards in orbitofrontal cortex is independent of value representation. Neuron **51:** 509–520.
17. ROLLS, E.T. et al. 1999. Responses to the sensory properties of fat of neurons in the primate orbitofrontal cortex. J. Neurosci. **19:** 1532–1540.
18. BALLEINE, B.W. & A. DICKINSON. 1998. Goal-directed instrumental action: contingency and incentive learning and their cortical substrates. Neuropharmacology **37:** 407–419.
19. DICKINSON, A. & B.W. BALLEINE. 1993. Actions and responses: the dual psychology of behaviour. In Spatial Representation. N. Eilan, R. McCarthy & M.W. Brewer, Eds.: 277–293. Basil Blackwell Ltd. Oxford.
20. HULL, C.L. 1943. Principles of Behavior. Appleton. New York.
21. HOLLAND, P.C. & J.J. STRAUB. 1979. Differential effects of two ways of devaluing the unconditioned stimulus after Pavlovian appetitive conditioning. J. Exp. Psychol. Anim. Behav. Process **5:** 65–78.

22. COLWILL, R.M. & D.K. MOTZKIN. 1994. Encoding of the unconditioned stimulus in Pavlovian conditioning. Anim. Learn. Behav. **22:** 384–394.
23. HOLLAND, P.C. 1979. Differential effects of omission contingencies on various components of Pavlovian appetitive conditioned responding in rats. J. Exp. Psychol. Anim. Behav. Process **5:** 178–193.
24. DELAMATER, A.R. 1995. Outcome-selective effects of intertrial reinforcement in Pavlovian appetitive conditioning. Anim. Learn. Behav. **23:** 31–39.
25. DURLACH, P.J. & D.O. SHANE. 1993. The effect of intertrial food presentations on anticipatory goal-tracking in the rat. Q. J. Exper. Psychol. B. **46:** 289–318.
26. FARWELL, B.J. & J.J. AYRES. 1979. Stimulus-reinforcer and response-reinforcer relations in the control of conditioned appetitive headpoking (goal tracking) in rats. Learn. Motiv. **10:** 295–312.
27. DICKINSON, A. *et al.* 1998. Omission learning after instrumental pretraining. Q. J. Exper. Psychol. B. **51:** 271–286.
28. UHL, C.N. 1974. Response elimination in rats with schedules of omission training, including yoked and response-independent reinforcement comparisons. Learn. Motiv. **5:** 511–531.
29. BALLEINE, B.W. 2005. Neural bases of food-seeking: affect, arousal and reward in corticostriatolimbic circuits. Physiol. Behav. **86:** 717–730.
30. HAMMOND, L.J. 1980. The effect of contingency upon the appetitive conditioning of free-operant behavior. J. Exp. Anal. Behav. **34:** 297–304.
31. ADAMS, C.D. & A. DICKINSON. 1981. Instrumental responding following reinforcer devaluation. Q. J. Exp. Psychol. B. **33:** 109–121.
32. COLWILL, R.M. & R.A. RESCORLA. 1985. Postconditioning devaluation of a reinforcer affects instrumental responding. J. Exp. Psychol. Anim. Behav. Process **11:** 120–132.
33. OSTLUND, S.B. & B.W. BALLEINE. 2007. Orbitofrontal cortex mediates outcome encoding in Pavlovian but not instrumental conditioning. J. Neurosci. **27:** 4819–4825.
34. HATFIELD, T. *et al.* 1996. Neurotoxic lesions of basolateral, but not central, amygdala interfere with Pavlovian second-order conditioning and reinforcer devaluation effects. J. Neurosci. **16:** 5256–5265.
35. BALLEINE, B.W. & S. KILLCROSS. 2006. Parallel incentive processing: an integrated view of amygdala function. Trends Neurosci. **29:** 272–279.
36. KITA, H. & S.T. KITAI. 1990. Amygdaloid projections to the frontal cortex and the striatum in the rat. J. Comp. Neurol. **298:** 40–49.
37. KRETTEK, J.E. & J.L. PRICE. 1977. Projections from the amygdaloid complex to the cerebral cortex and thalamus in the rat and cat. J. Comp. Neurol. **172:** 687–722.
38. MCDONALD, A.J. 1991. Organization of amygdaloid projections to the prefrontal cortex and associated striatum in the rat. Neuroscience **44:** 1–14.
39. MCDONALD, A.J., F. MASCAGNI & L. GUO. 1996. Projections of the medial and lateral prefrontal cortices to the amygdala: a *Phaseolus vulgaris* leucoagglutinin study in the rat. Neuroscience **71:** 55–75.
40. BAXTER, M.G. *et al.* 2000. Control of response selection by reinforcer value requires interaction of amygdala and orbital prefrontal cortex. J. Neurosci. **20:** 4311–4319.
41. MALKOVA, L., D. GAFFAN & E.A. MURRAY. 1997. Excitotoxic lesions of the amygdala fail to produce impairment in visual learning for auditory secondary reinforcement but interfere with reinforcer devaluation effects in rhesus monkeys. J. Neurosci. **17:** 6011–6020.

42. IZQUIERDO, A., R.K. SUDA & E.A. MURRAY. 2004. Bilateral orbital prefrontal cortex lesions in rhesus monkeys disrupt choices guided by both reward value and reward contingency. J. Neurosci. **24:** 7540–7548.

43. IZQUIERDO, A. & E.A. MURRAY. 2004. Combined unilateral lesions of the amygdala and orbital prefrontal cortex impair affective processing in rhesus monkeys. J. Neurophysiol. **91:** 2023–2039.

44. SCHOENBAUM, G., A.A. CHIBA & M. GALLAGHER. 1998. Orbitofrontal cortex and basolateral amygdala encode expected outcomes during learning. Nat. Neurosci. **1:** 155–159.

45. MCDANNALD, M.A. et al. 2005. Lesions of orbitofrontal cortex impair rats' differential outcome expectancy learning but not conditioned stimulus-potentiated feeding. J. Neurosci. **25:** 4626–4632.

46. ASRATYAN, E.A. 1974. Conditioned reflex theory and motivational behavior. Acta Neurobiol. Exp. **34:** 15–31.

47. BOLLES, R.C. 1972. Reinforcement, expectancy, and learning. Psychol. Rev. **79:** 394–409.

48. RESCORLA, R.A. & R.L. SOLOMON. 1967. Two-process learning theory: relationships between Pavlovian conditioning and instrumental training. Psychol. Rev. **74:** 151–183.

49. ESTES, W.K. 1943. Discriminative conditioning. I: a discriminative property of conditioned anticipation. J. Exp. Psychol. **32:** 150–155.

50. COLWILL, R.M. & R.A. RESCORLA. 1988. Associations between the discriminative stimulus and the reinforcer in instrumental learning. J. Exp. Psychol. Anim. Behav. Process **14:** 155–164.

51. KRUSE, J.M. et al. 1983. Pavlovian conditioned stimulus effects on instrumental choice behavior are reinforcer specific. Learn. Motiv. **14:** 165–181.

52. BALLEINE, B.W., A.S. KILLCROSS & A. DICKINSON. 2003. The effect of lesions of the basolateral amygdala on instrumental conditioning. J. Neurosci. **23:** 666–675.

53. BLUNDELL, P., G. HALL & S. KILLCROSS. 2001. Lesions of the basolateral amygdala disrupt selective aspects of reinforcer representation in rats. J. Neurosci. **21:** 9018–9026.

54. CORBIT, L.H. & B.W. BALLEINE. 2005. Double dissociation of basolateral and central amygdala lesions on the general and outcome-specific forms of pavlovian-instrumental transfer. J. Neurosci. **25:** 962–970.

55. OSTLUND, S.B. & B.W. BALLEINE. 2005. Lesions of the orbitofrontal cortex disrupt Pavlovian, but not instrumental, outcome encoding. Soc. Neuro. Abstracts Program No. 71.2.

56. CORBIT, L.H. & B.W. BALLEINE. 2003. The role of prelimbic cortex in instrumental conditioning. Behav. Brain Res. **146:** 145–157.

57. FEDORCHAK, P.M. & R.C. BOLLES. 1986. Differential outcome effect using a biologically neutral outcome difference. J. Exp. Psychol. Anim. Behav. Process **12:** 125–130.

58. COLWILL, R.M. & R.A. RESCORLA. 1990. Effect of reinforcer devaluation on discriminative control of instrumental behavior. J. Exp. Psychol. Anim. Behav. Process **16:** 40–47.

59. HOLLAND, P.C. 2004. Relations between Pavlovian-instrumental transfer and reinforcer devaluation. J. Exp. Psychol. Anim. Behav. Process **30:** 104–117.

60. RESCORLA, R.A. 1994. Transfer of instrumental control mediated by a devalued outcome. Anim. Learn. Behav. **22:** 27–33.

61. BALLEINE, B.W. & S.B. OSTLUND. 2007. Still at the choice-point: action selection and initiation in instrumental conditioning. Ann. N. Y. Acad. Sci. **1104:** 147–171.
62. TRAPOLD, M.A. & J.B. OVERMIER. 1972. The Second Learning Process in Instrumental Learning. Appleton-Century-Crofts. New York.
63. RESCORLA, R.A. 1999. Learning about qualitatively different outcomes during a blocking procedure. Learn. Behav. **27:** 140–151.
64. CHUDASAMA, Y. & T.W. ROBBINS. 2003. Dissociable contributions of the orbitofrontal and infralimbic cortex to pavlovian autoshaping and discrimination reversal learning: further evidence for the functional heterogeneity of the rodent frontal cortex. J. Neurosci. **23:** 8771–8780.
65. PADOA-SCHIOPPA, C. & J.A. ASSAD. 2006. Neurons in the orbitofrontal cortex encode economic value. Nature **441:** 223–226.
66. ONGUR, D. & J.L. PRICE. 2000. The organization of networks within the orbital and medial prefrontal cortex of rats, monkeys and humans. Cereb. Cortex **10:** 206–219.

Neural Encoding in the Orbitofrontal Cortex Related to Goal-Directed Behavior

TOMOYUKI FURUYASHIKI AND MICHELA GALLAGHER

Johns Hopkins University, Department of Psychological and Brain Sciences, Baltimore, Maryland 21218, USA

ABSTRACT: Research using laboratory animals, alongside clinical studies of human patients, support a role for the orbitofrontal cortex (OFC) in adaptive decision-making and goal-directed behavior. The functions of OFC neurons within this domain have been studied extensively in both rats and primates. Electrophysiological recordings during performance of relevant behavioral tasks provide a coherent portrait of OFC encoding that is reward related. OFC neurons represent associative relationships between events, encoding information that is predictive of outcome value. That encoding can be understood as a neural basis for deficits seen after OFC damage in the use of outcome expectancy to guide performance. There is less agreement, however, on whether OFC itself plays a role in translating information on outcome expectancy into the actual guidance of overt behavioral responding. New findings indicate that rat OFC neurons prominently encode additional task-related information and events related to goal-directed action. This encoding can occur in populations of OFC neurons that are independent of the OFC neurons representing reward value. The significance of this emerging evidence may require studies that address the larger scale network through which OFC integrates expected outcome information with behavioral control.

KEYWORDS: orbitofrontal cortex; behavioral response; reward

INTRODUCTION

Research conducted in recent years has forged a broad consensus on the orbitofrontal cortex (OFC) as part of a neurocognitive system that is critical for behavioral guidance based on outcome expectancy.[1–9] As such, the OFC plays an important role in the prospective use of information about predicted rewarding and aversive events. This function is revealed in deficits observed

Address for correspondence: Tomoyuki Furuyashiki, Johns Hopkins University, Department of Psychological and Brain Sciences, Ames Hall, 3400 North Charles Street, Baltimore, MD 21218. Voice: 410-516-0167; fax: 410-516-0494.
   tfuruya1@jhu.edu

Ann. N.Y. Acad. Sci. 1121: 193–215 (2007). © 2007 New York Academy of Sciences.
doi: 10.1196/annals.1401.037

after OFC damage, with remarkable similarity in the profile of behavioral impairments in primates and rodents. In many respects the findings in laboratory animals are also consistent with abnormalities seen after frank prefrontal damage involving corresponding cortical regions in humans and further point to OFC dysfunction as a basis for certain symptomatic features in neuropsychiatric illnesses.

A hallmark feature of OFC damage, widely observed across species, is impairment in reversal learning. In such settings subjects have difficulty in altering behavioral responding when a previously established contingency between events, such as a stimulus-outcome or response-outcome association, is reversed.[10–19] Likewise, OFC damage consistently impairs the ability of animals to adapt in other settings when the identity of the associated events, such as a stimulus and outcome, remains the same but the value of the predicted outcome is altered.[17,20–23] In such reinforcer devaluation tasks, an internally generated outcome expectancy, updated for current value, is critical for normal behavioral guidance. Although less widely used in studies of OFC function, impairment is also seen after OFC damage in tasks using differential outcome expectancy (DOE) as a basis for performance.[24] Here the identity of different reinforcers, such as different flavored sucrose solutions, can contribute to greater accuracy in discriminative performance even when the incentive properties of those different outcomes are similar. Notably, this benefit of DOE is not seen with OFC damage, again indicating a failure to use outcome information to guide performance. In parallel, clinical evidence with the Iowa gambling task has accumulated to demonstrate that human patients with ventromedial prefrontal cortex including OFC cannot adjust their performance according to the risk and benefit of outcomes associated with each behavioral choice.[25,26] Altogether, this profile is consistent with the general view of OFC's contribution to behavioral guidance on the basis of outcome information.

Our current understanding of the nature of information specifically processed within the OFC region, which supports performance in settings, such as those described above, has come from recording the activity of single neurons while animals perform complex behavioral tasks.[27–54] Such research, again spanning studies in monkeys and rats, is providing key insights into the particular contribution of OFC to the adaptive control of behavior. For example, neural correlates in OFC are seen during recording studies in the context of reversal learning[29,32,35,44] and during the selective manipulation of reward values.[30,33,37] In such studies OFC encoding of rewarding events themselves, or cues that predict them, are regularly found. That encoding is particularly attuned to the relative motivational value of reward. Further, neural activity within the OFC occurs in anticipation of outcomes after the sampling of predictive cues, a feature that is consistent with the widely accepted view of this region's role in the internal representation of outcome expectancy.[29–35,37,38,40,41,43–46,48–51,53,54] Indeed, evidence for encoding of outcome expectancy exists in the activity of OFC neurons while subjects await outcome delivery after a response is made and in the neural encoding activated by predictive cues before action is taken (e.g., Refs. 37, 44). Encoding of the latter sort would be particularly useful in guiding an animal's behavioral response, as specifically assessed in reinforcer devaluation and DOE tasks.

Thus findings on the effects of OFC lesions and on the encoding properties of OFC neurons provide complementary evidence and coherent support of OFC's role in settings that depend on the processing and use of outcome information in adaptive behavior. Especially given previous primate studies that have emphasized the role of OFC for encoding the properties of expected outcomes, the hypothesis has emerged that OFC may generate outcome expectancy and provide such information to other brain areas for decision and response selection.[8,45,55] Interestingly, recent studies with rats have consistently reported that neurons in OFC encode the behavioral response or its correlates in addition to outcome encoding.[52–54] While these data might encourage a new look at how OFC itself may play a role in translating information on outcome expectancy into the actual guidance of overt behavioral responding, those findings would appear to be inconsistent with much of the evidence in previous primate studies.[37,38,45,48,50] In the remainder of this chapter we will first consider several possible accounts for discrepancies in the existing data. Then we will further consider what the neural correlates of behavioral responding, when such correlates are observed, teach us about OFC function and, finally, how this region may interact with other prefrontal and posterior associational cortical circuits in forming a neurocognitive system to organize and select goal-directed action.

THE FINDINGS

Tremblay and Schultz[37,38] first critically addressed whether OFC neurons encoded behavioral actions in addition to the representation of rewards. They trained monkeys to emit different behavioral responses to obtain the same reward or to emit the same behavioral action, which was either rewarded or not, depending on preceding visual cues. In these experiments, they elegantly showed that most OFC neurons encode the properties of expected outcomes but are indifferent to the behavioral actions for obtaining them. This apparent absence or scarcity of OFC correlates of behavioral responding during task performance was similarly observed in monkeys by other investigators.[45,48,50]

By contrast, a number of single unit recording studies, all involving rodents, have observed selectivity in OFC related to the behavioral response or its behavioral correlates.[52–54] In each of these investigations such encoding was observed while rats were selecting one of two choices to obtain rewards in odor-discrimination tasks. In those settings, behavioral correlates were robust, comprising a large population of OFC neurons. Moreover, in one such study the task contingencies allowed a separate analysis of outcome- and

response-related correlates, revealing largely distinct populations of OFC neurons with response selectivity and outcome selectivity, respectively, each with
different firing properties in relation to trial performance.[54] These findings are
compelling but clearly differ from those reported in other settings as described
above.

ACCOUNTS FOR THE EXISTING DATA

The studies that have shown activity selective for the behavioral response
differ in multiple ways from those that failed to identify such correlates in
OFC. An adequate understanding of the basis for this discrepancy could have
significant implications for better defining OFC function. Given that correlates of behavioral responses have been reported so far only in studies with
rodents,[52–54] a possible species difference first needs to be considered.

While our introduction highlighted many notable similarities across species
in recent OFC research, considerable uncertainty has historically attended the
definition of prefrontal cortical regions across the primate and rodent brain.
According to strict cytoarchitectonic criteria, the OFC in primates has no correspondence to a specific subdivision in rodent cortex. Functional homology
observed in lesion studies, however, has served as a basis for designating
the dorsal bank of the rhinal sulcus as the rodent counterpart of primate
OFC.[10–23,56–61] Primate OFC and the dorsal bank of the rodent rhinal sulcus
also share features of connectional anatomy with mediodorsal thalamus and
certain limbic structures.[62–79] Against that background, the possibility that the
designated OFC differs functionally, to some degree, in monkeys and rodents
could have important implications for defining the neural system basis of
behavioral guidance, including decision-making processes.

At the same time, because relevant species comparisons at a more refined
level of analysis are lacking, differences observed in OFC neural correlates
in recent investigations could be more apparent than real, coinciding with
the subregion surveyed within the OFC. Much anatomical evidence indicates
a heterogeneity of anatomical connections within the OFC both in primates
and in rodents.[62–85] While behavioral studies of monkeys with small lesions
have revealed that the orbital surface of the primate brain is comprised of
two functionally segregated subdivisions: the inferior convexity located laterally (mostly Walker's area 12) and so-called "orbitofrontal cortex" located
medially (mostly Walker's area 11/13/14),[10,11] this distinction has no clearly
demonstrated parallel in rodent OFC. In that context, it is perhaps notable that
single units from Walker's area 11, 13, or 14, but not from lateral OFC (the
orbital surface of Walker's area 12) were examined in those studies that failed
to observe response encoding in monkeys.[37,38,45,48,50] Recordings in the monkey lateral orbital region during behavioral task performance would address
this possible basis for differences in the existing data if behavioral response
correlates were found in area 12.

Other notable differences distinguish the investigations with monkeys and rodents. The first consistent difference is in the relationship of the behavioral response to the location of reward. In the studies that have indicated response encoding in OFC, rats were trained to perform an odor-discrimination instrumental task.[52-54] There were two fluid wells, and a rat had to make a correct behavioral response to either the left or right fluid well to obtain the fluid reward. A response to the opposite fluid well yielded no reward. Hence, when rats performed accurately the behavioral response was directed to the location of reward delivery. In contrast, in studies reporting the absence of response encoding in OFC the reward itself was delivered at a constant site (e.g., a spout connecting with the mouth, a food box).[37,38,45,48,50] Here the monkeys were trained to make a behavioral response, typically an eye saccade or arm reaching, to an informative visual cue that could occur at one of multiple spatial locations. Features of the visual cue, such as shape or color, predicted different identities or amounts of rewards. Thus, the location of the predicted outcome, e.g., the reward itself, would not be used to direct the behavioral response. In such tasks, many OFC neurons encoded the properties of expected outcomes, but not the behavioral response or its correlates (e.g., the spatial location of the visual cue).[37,38,45,48,50] Thus, the possibility that OFC encodes the behavioral action (or its correlates), only when the behavioral response is explicitly goal directed, e.g., spatially guided by the location of expected outcome, is an interesting distinction between the studies that have reported different results. Differences in response encoding across studies might also be due to an even more fundamental difference in the behavioral demands in rodent and primate studies. Thus, the behavioral response in the rodent studies typically involves whole body movement, including head direction (e.g., nose poke to a fluid well), whereas responses used in the primate studies are more delimited (e.g., eye saccades, arm reaching, lever manipulation). Such differences might affect OFC encoding of sensory, proprioceptive, and spatial stimuli triggered by the behavioral response.

In addition to differences in the nature of the movement and the mapping of the behavioral response and reward, previous studies also differ in the relationship between the predictive cue and behavioral action. As just mentioned, in most studies suggestive of no action encoding in OFC,[37,45,48,50] the behavioral response was directed to the informative visual cue itself (by reaching or saccade) such that its presence could be used to direct the correct response choice. In contrast, in those studies reporting behavioral correlates,[52-54] the informative cues differed only in identity (distinct odors at the same sampling port) with responses directed to a different location (one of two fluid wells), such that the predictive cues, themselves, would not direct behavioral actions. A correct behavioral response in this case could be based on a conditional rule between the stimulus and the correct response or, alternatively, could depend on an activated representation of the expected outcome, including its spatial location. Together these differences in behavioral tasks might indicate that

OFC encoding of behavioral responding only occurs when the response has to be internally retrieved, either based on a conditional rule or as a function of information tied to the representation of the expected outcome. The latter basis may be more likely considering all the available evidence. Notably, one study with primates conducted by Tremblay and Schultz[38] used a go/no-go task that was symmetrically reinforced such that correct go and no-go responses were both rewarded. A visual cue indicated whether the correct response was either lever touch or its withholding. Because the correct response choice was not directed by the visual cue in this case, similar to the rodent studies, retrieval of a conditional rule is required to guide performance. The account that OFC encodes the behavioral response only when the animal relies on a conditional rule is at odds with the absence of behavioral correlates reported by Tremblay and Schultz[38] in their study.

A third difference in studies of behavioral response correlates in OFC is in the sensory modality of the informative cues used in the behavioral tasks. Thus, the studies suggesting action correlates in OFC have exclusively used odor stimuli, while studies not suggestive of action encoding used visual cues. Perhaps this difference is significant, given the fact that association sensory cortices of different modalities connect with distinctive subdivisions of primate OFC.[82–84] Specifically, temporal lobe visual cortices project preferentially, but not exclusively, to the lateral part of primate OFC,[84,86] while olfactory and gustatory cortices connect with its posteromedial parts.[72,82,83] Previous studies that failed to identify response encoding in primate OFC analyzed single units mainly from the region medial to the lateral orbital sulcus,[37,38,45,48,50] thus not including neurons in lateral orbital cortex which receive strong input from association visual cortices in the temporal lobe. Thus, in primates, it might be the case that the behavioral response is only encoded in specific subdivisions of OFC corresponding to the sensory cue of a behaviorally relevant modality. It is also recognized that prior exposure to sensory stimuli in a behavioral task, which may considerably vary across studies, can affect neuronal firings in primate prefrontal cortex including OFC.[47,87,88] However, this factor does not seem to affect the proportion of response-selective encoding in primate OFC.[87]

Although few studies have examined OFC neurons with sensory stimuli of different modalities, in one rare case,[32] the distribution of neurons responsive to visual cues or olfactory cues were preferentially found in lateral and medial OFC, respectively. In contrast, Yonemori et al.[41] reported that neurons in rodent OFC that are responsive to reward-predictive cues of various modalities (i.e., olfactory, visual, auditory, somatosensory) are intermingled without apparent topography, suggesting less regional differentiation of rodent OFC. A second modality difference observed in the study by Rolls et al.[32] was that changes in the activities of OFC neurons in reversal learning differed depending on whether visual or olfactory stimuli were used as cues in a go/no-go task. In the case of visual cues, cue-selective firings in OFC rapidly changed, with nearly complete reversal, after the stimulus-outcome contingencies were altered. In contrast, in a task with olfactory cues, not all cue-selective neurons in OFC showed reversal of selectivity: neurons that were cue selective during initial acquisition showed reversal, no change, or even extinction/absence of firing. These findings suggest that, at least in primate OFC, information in different sensory modalities may indeed be subject to somewhat different processing functions. While such direct comparisons with different modalities do not exist in the rodent research, a pattern of changes upon reversal quite similar to that seen in the primate was reported in the case of olfactory cues in a go/no-go task with rats.[35]

WHAT CONTENT DOES RESPONSE-SELECTIVE ACTIVITY IN OFC REPRESENT?

A need for behavioral control occurs in settings with multiple response options. Here we are concerned with how encoding in OFC may be related to the guidance of action, including overt responses that occur in goal-directed behavior. It is possible that OFC, itself, does not participate in behavioral control at the level of action, as suggested by some of the studies we have considered.[37,38,45,48,50] Behavioral guidance, including selection of response and execution of performance, may be a function of other components of a system that relies on outcome (reward-related) information provided by OFC. Until recently, the data supported a view that OFC, itself, is not involved in the integration of behavioral- and reward-related information.[8,45,55] On the other hand, the existence of response correlates in OFC, now observed in some settings, may point to a more direct contribution of OFC processing to encoding that is related to the control and execution of action.

Feierstein et al.[52] designed a study to explicitly examine OFC encoding in relation to behavioral performance while the outcome of each correct response option was equated. In their two-alternative choice task, the odor cue presented on a trial specified the location of reward, which always consisted of water delivery. In this setting over half of OFC neurons encoded the direction of response, corresponding to the location of the goal. That finding alone counters the view that OFC encodes the relative motivational value of different rewards independent of other aspects of task demands and performance. Additional analyses were performed by Feierstein et al.[52] to determine the significance of the correlates they observed. Because the odor cue presented on a trial predicted the behavioral response that would be rewarded, they employed an analysis of neural activity on error trials in order to determine if selective activity during execution of movement was tied to the actual behavioral response rather than the prior sensory cue. They found that a significant portion of neurons with selective activity in correct trials with one response option were also similarly activated in error trials with the same response option following different odor cues. Thus they found support for encoding of the actual behavioral response or its behavioral correlate (spatial attributes of expected outcomes), independent of the cue sampled in the trial, a finding also observed for correlates of the behavioral response more recently reported by Furuyashiki et al.[54] Indeed, all reports thus far indicate that response direction selectivity, at least from the time of response initiation, is largely tied to the chosen behavioral response irrespective of preceding odor stimuli.[52-54]

The encoding in OFC related to the behavioral response observed by Roesch et al.[53] occurred in a study not explicitly designed for the purpose of such analysis. In their task, the location of the reward predicted whether the delay preceding reward delivery would be a short or long duration. The primary interest in this study was to assess the activity of OFC neurons in relation to reward discounting as a function of delay, as well as the value of the reward as a function of its magnitude. In their survey of the effect of these reward-related variables they found that substantial numbers of OFC neurons had a preferred direction (left versus right) in this task. Further, they found that the population of neurons with selectivity for delay did not similarly exhibit selectivity as a function of reward magnitude (differences in size of reward at the same delay). This result led to the conclusion that reward-related activity in OFC is not encoded as a common 'value' currency. While many response-selective neurons showed some influence of reward-related variables, given that the contingency between the behavioral response and the reward remained constant in a substantial block of trials, the behavioral response itself would provide a cue for the expected outcome. Thus response-outcome associations could provide a basis for correlates in this task.

Our recent study[54] adds considerable additional support to the view that the behavioral response or its correlate (e.g., location associated with the response) is represented by OFC neurons independent of the encoding of reward-related features of the outcomes. The task design in this case allowed separate analyses of outcome-selective and response-selective activity. For this purpose, four different odor cues were used in a two choice paradigm, such that each odor signaled a unique combination of response (left or right) and outcome (sucrose or water). Many neurons selectively encoded outcome (preferred activity for sucrose or water) independent of the response made in obtaining reward. A largely separate population had preferred activity for left or right responses, independent of the reward received as a consequence. Unlike the study by Roesch et al.,[53] response direction here was not a consistent predictor of reward value; rats received either preferred sucrose or water equally often after responding at each location in trials that were interleaved during performance of the task. Unlike Feierstein et al.,[52] odor cues signaled not only the correct location (left versus right) for the behavioral response but also the identity of the rewarding outcome (sucrose versus water), but response correlates independent of the associated outcome were still strongly represented in OFC. Indeed the response-selective population we observed was at least as large as the outcome-selective population within each phase of trial performance (odor sampling, response execution, reward anticipation). Thus, largely separate populations had outcome selectivity and response selectivity. However, it is noteworthy that a smaller, but significant, subset of OFC neurons had interesting features of combined selectivity. Given much evidence that the relative value of reward is strongly represented in the encoding properties of OFC neurons to discrete predictive cues, the encoding of the behavioral response largely apart from outcome encoding is quite interesting and might imply that directional response selectivity plays a different role in behavioral guidance from the outcome encoding associated with predictive cues. In the case of discrete predictive cues, the encoding of relative value or motivation significance would be informative for response selection. In the case of encoding that emerges during response execution or at response completion, relative value would not be useful for selecting among response options.

As we already noted, a common aspect of these studies is the relationship between the execution of a behavioral response and reward location.[52-54] In all cases, when rats perform accurately, the choice response is directed to the site where reward is delivered. Thus, correlates have been variously described as response selective, direction selective, or location selective. In these designations the difficulty becomes apparent in separating the response (either left or right movement) from the spatial site that is the target of the response (left or right well). Some insight into the nature of OFC encoding with reference to the response itself or the target of the response might be achieved by isolating analysis within different behavioral epochs of the trials. In an epoch defined according to the execution of movement (exit from the cue sampling port until entry at the reward location), selectivity is seen during the actual response phase[52,54] but a separate neuronal population strongly encodes selectivity for left versus right after response completion. This latter selectivity has been observed in a phase of the task that includes both a delay interval of waiting for reward[53,54] and during reward delivery itself.[52,53] Those correlates in OFC after completion of the choice response are reasonable candidates for encoding spatial location. Much as neural activity in OFC associatively encodes discrete cues (visual, olfactory) that predict reward, the spatial position of the fluid well, left or right, could be encoded as a location associated with reward.

As in the discussion of the encoding observed after response completion, and in parallel with other encoding properties in OFC, response-selective correlates observed during response execution could internally represent the expected 'location' of reward, analogous to representation of the expected reward itself, in outcome-selective activity. If that were the case, then those correlates might not encode behavioral responses but rather information specifically used to guide responding. While Feierstein et al.[52] suggested that the correlates of behavioral responses represent such spatial goals, they also argued that correlates in OFC are not strictly confined to reward location per se. They reported that a subset (19%) of the OFC neurons that were response selective during movement to the reward location also exhibited selectivity when the same movement, directionally defined, occurred to a different location during another (non-rewarded) phase of trial performance.

At the same time, other evidence indicates that correlates in OFC are tightly linked to behavioral events as described by Furuyashiki et al.[54] Notably, selectivity in the population of neurons encoding response (left or right) is synchronized to behavioral events both at the level of single units and within that population as a whole, particularly during response execution (see FIG. 1A). This profile is unlike the pattern of activity observed for OFC units that selectively encode outcome (sucrose versus water). As reported elsewhere, we found that activity related to outcome encoding is largely maintained from cue sampling until reward delivery. In contrast, the vast majority of units that had response selectivity during the phase of response execution in the task did not maintain selectivity after completion of the response (73 of 90 units that were response selective during the response phase). On the other hand, units that exhibited selectivity after the response was executed — with preferred activity at either the left or right fluid well — more typically maintained that selective activity until reward delivery, a profile that was also evident in the population (FIG. 1B). As such, encoding in OFC would appear to consist of different subsets of neurons with patterns of activity linked to response execution and to the location of reward delivery, respectively.

OFC AS A COMPONENT OF A NEUROCOGNITIVE SYSTEM FOR GOAL-DIRECTED BEHAVIOR

The anatomical connectivity of OFC with other information processing and motor control systems is extensive, as reviewed in contributions to this volume. Here we will consider the new findings on correlates in OFC related to behavioral responses in the context of a more mature line of research on OFC correlates of reward and outcome expectancy. We will consider how strategies that have led to progress in understanding that OFC function could usefully be applied to this newer topic of its role in the control and execution of action.

Behavioral control is adaptively organized to ensure survival. For example, a hungry animal disengages from foraging activities in the face of a predator. Learning and memory greatly augment the ability to respond adaptively, with related cognitive functions serving a particularly key role in behavioral guidance. Expected outcomes, based on predictive relationships experienced in the past, are especially relevant for choosing a current course of action. In addition, the need to integrate information from multiple sources can be especially critical in choosing among response options. Devaluation paradigms, as used in much research on OFC function,[17,20–23] provide an illustrative example. While

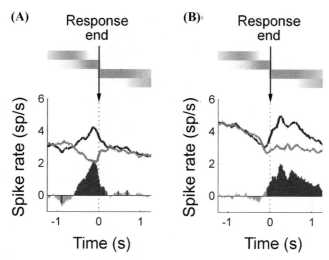

FIGURE 1. Activity profiles of neuronal correlates of the behavioral response in rat OFC during two different behavioral epochs. Figure shows population perievent spike-rate histograms of rat OFC units selective to the behavioral response during an instrumental, odor-discrimination task. In this task, after sampling an odor cue (odor presentation phase), a rat had to make a nosepoke to one of two fluid wells, either left or right (response phase). If the behavioral response was correct, either sucrose or water solution was delivered as fluid reward after a variable delay interval (reward-waiting phase), followed by its consumption (consumption phase). Average duration of each behavioral phase is indicated by horizontal bars above each panel. From left/right and top/bottom the four horizontal bars represent durations of the odor presentation phase, the response phase, the reward-waiting phase, and the consumption phase. Histograms in both panels were generated with activity synchronized to the time of response completion. Each panel shows the histograms for a population of rat OFC neurons with selective activity for response (left versus right) in a specific phase of behavioral performance. The panel on the left shows the response phase (**A**) and the right panel shows the reward-waiting phase (**B**). Dark-gray and light-gray lines in each panel indicate averaged activities for each population in trials with preferred and non-preferred response option, respectively. A difference between those activities at each time bin was averaged across neurons in each population, and displayed in bar histograms at the bottom of each panel. Dark portions of these bar histograms indicate time bins where the difference between preferred and non-preferred activities was statistically significant. Note that the activity of each population was mostly confined within its corresponding behavioral phase, keyed to salient behavioral events (e.g., response end, reward delivery). These profiles were not observed in neuronal correlates to the expected outcome, as described in the text (data not shown).

cues gain the ability to signal a desirable outcome during initial associative learning in one training environment, a subsequent experience is devised to render that outcome undesirable, e.g., illness induced after consumption in a different environment. The activation of a representation of the outcome by the initially trained cue now becomes sufficient to alter behavioral action, which is no longer eagerly directed to the original goal. This behavioral control is based on the outcome's internal representation alone, because in the critical test no outcome is present but only the cue that signals it.

The well-recognized role of OFC in the associative representation of outcome information, as indicated by both information encoding in OFC neurons and deficits after OFC damage, positions OFC within a neurocognitive system for behavioral guidance and decision-making processes. The circuitry that governs this role of OFC in outcome encoding critically depends on the cooperative function of additional components of a larger network. Indeed, significant progress has been in understanding the role of OFC in outcome expectancy by a circuit analysis that has focused on the interactions between OFC and the basolateral amygdala (ABL), which share strong reciprocal connections.

Now a large body of evidence, including the use of lesions that disconnect these structure, indicates that OFC-ABL is critically needed to establish cue-outcome associations, and, at least in some circumstances, is also needed for updating and retrieving outcome expectancy used in goal-directed behavior.[10-24,89-95] In this work, largely consistent findings have been obtained for both non-human primates and rodents, with experimental and clinical evidence supporting the existence of a similar functional OFC-ABL circuit in the human brain (for review see Ref. 9).

Encoding in OFC specifically related to response, direction, or location independent of outcome selectivity suggests the importance of other OFC networks, apart from its connectivity with the amygdala. For example, the possibility that goal location is a feature of OFC encoding, as discussed in the previous section, directs attention to neuroanatomical connectivity of the OFC with the hippocampal formation, which is specialized in the processing of spatial information. Direct connections from the intermediate part and the ventral and temporal part of the hippocampus and subiculum target the lateral OFC in rats.[96] While this direct projection from hippocampus to OFC is relatively sparse,[96,97] indirect pathways are more extensive. One prominent pathway exists via projections from parahippocampal regions, such as entorhinal, perirhinal, and postrhinal cortices, to OFC.[67,70] A hallmark of hippocampal neurons is location-specific encoding, so-called 'place fields'[98-101] and features of spatial encoding are also observed in the parahippocampal region.[101-105] An additional indirect pathway connects the ventral and temporal part of the hippocampus and subiculum with lateral OFC via prelimbic (PrL) and infralimbic (IL) cortices.[76,96,97,106-110] Interestingly, Hok et al.[111] reported that PrL and IL neurons encode the spatial location of a behavioral goal. Other studies have suggested that PrL/IL neurons are spatially attuned primarily because selective activation occurs as a function of behavioral sequence during navigation.[112-114] Whether OFC encoding, including features of reward location and goal-directed action, depend on these connections could be subjected to analysis modeled on studies of OFC-ABL interactions.

Behavioral response correlates of OFC neurons may be important to consider in an even broader network of association cortices. In particular, OFC is connected with medial precentral cortex (PrC_m) and posterior parietal cortex (PPC) in rats,[76,109,115–120] a network that is proposed to serve a crucial role in directing spatial attention.[76,121] Damage to these areas causes behavioral deficits in spatial orienting and learning based on such spatial information.[120–132] More specifically, PPC neurons encode specific types of movements (e.g., left or right rotation, forward) or head direction,[133,134] and PPC encoding of movement and head direction in rats varies according to a number of relevant factors, such as active or passive movement, and spatial context.[133–135] Thus a network that includes OFC-PPC could also contribute to the encoding characteristics of OFC neurons.

An experimental analysis of the networks contributing to OFC correlates of response/location could be modeled after some of the most informative studies on the OFC-ABL circuit. A powerful approach used for investigations of the OFC-ABL circuit entailed examination of the encoding properties in one component of the circuit under experimental manipulation of the other component. As a result, impairment in reward devaluation performance after OFC damage can be understood as a network failure; OFC neurons do not develop critical cue-activated representations of outcome information when ABL is functionally removed during learning.[44] This role for the OFC-ABL circuit is largely consistent with the accepted view that the amygdala is critical in associative learning, whereby cues acquire motivational value, but additionally connects that function to the representational capacity of a cortical system. Moreover, influences between OFC and ABL are reciprocal; specific features of encoding in ABL that normally emerge during learning are impaired when the OFC is offline.[136] These studies are a potential template for future work to illuminate the basis of other information encoding functions of OFC, such as those that might depend on the medial temporal lobe, PrL/IL, and PPC circuits. Indeed, Ramus et al.[137] in a different chapter in this volume describes such an example where OFC encoding of prospective odor cues was impaired in rats with hippocampal lesions. For this purpose, the specific method used earlier is especially well-suited to the problem of behavioral correlates. In studies of the OFC-ABL circuit, a unilateral manipulation of the amygdala (or OFC) was sufficient to reveal substantial changes in the encoding function of the interconnected region. The advantage here is that a unilateral intervention, whether lesion or reversible inactivation, is insufficient to alter task performance so that information processing at ipsilateral recording sites can be studied and compared to the intact brain without behavioral confounds. In this manner, a number of interesting hypotheses concerning the encoding of behavioral correlates in OFC could be tested.

Similar to research on the function of the OFC-ABL circuit, studies of other brain regions that interface with OFC are also amenable to comparative investigation across species. For example, in primates similar reciprocal connections exist between OFC and PPC[84,138,139] to those described in rodents with some demonstrated functional homology (e.g., Refs. 58 and 120). Further, PPC neurons in primates, which exhibit selective activity for spatial locations that are the target of behavioral responses, were recently observed to be modulated by expected reward value, e.g., amount and probability,[140,141] suggesting that OFC may contribute to reward-dependent modulation in PPC. Just as the components of the OFC-ABL circuit have reciprocal influences, the functional interactions between PPC and OFC are also likely to be reciprocal.

To complete a network in which OFC can effectively participate in overt behavioral responding, some connection between OFC and motor-related areas, either direct or indirect, is necessary. In primate, although direct connections exist between OFC and motor-related areas, they are much more sparse than those from sensory-related areas.[84] However, OFC can gain an indirect access to motor cortices via other prefrontal areas, such as DLPFC.[72,81,142] According to Fuster,[143,144] DLPFC, as a high level component in the motor hierarchy, provides the executive network to temporally integrate and organize information and preparatory sets for behavioral actions. In primates, Wallis and Miller[45] found that outcome expectancy is evident earlier in OFC than in DLPFC but that action correlates are then only observed in DLPFC. This finding supports the notion that OFC may generate outcome expectancy and provide such information to other brain areas, such as DLPFC, for decision and response selection.[8,45,55] By this account, correlates in OFC would provide a representation of behavioral responses useful in guiding performance but not essential for behavioral choice. The relevance of the research on primate DLPFC and OFC interactions to the rodent is not straightforward. Although still controversial, it has been proposed that rat medial prefrontal cortex (MPFC), including PrL/IL, anterior cingulate cortex, and PrC_m, shares functional homology with DLPFC in the primate brain.[145,146] In support of that idea, lesions of rat MPFC reveal some deficits that resemble those produced by lesions of primate DLPFC, for example, in spatial and temporal processing, working memory and monitoring, strategy selection, and flexible switching.[124,128,130,131,143,144,147–154] Nonetheless, research that is more closely modeled on the primate studies of DLPFC-OFC, including task intervals in which response preparation can be isolated, will be needed to better define the network for choice and decision making in the rodent brain, including pathways through which OFC plays a role.

CONCLUDING REMARKS

The role of OFC processing in behavioral guidance is not limited to encoding of outcome expectancy and reward-related information in behavioral tasks. We discuss the recently described features of OFC neurons that appear related to encoding for location, or the specification of movement to get there. Although the content of these correlates is currently difficult to characterize with certainty, it is clear that parallel and largely independent populations of neurons exhibit outcome- and response-related selectivity within OFC. Such independence of encoding might allow for more flexible use of associative information in behavioral guidance. This encoding also points to a large-scale neurocognitive network, involving OFC, for the spatiotemporal organization of goal-directed behavior.

ACKNOWLEDGMENTS

This article was supported by the grant to M.G. from the NIMH (R01-MH060 179) and a research fellowship to T.F. from the Uehara Memorial Foundation in Japan.

REFERENCES

1. BECHARA, A., H. DAMASIO & A.R. DAMASIO. 2000. Emotion, decision making and the orbitofrontal cortex. Cereb. Cortex **10:** 295–307.
2. ROLLS, E.T. 2000. The orbitofrontal cortex and reward. Cereb. Cortex **10:** 284–294.
3. BAXTER, M.G. & E.A. MURRAY. 2002. The amygdala and reward. Nat. Rev. Neurosci. **3:** 563–573.
4. HOLLAND, P.C. & M. GALLAGHER. 2004. Amygdala-frontal interactions and reward expectancy. Curr. Opin. Neurobiol. **14:** 148–155.
5. ROBERTS, A.C. 2006. Primate orbitofrontal cortex and adaptive behavior. Trends Cogn. Sci. **10:** 83–90.
6. SCHOENBAUM, G., M.R. ROESCH & T.A. STALNAKER. 2006. Orbitofrontal cortex, decision-making and drug addiction. Trends Neurosci. **29:** 116–124.
7. SCHULTZ, W. 2006. Behavioral theories and the neurophysiology of reward. Annu. Rev. Psychol. **57:** 87–115.
8. WALLIS, J.D. 2007. Orbitofrontal cortex and its contribution to decision-making. Annu. Rev. Neurosci. **30:** 31–56.
9. DOLAN, R.J. 2007. The human amygdala and orbital prefrontal cortex in behavioural regulation. Phil. Trans. R. Soc. B **362:** 787–799.
10. BUTTER, C.M. 1969. Perseveration in extinction and in discrimination reversal tasks following selective frontal ablations in macaca mulatta. Physiol. Behav. **4:** 163–171.
11. IVERSEN, S.D. & M. MISHKIN. 1970. Perseverative interference in monkeys following selective lesions in the inferior prefrontal convexity. Exp. Brain Res. **11:** 376–386.
12. DIAS, R., T.W. ROBBINS & A.C. ROBERTS. 1996. Dissociation in prefrontal cortex of affective and attentional shifts. Nature **380:** 69–72.
13. SCHOENBAUM, G., S.L. NUGENT, M.P. SADDORIS, *et al.* 2002. Orbitofrontal lesions in rats impair reversal but not acquisition of go, no-go odor discriminations. Neuroreport **13:** 885–890.

14. SCHOENBAUM, G., B. SETLOW, S.L. NUGENT, *et al.* 2003. Lesions of orbitofrontal cortex and basolateral amygdala complex disrupt acquisition of odor-guided discriminations and reversals. Learn. Mem. **10:** 129–140.
15. CHUDASAMA, Y. & T.W. ROBBINS. 2003. Dissociable contributions of the orbitofrontal and infralimbic cortex to Pavlovian autoshaping and discrimination reversal learning: Further evidence for the functional heterogeneity of the rodent frontal cortex. J. Neurosci. **23:** 8771–8780.
16. MCALONAN, K. & V.J. BROWN. 2003. Orbital prefrontal cortex mediates reversal learning and not attentional set shifting in the rat. Behav. Brain Res. **146:** 97–103.
17. IZQUIERDO, A., R.K. SUDA & E.A. MURRAY. 2004. Bilateral orbital prefrontal cortex lesions in rhesus monkeys disrupt choices guided by both reward value and reward contingency. J. Neurosci. **24:** 7540–7548.
18. KIM, J. & M.E. RAGOZZINO. 2005. The involvement of the orbitofrontal cortex in learning under changing task contingencies. Neurobiol. Learn. Mem. **83:** 125–133.
19. BOULOUGOURIS, V., J.W. DALLEY & T.W. ROBBINS. 2007. Effects of orbitofrontal, infralimbic and prelimbic cortical lesions on serial spatial reversal learning in the rat. Behav. Brain Res. **179:** 219–228.
20. GALLAGHER, M., R.W. MCMAHAN & G. SCHOENBAUM. 1999. Orbitofrontal cortex and representation of incentive value in associative learning. J. Neurosci. **19:** 6610–6614.
21. BAXTER, M.G., A. PARKER, C.C. LINDNER, *et al.* 2000. Control of response selection by reinforcer value requires interaction of amygdala and orbital prefrontal cortex. J. Neurosci. **20:** 4311–4319.
22. PICKENS, C.L., M.P. SADDORIS, B. SETLOW, *et al.* 2003. Different roles for orbitofrontal cortex and basolateral amygdala in a reinforcer devaluation task. J. Neurosci. **23:** 11078–11084.
23. PICKENS, C.L., M.P. SADDORIS, M. GALLAGHER, *et al.* 2005. Orbitofrontal lesions impair use of cue-outcome associations in a devaluation task. Behav. Neurosci. **119:** 317–322.
24. MCDANNALD, M.A., M.P. SADDORIS, M. GALLAGHER, *et al.* 2005. Lesions of orbitofrontal cortex impair rats' differential outcome expectancy learning but not conditioned stimulus-potentiated feeding. J. Neurosci. **25:** 4626–4632.
25. BECHARA, A., H. DAMASIO, D. TRANEL, *et al.* 1997. Deciding advantageously before knowing the advantageous strategy. Science **275:** 1293–1295.
26. BECHARA, A., H. DAMASIO, A.R. DAMASIO, *et al.* 1999. Different contributions of the human amygdala and ventromedial prefrontal cortex to decision-making. J. Neurosci. **19:** 5473–5481.
27. NIKI, H., M. SAKAI & K. KUBOTA. 1972. Delayed alternation performance and unit activity of the caudate head and medial orbitofrontal gyrus in the monkey. Brain Res. **38:** 343–353.
28. ROSENKILDE, C.E., R.H. BAUER & J.M. FUSTER. 1981. Single cell activity in ventral prefrontal cortex of behaving monkeys. Brain Res. **209:** 375–394.
29. THORPE, S.J., E.T. ROLLS & S. MADDISON. 1983. The orbitofrontal cortex: neuronal activity in the behaving monkey. Exp. Brain Res. **49:** 93–115.
30. ROLLS, E.T. 1989. Information processing in the taste system of primates. J. Exp. Biol. **146:** 141–164.
31. SCHOENBAUM, G. & H. EICHENBAUM. 1995. Information coding in the rodent prefrontal cortex. I. Single-neuron activity in orbitofrontal cortex compared with that in pyriform cortex. J. Neurophys. **74:** 733–750.

32. ROLLS, E.T., H.D. CRITCHLEY, R. MASON, *et al.* 1996. Orbitofrontal cortex neurons: role in olfactory and visual association learning. J. Neurophys. **75:** 1970–1981.

33. CRITCHLEY, H.D. & E.T. ROLLS. 1996. Hunger and satiety modify the responses of olfactory and visual neurons in the primate orbitofrontal cortex. J. Neurophys. **75:** 1673–1686.

34. SCHOENBAUM, G., A.A. CHIBA & M. GALLAGHER. 1998. Orbitofrontal cortex and basolateral amygdala encode expected outcomes during learning. Nat. Neurosci. **1:** 155–159.

35. SCHOENBAUM, G., A.A. CHIBA & M. GALLAGHER. 1999. Neural encoding in orbitofrontal cortex and basolateral amygdala during olfactory discrimination learning. J. Neurosci. **19:** 1876–1884.

36. LIPTON, P.A., P. ALVAREZ & H. EICHENBAUM. 1999. Crossmodal associative memory representations in rodent orbitofrontal cortex. Neuron **22:** 349–359.

37. TREMBLAY, L. & W. SCHULTZ. 1999. Relative reward preference in primate orbitofrontal cortex. Nature **398:** 704–708.

38. TREMBLAY, L. & W. SCHULTZ. 2000. Reward-related neuronal activity during go-nogo task performance in primate orbitofrontal cortex. J. Neurophys. **83:** 1864–1876.

39. RAMUS, S.J. & H. EICHENBAUM. 2000. Neural correlates of olfactory recognition memory in the rat olfactory cortex. J. Neurosci. **20:** 8199–8208.

40. HIKOSAKA, K. & M. WATANABE. 2000. Delay activity of orbital and lateral prefrontal neurons of the monkey varying with different rewards. Cereb. Cortex **10:** 263–271.

41. YONEMORI, M., H. NISHIJO, T. UWANO, *et al.* 2000. Orbital cortex neuronal responses during an odor-based conditioned associative task in rats. Neuroscience **95:** 691–703.

42. WALLIS, J.D. & E.K. MILLER. 2001. Single neurons in prefrontal cortex encode abstract rules. Nature **411:** 953–956.

43. ALVAREZ, P. & H. EICHENBAUM. 2002. Representations of odors in the rat orbitofrontal cortex change during and after learning. Behav. Neurosci. **116:** 421–433.

44. SCHOENBAUM, G., B. SETLOW, M.P. SADDORIS, *et al.* 2003. Encoding predicted outcome and acquired value in orbitofrontal cortex during cue sampling depends upon input from basolateral amygdala. Neuron **39:** 855–867.

45. WALLIS, J.D. & E.K. MILLER. 2003. Neuronal activity in primate dorsolateral and orbital prefrontal cortex during performance of a reward preference task. Eur. J. Neurosci. **18:** 2069–2081.

46. ROESCH, M.R. & C.R. OLSON. 2004. Neuronal activity related to reward value and motivation in primate frontal cortex. Science **304:** 307–310.

47. XIANG, J.-Z. & M.W. BROWN. 2004. Neuronal responses related to long-term recognition memory processes in prefrontal cortex. Neuron **42:** 817–829.

48. ROESCH, M.R. & C.R. OLSON. 2005. Neuronal activity in primate orbitofrontal cortex reflects the value of time. J. Neurophys. **94:** 2457–2471.

49. HOSOKAWA, T., K. KATO, M. INOUE, *et al.* 2005. Correspondence of cue activity to reward activity in the macaque orbitofrontal cortex. Neuroreport **389:** 146–151.

50. PADOA-SCHIOPPA, C. & J.A. ASSAD. 2006. Neurons in the orbitofrontal cortex encode economic value. Nature **441:** 223–226.

51. ICHIHARA-TAKEDA, S. & S. FUNAHASHI. 2006. Reward-period activity in primate dorsolateral prefrontal and orbitofrontal neurons is affected by reward schedules. J. Cogn. Neurosci. **18:** 212–226.
52. FEIERSTEIN, C.E., M.C. QUIRK, N. UCHIDA, et al. 2006. Representation of spatial goals in rat orbitofrontal cortex. Neuron **51:** 495–507.
53. ROESCH, M.R., A.R. TAYLOR & G. SCHOENBAUM. 2006. Encoding of time-discounted rewards in orbitofrontal cortex is independent of value representation. Neuron **51:** 509–520.
54. FURUYASHIKI, F., A.T. EHRLICH, P.C. HOLLAND & M. GALLAGHER. 2007. The rodent orbitofrontal cortex maintains outcome expectancy, while transiently encoding the stimulus and the behavioral response, during goal-directed behavior [abstract]. Soc. Neurosci. Abstracts.
55. HOLLERMAN, J.R., L. TREMBLAY & W. SCHULTZ. 2000. Involvement of basal ganglia and orbitofrontal cortex in goal-directed behavior. Prog. Brain Res. **126:** 193–215.
56. KOLB, B., A.J. NONNEMAN & R.K. SINGH. 1974. Double dissociation of spatial impairments and perseveration following selective prefrontal lesions in rats. J. Comp. Physiol. Psychol. **87:** 772–780.
57. EICHENBAUM, H., R.A. CLEGG & A. FEELEY. 1983. Reexamination of functional subdivisions of the rodent prefrontal cortex. Exp. Neurol. **79:** 434–451.
58. KOLB, B. 1984. Functions of the frontal cortex of the rat: A comparative review. Brain Res. Rev. **8:** 65–98.
59. OTTO, T. & H. EICHENBAUM. 1992. Complementary roles of the orbital prefrontal cortex and the perirhinal-entorhinal cortices in an odor-guided delayed-nonmatching-to-sample task. Behav. Neurosci. **106:** 762–775.
60. MISHKIN, M. & F.J. MANNING. 1978. Non-spatial memory after selective prefrontal lesions in monkeys. Brain Res. **143:** 313–323.
61. MEUNIER, M., J. BACHEVALIER & M. MISHKIN. 1997. Effects of orbital frontal and anterior cingulate lesions on object and spatial memory in rhesus monkeys. Neuropsychologia **35:** 999–1015.
62. KRETTEK, J.E. & J.L. PRICE. 1977. The cortical projections of the mediodorsal nucleus and adjacent thalamic nuclei in the rat. J. Comp. Neurol. **171:** 157–192.
63. DEACON, T.W., H. EICHENBAUM, P. ROSENBERG, et al. Afferent connections of the perirhinal cortex in the rat. J. Comp. Neurol. **220:** 168–190.
64. GROENEWEGEN, H.J. 1988. Organization of the afferent connections of the mediodorsal thalamic nucleus in the rat, related to the mediodorsal-prefrontal topography. Neuroscience **24:** 379–431.
65. PRICE, J.L., B.M. SLOTNICK & M.-F. REVIAL. 1991. Olfactory projections to the hypothalamus. J. Comp. Neurol. **306:** 447–461.
66. RAY, J.P. & J.L. PRICE. 1992. The organization of the thalamocortical connections of the mediodorsal thalamic nucleus in the rat, related to the ventral forebrain-prefrontal cortex topography. J. Comp. Neurol. **323:** 167–197.
67. INSAUSTI, R., M.T. HERRERO & M.P. WITTER. 1997. Entorhinal cortex of the rat: cytoarchitectonic subdivisions and the origin and distribution of cortical efferents. Hippocampus **7:** 146–183.
68. MCDONALD, A.J. 1998. Cortical pathways to the mammalian amygdala. Prog. Neurobiol. **55:** 257–332.
69. BURWELL, R.D. & D.G. AMARAL. Cortical afferents of the perirhinal, postrhinal, and entorhinal cortices of the rat. J. Comp. Neurol. **398:** 179–205.

70. DELATOUR, B. & M.P. WITTER. 2002. Projections from the parahippocampal region to the prefrontal cortex in the rat: evidence of multiple pathways. Eur. J. Neurosci. **15:** 1400–1407.

71. BARBAS, H. & J. DE OLMOS. 1990. Projections from the amygdala to basoventral and mediodorsal prefrontal regions in the rhesus monkey. J. Comp. Neurol. **300:** 549–571.

72. MORECRAFT, R.J., C. GEULA & M.-M. MESULAM. 1992. Cytoarchitecture and neural afferents of orbitofrontal cortex in the brain of the monkey. J. Comp. Neurol. **323:** 341–358.

73. RAY, J.P. & J.L. PRICE. 1993. The organization of projections from the mediodorsal nucleus of the thalamus to orbital and medial prefrontal cortex in macaque monkeys. J. Comp. Neurol. **337:** 1–31.

74. SUZUKI, W.A. & D.G. AMARAL. 1994. Perirhinal and parahippocampal cortices of the macaque monkey: Cortical afferents. J. Comp. Neurol. **350:** 497–533.

75. CARMICHAEL, S.T. & J.L. PRICE. 1995. Limbic connections of the orbital and medial prefrontal cortex in macaque monkeys. J. Comp. Neurol. **363:** 615–641.

76. REEP, R.L., J.V. CORWIN & V. KING. 1996. Neuronal connections of orbital cortex in rats: topography of cortical and thalamic afferents. Exp. Brain Res. **111:** 215–232.

77. REMPEL-CLOWER, N.L. & H. BARBAS. 1998. Topographic organization of connections between the hypothalamus and prefrontal cortex in the rhesus monkey. J. Comp. Neurol. **398:** 393–419.

78. LAVENEX, P., W.A. SUZUKI & D.G. AMARAL. 2002. Perirhinal and parahippocampal cortices of the macaque monkey: Projections to the neocortex. J. Comp. Neurol. **447:** 394–420.

79. GHASHGHAEI, H.T. & H. BARBAS. 2002. Pathways for emotion: interactions of prefrontal and anterior temporal pathways in the amygdala of the rhesus monkey. Neuroscience **115:** 1261–1279.

80. BARBAS, H. 1988. Anatomic organization of basoventral and mediodorsal visual recipient prefrontal regions in the rhesus monkey. J. Comp. Neurol. **276:** 313–342.

81. BARBAS, H. & D.N. PANDYA. 1989. Architecture and intrinsic connections of the prefrontal cortex in the rhesus monkey. J. Comp. Neurol. **286:** 353–375.

82. BARBAS, H. 1993. Organization of cortical afferent input to orbitofrontal areas in the rhesus monkey. Neuroscience **56:** 841–864.

83. CARMICHAEL, S.T., M.-C. CLUGNET & J.L. PRICE. 1994. Central olfactory connections in the macaque monkey. J. Comp. Neurol. **346:** 403–434.

84. CARMICHAEL, S.T. & J.L. PRICE. 1995. Sensory and premotor connections of the orbital and medial prefrontal cortex of macaque monkeys. J. Comp. Neurol. **363:** 642–664.

85. CARMICHAEL, S.T. & J.L. PRICE. 1996. Connectional networks within the orbital and medial prefrontal cortex of macaque monkeys. J. Comp. Neurol. **371:** 179–207.

86. WEBSTER, M.J., J. BACHEVALIER & L.G. UNGERLEIDER. 1994. Connections of inferior temporal areas TEO and TE with parietal and frontal cortex in macaque monkeys. Cereb. Cortex **5:** 470–483.

87. TREMBLAY, L. & W. SCHULTZ. 2000. Modifications of reward expectation-related neuronal activity during learning in primate orbitofrontal cortex. J. Neurophys. **83:** 1877–1885.

88. RAINER, G. & E.K. MILLER. 2000. Effects of visual experience on the representation of objects in the prefrontal cortex. Neuron **27:** 179–189.
89. HATFIELD, T., J.-S. HAN, M. CONLEY, *et al.* 1996. Neurotoxic lesions of basolateral, but not central, amygdala interfere with Pavlovian second-order conditioning and reinforcer devaluation effects. J. Neurosci. **16:** 5256–5265.
90. MÁLKOVÁ, L., D. GAFFAN & E.A. MURRAY. 1997. Excitotoxic lesions of the amygdala fail to produce impairment in visual learning for auditory secondary reinforcement but interfere with reinforcer devaluation effects in rhesus monkeys. J. Neurosci. **17:** 6011–6020.
91. BLUNDELL, P., G. HALL & S. KILLCROSS. 2001. Lesions of the basolateral amygdala disrupt selective aspects of reinforcer representation in rats. J. Neurosci. **21:** 9018–9026.
92. CORBIT, L.H. & B.W. BALLEINE. 2005. Double dissociation of basolateral and central amygdala lesions on the general and outcome-specific forms of Pavlovian-instrumental transfer. J. Neurosci. **25:** 962–970.
93. WELLMAN, L.L., K. GALE & L. MÁLKOVÁ. 2005. GABAA-mediated inhibition of basolateral amygdala blocks reward devaluation in macaques. J. Neurosci. **25:** 4577–4586.
94. OSTLUND, S.B. & B.W. BALLEINE. 2007. Orbitofrontal cortex mediates outcome encoding in Pavlovian but not instrumental conditioning. J. Neurosci. **27:** 4819–4825.
95. STALNAKER, T.A., T.M. FRANZ, T. SINGH, *et al.* 2007. Basolateral amygdala lesions abolish orbitofrontal-dependent reversal impairments. Neuron **54:** 51–58.
96. VERWER, R.W., R.J. MEIJER, H.F. VAN UUM, *et al.* 1997. Collateral projections from the rat hippocampal formation to the lateral and medial prefrontal cortex. Hippocampus **7:** 397–402.
97. JAY, T.M. & M.P. WITTER. 1991. Distribution of hippocampal CA1 and subicular efferents in the prefrontal cortex of the rat studied by means of anterograde transport of *Phaseolus vulgaris*-Leucoagglutinin. J. Comp. Neurol. **313:** 574–586.
98. O'KEEFE, J. 1979. A review of the hippocampal place cells. Prog. Neurobiol. **13:** 419–439.
99. MULLER, R. 1996. A quarter of a century of place cells. Neuron **17:** 979–990.
100. KNIERIM, J.J., I. LEE & E.L. HARGREAVES. 2006. Hippocampal place cells: parallel input streams, subregional processing, and implications for episodic memory. Hippocampus **16:** 755–764.
101. MCNAUGHTON B.L., F.P. BATTAGLIA, O. JENSEN, *et al.* 2006. Path integration and the neural basis of the 'cognitive map'. Nat. Rev. Neurosci. **7:** 663–678.
102. FRANK, L.M., E.N. BROWN & M. WILSON. 2000. Trajectory encoding in the hippocampus and entorhinal cortex. Neuron **27:** 169–178.
103. HARGREAVES, E.L., G. RAO, I. LEE, *et al.* 2005. Major dissociation between medial and lateral entorhinal input to dorsal hippocampus. Science **308:** 1792–1794.
104. HAFTING, T., M. FYHN, S. MOLDEN, *et al.* 2005. Microstructure of a spatial map in the entorhinal cortex. Nature **436:** 801–806.
105. SARGOLINI, F., M. FYHN, T. HAFTING, *et al.* 2007. Conjunctive representation of position, direction, and velocity in entorhinal cortex. Science **312:** 758–762.
106. SWANSON, L.A. 1981. A direct projection from Ammon's horn to prefrontal cortex in the rat. Brain Res. **217:** 150–154.

107. SESACK, S.R., A.Y. DEUTCH, R.H. ROTH, *et al.* 1989. Topographical organization of the efferent projections of the medial prefrontal cortex in the rat: an antero-grade tract-tracing study with *Phaseolus vulgaris* leucoagglutinin. J. Comp. Neurol. **290:** 213–242.

108. TAKAGISHI, M. & T. CHIBA. 1991. Efferent connections of the infralimbic (area 25) region of the medial prefrontal cortex in the rat: an anterograde tracer PHA-L study. Brain Res. **566:** 26–39.

109. CONDÉ, F., E. MAIRE-LEPOIVRE, E. AUDINAT, *et al.* 1995. Afferent connections of the medial frontal cortex of the rat. II. Cortical and subcortical afferents. J. Comp. Neurol. **352:** 567–593.

110. THIERRY, A.-M., Y. GIOANNI, E. DÉGÉNÉTAIS, *et al.* 2000. Hippocampo-prefrontal cortex pathways: anatomical and electrophysiological characteristics. Hippocampus **10:** 411–419.

111. HOK, V., E. SAVE, P.P. LENCK-SANTINI, *et al.* 2005. Coding for spatial goals in the prelimbic/infralimbic area of the rat frontal cortex. Proc. Natl. Acad. Sci. USA **102:** 4602–4607.

112. POUCET, B. 1997. Searching for spatial unit firing in the prelimbic area of the rat medial prefrontal cortex. Behav. Brain Res. **84:** 151–159.

113. JUNG, M.W., Y. QIN, B.L. MCNAUGHTON, *et al.* 1998. Firing characteristics of deep layer neurons in prefrontal cortex in rats performing spatial working memory tasks. Cereb. Cortex **8:** 437–450.

114. PRATT, W.E. & S.J. MIZUMORI. 2001. Neurons in rat medial prefrontal cortex show anticipatory rate changes to predictable differential rewards in a spatial memory task. Behav. Brain Res. **123:** 165–183.

115. REEP, R.L., J.V. CORWIN, A. HASHIMOTO, *et al.* 1984. Afferent connections of medial precentral cortex in the rat. Neurosci. Lett. **44:** 247–252.

116. REEP, R.L., J.V. CORWIN, A. HASHIMOTO, *et al.* 1987. Efferent connections of the rostral portion of medial agranular cortex in rats. Brain Res. Bull. **19:** 203–221.

117. REEP, R.L., G.S. GOODWIN & J.V. CORWIN. 1990. Topographic organization in the corticocortical connections of medial agranular cortex in rats. J. Comp. Neurol. **294:** 262–280.

118. REEP, R.L., H.C. CHANDLER, V. KING, *et al.* 1994. Rat posterior parietal cortex: topography of corticocortical and thalamic connections. Exp. Brain Res. **100:** 67–84.

119. MILLER, M.W. & B.A. VOGT. 1984. Direct connections of rat visual cortex with sensory, motor, and association cortices. J. Comp. Neurol. **226:** 184–202.

120. KOLB, B. & J. WALKEY. 1987. Behavioural and anatomical studies of the posterior parietal cortex in the rat. Behav. Brain Res. **23:** 127–145.

121. BURCHAM, K.J., J.V. CORWIN, M.L. STOLL, *et al.* 1997. Disconnection of medial agranular and posterior parietal cortex produces multimodal neglect in rats. Behav. Brain Res. **86:** 41–47.

122. CROWNE, D.P. & M.N. PATHRIA. 1982. Some attentional effects of unilateral frontal lesions in the rat. Behav. Brain Res. **6:** 25–39.

123. CROWNE, D.P., C.M. RICHARDSON & K.A. DAWSON. 1986. Parietal and frontal eye field neglect in the rat. Behav. Brain Res. **22:** 227–231.

124. KESNER, R.P., G. FARNSWORTH & B.V. DIMATTIA. 1989. Double dissociation of egocentric and allocentric space following medial prefrontal and parietal cortex lesions in the rat. Behav. Neurosci. **103:** 956–961.

125. KING, V.R. & J.V. CORWIN. 1992. Spatial deficits and hemispheric asymmetries in the rat following unilateral and bilateral lesions of posterior parietal or medial agranular cortex. Behav. Brain Res. **50:** 53–68.

126. KING, V.R. & J.V. CORWIN. 1993. Comparisons of hemi-inattention produced by unilateral lesions of the posterior parietal cortex or medial agranular prefrontal cortex in rats: neglect, extinction, and the role of stimulus distance. Behav. Brain Res. **54:** 117–131.

127. CORWIN, J.V., M. FUSSINGER, R.C. MEYER, et al. 1994. Bilateral destruction of the ventrolateral orbital cortex produces allocentric but not egocentric deficits in rats. Behav. Brain Res. **61:** 79–86.

128. KOLB, B., K. BUHRMANN, R. MCDONALD, et al. 1994. Dissociation of the medial prefrontal, posterior parietal, and posterior temporal cortex for spatial navigation and recognition memory in the rat. Cereb. Cortex **6:** 664–680.

129. SAVE, E. & M. MOGHADDAM. 1996. Effects of lesions of the associative parietal cortex on the acquisition and use of spatial memory in egocentric and allocentric navigation tasks in the rat. Behav. Neurosci. **110:** 74–85.

130. KESNER, R.P., M.E. HUNT, J.M. WILLIAMS, et al. 1996. Prefrontal cortex and working memory for spatial response, spatial location, and visual object information in the rat. Cereb. Cortex **6:** 311–318.

131. RAGOZZINO, M.E. & R.P. KESNER. 2001. The role of rat dorsomedial prefrontal cortex in working memory for egocentric responses. Neurosci. Lett. **308:** 145–148.

132. VAFAEI, A.A. & A. RASHIDY-POUR. 2004. Reversible lesion of the rat's orbitofrontal cortex interferes with hippocampus-dependent spatial memory. Behav. Brain Res. **149:** 61–68.

133. MCNAUGHTON, B.L., S.J. MIZUMORI, C.A. BARNES, et al. 1994. Cortical representation of motion during unrestrained spatial navigation in the rat. Cereb. Cortex **4:** 27–39.

134. CHEN, L.L., L.-H. LIN, E.J. GREEN, et al. 1994. Head-direction cells in the rat posterior cortex. I. Anatomical distribution and behavioral modulation. Exp. Brain Res. **101:** 8–23.

135. NITZ, D.A. 2006. Tracking route progression in the posterior parietal cortex. Neuron **49:** 747–756.

136. SADDORIS, M.P., M. GALLAGHER & G. SCHOENBAUM. 2005. Rapid associative encoding in basolateral amygdala depends on connections with orbitofrontal cortex. Neuron **46:** 321–331.

137. RAMUS, S.J., J.B. DAVIS, R.J. DONAHUE, et al. 2007. Interactions between the orbitofrontal cortex and hippocampal memory system during the storage of long-term memory. Ann. N.Y. Acad. Sci. This volume.

138. CAVADA, C. & P.S. GOLDMAN-RAKIC. 1989. Posterior parietal cortex in rhesus monkey: II. Evidence for segregated corticocortical networks linking sensory and limbic areas with the frontal lobe. J. Comp. Neurol. **287:** 422–445.

139. ANDERSEN, R.A., C. ASANUMA, G. ESSICK, et al. 1990. Corticocortical connections of anatomically and physiologically defined subdivisions within the inferior parietal lobule. J. Comp. Neurol. **296:** 65–113.

140. PLATT, M.L. & P.W. GLIMCHER. 1999. Neural correlates of decision variables in parietal cortex. Nature **400:** 233–238.

141. SUGRUE, L.P., G.S.CORRADO & W.T. NEWSOME. 2004. Matching behavior and the representation of value in the parietal cortex. Science **304:** 1782–1787.

142. PANDYA, D.N. & E.H. YETERIAN. 1990. Prefrontal cortex in relation to other cortical areas in rhesus monkey: architecture and connections. Prog. Brain Res. **85:** 63–94.

143. FUSTER, J.M. 1997. The Prefrontal Cortex: Anatomy, Physiology, and Neuropsychology of the Frontal Lobe, 3rd ed. Lippincott-Raven. Philadelphia.

144. FUSTER, J.M. 2001. The prefrontal cortex—an update: time is of essence. Neuron **30**: 319–333.
145. UYLINGS, H.B., H.J. GROENEWEGEN & B. KOLB. 2003. Do rats have a prefrontal cortex? Behav. Brain Res. **146**: 3–17.
146. VERTES, R.P. 2006. Interactions among the medial prefrontal cortex, hippocampus and midline thalamus in emotional and cognitive processing in the rat. Neuroscience **142**: 1–20.
147. RAGOZZINO, M.E., S. DETRICK & R.P. KESNER. 1999. Involvement of the prelimbic-infralimbic areas of the rodent prefrontal cortex in behavioral flexibility for place and response learning. J. Neurosci. **19**: 4585–4594.
148. BIRRELL, J.M. & V.J. BROWN. 2000. Medial frontal cortex mediates perceptual attentional set shifting in the rat. J. Neurosci. **20**: 4320–4324.
149. RAGOZZINO, M.E., S. DETRICK & R.P. KESNER. 2002. The effects of prelimbic and infralimbic lesions on working memory for visual objects in rats. Neurobiol. Learn. Mem. **77**: 29–43.
150. HANNESSON, D.K., J.G. HOWLAND & A.G. PHILLIPS. 2004. Interaction between perirhinal and medial prefrontal cortex is required for temporal order but not recognition memory for objects in rats. J. Neurosci. **24**: 4596–4604.
151. MISHKIN, M. 1964. Perseveration of central sets after frontal lesions in monkeys. *In* The Frontal Granular Cortex and Behavior. J.M. Warren & K. Akert, Eds.: 219–241. McGraw-Hill. New York.
152. GOLDMAN-RAKIC, P.S. 1996. The prefrontal landscape: implications of functional architecture for understanding human mentation and the central executive. Phil. Trans. R. Soc. Lond. B **351**: 1445–1453.
153. SHALLICE, T. & P. BURGESS. 1996. The domain of supervisory process and temporal organization of behavior. Phil. Trans. R. Soc. Lond. B **351**: 1405–1412.
154. PETRIDES, M. 2005. Lateral prefrontal cortex: architectonic and functional organization. Phil. Trans. R. Soc. B **360**: 781–795.

Interactions between the Orbitofrontal Cortex and the Hippocampal Memory System during the Storage of Long-Term Memory

SETH J. RAMUS,[a,b] JENA B. DAVIS,[a] RACHEL J. DONAHUE,[a] CLAIRE B. DISCENZA,[a] AND ALISSA A. WAITE[a]

[a]*Program in Neuroscience and* [b]*Department of Psychology, Bowdoin College, Brunswick, Maine 04011, USA*

ABSTRACT: It has been proposed that long-term declarative memories are ultimately stored through interactions between the hippocampal memory system and the neocortical association areas that initially processed the to-be-stored information. One association neocortex, the orbitofrontal cortex (OFC) is strongly and reciprocally connected with the hippocampal memory system and plays an important role in odor recognition memory in rats. We will report data from two studies: one that examined the firing of neurons in a task dependent on the parahippocampal region (PHR; including the perirhinal, postrhinal, and entorhinal cortices), and one examined the firing of OFC neurons performing a task that is presumably dependent on the hippocampus. In the first study, we examined the role of OFC neurons in the continuous odor-guided nonmatching to sample task. While the firing of neurons in the PHR and OFC are similar in this task, there are several notable differences that are consistent with the idea that OFC is a high-order association cortex which interacts extensively with the PHR to store declarative memories. In the second study, we characterized the firing patterns of neurons in the OFC rats performing a passive, 8-odor-sequence memory task. Most interesting were neurons that fired selectively in anticipation of specific odors. We found that hippocampal lesions abolished the anticipatory firing in OFC, suggesting that these anticipatory responses (memory) were in fact dependent on the hippocampus, further supporting the view that the OFC interacts with the hippocampal memory system to store long-term, declarative memories.

KEYWORDS: rat; orbitofrontal cortex; neurophysiology; hippocampus; parahippocampal region; declarative memory

Address for correspondence: Seth J. Ramus, 6900 College Station, Brunswick, ME 04011. Voice: (207)725-3624; fax: (207)725-3892.
sramus@bowdoin.edu

Ann. N.Y. Acad. Sci. 1121: 216–231 (2007). © 2007 New York Academy of Sciences.
doi: 10.1196/annals.1401.038

In this chapter, we will present an approach to understanding the function of the orbitofrontal cortex (OFC) that is unique in this volume—we will examine how the OFC interacts with the hippocampus and surrounding parahippocampal region (PHR) during the acquisition and storage of long-term declarative memories in the rat. As noted in many chapters in this volume, the OFC is important for many kinds of learning including affective learning, discrimination learning, and rule learning. Further, the OFC is widely connected with many learning systems including the amygdala, basal ganglia and PHR, as well as widespread somatosensory and motor areas. Thus, the OFC can be viewed as a nexus for the integration of abstract information about cues, including their affective value, with behavioral outcomes. It should therefore not be surprising that the OFC also participates in the acquisition and storage of long-term declarative memories. In this chapter, we will first review evidence that the association neocortex should be considered part of a broader system for declarative memory. We will then present evidence from our laboratory that the OFC (an olfactory association neocortex in the rat) normally interacts with the PHR and the hippocampus during acquisition and performance of long-term memory tasks.

A BROADER SYSTEM FOR DECLARATIVE MEMORY

Long-term, declarative memory is mediated by a network of brain structures including the hippocampus, the PHR (including the entorhinal, perirhinal, and parahippocampal/postrhinal cortex), and widespread neocortical association areas.[1-3] Declarative memory is memory for facts and events, which are stored explicitly so that they are later available to conscious recollection.[4] This kind of memory has also been termed *episodic*[5] or *explicit* memory.[6] Despite the variety of terminology used to characterize this form of memory, there is consensus that the medial temporal lobes are important for the rapid formation and representation of episodes within a general semantic framework. These memories are available to conscious recollection and are able to be expressed 'flexibly,' that is, in a variety of contexts outside repetition of the learning event.[7,8] Recently, Ramus and Eichenbaum[3] have argued that the functions of the association neocortex are critical for normal declarative memory, and thus, should me considered part of the memory system.

The anatomical connectivity between areas of this memory network is illustrated in FIGURE 1. Understanding the connectivity of these regions has been extremely helpful in determining how the individual components of the system contribute to memory, and how they interact with one another. A large body of neuroanatomical tracer studies has outlined the neural pathways through the hippocampal memory system.[9-16] The pathways through this system are largely similar in rats and primates. Broadly outlined, information flow through the hippocampal memory system is marked by hierarchical stages of

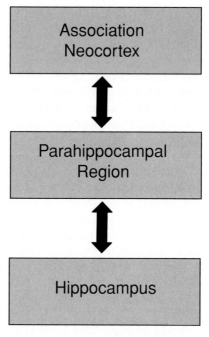

FIGURE 1. A schematic of a Broader Hippocampal Memory System. Widespread neocortical association areas (including the OFC and area TE) project to the PHR, which in turn provides the majority of the cortical input to the hippocampus. As the bi-directional arrows indicate, the hippocampus projects back to the association cortex via the PHR.

processing, involving convergence of information from neocortex to the PHR, then to the hippocampus. A corresponding set of back projections involves divergent projections from the hippocampus, returning to the PHR, which in turn sends major projections back to a several areas of the neocortex.[17] The projections to the PHR arise from virtually every neocortical association area[15,16] importantly including the OFC[13,18] (also see other chapters in this volume). Each of these cortical outputs projects to one or more subdivisions of the PHR.[19,20] All of the areas of the PHR in turn project to multiple subdivisions of the hippocampus itself, including the dentate gyrus, CA3, CA1, and subiculum. Thus, the PHR serves as a convergence site for cortical input and distributes these inputs within the hippocampus. The hippocampus supports mechanisms of plasticity that could mediate the rapid coding of new conjunctions of information[21] within its broadly convergent and divergent intrinsic connections.[22] The output from the hippocampus is directed back to the entire PHR and then to the same neocortical association areas from which the input originated.[15,16] This pattern of neuroanatomical pathways is consistent with the idea that there is a broad convergence of sensory information onto the hippocampal system. Furthermore, through back projections, the hippocampus and PHR are positioned to alter the nature, persistence, and organization of memory representations within the neocortex.

Several additional recent lines of evidence indicate that association neocortex should also be considered a part of this memory network.[3] First, recent human neuroimaging studies have suggested that the neocortex may normally interact with medial temporal lobe structures in memory storage and retrieval.[23–26] Notably, Gottfried *et al.*[27] have reported activation in both the anterior hippocampus and the piriform cortex during the successful retrieval of objects in an object-olfactory cross-modal recognition memory task. Second, damage to the hippocampus or PHR prevents the ability to form new long-term memories (anterograde amnesia), but spares short-term or immediate memory.[28] It is generally believed that the neocortical areas that send inputs to the hippocampus and PHR mediate this capacity for short-term memory and provide the gateway to the hippocampal system. Finally, damage to the hippocampus and PHR also results in a retrograde memory loss in humans and animals.[1,29,30] This temporally graded retrograde amnesia is characterized by impaired memory for recently acquired information with relative sparing of memories acquired a longer time before brain injury. This observation indicates that the hippocampus and PHR are not the final repository of memories. Rather, these regions must be considered as critical for the formation of long-term memories, but not as the final storage site. By this view, the role of the hippocampus and PHR is to facilitate the gradual establishment of long term memories elsewhere in the brain—a process called memory consolidation. The proposed ultimate storage site for long-term memory is the neocortical association areas that initially processed the information.[1,31]

Together, these findings suggest a functional organization for the broader hippocampal memory system, with three distinct but related levels of processing, specifically in the hippocampus, the PHR, and the association neocortex. According to the model proposed by Eichenbaum and others[1–3] the association neocortex is involved in the initial processing of memory information, including the brief maintenance of sensory representations. The PHR maintains these short-lived neocortical representations for an intermediate period of time via its direct bi-directional connections with the neocortex. Through these interconnections, persistent parahippocampal representations could likewise alter neocortical processing to reflect associations between events that are processed separately in different neocortical areas, or that are separated in time. The hippocampus, through its bi-directional connections with the PHR, is also privy to these sustained representations, as well as to the integration of information across time and functional domains of cortical processing. The hippocampus, in turn, contains the neural mechanisms for rapidly encoding the sequences of events that comprise episodic memory, linking these episodes by their common elements, which allows generalization between events and for representations to be linked over long periods of time. In other words, the neocortex itself can represent items for very brief periods. When the task demands that the item be remembered across a delay or distraction (e.g., in the delayed nonmatching to sample (DNMS) task, see below) the PHR is engaged. Finally, the hippocampus serves to bind multiple representations across space and time.

Our laboratory has sought to find evidence for this model of a broader hippocampal memory system. We have therefore examined the role of the OFC—a high-order olfactory association cortex in the rat—as a model of neocortical–hippocampal memory system interactions. The OFC in the rat plays a role in the representation and acquisition of odor memories[32,33] and in the representation of odors and their significance.[34–37] In the first section below, we will describe a study that examined the interactions between the OFC and PHR in the odor-guided DNMS task. In the next section, we will describe preliminary results from a study that examined the interaction between the OFC and the hippocampus in an odor-sequence learning task.

INTERACTIONS BETWEEN THE OFC AND PHR IN THE STORAGE OF LONG-TERM MEMORY

In the first series of studies[33] we examined the role of the OFC in the DNMS task, a task that depends on the PHR. The DNMS[38,39] has become a benchmark task of visual recognition memory in the monkey and has been especially important for understanding that the PHR has a role distinct in memory from that of the hippocampus.[28] Briefly, this task requires an animal to remember a 'sample' stimulus across a variable delay, and then to decide whether a 'choice' stimulus matches the 'sample.' Animals are initially trained at short delay intervals, and after reaching criterion-level performance are tested at progressively longer delays. Typically, monkeys with damage to all or part of the PHR do well remembering the sample when the memory delay interval is relatively short. However, when the delay is lengthened to increase memory demands, severe deficits emerge.[40,41]

Importantly, the pattern of deficits in DNMS performance is different following lesions of the PHR, the hippocampus, or the neocortex. In monkeys, deficits following PHR damage are more severe than those following damage limited to the hippocampus [42,43] or its primary subcortical input, the fornix.[44] By contrast, damage to visual association cortex (area TE) impairs learning of the task, even at the briefest of delays.[45] This latter finding suggests that area TE is involved in perceptual processes or short-term memory that are important for the performance of the DNMS rather than in long-term memory per se.

A similar pattern of results has been observed in parallel studies in rats using a continuous, odor-guided version of the DNMS. In these studies, rats with lesions of the PHR were able to learn the task at the normal rate and continued to perform well at the briefest delay intervals. However, these rats were impaired when the delay between sample and choice was lengthened beyond a few seconds, indicating a deficit in their ability to maintain the memory for the sample stimulus. Also, in rats, as in monkeys, damage to the hippocampus produces little or no deficit on nonspatial versions of the DNMS.[46–48] By contrast, rats with lesions of the OFC (here considered as an olfactory association neocortex) were impaired on the acquisition of the DNMS rule at the shortest delay intervals.[32] Taken together, these findings from monkeys and rats are consistent with the idea that the PHR maintains persistent representations for single items in memory during the delay interval, a central requirement for performance on the DNMS task. By contrast, the OFC (and TE in monkeys) are important for the acquisition of the basic DNMS rule. Thus, the DNMS is an ideal task for examining the interactions between the OFC and the PHR in recognition memory.

In the first study, we implanted stereotrode electrodes bilaterally into the OFC of rats (dorsal agranular insula, just dorsal to the rhinal fissure), and recorded while the animals learned and performed the 8-odor continuous version of DNMS.[33] Consistent with the idea that the OFC is important for DNMS performance, we found that nearly all of the cells recorded in the OFC (95.6% of the 276 neurons) fired in relation to one or more task events. The majority, 73% of neurons, were responsive during the delivery of water reward.

But we also found cells with both sensory and memory-related firing. Approximately 16% of the cells fired differentially during the odor-sampling period to each of the 8 odors used in the task. An example of an odor-specific, sensory response is illustrated in FIGURE 2. In addition, we found two types of memory-related responses. First, about half (49%) of the odor-selective cells also fired differently on match and nonmatch trials. In other words, the odor-specific response was modulated when the odor was repeated. Examples of odor-specific match enhancement and match suppression cells are shown in FIGURE 3. Thus, the neurons in the OFC are privy to whether an odor is the same as, or different than the previous odor. Second, about 5% of the cells recorded in OFC showed sustained, odor-specific firing during the delay interval, and an example of this kind of cell is shown in FIGURE 4. These cells therefore maintain a representation of the sample odor during the delay interval. Thus, the firing of OFC neurons reflect all of the critical elements for performance of the DNMS task—the identity of the odor cue, the identity of the previous odor, and the reward. In addition, we found cells that represented behavioral outcomes. For example, one relatively infrequent group of cells fired differentially when the rat was about to make an error of commission (*i.e.*, the cell "knew" that the odor was a match and that the rat was going to make an incorrect behavioral response).

Given that the OFC is highly and reciprocally interconnected with the PHR, it is not surprising that the sensory and memory responses described in the

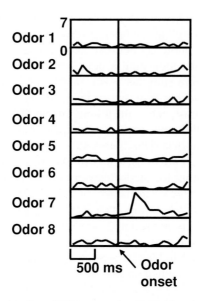

FIGURE 2.   Example of an OFC neuron that is highly odor-selective (sensory response). Activity of cell from 1 s before to 1.5 s after the odor onset for each of the 8 odors. Each box illustrates the average firing rate (spikes per second) of the cell to one of the 8 odors. This cell fires more strongly to odor 7 than to any of the other 7 odors. Adapted from Ramus and Eichenbaum.[33]

previous paragraph have also be described in the PHR during the same continuous odor-guided version of DNMS,[49] and long-lasting stimulus-specific suppression of neuronal firing to repeated stimuli have also been found in other studies.[50,51] Further, sustained delay activity and match enhancement and suppression have also been observed in the PHR of monkeys performing a visual delayed *matching* to sample task.[52,53] However, in this case, differences between the specific tasks used in rat and monkey studies (especially visual versus olfactory modality) make more direct comparisons difficult.[17]

However, there were two key differences between the firing of neurons in the OFC and PHR of rats of rats trained on the odor-guided DNMS, and these differences are illustrated in FIGURE 5. First, we found twice as many cells in the PHR that demonstrated sustained delay firing than we found in the OFC. By contrast, there were about twice as many cells in the OFC that demonstrated stimulus-selective match suppression or enhancement. Further, the proportion of these cells in OFC that displayed match suppression or match enhancement increased with increasing performance as the rat learned the DNMS task. Together with the finding that OFC lesions impair acquisition of the DNMS task,[32] the finding that OFC neurons prominently code the critical match/nonmatch judgment suggests that the OFC may play a key role in the abstraction and representation of the nonmatching rule.

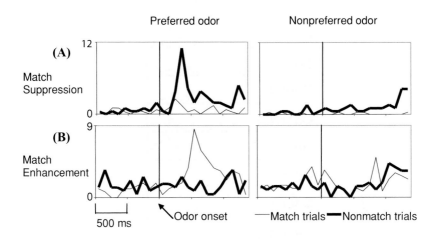

FIGURE 3. Two examples of OFC neurons that shows odor-specific modulation of firing when an odor is repeated (memory response). (**A**) Match Supression cell. This cell fires more robustly to the preferred odor on nonmatch trials than on match trials (*left*), but shows no modulation for a nonpreferred odor (*right*). (**B**) Match Enhancement cell. This cell fires more robustly to the preferred odor on match trials than on non-match trials (*left*), but shows no modulation for a nonpreferred odor. These cells represent the critical match/nonmatch judgment for the DNMS task. Adapted from Ramus and Eichenbaum.[33]

Second, the firing of cells in the OFC was more complex than the firing of cells recorded in the PHR—cells fired in relation to more task events or to complex behavioral states of the rat. Together, these findings from OFC neurons are consistent with the idea that the OFC is a "mixing pot" for sensory signals originating from piriform cortex and memory signals arising in the PHR. In fact, several neuroimaging reports suggest that the piriform cortex itself has interacts with the hippocampal memory system during cross-modal olfactory recognition memory tasks,[27,54] either through its indirect connections through the OFC or through direct inputs to components of the PHR. It would therefore be interesting to compare the firing patterns of piriform neurons to those recorded in OFC during the DNMS task (and also during the odor-sequence learning task described in the next section).

Taken together, our findings suggest that the OFC participates both in the memory representations for specific stimuli, and in the acquisition and application of task rules. Similar findings have been reported in the monkey lateral prefrontal cortex.[55] Although task and species differences make direct comparison to the rodent work difficult, Miller has come to similar conclusions about the role of prefrontal cortex in recognition memory performance.[56] Our work further supports the idea that the OFC normally interacts with the PHR during the acquisition and storage of long-term memories

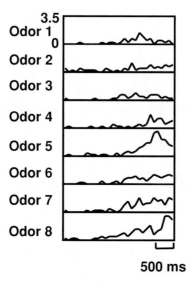

FIGURE 4. Example of an OFC neuron that shows sustained odor-specific delay activity (memory response). Activity of cell during final 3 s of delay interval. Each box illustrates the average firing rate (spikes per second) of the cell during the interval following one of the 8 odors. This cell fires differently following each odor. Adapted from Ramus and Eichenbaum.[33]

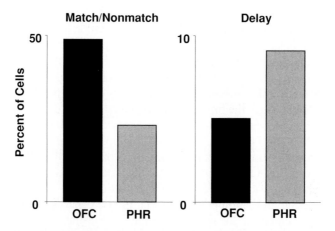

FIGURE 5. Differences in the proportions of cells in OF and PHR that represent the nonmatching rule (Match/Nonmatch e.g., cells illustrated in Fig. 3) and the memory of the stimulus (Delay; e.g., the cell illustrated in Fig. 4) during performance of the DNMS task. Consistent with the interconnectivity of these regions, neurons in both the OFC and the PHR display sensory-specific firing, firing that reflects the nonmatching rule, and mnemonic firing. However, more cells in the OFC than PHR represent the task rule, while more cells in the PHR represent the memory for the stimulus odor.

and therefore also support the role of the OFC as an association neocortex in the model of the broader memory system outlined in the first section of this chapter.

This model is further supported in a similar series of studies in monkeys looking at the interaction between another neocortical area (area TE, a visual association neocortex) in a visual paired associates task. Sakai and Miyashita[57] found stimulus-selective cells in anterior inferotemporal cortex with two memory properties. The first type of cell, 'pair-coding' neurons, fired maximally to presentations of either of two paired-associates, but not to any of the other stimuli involved in other pairings (i.e., the firing of cells became highly correlated for the items in each paired-associate). The second type of cell, 'pair-recall' neurons, showed sustained firing during the delay when the paired-associate of the cell's optimal stimulus was used as the sample; however, these two types of cells were found in both the PHR *and* in area TE. To examine the origin of these memory signals Higuchi and Miyashita[58] trained monkeys on the paired-associate task, and then recorded from TE neurons in monkeys with and without unilateral lesions of the PHR. Observing the electrophysiological properties of the cells in TE on the lesioned side of the brain, Higuchi and Miyashita found that cells maintained their responsiveness to visual stimuli. However, the responses to paired stimuli were no longer highly correlated. Thus, the authors concluded that lesions of the PHR disrupted the associative code in area TE without impairing the visual responsiveness to the stimuli.

A more recent study from the same laboratory extended these conclusions by examining the time-course of sensory and memory signals in association cortex and the PHR. Simultaneously recordings in TE and in perirhinal cortex revealed that the latency of the visual response was shorter in TE than in they perirhinal cortex, confirming the forward propagation of these sensory signals. Conversely, pair-recall cells showed increases in firing rate with a shorter latency in perirhinal cortex than in area TE, confirming the backward propagation of the memory signal from the PHR to association neocortex.[59]

These findings from the Miyashita lab lend additional support to our view that sensory signals arising in neocortex (whether OFC or TE) propagate through the hippocampal memory system, where they are attached with mnemonic information. These mnemonic signals then propagate backwards through the network to the association areas that originally processed the information. This accounting is consistent with the expectation that both sensory and memory information would be represented by cells in the association neocortex. Finally, all these findings are consistent with the idea that association cortex and the PHR contribute to memory in different, but complementary ways. In the next series of studies, we further extend this interaction to the hippocampus itself.

INTERACTIONS BETWEEN THE OFC AND HIPPOCAMPUS IN THE STORAGE OF LONG-TERM MEMORY

To examine the interactions between the OFC and hippocampus, we needed to find a task that would tap hippocampal function, since hippocampal lesions produce mild (if any) impairment on DNMS in either monkeys or rats.[42,43,46-48] However, when the basic design of the DNMS task is altered such that the rats need to remember the order of odors rather than to make a familiarity judgment, then the hippocampus becomes critical for performance of the task.[60] Further, hippocampal lesions impair a rat's ability to disambiguate overlapping sequences of odors.[61] We therefore characterized the firing of neurons in the OFC during a passive 8-odor sequence learning task.[62,63]

As in our previous recording study[33] we found that almost all of the cells in OFC fire in relation to at least one task event, including trial initiation, delivery of the water reward, and delivery of the odor stimulus. Sixty-seven percent ($n = 269/400$ cells from 4 rats) of the cells recorded in OFC showed changes in firing relative to base line in response to presentation of the odor (i.e., are odor responsive). Of these odor-responsive cells, 56% ($n = 150/269$) show odor-selective firing during the odor-sampling period.

Most interesting, however, is the new finding that 29% ($n = 79/269$) of the odor-responsive cells recorded from OFC showed odor-selective firing *in anticipation* of the presented odor. Typically, this anticipatory firing was observed between 200–400 ms *prior* to the onset of the odor. An example of an anticipatory cell is illustrated in FIGURE 6. This sort of neuronal firing in anticipation of an odor has been observed when an odor was predictably repeated during an 8-odor discrimination task[34] and when a place predicted the upcoming odor.[64] In our study, the anticipatory firing observed in OFC appears to code memory for the sequence of odors, and in fact the anticipatory firing was not found in 3 rats trained on the same odors, but with no predictable sequence ($n = 5/117$, 4.3%; note: because we used a statistical criterion we would expect to see some anticipatory responses by chance). Finally, we have further isolated 54 cells from the OFC of two rats with bilateral electrolytic lesions of hippocampus. Of these, only one (2.3%) of the odor-responsive cells showed anticipatory firing. These findings strongly suggest that the anticipatory response we observed in the OFC reflects a memory representation of the odor sequence, which is in turn dependent on the hippocampus. These findings further support the idea that the OFC is important for the formation and storage of long-term memory, and that the OFC is part of a broader hippocampal memory system for the storage of olfactory memories.

CONCLUSIONS

The studies outlined above provide evidence for a broader hippocampal memory system that critically includes the functions of association neocortex.

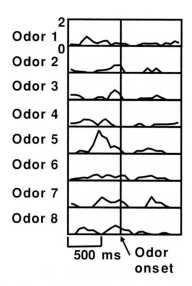

FIGURE 6. Example of an OFC neuron with an anticipatory response (memory) during the 8-odor sequence learning task. Activity of cell from 700 ms before to 700 ms after the odor onset for each of the 8 odors. Each box illustrates the average firing rate (spikes per second) of the cell to one of the 8 odors. This cell shows an increase in firing ~400 ms before the onset of odor 5 but not before the onset of any of the other 7 odors.

By this view, sensory information is initially processed in widespread neocortical association areas. This processed sensory information is then propagated through the PHR to the hippocampus. Through back projections, memory information is sent from the hippocampus to the PHR and then to the association neocortex, which forms the ultimate repository for these memories. Our work shows that the OFC interacts with both the PHR and the hippocampus during the storage of long-term memories, consistent with the model of a broader hippocampal memory system. By this view, the OFC serves as a high-order association neocortex for olfactory information that plays a role in the representation of memories for specific stimuli and in the application of task rules.

REFERENCES

1. SQUIRE, L.R. & P. ALVAREZ. 1995. Retrograde amnesia and memory consolidation: a neurobiological perspective. Current Opinion in Neurobiology **5:** 169–177.
2. EICHENBAUM, H. 2000. A cortical-hippocampal system for declarative memory. Nature Reviews Neuroscience **1:** 41–50.
3. RAMUS, S.J. & H. EICHENBAUM. 2007. A brain system for declarative memory. *In* Topis in Integrative Neuroscience: From Cells to Cognition. J. Pomerantz, Ed. Cambridge University Press. In press.

4. COHEN, N. & L. SQUIRE. 1980. Preserved learning and retention of a pattern-analylizing skill in amnesia: dissociation of knowing how and knowing that. Science **210:** 207–210.
5. TULVING, E. 1993. What is episodic memory? Current Dirctions in Psychological Science **2:** 67–70.
6. GRAF, P. & D. SCHACTER. 1985. Implicit and explicit memory for new associations in normal and amnesic subjects. Journal of Experimental Psychology. Learning, Memory and Cognition **11:** 501–518.
7. COHEN, N. & H. EICHENBAUM. 1993. Memory, Amnesia, and the Hippocampal System. MIT Press. Cambridge, MA.
8. SCHACTER, D. & E. TULVING. 1994. Whater are the memory systems of 1994? *In* Memory Systems 1994. D. Schacter & E. Tulving, Eds.: 341–380. Guilford Press. New York.
9. VAN HOESEN, G., D. PANDYA & N. BUTTERS. 1972. Cortical afferents to the entorhinal cortex of the rhesus monkey. Science **175:** 1471–1473.
10. VAN HOESEN, G., D. PANDYA & N. BUTTERS. 1975. Some connections of the entorhinal (area 28) and perirhinal (area 35) cortices of the rhesus monkey. II. Frontal lobe afferents. Brain Research **95:** 25–38.
11. VAN HOESEN, G. & D. PANDYA. 1975. Some connections of the entorhinal (area 28) and perirhinal (area 35) cortices of the rhesus monkey. I. Temporal lobe afferents. Brain Research **95:** 1–24.
12. VAN HOESEN, G. & D. PANDYA. 1975. Some connections of the entorhinal (area 28) and perirhinal (area 35) cortices of the rhesus monkey. III. Efferent connection. Brain Research **95:** 48–67.
13. DEACON, T. *et al.* 1983. Afferent connections of the perirhinal cortex in the rat. Journal of Comparative Neurology **220:** 168–190.
14. MARTIN-ELKINS, C.L. & J.A. HOREL. 1992. Cortical afferents to behaviorally defined regions of the inferior temporal and parahippocampal gyri as demonstrated by WGA-HRP. Journal of Comparative Neurology **321:** 177–192.
15. SUZUKI, W.A. & D.G. AMARAL. 1994. Perirhinal and parahippocampal cortices of the macaque monkey: cortical afferents. Journal of Comparative Neurology **350:** 497–533.
16. BURWELL, R.D. & D.G. AMARAL. 1998. Cortical afferents of the perirhinal, postrhinal, and entorhinal cortices of the rat. Journal of Comparative Neurology **398:** 179–205.
17. SUZUKI, W.A. & H. EICHENBAUM. 2000. The neurophysiology of memory. Annals of the New York Academy of Sciences **911:** 175–191.
18. PRICE, J.L. *et al.* 1991. Olfactory input to the prefrontal cotex. *In* Olfaction: a Model System for Computational Neuroscience. J. Davis & H. Eichenbaum, Eds. MIT Press. Cambridge, MA.
19. BURWELL, R.D., M.P. WITTER & D.G. AMARAL. 1996. Perirhinal and postrhinal cortices of the rat: a review of the neuroanatomical literature and comparison with findings from the monkey brain. Hippocampus **5:** 390–408.
20. SUZUKI, W.A. 1996. Neuroanatomy of the monkey entorhinal,perirhinal and parahippocampal cortices: organization of cortical inputs and interconnections with amygdala and striatum. Neuroscience **8:** 3–12.
21. BLISS, T.V. & G.L. COLLINGRIDGE. 1993. A synaptic model of memory: long-term potentiation in the hippocampus. Nature **361:** 31–39.
22. AMARAL, D.G. & M.P. WITTER. 1989. The three-dimensional organization of the hippocampal formation: a review of anatomical data. Neuroscience **31:** 571–591.

23. NYBERG, L. *et al.* 2000. Reactivation of encoding-related brain activity during memory retrieval. Proceedings of the National Academy of Sciences of the United States of America **97:** 11120–11124.
24. WHEELER, M.E., S.E. PETERSEN & R.L. BUCKNER. 2000. Memory's echo: vivid remembering reactivates sensory-specific cortex. Proceedings of the National Academy of Sciences of the United States of America **97:** 11125–11129.
25. BUCKNER, R.L. & M.E. WHEELER. 2001. The cognitive neuroscience of remembering. Nature Reviews Neuroscience **2:** 624–634.
26. FLETCHER, P., C. FRITH & M. RUGG. 1997. The functional neuroanatomy of episodic memory. Trends in Neuorscience **20:** 213–218.
27. GOTTFRIED, J.A. *et al.* 2004. Rememberance of odors past: human olfactory cortex in cross-modal recognition memory. Neuron **42:** 687–695.
28. EICHENBAUM, H., P. ALVAREZ & S. RAMUS. 2000. Animal models of amnesia. *In* Handbook of Neuorpsychology, Vol. 2: memory Disorders. L. Cermak, Ed.: 1–24. Elsevier Science. Amsterdam.
29. CORKIN, S. 1984. Lasting consequences of bilateral medial temporal lobectomy: clinical course and experimental findings in H.M. Seminars in Neurology **4:** 249–259.
30. SQUIRE, L.R., B. KNOWLTON & G. MUSIN. 1993. The structure and organization of memory. Annual Review of Psychology **44:** 453–495.
31. ALVAREZ, P. & L.R. SQUIRE. 1994. Memory consolidation and the medial temporal lobe: a simple network model. Proceedings of the National Academy of Sciences of the United States of America **91:** 7041–7045.
32. OTTO, T. & H. EICHENBAUM. 1992. Complementary roles of orbital prefrontal cortex and the perirhinal-entorhinal cortices in an odor-guided delayed non-matching to sample task. Behavioral Neuroscience **106:** 763–776.
33. RAMUS, S.J. & H. EICHENBAUM. 2000. Neural correlates of olfactory recognition memory in the rat orbitofrontal cortex. Journal of Neuroscience **20:** 8199–8208.
34. SCHOENBAUM, G. & H. EICHENBAUM. 1995. Information coding in the rodent prefrontal cortex. I. Single-neuron activity in orbitofrontal cortex compared with that in pyriform cortex. Journal of Neurophysiology **74:** 733–750.
35. SCHOENBAUM, G. & H. EICHENBAUM. 1995. Information coding in the rodent prefrontal cortex. II. Ensemble activity in orbitofrontal cortex. Journal of Neurophysiology **74:** 751–762.
36. SCHOENBAUM, G., A.A. CHIBA & M. GALLAGHER. 1998. Orbitofrontal cortex and basolateral amygdala encode expected outcomes during learning. Nature Neuroscience **1:** 155–159.
37. ALVAREZ, P. & H. EICHENBAUM. 2002. Representations of odors in the rat orbitofrontal cortex change during and after learning. Behavioral Neuroscience **116:** 421–433.
38. GAFFAN, D. 1974. Recognition impaired and association intact in the memory of monkeys after transection of the fornix. J. Comp. Physiol. Psychol. **86:** 1100–1109.
39. MISHKIN, M. & J. DELACOUR. 1975. An analysis of short-term visual memory in the monkey. J. Exp. Psychol. Anim. Behav. Process **1:** 326–334.
40. ZOLA-MORGAN, S. *et al.* 1989. Lesions of perirhinal and parahippocampal cortex that spare the amygdala and hippocampal formation produce severe memory impairment. Journal of Neuroscience **9:** 4355–4370.
41. MEUNIER, M. *et al.* 1993. Effects on visual recognition of combined and separate ablations of the entorhinal and perirhinal cortex in rhesus monkeys. Journal of Neuroscience **13:** 5418–5432.

42. MURRAY, E. & M. MISHKIN. 1998. Object recognition and location memory in monkeys with excitotoxic lesions of the amygdala and hippocampus. The Journal of Neuroscience **18:** 6568–6582.
43. ZOLA, S.M. *et al.* 2000. Impaired recognition memory in monkeys after damage limited to the hippocampal region. The Journal of Neuroscience **20:** 451–463.
44. GAFFAN, D. 1994. Scene-specific memory of objects: a model of episodic memory impairment in monkeys with fornix transection. Journal of Cognitive Neurology **6:** 305–320.
45. BUFFALO, E.A. *et al.* 2000. Perception and recognition memory in monkeys following lesions of area TE and perirhinal cortex. Learning and Memory **7:** 375–382.
46. ROTHBLAT, L.A. & L.F. KROMER. 1991. Object recognition memory in the rat: the role of the hippocampus. Behavioral Brain Research **42:** 25–32.
47. MUMBY, D.G., E.R. WOOD & J.P.L. PINEL. 1992. Object-recognition memory is only mildly impaired in rats with lesions of the hippocampus and amygdala. Psychobiology **20:** 18–27.
48. OTTO, T. & H. EICHENBAUM. 1992. Neuronal activity in the hippocampus during delayed non-match to sample performance in rats: evidence for hippocampal processing in recognition memory. Hippocampus **2:** 323–334.
49. YOUNG, B.J. *et al.* 1997. Memory representation within the parahippocampal region. The Journal of Neuroscience **17:** 5183–5195.
50. FAHY, F.L., I.P. RICHES & M.W. BROWN. 1993. Neuronal activity related to visual recognition memory: long-term memory and encoding of recency and familiarity information in the primate anterior and medial inferior temporal and rhinal cortex. Experimental Brain Research **96:** 457–472.
51. XIANG, J.Z. & M.W. BROWN. 1988. Differential neuronal encoding of novelty, familiarity and recency in regions of the anterior temporal lobe. Neuropharmacology **37:** 657–676.
52. MILLER, E.K., L. LI & R. DESIMONE. 1991. A neural mechanism for working and recognition memory in inferior temporal cortex. Science **254:** 1377–1379.
53. SUZUKI, W.A., E.K. MILLER & R. DESIMONE. 1997. Object and place memory in the macaque entorhinal cortex. Journal of Neurophysiology **78:** 1062–1081.
54. CERF-DUCASTEL, B. & C. MURPHY. 2006. Neural substrates of cross-modal olfactory recognition memory: an fMRI study. NeuroImage **31:** 386–396.
55. MILLER, E.K., C.A. ERICKSON & R. DESIMONE. 1996. Neural mechanism of visual working memory in prefrontal cortex of the macaque. The Journal of Neuroscience **16**.
56. MILLER, E.K. 2000. The prefrontal cortex and cognitive control. Nature Reviews Neuroscience **1:** 9–65.
57. SAKAI, K. & Y. MIYASHITA. 1991. Neural organization for the long-term memory of paired associates. Nature **354:** 152–155.
58. HIGUCHI, S. & Y. MIYASHITA. 1996. Formation of mnemonic neural responses to visual paired associations in inferotemporal cortex is impaired by perirhinal and entorhinal lesions. Proceedings of the National Academy of Sciences of the United States of America **93:** 739–743.
59. NAYA, Y., M. YOSHIDA & Y. MIYASHITA. 2001. Backward spreading of memory-retrieval signal in the primate temporal cortex. Science **291:** 661–664.
60. FORTIN, N., K. AGSTER & H. EICHENBAUM. 2002. Critical role of the hippocampus in memory for sequences of events. Nature Neuroscience **5:** 458–462.
61. AGSTER, K.L., N.J. FORTIN & H. EICHENBAUM. 2002. The hippocampus and disambiguation of overlapping sequences. J. Neurosci. **22:** 5760–5768.

62. DISCENZA, C.B. *et al.* 2005. Anticipatory neuronal firing in the orbitofrontal cortex of rats learning an odor-sequence memory task. Abstracts of the Society for Neuroscience 66.15.
63. DAVIS, J.B. *et al.* 2006. Hippocampal-dependence of anticipatory neuronal firing in the orbitofronal cortex fo rats learning an odor-sequence memory task. Abstracts of the Society for Neuroscience 66.7.
64. LIPTON, P.A., P. ALVAREZ & H. EICHENBAUM. 1999. Crossmodal associative memory representations in rodent orbitofrontal cortex. Neuron **22:** 349–359.

Orbitofrontal Cortex and the Computation of Economic Value

CAMILLO PADOA-SCHIOPPA

Department of Neurobiology, Harvard Medical School, Boston, Massachusetts 02115, USA

ABSTRACT: Economic choice is the behavior observed when individuals select one of many available options solely based on subjective preferences. Behavioral evidence suggests that economic choice entails two mental processes: values are first assigned to the available options, and a decision is subsequently made between these values. Numerous reports show that lesions to the orbitofrontal cortex (OFC) lead to choice deficits in various domains, and imaging studies indicate that the OFC activates when people make choices. In this chapter, we review evidence from single cell recordings linking the OFC more specifically to valuation. Individual neurons in the OFC encode the value that monkeys assign to different beverages when they choose between them. These neurons encode economic value as a subjective quantity. Most importantly, neurons in the OFC encode economic value *per se*, not as a modulation of sensory or motor processes. This trait distinguishes the value representation in the OFC from that observed in other brain areas. That OFC neurons encode economic value independently of visuomotor contingencies suggests that economic choice is fundamentally a choice between goods (good-based model) rather than a choice between actions (action-based model).

KEYWORDS: neuroeconomics; economic choice; decision making; subjective value; monkey

INTRODUCTION

Economic choice is the behavior observed when choices are based on subjective preferences. It is a behavior we engage in frequently, for example, when we select an item from a restaurant menu, when we choose among different financial investments, or when we choose between a job that will pay better and one that we might enjoy more. It is called economic choice because this behavior has been traditionally the object of economic theory.[1,2] However, economic

Address for correspondence: Camillo Padoa-Schioppa, Ph.D., Department of Neurobiology, Harvard Medical School, 220 Longwood Avenue, Boston, MA 02115. Voice: 617-432-2805; fax: 617-734-7557.
camillo@alum.mit.edu

Ann. N.Y. Acad. Sci. 1121: 232–253 (2007). © 2007 New York Academy of Sciences.
doi: 10.1196/annals.1401.011

choice has also been studied in psychology[3,4]; an extensive literature (behavioral economics) shows how human choices are often affected by "fallacies," such as hyperbolic discounting or loss aversion, that ultimately result in non-rational behavior.[5-7] Economic choice is also relevant from medical and clinical perspectives. Indeed, many disorders that affect the frontal lobe, such as frontotemporal dementia[8-11] and obsessive compulsive disorder,[12,13] can be characterized as patients making poor choices. Moreover, drug addiction can be thought of as an extreme case of dysfunctional choice behavior.[13,14] This review focuses on the cognitive and neuronal mechanisms of economic choice. As we will see, recent evidence indicates that the orbitofrontal cortex (OFC) participates in the computation of economic value, a process necessary for choice.[15,16]

ECONOMIC CHOICE, A DISTINCT MENTAL PROCESS

Consider a person sitting in a restaurant and choosing among different items on the menu. That choice can sometimes prove difficult—should she order the tuna tartare or the fried calamari? The Pinot Noir or the Nebbiolo? In these situations, the difficulty is not in comprehending what options are available, or in communicating our decision to the waiter. Sensory processing and motor control are both complex operations, but solving them successfully does not amount to choosing. The difficulty when choosing among different dishes or different wines on the menu is in introspecting, pondering options, and selecting the one that best satisfies our current desires. These mental processes and the resulting behavior are "economic choice."

In the following sections, we will describe recent results showing that when monkeys engage in economic choice, neurons in the OFC encode the value that animals assign to different goods. Before doing so, however, it is useful to distinguish the mental processes underlying economic choice from other mental processes examined in experiments that also encompass a "choice." Indeed, a number of papers in the past 10 years described neuronal activity related to values and decisions.

Ultimately, the mental processes of economic choice are distinct from the mental processes dissected by other behavioral tasks that can be construed as requiring a choice.[3] For example, some experiments present monkeys with perceptually ambiguous sensory stimuli and ask them to "choose" between two possible reports. In such cases, monkeys are not asked to introspect and decide what they *want*—no doubt they want the juice. Instead, monkeys are asked to report what they *perceive*. The mental process taking place in this kind of task has been referred to as a perceptual decision.[17,18] Conceptually, the demands of these tasks are very different from those we face, for example, when presented with a restaurant menu. Analogously, many experiments require monkeys to "choose" among multiple possible responses of which one is intrinsically correct. For example, two perceptually unambiguous stimuli might be associated with two different quantities of the same juice.[19–26] Alternatively, two stimuli might be associated with a fixed amount of juice delivered with different probabilities.[22,27] In both cases, once monkeys have learned the association between the stimuli and the expected quantity of juice, "choices" reduce to trivial responses. It can thus be said that these tasks do not ask monkeys to decide what they want, but simply to demonstrate whether they remember the correct answer.

More recent experiments set monkeys in more complex situations in which there is no strictly correct answer in any particular trial, but there is an overall optimal strategy across trials. In the simplest of such cases, monkeys play the game "matching pennies," in which the ideal strategy for a subject playing against an infinitely intelligent opponent (reasonably approximated by a computer program) is to select one of two possible responses randomly and with equal probability in every trial.[28] In other games, the optimal strategy is to choose unpredictably but with unequal (and sometimes changing) probabilities.[29] Finally, other experiments (matching tasks) set monkeys in somewhat intermediate situations, in the sense that there is a locally (and statistically) correct answer, but the correct answer changes from trial to trial depending on previous choices and outcomes.[30] In all these tasks, however, the demand on the monkeys is always to *infer* the best possible response necessary to receive a given amount of juice, not to introspect and to decide what they want. In other words, these tasks tackle monkeys' intelligence, or ability to learn, not their will. In contrast, the experiments described here focus on mental processes that take place when monkeys choose among different goods with no correct answer or strategy, on the basis of only their subjective preferences.

ECONOMIC CHOICE, A MULTISTAGE MENTAL PROCESS

Behavioral studies on economic choice have often been concerned with complex choices and with choice "fallacies."[5–7] But in fact, relatively little is known about the cognitive and brain processes underlying even simple choices, such as choices between two foods. Consider, for example, the situation illustrated in FIGURE 1. In this experiment, capuchin monkeys (*Cebus apella*) chose between different foods offered in variable amounts.[15] In this particular session, a monkey chose between raisins (food A, preferred) and 1-g pieces of apple (food B). The *x* axis in the figure represents different offer types, and the *y* axis represents the percentage of times the monkey chose food B. When offered the choice between 1A and 1B, the monkey always chose 1A. However, when B was offered in sufficiently large amounts, the monkey chose it. For example, the monkey chose 4B over 1A and 3B over 1A. When offered 2B versus 1A, the monkey chose B roughly half of the time. In other words, the monkey was indifferent between 1A and 2B.

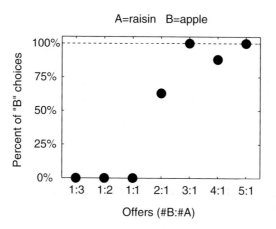

FIGURE 1. Food choice in capuchins. In this session, a capuchin monkey chose between raisins and 1-g pieces of apple. From Ref. 15.

The choice pattern illustrated in FIGURE 1 can be described in terms of relative values of the two foods. In this case, since the monkey was indifferent between 1A and 2B, the value of 1A is roughly equivalent to the value of 2B. But what psychological processes underlie this behavior?

One possibility is that monkeys' choices are simple associations between stimuli (for example, the offer 1A:3B) and responses (in this case, the choice 3B) acquired through experience. According to this view, in early encounters with foods A and B, a monkey chooses randomly, and feedback mechanisms measure its welfare after any given choice. Through multiple encounters with foods A and B, by trial and error, the monkey gradually learns to select 2A over 1B, 1A over 1B, 3B over 1A, etc. This associative model, originally proposed by Skinner,[31,32] represents the simplest possible psychological account of economic choice because it entails a single mental operation (an association). Interestingly, this model is a sufficient assumption from the point of view of standard economic theory.[33] The problem, however, is that human and animal choices often violate the main prediction of the associative model, namely that learning to choose takes time. For example, it was observed that monkeys choose between novel pairs of foods (i.e., pairs of foods that they never encountered together before) as effectively as they choose between familiar pairs of foods.[15] Remarkably, monkeys do so from the very first trial, a result inconsistent with choices being stimulus–response associations acquired by trial and error.[15] Hence, economic choice requires a more elaborate psychological account.

The next level of complexity is referred to as the cognitive model of choice. According to this hypothesis, economic choice results from a two-stage mental process: values are first assigned to the available options, and a decision is consequently made between these values.[15,34,35]

Notably, in spite of its intuitive appeal and relative simplicity, the cognitive model of choice cannot be tested directly based on behavior alone. The two mental operations of value assignment and decision making cannot be dissociated at the behavioral level because values cannot be measured behaviorally independently of choice. To appreciate this point, consider a simple example. Most people, given the choice between $1000 and a glass of water, will choose the money. Now suppose that one day you encounter Victoria, you offer her the choice between $1000 and a glass of water, and she chooses the water. One reason for her surprising behavior might be that her neurocognitive choice mechanisms malfunction, perhaps because she recently suffered a brain lesion. Another possibility is that Victoria's brain functions perfectly well, and she is so thirsty at that particular time that she would rather drink the water than take the money. The critical point is that it is impossible to distinguish between these two alternative hypotheses based on her choice alone.

That value cannot be measured behaviorally independently of choice implies that valuation and decision cannot be dissociated at the behavioral level. In fact, it can be argued that standard economic theory has historically resolved to such a rudimentary assumption as the associative model of choice precisely for this reason. On the other hand, value assignment and decision making could in principle be disentangled at the physiological level. For example, it is possible that the two mental operations are processed by distinct populations of neurons. In other words, in order to test whether values are actually assigned to the available options during economic choice, it is necessary to study the neuronal representation of economic value.

ECONOMIC CHOICE AND THE ORBITOFRONTAL CORTEX

Where in the brain does economic choice take place? Several lines of evidence point in particular to the OFC. For example, early clinical signs of frontotemporal dementia (a neurodegenerative disorder that initially affects the OFC)[8] include changes in eating habits, anorexia, and hyperorality.[9,10] When asked to exert simple preference judgments between foods, patients with OFC lesions make inconsistent or erratic choices significantly more often than either healthy subjects or patients with dorsolateral frontal lesions.[36] OFC patients also exhibit abnormal choice behavior in situations that involve uncertainty (enhanced risk-seeking)[11,37] and in social contexts (ultimatum game).[38] Damasio[39] refers to a deficit in "the ability to select an advantageous response among an array of available options." Interestingly, in multiattribute choice tasks, OFC patients present abnormal patterns of information acquisition.[40] Other deficits associated with OFC lesions include disrupted social behavior,[9,10] as exemplified by the famous case of Phineas Gage.[41] OFC patients also present perseveration in stimulus–reward association reversals.[42] In this case, subjects seemingly fail to reassign the proper value to a stimulus.

Lesion studies in monkeys provide consistent evidence, as OFC ablations result in abnormal eating patterns[43] and impairments in stimulus–reward association reversals.[44,45] Thus taken together, lesion studies in humans and monkeys suggest that the OFC may be a key neural substrate for choice behavior.

A second line of evidence linking the OFC to economic valuation and choice comes from imaging experiments in humans. Many studies found higher activation in the OFC when subjects were presented with affectively pleasant sensory stimuli compared to neutral stimuli (reviewed by O'Doherty).[46] Preference-dependent activation was consistently obtained with multiple sensory modalities including olfactory,[47,48] gustatory,[49] visual,[50,51] auditory,[52] and somatosensory,[53] suggesting that the OFC might represent behavioral valence as a common currency.[54] Supporting this view, the OFC was also activated when subjects earned money,[55,56] an intrinsically abstract stimulus. In all these studies, subjects were not asked to make choices. However, in the experiments of Arana and colleagues,[57] subjects did in fact make choices from a restaurant menu in a 2×2 design. Items in the menu had high or low incentive; in some cases, subjects were simply shown items on the menu, and in other cases they were asked to make a choice. Most interestingly, the medial OFC was significantly more activated in the choice condition compared to the no-choice condition. The same area was also more activated by high incentives compared to low incentives. In comparison, neural activation in the amygdala varied depending on the incentive level, but did not vary with task demands. A subsequent study found consistent results.[58]

With respect to the activity of individual OFC neurons, several studies used neurophysiological recordings in nonhuman primates to analyze neuronal responses associated with the expectation or the delivery of foods or beverages. While these experiments typically did not focus on choice behavior, several results are consistent with the hypothesis that OFC neurons might be a substrate for economic valuation. In an early study, Thorpe and colleagues[59] observed that neurons in the OFC responded to the presentation of visual stimuli in a way that was not purely sensory. For example, the response of one neuron to the visual presentation of a liquid-filled syringe depended on whether in previous trials the liquid was apple juice or salted water, even though the syringe was visually indistinguishable in the two conditions. Rolls and colleagues subsequently found that the activity of OFC neurons responding to a particular taste could be modulated by hunger and satiety, a modulation not observed in the primary taste area.[60] In summary, these results indicated that the activity of OFC neurons is modulated both by physical stimuli and by the motivational state of the animal.

In another study, Tremblay and Schultz (T&S) delivered to monkeys one of three types of juice (A, B, and C, in decreasing order of preference) in a fixed amount.[61] In their experiment, trials were blocked, with only one pair of juices employed in each block. T&S found OFC neurons that responded to juice A but not to juice B during A:B blocks, and to juice B but not to juice

C in B:C blocks. T&S interpreted this as neurons reflecting juice *preference* (i.e., ordinal ranking). However, subsequent work showed that OFC neurons encode juice *value* in a cardinal (i.e., numberlike) sense.[16,62] T&S's results thus suggest that the value representation may vary depending on the behavioral context.[63]

Other studies found that the activity of neurons in the OFC can be modulated by the amount of juice delivered to the monkey.[21,64,65] Roesch and Olson (R&O) also found that OFC neuronal activity varied depending on the duration of a time delay intervening before juice delivery.[64,65] Interestingly, there was an inverse correlation between the effects of juice amount and the effects of time delay. Under the assumption that the neurons recorded by R&O encode the subjective value at stake in any trial, one possible interpretation of this result is that the delay represents a cost to the monkey and that OFC neurons encode cost-affected values.

Taken together, the results reviewed above suggest that individual neurons in the OFC might represent the behavioral valence of goods. However, in the experiments with monkeys, the animals were never asked to choose based on their own preferences. Rather, monkeys were either simply delivered juice, or they were asked to select between two options, one of which was intrinsically correct. Consequently, these tasks could not distinguish value from the objective properties of the to-be-delivered juice (e.g., juice quantity, probability, and delivery time). In contrast, the behavioral paradigm described in FIGURE 1 does provide an operational measure for the subjective value monkeys assign to the food (or juice). In the experiments described in the following sections, this behavioral paradigm was employed to study the relationship between the activity of OFC neurons and economic value.

NEURONS IN ORBITOFRONTAL CORTEX ENCODE ECONOMIC VALUE

Electrophysiological experiments were conducted in rhesus macaques (*Macaca mulatta*).[16] The behavioral paradigm was similar to that illustrated in FIGURE 1, but in this case monkeys chose between different beverages. During the experiments, monkeys sat in front of a computer monitor in an electrically isolated enclosure with their heads restrained. Their eye positions were monitored through a scleral eye coil.[66] Every trial began with the monkey fixating on a small dot at the center of the monitor (FIG. 2A). After 1.5 s, two sets of squares appeared on opposite sides of the fixation point (*offer*). The colors of the squares indicated the juice type, and the number of squares indicated the juice amount. For example, a monkey offered 3 red squares versus 1 blue square chose between 3 drops of unsweetened Kool-Aid and 1 drop of water. After a randomly variable delay (1–2 s), two saccade targets appeared near the offers (*go* signal). The monkey indicated its choice with an eye move-

(A)

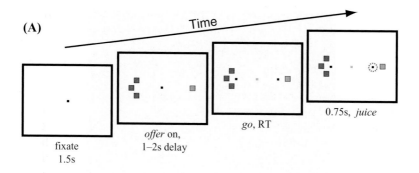

fixate
1.5s

offer on,
1–2s delay

go, RT

0.75s, *juice*

(B)

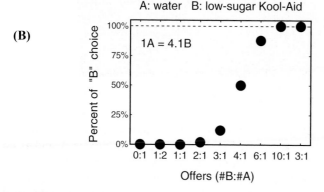

FIGURE 2. Experimental design (**A**) and choice pattern (**B**) in neurophysiology experiments. Adapted from Ref. 16.

ment and, after 0.75 s, the chosen juice was delivered (*juice*). In different sessions, we used a variety of different juices; in any given session, we referred to the preferred juice as juice A and to the less-preferred juice as juice B. The amounts of the two juices (0–10 drops) offered in any given trial varied pseudorandomly, and offer types included "forced choices" (such as 0B:1A or 2B:0A). For a given offer type, left/right positions were counterbalanced (e.g., the monkey could be offered 3B on the left and 1A on the right, or vice versa).

As shown in FIGURE 2B, the basic behavioral result obtained with solid foods was reproduced with beverages. To estimate the relative value of two juices in a given session, we fit the choice pattern with a sigmoid, and we determined the relative value from the flex point. Indicating with V(X) the value of X, for the session in FIGURE 2, we obtained $V(1A) = V(4.1B)$. In the analysis we assumed linear value functions, from which we obtained the equation $V(1A) = 4.1V(1B)$.

Like apples and oranges, A and B are different goods that in principle are not easy to compare. From the psychological point of view, value represents a

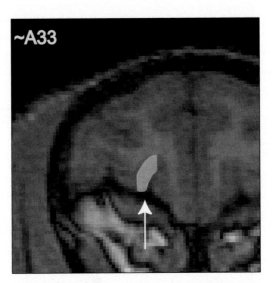

FIGURE 3. Recording sites were tentatively identified with area 13m.

common unit to make that comparison. For our analysis, the equation obtained from the choice pattern allowed us to measure quantities of A and B on a common value scale. We conventionally expressed values in units of V(B). We thus computed, for each trial, the value of the juice chosen by the monkey. For the session in FIGURE 2, the chosen value was ≈4 when the monkey chose 1A and when it chose 4B. When the monkey chose 2A, the chosen value was ≈8. When the monkey chose 6B, 10B, and 3B, the chosen value was respectively equal to 6, 10, and 3. In any session, we thus computed the variable chosen value. Similarly, we defined and computed other value-related variables.[16]

Neuronal recordings focused on the lateral bank of the medial orbital sulcus and the medial part of the posterior orbital gyrus (FIG. 3; presumably area 13m).[67,68] We recorded and analyzed the activity of 931 cells.[16]

As illustrated in FIGURE 4, OFC responses typically did not depend on the spatial configuration of the visual stimuli on the monitor (i.e., whether A was presented on the left and B on the right, or vice versa). Likewise, neuronal activity did not depend on the motor response used by the monkey to indicate its choice (i.e., a leftward or a rightward saccade). Overall, the activity of over 95% of OFC cells was independent of the spatial configuration and the motor response. However, the activity of neurons in OFC was often modulated by the offer type.

We defined seven 0.5-s time windows aligned with the *offer*, with the *go*, and with the *juice* delivery, and we analyzed the response of each neuron in each time window. In total, 1379 responses were significantly modulated by the offer type (ANOVA, $P < 0.001$), and 54% of cells were modulated in at least one time window. We analyzed further only responses modulated by the

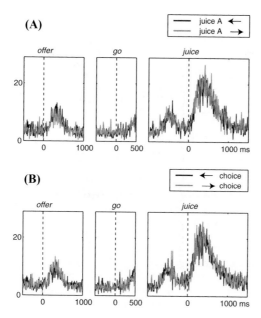

FIGURE 4. OFC responses are independent of visuomotor contingencies. **(A)** The two traces depict the activity of one representative neuron recorded when juice A was presented on the left and juice B on the right (dark trace) and with the reverse contingency (light trace). **(B)** In this case, the two traces depict the activity recorded when the monkey indicated its choice with a saccade to the left (dark trace) and with a saccade to the right (light trace). Adapted from Ref. 16.

offer type.

FIGURE 5 illustrates the activity of one representative neuron. In this session, the monkey chose between grape juice (A) and diluted cranberry juice (B). From the behavioral choice pattern (FIG. 5A, black symbols), we inferred $V(A) = 3.0 \ V(B)$. The response of the cell (FIG. 5A, gray symbols) had a characteristic U shape, similar to what we would expect if the neuron encoded the value chosen by the monkey in any given trial. Indeed, the activity of the cells was low when the monkey chose 1A and when it chose 3B (in units of $V(B)$, *chosen value* = 3); it was higher when the monkey chose 2A and when it chose 6B (*chosen value* = 6); and it was highest when the monkey chose 3A and when it chose 10B (*chosen value* $\approx$ 10). Plotted as a linear function of the numbers of A and B chosen (FIG. 5B), the U shape was asymmetrical. A linear regression of the response on the variable *chosen value* (FIG. 5C) provided $R^2 = 0.90$.

U-shaped responses seemingly encoding the *chosen value* were frequent in the OFC. In total, 54% of OFC neurons were modulated in the task, and about one-third of these (18% of the total) encoded the *chosen value* in at least one time window.

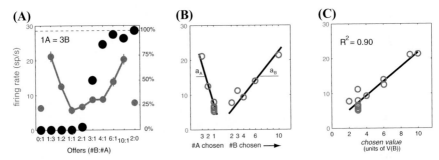

FIGURE 5. Activity of one OFC neuron encoding the *chosen value*. (**A**) Black symbols represent the behavioral choice pattern (with the *y* axis indicating the percent of B choices), and gray symbols indicate the firing rate. We conventionally express values in units of V(B). The cell activity is low when the monkey chooses 1 A and when it chooses 3B (offer types 1B:1A, 2B:1A, 3B:1A; *chosen value* = 3); it is higher when the monkey chooses 2A and when it chooses 6B (offer types 1B:2A, 6B:1A; *chosen value* = 6); and it is highest when the monkey chooses 3A and when it chooses 10B (offer types 1B:3A, 10B:1A; *chosen value* ≈ 10). (**B**) Same neuronal response plotted against the number of A and B chosen (linear scale). (**C**) Same neuronal responses plotted against the variable *chosen value* (expressed in units of V(B)). A linear regression provides $R^2 = 0.90$.

We also found other types of responses. For example, neuronal responses often encoded the *offer value*, that is, the value of one of the two juices alone. FIGURE 6A and B shows two neuronal responses encoding, respectively, *offer value A* and *offer value B*. Other frequently observed responses varied in a binary fashion depending on the type of juice chosen by the monkey, independently of the amount (FIG. 6C). We labeled these responses as encoding the juice *taste*.

Many OFC responses seemed to encode the variables *chosen value, offer value,* or *taste*. However, the relationship between the neuronal responses and these three variables could be subordinate to a correlation with other behavioral variables. For example, neurons in the OFC might encode the number of squares on the monitor (or variables proportional to the number, such as juice volume) or the variable *total value* (i.e., the value sum of the chosen juice and the other juice). In addition, OFC responses might encode other variables, such as the *value difference*. We examined quantitatively a total of 19 variables. Multiple procedures for variable selection all unequivocally identified *chosen value, offer value,* and *taste* as the three variables that best describe the population of responses. These three variables accounted for nearly 80% of OFC responses (mean $R^2 = 0.63$).[16]

Notably, the three types of responses are found in different proportions in different time windows. Comparing, in particular, the post-*offer* and post-*juice* time windows (corresponding, respectively, to the 0.5 s following the *offer* and the *juice*), we noted that *taste* responses were much more frequent at the time

(A)   **(B)**   **(C)**

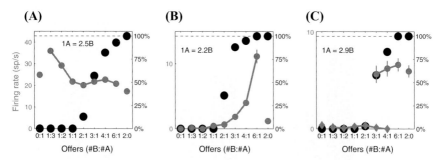

FIGURE 6. Activity of three neurons encoding the variables *offer value A* (**A**), *offer value B* (**B**), and *taste* (**C**). All conventions are as in FIGURE 5A. Adapted from Ref. 16.

of juice delivery than during the delay (FIG. 7). Also, *offer value* responses were most prevalent in the post-*offer* time window, consistent with the idea that, in order to choose, the monkey had to assign values to the two juices separately. This suggests the hypothesis that choices may be based upon the activity of *offer value* responses.

COMPARING BEHAVIORAL AND NEURONAL MEASURES OF ECONOMIC VALUE

Conceptually, responses encoding the *chosen value* are particularly interesting because, in addition to being independent of visuomotor contingencies, they are also independent of the specifics of the good (i.e., juice type and juice amount). A further analysis confirms that U-shaped responses encode the subjective value assigned by the monkeys as opposed to any physical property of the juices. Referring again to FIGURE 5B, we regress the activity of the neuron separately on the number of A chosen (#A) and on the number of B chosen (#B), and we obtain the two slopes a_A and a_B. The hypothesis that the response encodes the *chosen value* leads to a simple prediction regarding slopes a_A and a_B. Specifically, a_A should be proportional to the value of A, a_B should be proportional to the value of B, and the ratio $k^* \equiv a_A/a_B$ should be equal to the value ratio $V(A)/V(B)$. In other words, the slope ratio (k^*) provides a neuronal measure of the relative value of the two juices, independent of the behavioral measure of relative value (n^*), which represents the indifference point and which we obtain from the sigmoid fit. If U-shaped responses indeed encode the *chosen value*, we predict the identity $k^* = n^*$.

For the cell in FIGURE 5, this identity holds true. Indeed, from the two linear regressions, we obtain $k^* = 2.8$ (± 0.7), which is statistically indistinguishable from the behavioral measure $n^* = 3.0$. The following analysis shows that the identity $k^* = n^*$ holds true in general.

During the experiments, we used a large number of different juices and a total of 25 juice pairs.[16] Relative values were generally stable within any recording

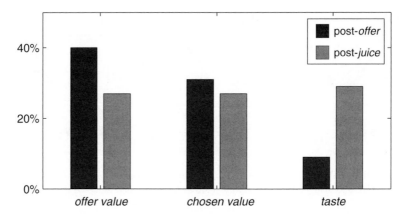

FIGURE 7. Class prevalence in different time windows. In the post-*offer* time window, a total of 284/931 (31%) of cells passed the ANOVA criterion. Of these, 40%, 31%, and 9% were classified as encoding, respectively, the *offer value*, *chosen value*, and *taste*. In the post-*juice* time window, a total of 332/931 (36%) of cells passed the ANOVA criterion. Of these, 27%, 27%, and 29% were classified as encoding, respectively, the *offer value*, *chosen value*, and *taste*.

session. However, the relative value of any given pair of juices could vary from day to day. For example, the relative value of apple juice versus peppermint tea varied between 1.5 and 3. This variability can be exploited to test the prediction $k^* = n^*$, in the sense that the slope ratio k^* should covary with the behavioral measure of relative value n^*. We identify U-shaped responses as those for which both regression slopes a_A and a_B (FIG. 2B) are significantly nonzero ($P < 0.01$), and we analyze neuronal data from each juice pair separately. For example, FIGURE 8 illustrates all U-shaped responses recorded with apple juice and peppermint tea. In the figure, the x axis represents the behavioral measure of relative value (n^*), the y axis represents the neuronal measure (k^*), and each dot represents one U-shaped response. Different responses were recorded from different cells on different days. A linear relationship between the two variables can be observed in the figure. The linear regression $k^* = b_0 + b_1 n^*$ provides $b_0 = 0.08$ and $b_1 = 1.18$. Averaging the two coefficients across juice pairs, we obtain $\bar{b}_0 = -0.13$ (± 0.15) and $\bar{b}_1 = 1.05$ (± 0.15), a result consistent with the identity $k^* = n^*$.

The result illustrated in FIGURE 8 demonstrates that U-shaped responses indeed encode value as a subjective quantity, as opposed to any physical property of the juices. To appreciate this point, consider for example the hypothesis that U-shaped responses encode a physical property such as the quantity of one particular ingredient (e.g., sugar). If that were the case, for any given pair of juices, U shapes should not vary from session to session depending on the relative value the monkey assigns to the juices in that particular session. In other words, if U-shaped responses encoded a physical property of the juices,

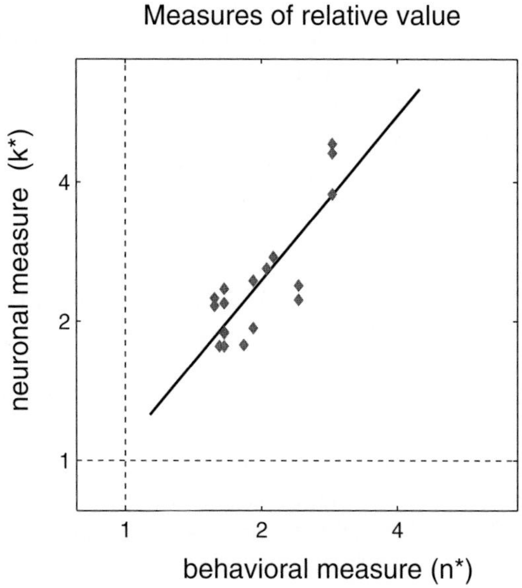

Measures of relative value

FIGURE 8. Measures of relative value. In the scatterplot, each data point represents one response, and all U-shaped responses recorded with apple juice and peppermint tea are shown. From the linear regression, we obtain $k^* = 0.08 + 1.18\ n^*$. Adapted from Ref. 16.

neuronal data should lie on a horizontal line in FIGURE 8, contrary to what we observe. We thus conclude that U-shaped responses indeed encode the value monkeys assign to the juice they choose to consume.[16]

REPRESENTATIONS OF VALUE IN ORBITOFRONTAL CORTEX AND OTHER BRAIN AREAS

A number of papers in recent years described how the activity of individual neurons in various brain areas can be modulated by value. Value-related activity has been documented in the lateral intraparietal area,[22,29,30] dorsolateral prefrontal cortex,[21,24,28] dorsal anterior cingulate,[69,70] ventral anterior cingulate,[71] posterior cingulate,[27] premotor cortex,[23] frontal eye fields,[23] supplementary eye fields,[23,72] superior colliculus,[19] basal ganglia,[20,25] amygdala,[73] and centromedian nucleus of the thalamus.[26] As a caveat, it should be noted that, at least in some cases, modulations described as related to value may also be explained in terms of visual attention, because most paradigms employed to study value-related phenomena fail to dissociate between these two alternative hypotheses.[74]

What distinguishes the representation of value found in the OFC is the fact that neurons in this area encode economic value *per se*, independently of the visuomotor contingencies of choice (FIG. 4). In contrast, in many other brain areas, value modulates responses that are sensory or motor in nature. Notably, the phenomena observed in the OFC cannot be interpreted in terms of attention, because attention is usually thought of as modulating a sensory process, not as a quantity neurons would encode *per se*. As discussed next, the phenomena observed in the OFC might have important implications regarding possible psychological models of economic choice.

COGNITIVE MODELS OF ECONOMIC CHOICE: GOOD BASED VERSUS ACTION BASED

The fact that many brain areas where neuronal activity is modulated by value are indirectly or directly involved in the generation of movements led to the proposal that economic choices may ultimately be choices between actions.[35] Consider, for example, the lateral intraparietal area (LIP). Neurons in this area have a response field—they activate when a visual stimulus is placed in a particular region of the visual field and when monkeys plan the corresponding saccade. Several studies found that these neurons' activity is enhanced if the saccade is associated with higher value.[22,29,30] Different neurons in the LIP represent different saccades, and neurons in other areas of the parietal lobe represent other types of movements.[75] The LIP and other parietal areas can thus be thought of as forming maplike structures representing all possible courses of action.[35] Within this framework, one possible function of value-related modulations is that they may subserve action selection, which could unfold through a winner-take-all process.[35] Most relevant to our focus, it was proposed that these parietal areas provide a common pathway for decision making, and that they are the substrate upon which choice is actually generated.[35] In other words, according to this action-based model, economic choice is fundamentally choice between actions.

That neurons in the OFC encode economic value *per se*, and not as a modulation of sensorimotor processes, suggests an alternative good-based model, according to which economic choice is fundamentally choice between goods.[16] In this view, economic choice is first made between different goods, and a suitable motor action is subsequently planned and executed.

In principle, the good-based model and the action-based model of economic choice are both legitimate hypotheses, and their merits should be established on empirical ground. Here we present three arguments in favor of the good-based model.

The first argument is that the action-based model violates a simple principle of modularity.[76–78] According to the action-based model, the physiological substrate of economic choice depends on the modality of the motor act employed to reveal the choice. For example, suppose that you are having lunch in a restaurant and that you have to choose, from the menu, between pizza and salad. According to the action-based model, the way you choose between pizza and salad depends on whether you indicate your choice with a left arm movement or with a right arm movement. If you indicate your choice verbally, the way you choose what to have for lunch depends on precisely what words you use to communicate with the waiter, because different sequences of words, which represent distinct courses of action, are processed and evaluated separately by the nervous system. In fact, according to the action-based model, as you choose between pizza and salad, many possible motor acts (different arm movements, different sequences of words, etc.) all representing the same food choice (e.g., salad) compete with each other.

The action-based hypothesis violates a principle of modularity because the nervous system could certainly break down the complex operation [choosing & moving] into two separate and simpler operations, [choosing] and [moving]. From a computational point of view, a modular organization offers tremendous advantages.[76] Controlling even a simple voluntary motor act, such as an arm reaching, is a challenging operation that involves many degrees of freedom and requires resolving multiple problems with infinite solutions.[79,80] If convolving the control of any motor act with economic choice requires even a minimal extra computational power, the great redundancy of the motor systems would make a nonmodular design ([choosing & moving]) enormously more expensive than a modular design ([choosing] and [moving]). For this reason, the good-based hypothesis is in principle more parsimonious.

Of course, natural selection does not always find optimal solutions. It is possible that primates may have evolved to make action-based economic choices, even though it is a costly way to function. After all, neurons in the parietal lobe and other premotor areas *are* modulated by value. If neurons encoding the value of goods independently of motor acts were not found in any brain area, the action-based model should certainly remain a leading hypothesis. In this sense, the results reviewed in previous sections provide an existence proof that directly supports the good-based model. Indeed, neurons in the OFC encode the value of offered and chosen goods *per se*, independently of visuomotor contingencies. In other words, they encode the variables necessary for efficient, good-based economic choices.

Another argument against the action-based model—and specifically against the idea that areas in the parietal lobe are the substrate upon which choice is generated—comes from common observations in neuropsychology. Typically, lesions of the parietal cortex result in visuospatial deficits, such as hemineglect and Balint's syndrome.[81,82] In contrast, economic choices are typically affected by orbitofrontal lesions.[9–11,36–38,40] Hence, unlike the OFC, parietal areas are not strictly necessary for economic choice behavior.

The results reviewed here, together with other lines of evidence, thus support the good-based model of economic choice. What, then, might be the functional significance of value-related modulations observed in sensory and motor areas? Two hypotheses (mutually nonexclusive) can be considered. First, value modulations in motor areas might indeed subserve action selection—as a distinct process, computationally downstream of economic choice. In other words, while economic choice is likely good based, action selection is likely action based. Second, it is certainly possible that information about the value assigned to objects flows from the frontal lobe to other sensory and motor areas, perhaps to increase the accuracy of the neuronal processes taking place in these areas. In the sensory domain, value modulations could serve perceptual attention. In the motor domain, value modulations could similarly serve a function of motor attention to increase motor accuracy. Verifying the merits of these hypotheses is an important goal for future research.

COMPARISON WITH OTHER SPECIES

From an evolutionary perspective, it is interesting to notice that there is a qualitative difference between OFC responses observed in monkeys and those observed in rodents. Two recent studies found that the activity of OFC neurons in rats actually does depend on spatial or motor contingencies.[83,84] Moreover, using behavioral paradigms that involve time discounting, researchers observed that value and time are represented separately in the rat OFC.[84] In contrast, in monkeys, OFC neurons reflect time-discounted values.[65]

Although it is possible that the recording region in rats was not exactly homologous to that in monkeys, these studies suggest that the representation of economic value in primates may be substantially more abstract than the representation in rodents.[85] With respect to the preceding discussion, this observation suggests that good-based choices may have emerged relatively late in the course of evolution. Importantly, this hypothesis is contingent upon future research, necessary to establish whether any abstract representation of value actually exists in the rat brain. Conversely, it remains to be determined whether OFC responses in rodents actually encode economic value in the sense defined in this chapter, as opposed to physical properties of appetitive stimuli (e.g., food volume or weight).

CONCLUSION

In summary, we defined economic choice and we described an experimental paradigm to study this behavior in nonhuman primates. Behavioral evidence indicates that choices cannot be explained as simple stimulus–response associations. According to a cognitive model, economic choice entails assigning values to the available options and deciding consequently. A rich literature from lesion studies, functional imaging, and primate neurophysiology suggests that critical mechanisms for economic choice might take place in the OFC. More specifically, recent results from single cell recordings in monkeys link the OFC to the computation of economic value. We showed that the value representation in the OFC reflects the subjective nature of economic value, and that neurons in this area encode value *per se*, independently of the visuomotor contingencies of choice. Finally, we discussed the implications of this result for possible cognitive models of choice, and we advocated the hypothesis that economic choices are fundamentally choices between goods rather than choices between actions.

A number of important issues remain open. For example, it is not clear whether the same neuronal population described here encodes the value of other types of commodities (e.g., socially valuable commodities).[86] The neuronal mechanisms by which values are compared (i.e., by which decisions are made) are also currently unknown. Research in the coming years will hopefully shed light on these fundamental questions.

ACKNOWLEDGMENTS

The studies described here were conducted in collaboration with John Assad, whom I thank for his advice and support. My research was founded by a postdoctoral fellowship from the Harvard Mind/Brain/Behavior Initiative and by a Pathway to Independence Award (K99-MH-080852) from the National Institute of Mental Health.

REFERENCES

1. KREPS, D.M. 1990. A Course in Microeconomic Theory. 850. Princeton University Press. Princeton, NJ.
2. ALLINGHAM, M. 2002. Choice Theory: a Very Short Introduction. 127. Oxford University Press. Oxford, UK; New York, NY.
3. LUCE, R.D. 1959. Individual Choice Behavior; a Theoretical Analysis. 153. Wiley. New York, NY.
4. KAGEL, J.H., R.C. BATTALIO & L. GREEN 1995. Economic Choice Theory: an Experimental Analysis of Animal Behavior, xii. 230. Cambridge University Press. Cambridge, UK; New York, NY.
5. AINSLIE, G. 1992. Picoeconomics: the Strategic Interaction of Successive Motivational States Within the Person, xvi. 440. Cambridge University Press. Cambridge, UK; New York, NY.
6. KAHNEMAN, D. & A. TVERSKY, Eds. 2000. Choices, Values and Frames, xx. 840. Russell Sage Foundation—Cambridge University Press. Cambridge, UK; New York, NY.
7. CAMERER, C. 2003. Behavioral Game Theory: experiments in Strategic Interaction. Russell Sage Foundation—Princeton University Press. Princeton, NJ.
8. ROSSOR, M.N. 2001. Pick's disease: a clinical overview. Neurology 56: S3–S5.
9. PASQUIER, F. & H. PETIT. 1997. Frontotemporal dementia: its rediscovery. Eur. Neurol. 38: 1–6.

10. HODGES, J.R. 2001. Frontotemporal dementia (Pick's disease): clinical features and assessment. Neurology **56:** S6–S10.
11. RAHMAN, S., B.J. SAHAKIAN, J.R. HODGES, *et al.* 1999. Robbins specific cognitive deficits in mild frontal variant of frontotemporal dementia. Brain **122**(Pt 8): 1469–1493.
12. SHAPIRO, D. 1965. Neurotic Styles, xii. 207. Basic Books. New York, NY.
13. EVERITT, B.J. & T.W. ROBBINS. 2005. Neural systems of reinforcement for drug addiction: from actions to habits to compulsion. Nat. Neurosci. **8:** 1481–1489.
14. VOLKOW, N.D. & T.K. LI. 2004. Drug addiction: the neurobiology of behaviour gone awry. Nat. Rev Neurosci. **5:** 963–970.
15. PADOA-SCHIOPPA, C., L. JANDOLO & E. VISALBERGHI. 2006. Multi-stage mental process for economic choice in capuchins. Cognition **99:** B1–B13.
16. PADOA-SCHIOPPA, C. & J.A. ASSAD. 2006. Neurons in orbitofrontal cortex encode economic value. Nature **441:** 223–226.
17. MAZUREK, M.E., J.D. ROITMAN, J. DITTERICH & M.N. SHADLEN. 2003. A role for neural integrators in perceptual decision making. Cereb. Cortex **13:** 1257–1269.
18. ROMO, R. & E. SALINAS. 2003. Flutter discrimination: neural codes, perception, memory and decision making. Nat. Rev. Neurosci. **4:** 203–218.
19. IKEDA, T. & O. HIKOSAKA. 2003. Reward-dependent gain and bias of visual responses in primate superior colliculus. Neuron **39:** 693–700.
20. KAWAGOE, R., Y. TAKIKAWA & O. HIKOSAKA. 1998. Expectation of reward modulates cognitive signals in the basal ganglia. Nat. Neurosci. **1:** 411–416.
21. WALLIS, J.D. & E.K. MILLER. 2003. Neuronal activity in primate dorsolateral and orbital prefrontal cortex during performance of a reward preference task. Eur. J. Neurosci. **18:** 2069–2081.
22. PLATT, M.L. & P.W. GLIMCHER. 1999. Neural correlates of decision variables in parietal cortex. Nature **400:** 233–238.
23. ROESCH, M.R. & C.R. OLSON. 2003. Impact of expected reward on neuronal activity in prefrontal cortex, frontal and supplementary eye fields and premotor cortex. J. Neurophysiol. **90:** 1766–1789.
24. LEON, M.I. & M.N. SHADLEN. 1999. Effect of expected reward magnitude on the response of neurons in the dorsolateral prefrontal cortex of the macaque. Neuron **24:** 415–425.
25. SAMEJIMA, K., Y. UEDA, K. DOYA & M. KIMURA. 2005. Representation of action-specific reward values in the striatum. Science **310:** 1337–1340.
26. MINAMIMOTO, T., Y. HORI & M. KIMURA. 2005. Complementary process to response bias in the centromedian nucleus of the thalamus. Science **308:** 1798–1801.
27. McCOY, A.N., J.C. CROWLEY, G. HAGHIGHIAN, *et al.* 2003. Saccade reward signals in posterior cingulate cortex. Neuron **40:** 1031–1040.
28. BARRACLOUGH, D.J., M.L. CONROY & D. LEE. 2004. Prefrontal cortex and decision making in a mixed-strategy game. Nat. Neurosci. **7:** 404–410.
29. DORRIS, M.C. & P.W. GLIMCHER. 2004. Activity in posterior parietal cortex is correlated with the relative subjective desirability of action. Neuron **44:** 365–378.
30. SUGRUE, L.P., G.S. CORRADO & W.T. NEWSOME. 2004. Matching behavior and the representation of value in the parietal cortex. Science **304:** 1782–1787.
31. SKINNER, B.F. 1953. Science and Human Behavior. 461. Macmillan. New York, NY.

32. SKINNER, B.F. 1981. Selection by consequences. Science **213:** 501–504.
33. ROSS, D. 2005. Economic Theory and Cognitive Science: microexplanation, x. 444. MIT Press. Cambridge, MA.
34. FELLOWS, L.K. 2004. The cognitive neuroscience of human decision making: a review and conceptual framework. Behav. Cogn. Neurosci. Rev. **3:** 159–172.
35. GLIMCHER, P.W., M.C. DORRIS & H.M. BAYER. 2005. Physiological utility theory and the neuroeconomics of choice. Games Econ. Behav. **52:** 213–256.
36. FELLOWS, L.K. & M.J. FARAH. 2007. The role of ventromedial prefrontal cortex in decision making: judgment under uncertainty or judgment per se? Cereb. Cortex **17:** 2669–2674.
37. BECHARA, A., A.R. DAMASIO, H. DAMASIO & S.W. ANDERSON. 1994. Insensitivity to future consequences following damage to human prefrontal cortex. Cognition **50:** 7–15.
38. KOENIGS, M. & D. TRANEL. 2007. Irrational economic decision-making after ventromedial prefrontal damage: evidence from the Ultimatum Game. J. Neurosci. **27:** 951–956.
39. DAMASIO, A.R. 1994. Descartes' Error: emotion, Reason, and the Human Brain, xix. 312. Putnam. New York, NY.
40. FELLOWS, L.K. 2006. Deciding how to decide: ventromedial frontal lobe damage affects information acquisition in multi-attribute decision making. Brain **129:** 944–952.
41. DAMASIO, H., T. GRABOWSKI, R. FRANK, et al. 1994. The return of Phineas Gage: clues about the brain from the skull of a famous patient. Science **264:** 1102–1105.
42. FELLOWS, L.K. & M.J. FARAH. 2003. Ventromedial frontal cortex mediates affective shifting in humans: evidence from a reversal learning paradigm. Brain **126:** 1830–1837.
43. BUTTER, C.M., J.A. MCDONALD & D.R. SNYDER. 1969. Orality, preference behavior, and reinforcement value of nonfood object in monkeys with orbital frontal lesions. Science **164:** 1306–1307.
44. DIAS, R., T.W. ROBBINS & A.C. ROBERTS. 1996. Dissociation in prefrontal cortex of affective and attentional shifts. Nature **380:** 69–72.
45. IZQUIERDO, A., R.K. SUDA & E.A. MURRAY. 2004. Bilateral orbital prefrontal cortex lesions in rhesus monkeys disrupt choices guided by both reward value and reward contingency. J. Neurosci. **24:** 7540–7548.
46. O'DOHERTY, J.P. 2004. Reward representations and reward-related learning in the human brain: insights from neuroimaging. Curr. Opin. Neurobiol. **14:** 769–776.
47. ANDERSON, A.K. et al. 2003. Dissociated neural representations of intensity and valence in human olfaction. Nat. Neurosci. **6:** 196–202.
48. ROLLS, E.T., M.L. KRINGELBACH & I.E. DE ARAUJO. 2003. Different representations of pleasant and unpleasant odours in the human brain. Eur. J. Neurosci. **18:** 695–703.
49. O'DOHERTY, J., E.T. ROLLS, S. FRANCIS, et al. 2001. Representation of pleasant and aversive taste in the human brain. J. Neurophysiol. **85:** 1315–1321.
50. AHARON, I. et al. 2001. Beautiful faces have variable reward value: fMRI and behavioral evidence. Neuron **32:** 537–551.
51. O'DOHERTY, J. et al. 2003. Beauty in a smile: the role of medial orbitofrontal cortex in facial attractiveness. Neuropsychologia **41:** 147–155.
52. BLOOD, A.J., R.J. ZATORRE, P. BERMUDEZ & A.C. EVANS. 1999. Emotional responses to pleasant and unpleasant music correlate with activity in paralimbic

brain regions. Nat. Neurosci. **2:** 382–387.

53. ROLLS, E.T. *et al.* 2003. Representations of pleasant and painful touch in the human orbitofrontal and cingulate cortices. Cereb. Cortex **13:** 308–317.

54. MONTAGUE, P.R. & G.S. BERNS. 2002. Neural economics and the biological substrates of valuation. Neuron **36:** 265–284.

55. O'DOHERTY, J., M.L. KRINGELBACH, E.T. ROLLS, *et al.* 2001. Abstract reward and punishment representations in the human orbitofrontal cortex. Nat. Neurosci. **4:** 95–102.

56. MCCLURE, S.M., D.I. LAIBSON, G. LOEWENSTEIN & J.D. COHEN. 2004. Separate neural systems value immediate and delayed monetary rewards. Science **306:** 503–507.

57. ARANA, F.S. *et al.* 2003. Dissociable contributions of the human amygdala and orbitofrontal cortex to incentive motivation and goal selection. J. Neurosci. **23:** 9632–9638.

58. BLAIR, K. *et al.* 2006. Choosing the lesser of two evils, the better of two goods: specifying the roles of ventromedial prefrontal cortex and dorsal anterior cingulate in object choice. J. Neurosci. **26:** 11379–11386.

59. THORPE, S.J., E.T. ROLLS & S. MADDISON. 1983. The orbitofrontal cortex: neuronal activity in the behaving monkey. Exp. Brain Res. **49:** 93–115.

60. ROLLS, E.T., Z.J. SIENKIEWICZ & S. YAXLEY. 1989. Hunger modulates the responses to gustatory stimuli of single neurons in the caudolateral orbitofrontal cortex of the macaque monkey. Eur. J. Neurosci **1:** 53–60.

61. TREMBLAY, L. & W. SCHULTZ. 1999. Relative reward preference in primate orbitofrontal cortex. Nature **398:** 704–708.

62. STUPHORN, V. 2006. Neuroeconomics: cardinal utility in the orbitofrontal cortex? Curr. Biol. **16:** R591–R593.

63. PADOA-SCHIOPPA, C. & J.A. ASSAD. 2006. Neurons in orbitofrontal cortex encode economic value independently of the "menu". Society for Neuroscience Meeting, [Abstract, Abstract number 571.14].

64. ROESCH, M.R. & C.R. OLSON. 2004. Neuronal activity related to reward value and motivation in primate frontal cortex. Science **304:** 307–310.

65. ROESCH, M.R. & C.R. OLSON. 2005. Neuronal activity in primate orbitofrontal cortex reflects the value of time. J. Neurophysiol. **94:** 2457–2471.

66. JUDGE, S.J., B.J. RICHMOND & F.C. CHU. 1980. Implantation of magnetic search coils for measurement of eye position: an improved method. Vision Res. **20:** 535–538.

67. CARMICHAEL, S.T. & J.L. PRICE. 1994. Architectonic subdivision of the orbital and medial prefrontal cortex in the macaque monkey. J. Comp. Neurol. **346:** 366–402.

68. ONGUR, D. & J.L. PRICE. 2000. The organization of networks within the orbital and medial prefrontal cortex of rats, monkeys and humans. Cereb. Cortex **10:** 206–219.

69. ITO, S., V. STUPHORN, J.W. BROWN & J.D. SCHALL. 2003. Performance monitoring by the anterior cingulate cortex during saccade countermanding. Science **302:** 120–122.

70. MATSUMOTO, K., W. SUZUKI & K. TANAKA. 2003. Neuronal correlates of goal-based motor selection in the prefrontal cortex. Science **301:** 229–232.

71. SHIDARA, M. & B.J. RICHMOND. 2002. Anterior cingulate: single neuronal signals related to degree of reward expectancy. Science **296:** 1709–1711.

72. STUPHORN, V., T.L. TAYLOR & J.D. SCHALL. 2000. Performance monitoring by the supplementary eye field. Nature **408:** 857–860.
73. PATON, J.J., M.A. BELOVA, S.E. MORRISON & C.D. SALZMAN. 2006. The primate amygdala represents the positive and negative value of visual stimuli during learning. Nature **439:** 865–870.
74. MAUNSELL, J.H. 2004. Neuronal representations of cognitive state: reward or attention? Trends Cogn. Sci. **8:** 261–265.
75. SNYDER, L.H., A.P. BATISTA & R.A. ANDERSEN. 1997. Coding of intention in the posterior parietal cortex. Nature **386:** 167–170.
76. SIMON, H.A. 1962. The architecture of complexity. Proc. Am. Phil. Soc. **106:** 467–482.
77. FODOR, J.A. 1983. The Modularity of Mind: an Essay on Faculty Psychology. 145. MIT Press. Cambridge, MA.
78. PINKER, S. 1997. How the Mind Works, xii. 660. Norton. New York, NY.
79. WOLPERT, D.M. & Z. GHAHRAMANI. 2000. Computational principles of movement Neuroscience. Nat. Neurosci. **3**(Suppl): 1212–1217.
80. MUSSA-IVALDI, F.A. & E. BIZZI. 2000. Motor learning through the combination of primitives. Philos. Trans. R. Soc. Lond. B Biol. Sci. **355:** 1755–1769.
81. COLBY, C.L. & C.R. OLSON. 1999. Spatial cognition. *In* Fundamental Neuroscience. M.J. Zigmond, F.E. Bloom, S.C. Landis, J.L. Roberts & L.R. Squire, Eds.: 1363–1383. Academic Press. San Diego, CA.
82. KANDEL, E.R., J.H. SCHWARTZ & T.M. JESSELL, Eds. 2000. Principles of Neural Science, xli. 1414. McGraw-Hill. New York, NY.
83. FEIERSTEIN, C.E., M.C. QUIRK, N. UCHIDA, *et al.* 2006. Representation of spatial goals in rat orbitofrontal cortex. Neuron **51:** 495–507.
84. ROESCH, M.R., A.R. TAYLOR & G. SCHOENBAUM. 2006. Encoding of time-discounted rewards in orbitofrontal cortex is independent of value representation. Neuron **51:** 509–520.
85. ZALD, D.H. 2006. The rodent orbitofrontal cortex gets time and direction. Neuron **51:** 395–397.
86. DEANER, R.O., A.V. KHERA & M.L. PLATT. 2005. Monkeys pay per view: adaptive valuation of social images by rhesus macaques. Curr. Biol. **15:** 543–548.

Lights, Camembert, Action! The Role of Human Orbitofrontal Cortex in Encoding Stimuli, Rewards, and Choices

JOHN P. O'DOHERTY

Computation and Neural Systems Program, California Institute of Technology, Pasadena, California 91125, USA

Division of Humanities and Social Sciences, California Institute of Technology, Pasadena, California 91125, USA

ABSTRACT: This review outlines some of the main conclusions about the contributions of the orbitofrontal cortex to reward learning and decision making arising from functional neuroimaging studies in humans. It will be argued that human orbitofrontal cortex is involved in a number of distinct functions: signaling the affective value of stimuli as they are perceived, encoding expectations of future reward, and updating these expectations, either by making use of prediction error signals generated in the midbrain, or by using knowledge of the rules or structure of the decision problem. It will also be suggested that this region contributes to the decision making process itself, by encoding signals that inform an individual about what action to take next. Evidence for functional specialization within orbitofrontal cortex in terms of valence will also be evaluated, and the possible contributions of the orbitofrontal cortex in representing the values of actions as well as that of stimuli will be discussed. Finally, some of the outstanding questions for future neuroimaging research of orbitofrontal cortex function will be highlighted.

KEYWORDS: fMRI; neuroimaging; learning; conditioning; decision making

INTRODUCTION

It is well established that damage to human orbitofrontal cortex (OFC) and adjacent medial prefrontal cortex can result in impairments on tasks probing the ability to make decisions for reward under uncertainty, as well as to flexibly modulate action selection in the face of changing contingencies.[1–4] However, the precise nature of the computations being implemented by this region that

Address for correspondence: John P. O'Doherty, Division of Humanities and Social Sciences, California Institute of Technology, 1200 E California Blvd, Pasadena, CA 91125. Voice: +1 626 395 5981; +1 626 793 8580.

jdoherty@caltech.edu

Ann. N.Y. Acad. Sci. 1121: 254–272 (2007). © 2007 New York Academy of Sciences.
doi: 10.1196/annals.1401.036

give rise to such deficits are much less well understood. In this paper we review evidence about the functions of human OFC garnered from functional neuroimaging studies in humans.

Insight into the functions of the OFC can be derived from its anatomical location and connectivity. It is highly interconnected with sub-cortical structures involved in affective processing such as the amygdala and ventral striatum,[5] consistent with a role for OFC in reward and affect related processing. On the other hand, the OFC as a part of prefrontal cortex is also highly interconnected with other sectors within prefrontal cortex.[6] Therefore, it is plausible that OFC will in addition to its role in reward and affect, share functional commonalities with these other parts of prefrontal cortex. Here, it will be argued that as a key component of the reward system, OFC is involved in representing stimulus-reward value as well as in encoding representations of future expected reward, functions which it may share in common with the amygdala and ventral striatum. In addition, OFC receives signals pertaining to errors in reward prediction, that may underlie learning of reward predictions. Much like other parts of the prefrontal cortex,[7] OFC and adjacent ventral medial prefrontal cortex may also play a role in encoding abstract rules, in this case by incorporating knowledge of the structure pertaining to the rules of the decision problem, and in applying knowledge of such rules to guide reward expectations. Finally, in common with the prefrontal cortex as a whole, this region also plays an important role in the flexible control of behavior,[8] by generating decision signals that inform an individual about what action to take next.

REPRESENTATIONS OF STIMULUS VALUE

One of the most established findings regarding the OFC is that it is involved in coding for the reward value of a stimulus, shown initially in single-unit recording studies in monkeys whereby neurons in this region were found to respond to a particular taste or odor when an animal was hungry but decreased their firing rate once the animal was satiated and the corresponding food was no longer rewarding.[9,10] Imaging studies in humans have not only confirmed these findings for olfactory and gustatory stimuli[11-16] but have also shown that BOLD responses in OFC correlate with the reward value of stimuli in other sensory modalities, such as in the somatosensory, auditory, and visual domains.[15-17] It has also been shown that OFC responds to abstract rewards not tied to a particular sensory modality, such as money or social praise.[18-20] These findings suggest that human OFC is involved in flexibly encoding the reward value of a wide variety of stimuli in diverse modalities. There is also considerable evidence to suggest that OFC responds not only to rewards but also to punishers.[13,17,18,21]

Regional Specialization within OFC: Rewards versus Punishers

This raises the question as to whether anatomically dissociable sub-regions within OFC are involved in responding to rewarding and punishing events respectively. Evidence in support of such a possibility was first provided by O'Doherty et al.,[21] who reported a medial versus lateral dissociation in OFC responses to rewards and punishers during performance of a task in which subjects could win or lose abstract monetary reward. Medial sectors of OFC were found to respond to monetary reward, and a part of lateral OFC was found to respond to monetary loss. Comparable results were obtained by Ursu and Carter[22] A similar dissociation was also found in an fMRI study of facial attractiveness in which both high and low attractiveness faces were presented to subjects while they performed an unrelated gender judgment task.[17] Faces high in attractiveness recruited medial OFC whereas low attractive faces recruited lateral OFC. Small and colleagues also reported a differential responses in medial and lateral OFC during the consumption of a chocolate meal to satiety.[23] Medial OFC responded during early stages of feeding, when the chocolate had high reward value, whereas enhanced lateral OFC activity was only evident when subjects were reaching satiety and the chocolate went from being pleasant to aversive. A number of imaging studies of olfaction have also reported a similar medial versus lateral dissociation, with medial OFC responding to pleasant odors and lateral to aversive odors.[11,12,15] More recently Kim and colleagues[24] reported that medial OFC was activated not only by receipt of a rewarding outcome but also by the successful avoidance of an aversive outcome, suggesting that successful avoidance in itself can act as an intrinsic reward (FIG. 1). On the other hand, more lateral areas of prefrontal cortex extending onto the orbital surface were found to respond both during receipt of an aversive outcome as well as following a failure to obtain reward.

While the above studies appear to support a medial vs lateral dissociation, a number of other studies have failed to report such a dissociation. For instance, Elliott and colleagues used a block fMRI design to measure neural responses to parametrically varied quantities of monetary gain and loss.[25] Significant activity was reported in both medial and lateral OFC to monetary gain and loss. Similarly, Breiter et al.[18] have also found that both medial and lateral regions of OFC responded equally to rewarding and punishing feedback. In a study of probabilistic reversal learning, monetary gains were associated with activity in both anterior medial and central OFC, whereas monetary loss recruited a part of posterior lateral OFC only if this was followed by a switch in behavioral strategy on the subsequent trial.[26] Furthermore, other studies have reported a role for the medial OFC in complex emotions such as regret which may contain both positive and negative affective components.[27] These discrepant findings suggest that the differential functions of medial and lateral OFC areas may be more complex than at first supposed. In order to understand

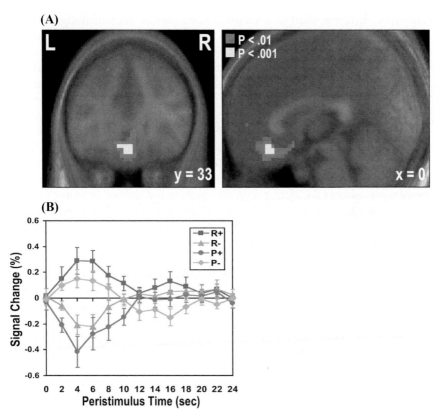

FIGURE 1. Responses to receipt of reward and successful avoidance of an aversive outcome in medial OFC. **(A)** Medial OFC showing a significant increase in activity after avoidance of an aversive outcome as well as after obtaining reward [x = 0, y = 33, z = −18, Z = 3.48, P < 0.05] (corrected for small volume using coordinates derived from a previous study). No other brain areas showed significant effects at P < 0.001, uncorrected. Voxels significant at P < 0.001 are shown in yellow. To illustrate the extent of the activation we also show voxels significant at P < 0.01 in red. **(B)** Time-course plots of peak voxels in the OFC for each of four different possible outcomes: receipt of reward (R+), avoidance of an aversive outcome (P−), missed reward (R−), and receipt of an aversive outcome (P+). The plots are arranged such that time 0 corresponds to the point of outcome delivery. These time courses are shown after adjusting for the effects of expected value and prediction error (i.e., removing those effects from the data). Data from Kim et al.[24] (In color in *Annals* online.)

the possible basis of such differences between studies it may be important to consider at least two factors.

First, some of the studies that have failed to report functional dissociations within OFC are complex gambling or decision making tasks in which a number of distinct processes are engaged besides coding outcome value, such as anticipation or expectation of reward, selection of appropriate behavioral responses, detecting change in contingencies, and/or implementing changes in behavioral strategy. Thus, the degree to which these different processes are engaged in a given task, and the extent to which these different processes are disambiguated from each other in the experimental design and analysis, could contribute to discrepancies in reported results between studies. In support of the this possibility, in the Kim *et al.*[24] study, it was found that both medial and central parts of OFC were engaged during expectation of reward, whereas only medial OFC was engaged following receipt of a rewarding outcome and avoidance of an aversive one. These findings suggest that a clear dissociation between responses may only be present in relation to the receipt but not the expectation of reward. However, a recent study found a medial versus lateral dissociation within OFC during *both* anticipation and receipt, such that medial OFC was more active when subjects were anticipating, receiving and evaluating monetary gains, and lateral OFC was more engaged under situations where subjects were anticipating, obtaining or evaluating monetary losses.[28]

The second factor likely to play a role in accounting for differences between studies is that monetary loss may differ from other more biologically relevant punishers in that the behavioral significance of a loss to an individual likely depends strongly on the context in which that outcome is presented. Contextual effects on decision making have long been demonstrated in the behavioral economics literature, such that for instance subjects respond differently to outcomes framed in a loss context than they do to the same outcomes framed in a gain context.[29] In most human imaging studies where feedback is obtained on a trial by trial basis, neural responses to monetary loss may depend on the degree to which those losses signal to the subjects that a change in their current behavior is warranted. In the case of more natural or primary reinforcers, such as pain or unpleasant taste, obtaining such an outcome may naturally lead to a change in behavior in order to avoid the outcome in the future. However, in some gambling or decision-making tasks, a monetary loss does not automatically signal that behavior should be altered. For example in the case of probabilistic reversal learning, the nature of the probabilistic contingencies imply that sometimes one receives a monetary loss for choosing the correct stimulus and sometimes a reward is obtained even when choosing the incorrect stimulus. This introduces an ambiguity into the meaning of a rewarding or punishing outcome. It is no longer the case that the reward or punisher itself is a straightforward cue as to what behavioral strategy should be adopted because a punishing outcome can occur following choice of the correct stimulus as well as following choice of the incorrect stimulus. This is the case in many other types of decision-making tasks besides reversal, such as in gambling tasks where it is advantageous to sustain monetary loss in the short term in order to gain monetarily in the long run. Thus, the context in which rewarding or punishing stimuli are presented, particularly monetary outcomes, may need to be taken into account when interpreting the degree to which different tasks result in varying recruitment of appetitive and aversive motivational systems.

RESPONSES RELATED TO PREDICTIONS
OF FUTURE REWARD

It is known from single-unit neurophysiology studies that neurons in OFC are involved not only in responding to the receipt of rewarding and punishing outcomes, but also respond in anticipation of the receipt of such outcomes in the future.[40,41,58] Consistent with these findings from animal studies, human neuroimaging studies have implicated OFC alongside other structures, such as amygdala and ventral striatum, in predicting future rewards. An example is a study by O'Doherty and colleagues,[30] where arbitrary fractal stimuli were presented and followed, after a variable interval, by either a pleasant taste (glucose), an affectively neutral taste (control tasteless solution), or by an aversive taste (saline). Significant effects were found in anterior OFC during anticipation, as well as receipt of, reward. These results have subsequently been confirmed in other paradigms, using different types of reward. For instance, in one study neural responses to cues associated with subsequent delivery of either a pleasant or aversive odor where each cue was followed on 50% of occasions by a specific odor.[31] Significant orbitofrontal responses (in anterior central OFC) were found to the predictive cues associated with the pleasant and aversive odors. These findings also implicate OFC in maintaining predictions for negatively as well as positively valenced stimuli.

The Content of Predictive Representations in OFC

The finding that predictive reward representations are present in OFC leaves open the question as to the content of these representations. In order to appreciate the importance of this question it is useful to consider the ultimate function of predictive representations. Predictions enable behavior to be organized prospectively so that an organism is prepared in advance for the occurrence of an affectively significant event. Many such responses can be considered to be reflexive, in they are automatically elicited by a conditioned stimulus (CS). The paradigmatic example of this is the conditioned salivatory response that Pavlov observed in his food conditioned dogs.[32] In this example as in others, the conditioned responses are identical to those elicited by the unconditioned stimulus (UCS). For example, Pavlov's dogs salivate to the food itself and then also come to salivate to the CS after learning. A central question in learning theory concerns the nature of the CS encoding. Pavlov proposed that a CS constitutes a 'stimulus substitute' for the UCS in that it elicits the same response that occurs following presentation of the UCS (see also Ref. 33). Stimulus substitution could be a very useful mechanism for enabling the animal to know *what* is predicted. However, not all conditioned responses are identical to those elicited by the UCS. For example, a CS for food reward can involve approach and orientation responses distinct from those produced by the UCS itself.[34–36] Consequently stimulus substitution may not be the only mechanism by which a CS acquires predictive value. Indeed it would be extremely useful for the animal to have a predictive mechanism that signals an impending behaviorally significant event without eliciting a representation of the event itself. In effect this would enable an animal to distinguish cues that predict a stimulus from the actual UCS itself. In many instances different behavioral responses are appropriate when anticipating a rewarding or punishing event than when experiencing it. If stimulus substitution were to be the only mechanism in place then a CS would be indistinguishable from the UCS from the point of view of the animal. Thus, a light cue predicting food would be treated as if it were the food itself and the animal would attempt to consume it. Intriguingly this type of behavior has been observed in some instances.[33] However, given that in many cases, animals (including humans) can distinguish a predictive cue from the UCS itself, as indicated by distinct behavioral responses in these two cases, it seems likely from that there are at least two distinct associative mechanisms in the brain, one based on stimulus substitution and the other uniquely signalling prediction.

With regard to the OFC there is some preliminary evidence to suggest that this region may be involved in maintaining both CS-specific and stimulus-substitution related predictions. Galvan et al.,[37] reported a region of lateral OFC that responded in anticipation of future rewards, but where responses did not occur initially following presentation of the reward, suggesting a CS-specific encoding in this area. In the Kim et al. study discussed previously,[24] a region of central OFC was found to respond during anticipation of reward but not during its receipt, again consistent with a CS-specific representation, whereas a region of medial OFC was found to respond both during expectation of reward and receipt of reward, suggestive of predictive responses based on stimulus-substitution. Moreover, Rolls et al.,[38] also reported activation in medial OFC during both anticipation and receipt of reward.

Another related question is to what feature of the UCS or reward stimulus does the prediction pertain? One form of predictive coding could be to simply elicit a representation of the sensory properties of the reward stimulus (e.g., its specific taste or flavor), without encoding its underlying hedonic value. Alternatively, such a representation could link directly to the underlying value of the reward stimulus. One way to discriminate between such possibilities is to change the value of the associated reward after the CS-reward association has been established and determine whether the associated CS representation changes as a function of devaluation or remains unchanged. If the CS representation were to access the underlying reward value of the UCS, the former result should be found, whereas if the CS accesses only the stimulus properties of the reward then the latter effect should be observed. To address this question, Gottfried and colleagues[39] performed a study in which predictive cues were associated with one of two food-related odors, and subjects were scanned while being presented with such cues before and after feeding to satiety on one of the corresponding foods, thereby selectively devaluing the odor of the food eaten. Predictive responses in anterior central OFC were found to track the specific value of the corresponding odors, indicating that the reward value and not the sensory properties of a stimulus is coded in this region.

Yet another distinction concerning the nature of predictive representations is whether such responses occur directly following presentation of a cue stimulus or whether such responses occur later in a trial in anticipation of the impending receipt of the subsequent outcome. Although some imaging studies have attempted to distinguish between these two possibilities, supporting a role for OFC in the latter,[37] limitations in the temporal resolution of fMRI has so far precluded definitive conclusions about the temporal characteristics of predictive representations in human OFC. However, as both types of predictive representations have been found to be present in OFC in single-unit recording studies in both rats and non-human primates,[40,41] it is reasonable to presume that both types of predictive signal will also be found in human OFC.

Stimulus or Action Values in Human OFC?

The vast majority of studies of reward prediction in both the animal neurophysiology and the human imaging literature have implicated OFC in stimulus bound predictions of future reward. That is, activity in OFC has been found to occur in response to the presentation of a cue (such as an odor or visual stimulus) that signals a future reward, or in the interval before a reward is delivered following presentation of such a cue. Although stimulus bound predictions provide information about whether a reward may be expected to occur, such predictions provide no information about what actions need to be performed in order to obtain it. For this, it is necessary to learn associations between stimuli, actions and outcomes, so that in a given context an animal can learn to perform a specific response in order to obtain reward. Evidence from animal learning studies suggests the process of action selection for reward may be implemented via two distinct learning processes, a goal-directed component which involves learning of associations between actions and the incentive value of outcomes (action-outcome or stimulus-action-outcome learning), and a habit learning component which involves learning associations between stimuli (or context) and actions (stimulus-response learning).[42] Substantial neurobiological evidence supports the existence of distinct goal-directed and habit learning systems in rats, implicating a part of the prefrontal cortex (prelimbic cortex) and dorsomedial striatum in the former and the dorsolateral striatum in the latter.[43-47] The finding that a part of rat prefrontal cortex contributes to action-outcome learning raises the question of whether there exists a homologous region of the primate brain performing a similar function.

To address this, Valentin and colleagues[48] scanned human subjects with fMRI while they learned to choose instrumental actions that were associated with the subsequent delivery of different food rewards (tomato juice, chocolate milk, and orange juice). Following training, one of these foods was devalued by feeding the subject to satiety on that food. The subjects were then scanned again, while being re-exposed to the instrumental choice procedure (in extinction). By testing for regions of the brain showing a change in activity during selection of the devalued action compared to that elicited during selection of the valued action from pre to post satiety, it was possible to test for regions showing sensitivity to the learned action-outcome associations. The regions found to show such a response profile were medial and central OFC (Fig. 2). These findings suggest that action-outcome information is present in OFC alongside stimulus–outcome representations, indicative of a role for OFC in encoding expectations of reward tied to specific actions above and beyond its role in encoding stimulus bound predictions. A number of recent single-unit neurophysiology studies in rats have also found evidence of response selectivity in OFC neurons, consistent with the findings of the Valentin et al.[48] study. However, in contradiction of the above findings, it has also been recently shown that lesions of OFC in rats do not produce impairments at goal-directed learning in contrast to the effects of lesions of the prelimbic area that do produce robust deficits in this capacity.[67]

The source of such discrepancies between studies remains to be determined, but one intriguing possibility is that rat and human OFC may not be entirely homologous in their entirety. It is interesting to note that in the previous stimulus-based devaluation study by Gottfried et al.,[39] modulatory effects of reinforcer devaluation were found in central, but not medial OFC areas, whereas in the Valentin et al.[48] study, evidence was found of instrumental devaluation effects in both central and medial areas. This raises the possibility that the medial OFC may be more involved in the goal-directed component of instrumental conditioning whereas central OFC may be more involved in pavlovian stimulus–outcome learning (as this area was found in both the Valentin et al.[48] study and in the previous pavlovian devaluation study). This speculation is consistent with the known anatomical connectivity of these areas in which central areas of OFC (Brodmann areas 11 and 13) receive input primarily from sensory areas, consistent with a role for these areas in stimulus–stimulus learning, whereas the medial OFC (areas 14 and 25) receives input primarily from structures on the adjacent medial wall of prefrontal cortex, such as cingulate cortex, an area often implicated in response selection and/or reward-based action choice.[49] It is also notable that although the majority of single-unit studies in monkeys have reported stimulus-related activity and not response-related selectivity in the OFC (e.g., Refs. 41, 50, 51) these studies have typically recorded from more lateral and central areas of the OFC (Brodmann areas 12/47 and 13, respectively), and not from more medial areas. It is therefore plausible that the more medial sectors of the OFC in humans correspond to regions considered part of medial prefrontal cortex in rats that have been more conclusively linked to goal-directed learning in the rat lesion studies.[44,45]

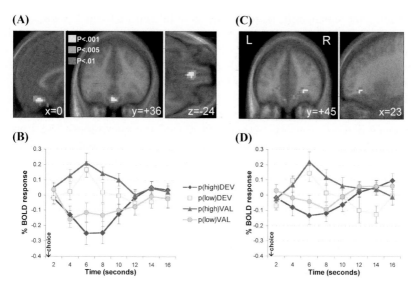

FIGURE 2. Regions of OFC exhibiting response properties consistent with action-outcome learning. Neural activity during action selection for reward in OFC showing a change in response properties as a function of the value of the outcome with each action. Choice of an action leading to a high probability of obtaining an outcome that had been devalued (p(high)DEV) led to a decrease in activity in these areas whereas choice of an action leading to a high probability of obtaining an outcome that was still valued by led to an increase in activity in the same areas. Devaluation was accomplished by means of feeding the subject to satiety on that outcome prior to the test period. **(A)** A region of medial OFC showing a significant modulation in its activity during instrumental action selection as a function of the value of the associated outcome [medial OFC; −3, 36, −24 mm, Z = 3.29, P < 0.001]. **(B)** Time-course plots derived from the peak voxel (from each individual subject) in the medial OFC during trials in which subjects chose each one of the four different actions (choice of the high vs low probability action in either the Valued or Devalued conditions). **(C)** A region of right central OFC also showing a significant interaction effect [24, 45, −6 mm, Z = 3.19, P < 0.001]. **(D)** Time-course plots from the peak voxel (from each individual subject) in the right central OFC. Data from Valentin et al.[48] Copyright 2007 The Society for Neuroscience.

PREDICTION ERROR SIGNAL INPUTS TO OFC

How does the OFC and indeed other brain regions acquire predictive value representations be they stimulus or action bound? Some contemporary models of animal learning consider that learning occurs via a prediction error which signals discrepancies between expected and actual reward (or punishment).[52] In one extension of this theory—temporal difference learning, predictions are formed about the expected future reward in a trial, and a prediction error reports differences in successive predictions of future reward.[53] Single-unit studies in non-human primates implicate phasic activity within dopaminergic neurons as a possible neural substrate of this signal.[54,55] Over the course of learning, the signal shifts its responses from the reward to the CS, unexpected omission of reward results in a decrease in activity from baseline (a negative prediction error), whereas unexpected presentation of reward results in an increase in activity (positive prediction error). Human neuroimaging studies of classical conditioning for reward report prediction error signals in prominent target areas of dopamine neurons, including the OFC.[56,57] Dopamine neurons could facilitate learning of value predictions in these areas by gating plastic changes between sensory, action, and reward representations. The finding that prediction error related responses are present in OFC and throughout the reward network, is consistent with the possibility that this mechanism is used to mediate flexible learning and updating of reward associations, a function often ascribed to the OFC.[58]

RESPONSES RELATED TO ABSTRACT RULES IN A DECISION PROBLEM

Theories of learning based on prediction errors provide an account of how expected reward representations in OFC can be updated on an incremental basis through experience. However, in at least some situations an error correcting learning mechanism may not be the only means by which reward expectations can be modulated. Many types of decision problems, may have abstract rules or structure, that impact on the rewards available following choice of a particular action or set of actions. An example of such structure is in probabilistic reversal learning whereby an anti-correlation exists between the rewards available following choice of either action such that when one action yields a high probability of reward, the other action offers a low probability of reward. Thus at any one time, when one action is a good prospect the other is a bad prospect. Knowledge of such rules would confer considerable advantage to an individual attempting to solve such a problem and maximize reward. In a recent study, Hampton et al.[59] showed that during performance of a reversal-learning task, responses related to expected reward in medial OFC and adjacent medial prefrontal cortex did indeed incorporate knowledge of the abstract structure of this task, by reflecting the anti-correlation in the rewards that could be obtained from choice of either action. Thus, expected reward representations in OFC are updated not only via prediction errors but also according to knowledge of the abstract structure in a given decision problem. For a more detailed discussion of this particular feature of OFC function see O'Doherty et al.[60]

DECISION SIGNALS IN OFC

Lesion studies of orbital and ventral medial prefrontal cortex suggest that OFC is necessary for adaptive decision making.[1-4] However, the precise

functional contribution of OFC to the decision-making process is not immediately clear on the basis of those lesion studies. Impairments in such patients
could be due to an inability to maintain representations of predicted reward
that are used to guide decision making processes elsewhere. Alternatively,
OFC could play a role in the actual decision-making process itself, that is, in
the actual comparison process between the expected values of different actions
and in the selection of a specific action.

As we have seen, there is now considerable evidence to implicate OFC in
maintaining predictions of future reward, consistent with the first possibility.
However, a study by O'Doherty and colleagues,[26] also provides evidence to
support the second possibility—a role for OFC in the actual decision-making
process itself. This study involved reversal learning, a task described previously, in which subjects must choose between two different actions that yield
rewards and punishers with different probabilities. One action is advantageous
in that choice of that action has a high probability of reward (70%) and a low
probability of punisher (30%), whereas the other action is disadvantageous
in that choice of that action yields reward with a low probability (30%) and
punisher with high probability (70%). Occasionally, the contingencies reverse
such that subjects must work out on a trial by trial basis if contingencies have
changed and switch their choice of action in order to perform adaptively. The
design of the study enabled responses to rewards and punishers to be dissociated from signals related to behavioral choice. In this task subjects can
make one of two decisions: maintain responding to the current stimulus or
switch their choice of stimulus. In order to separate out this decision process from rewarding and punishing feedback, trials in which a punisher is
obtained and followed by a switch in stimulus choice (punish_switch) were
evaluated separately from trials in which a punisher is obtained and subjects
maintain responding to the current stimulus (punish_noswitch). Regions involved in behavioral choice (stay versus switch) were identified by comparing
punish_switch trials to reward (no_switch) and/or punish (no_switch) trials.
A region of medial and anterior central OFC was found to respond on trials in
which the subject maintained responding on the subsequent trial (irrespective
of whether the outcome was a reward or a punisher) (see Fig. 3). A different
region of posterior lateral OFC (contiguous with anterior insula) was found to
respond following a punisher on trials in which subjects switched their choice
of stimulus on the subsequent trial, but not otherwise. These findings suggest
that OFC is involved in behavioral choice and that different sectors of OFC
signal the appropriateness of different behavioral strategies—some regions
signal that on-going behavior should be maintained, whereas other regions
signal that behavior should be changed. These findings suggest that OFC may
be involved in actively computing the decision about what action to take next,
or at least in reporting the consequences of that decision. It should be noted
that while OFC may contribute to this process it is certainly not the only region containing signals relevant to decision making. For example, by using a

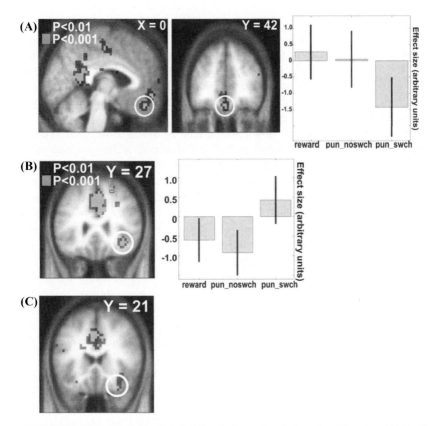

FIGURE 3.   Decision signals in OFC and adjacent ventral prefrontal cortex. **(A)** Sagittal and axial slices through a region of medial OFC that is involved in signaling that a behavioral response should be maintained. The plot of parameter estimates (*right of figure*) indicates that this region does not respond to rewards or punishments per se, but shows greater responses on rewarding and punishing trials if the subject does not switch their behavior compared to punishing trials followed by a switch in behavior (pun_swch). **(B)** Region of anterior insula extending into posterior lateral OFC that shows enhanced responses following a punishment if on the subsequent trial the subject switches their choice of stimulus (pun_swch) compared to rewarding or punishing trials were no such switch of behavior occurs. **(C)** Region of posterior lateral OFC that shows enhanced responses on punished trials following a switch in behavior compared to punished trials followed by no switch in behavior. Data from O'Doherty *et al.*[26] Copyright 2003 Society for Neuroscience.

classifier based approach, Hampton and O'Doherty[61] showed that information contained in three regions outside OFC: medial prefrontal cortex, ventral striatum, and anterior cingulate cortex were the most significant predictors of a subjects' subsequent decision out of all the regions studied (including OFC).

OUTSTANDING ISSUES

Considerable progress has been made in uncovering the functional contributions of human OFC since human neuroimaging became a mainstream tool for probing the functions of this brain area over 15 years ago. Yet, many outstanding questions remain. One such question is whether OFC contains a representation of common reward value. In order to make decisions between diverse types of reward it is reasonable to assume that somewhere in the brain a common currency for reward might be computed, such that the value of different rewards are encoded in the same relative scale.[62] Given the OFC's general role in encoding stimulus-reward value, this region would seem to be a strong candidate for encoding such a common currency. One possible mechanism by which such a common currency could be implemented at the neural level, is for information about the reward value of different types of reward to converge into the same brain region such that spatially overlapping neural representations would exist for the value of different rewards. As yet there is little evidence to either confirm or reject the possibility that OFC may play a role in encoding a common currency for reward, clearly an important direction for future research.

The precise nature of the functional anatomical specialization within OFC is also an unresolved issue. The OFC and adjacent medial prefrontal cortex is a vast area of cortex with over 22 different cytoarchitectonic sub-regions,[63] and therefore some degree of functional specialization within these areas is almost certainly going to be present. Here we have considered two possible sources for functional specialization: valence, or whether an outcome is rewarding or punishing; and the nature of the predictive associations being learned—whether they are stimulus or action bound. Another source of functional specialization not discussed in detail here is the nature of the reward itself, that is the sensory modality of the reward—whether it is conveyed in an auditory, visual, gustatory, olfactory, or somatosensory domain, and the associative history of that reward—whether it is a primary or secondary reinforcer. Future studies will be needed to evaluate these and other possibilities. It is likely that simple medial versus lateral or anterior-posterior dichotomies will provide an incomplete picture of the nature of the true functional heterogeneity in this area. Yet another issue for on-going research is the need to determine the differential contribution of OFC to reward-related learning and decision making compared to other interconnected brain regions, such as the amygdala, ventral striatum, and other sectors of prefrontal cortex, including the anterior cingulate cortex. Future studies will need to focus not only on the functions of each of these individual areas, but also on the nature of the interactions between them, mirroring recent progress being made along these lines in the animal literature.[40,64–66]

CONCLUSIONS

The OFC is both an integral part of the reward network and a part of prefrontal cortex. As a consequence, it simultaneously shares many functional commonalities with other parts of the reward system, and with other parts of prefrontal cortex. In this paper we have reviewed evidence primarily from functional neuroimaging studies in humans to suggest that OFC is involved in implementing at least five distinct functions, each of which are important for adaptive decision making. First of all, OFC encodes the value of stimuli as they are perceived. Such a basic valuation mechanism is necessary for the initial selection of goals, as stimuli perceived as having high reward value may be selected as items to be obtained in future, whereas stimuli perceived as having low or aversive significance may be selected as items to be avoided in future. Second, OFC is involved in maintaining representations of expected reward, both stimulus bound and action bound, computations that are necessary for providing information about the consequences that follow from taking particular courses of action or when choosing particular stimuli. Third, this region receives prediction error signals likely originating from dopamine neurons, an afferent signal that may underlie learning of reward predictions. Fourth, in addition to updating of expected value on the basis of prediction errors, OFC is also involved in using knowledge of the abstract structure of a decision problem to guide predictions of future reward. Finally, this region may also play a role in actually computing the decision itself, or at the very least in representing the consequences of that decision.

ACKNOWLEDGEMENTS

J.P.O. is supported by a Searle Scholarship, and by grants from the National Science Foundation, National Institute of Mental Health, and the Gordon and Betty Moore Foundation. The author would like to thank Peter Bossaerts, Alan Hampton, Hackjin Kim, Shin Shimojo, and Vivian Valentin at Caltech and Hugo Critchley, Peter Dayan, Ray Dolan, Jay Gottfried, Ben Seymour, and Joel Winston at UCL for their collaboration on many of the studies described here.

REFERENCES

1. BECHARA, A. *et al.* 1994. Insensitivity to future consequences following damage to human prefrontal cortex. Cognition **50:** 7–15.
2. FELLOWS, L.K. & M.J. FARAH. 2005. Different underlying impairments in decision-making following ventromedial and dorsolateral frontal lobe damage in humans. Cereb. Cortex **15:** 58–63.

3. HORNAK, J. *et al.* 2004. Reward-related reversal learning after surgical excisions in orbito-frontal or dorsolateral prefrontal cortex in humans. J. Cogn. Neurosci. **16:** 463–478.
4. ROLLS, E.T. *et al.* 1994. Emotion-related learning in patients with social and emotional changes associated with frontal lobe damage. J. Neurol. Neurosurg. Psychiatry **57:** 1518–1524.
5. CARMICHAEL, S.T. & J.L. PRICE. 1995. Limbic connections of the orbital and medial prefrontal cortex in macaque monkeys. J. Comp. Neurol. **363:** 615–641.
6. CARMICHAEL, S.T. & J.L. PRICE. 1996. Connectional networks within the orbital and medial prefrontal cortex of macaque monkeys. J. Comp. Neurol. **371:** 179–207.
7. WALLIS, J.D., K.C. ANDERSON & E.K. MILLER. 2001. Single neurons in prefrontal cortex encode abstract rules. Nature **411:** 953–956.
8. MILLER, E.K. & J.D. COHEN. 2001. An integrative theory of prefrontal cortex function. Annu. Rev. Neurosci. **24:** 167–202.
9. CRITCHLEY, H.D. & E.T. ROLLS. 1996. Hunger and satiety modify the responses of olfactory and visual neurons in the primate orbitofrontal cortex. J. Neurophysiol. **75:** 1673–86.
10. ROLLS, E.T., Z.J. SIENKIEWICZ & S. YAXLEY. 1989. Hunger modulates the responses to gustatory stimuli of single neurons in the caudolateral orbitofrontal cortex of the macaque monkey. Eur. J. Neurosci. **1:** 53–60.
11. ANDERSON, A.K. *et al.* 2003. Dissociated neural representations of intensity and valence in human olfaction. Nat. Neurosci. **6:** 196–202.
12. GOTTFRIED, J.A. *et al.* 2002. Functional heterogeneity in human olfactory cortex: an event-related functional magnetic resonance imaging study. J. Neurosci. **22:** 10819–10828.
13. O'DOHERTY, J. *et al.* 2001. Representation of pleasant and aversive taste in the human brain. J. Neurophysiol. **85:** 1315–1321.
14. O'DOHERTY, J. *et al.* 2000. Sensory-specific satiety-related olfactory activation of the human orbitofrontal cortex. Neuroreport **11:** 893–897.
15. ROLLS, E.T., M.L. KRINGELBACH & I.E. DE ARAUJO. 2003. Different representations of pleasant and unpleasant odours in the human brain. Eur. J. Neurosci. **18:** 695–703.
16. SMALL, D.M. *et al.* 2003. Dissociation of neural representation of intensity and affective valuation in human gustation. Neuron **39:** 701–711.
17. O'DOHERTY, J. *et al.* 2003. Beauty in a smile: the role of medial orbitofrontal cortex in facial attractiveness. Neuropsychologia **41:** 147–155.
18. BREITER, H.C. *et al.* 2001. Functional imaging of neural responses to expectancy and experience of monetary gains and losses. Neuron **30:** 619–639.
19. ELLIOTT, R., C.D. FRITH & R.J. DOLAN. 1997. Differential neural response to positive and negative feedback in planning and guessing tasks. Neuropsychologia **35:** 1395–1404.
20. KNUTSON, B. *et al.* 2001. Dissociation of reward anticipation and outcome with event-related fMRI. Neuroreport **12:** 3683–3687.
21. O'DOHERTY, J. *et al.* 2001. Abstract reward and punishment representations in the human orbitofrontal cortex. Nat. Neurosci. **4:** 95–102.
22. URSU, S. & C.S. CARTER. 2005. Outcome representations, counterfactual comparisons and the human orbitofrontal cortex: implications for neuroimaging studies of decision-making. Brain Res. Cogn. Brain Res. **23:** 51–60.
23. SMALL, D.M. *et al.* 2001. Changes in brain activity related to eating chocolate: from pleasure to aversion. Brain **124:** 1720–1733.

24. KIM, H., S. SHIMOJO & J.P. O'DOHERTY. 2006. Is avoiding an aversive outcome rewarding? Neural substrates of avoidance learning in the human brain. PLoS Biol. **4:** e233.

25. ELLIOTT, R. *et al.* 2003. Differential response patterns in the striatum and orbitofrontal cortex to financial reward in humans: a parametric functional magnetic resonance imaging study. J. Neurosci. **23:** 303–307.

26. O'DOHERTY, J. *et al.* 2003. Dissociating valence of outcome from behavioral control in human orbital and ventral prefrontal cortices. J. Neurosci. **23:** 7931–7939.

27. CORICELLI, G. *et al.* 2005. Regret and its avoidance: a neuroimaging study of choice behavior. Nat. Neurosci. **8:** 1255–1262.

28. LIU, X. *et al.* 2006. The involvement of the inferior parietal cortex in the numerical Stroop effect and the distance effect in a two-digit number comparison task. J. Cogn. Neurosci. **18:** 1518–1530.

29. TVERSKY, A. & D. KAHNEMAN. 1981. The framing of decisions and the psychology of choice. Science **211:** 453–458.

30. O'DOHERTY, J. *et al.* 2002. Neural responses during anticipation of a primary taste reward. Neuron **33:** 815–826.

31. GOTTFRIED, J.A., J. O'DOHERTY & R.J. DOLAN. 2002. Appetitive and aversive olfactory learning in humans studied using event-related functional magnetic resonance imaging. J. Neurosci. **22:** 10829–10837.

32. PAVLOV, I.P. 1927. Conditioned Reflexes. Oxford University Press. Oxford.

33. JENKINS, H.M. & B.R. MOORE. 1973. The form of the autoshaped response with food or water reinforcers. J. Exp. Anal. Behav. **20:** 163–181.

34. ZENER, K. 1937. The significance of behavior accompanying conditioned salivary secretion for theories of the conditioned response. Am. J. Psychol. **50:** 384–403.

35. HOLLAND, P.C. 1977. Conditioned stimulus as a determinant of the form of the Pavlovian conditioned response. J. Exp. Psychol. Anim. Behav. Process **3:** 77–104.

36. MACKINTOSH, N.J. 1983. Conditioning and Associative Learning. Clarendon Press. Oxford.

37. GALVAN, A. *et al.* 2005. The role of ventral frontostriatal circuitry in reward-based learning in humans. J. Neurosci. **25:** 8650–8656.

38. ROLLS, E.T., C. MCCABE & J. REDOUTE. 2007. Expected value, reward outcome, and temporal difference error representations in a probabilistic decision task. Cereb. Cortex Jun. 22 [Epub ahead of print].

39. GOTTFRIED, J.A., J. O'DOHERTY & R.J. DOLAN. 2003. Encoding predictive reward value in human amygdala and orbitofrontal cortex. Science **301:** 1104–1107.

40. SCHOENBAUM, G., A.A. CHIBA & M. GALLAGHER. 1998. Orbitofrontal cortex and basolateral amygdala encode expected outcomes during learning. Nat. Neurosci. **1:** 155–159.

41. TREMBLAY, L. & W. SCHULTZ. 1999. Relative reward preference in primate orbitofrontal cortex. Nature **398:** 704–708.

42. DICKINSON, A. 1985. Actions and habits: the development of a behavioural autonomy. Philos. Trans. R. Soc. Lond. B Biol. Sci. **308:** 67–78.

43. BALLEINE, B.W. & A. DICKINSON. 1998. Goal-directed instrumental action: contingency and incentive learning and their cortical substrates. Neuropharmacology **37:** 407–419.

44. Corbit, L.H. & B.W. Balleine. 2003. The role of prelimbic cortex in instrumental conditioning. Behav. Brain Res. **146:** 145–157.
45. Killcross, S. & E. Coutureau. 2003. Coordination of actions and habits in the medial prefrontal cortex of rats. Cereb. Cortex **13:** 400–408.
46. Yin, H.H., B.J. Knowlton & B.W. Balleine. 2004. Lesions of dorsolateral striatum preserve outcome expectancy but disrupt habit formation in instrumental learning. Eur. J. Neurosci. **19:** 181–189.
47. Yin, H.H. *et al.* 2005. The role of the dorsomedial striatum in instrumental conditioning. Eur. J. Neurosci. **22:** 513–523.
48. Valentin, V.V., A. Dickinson & J.P. O'Doherty. 2007. Determining the neural substrates of goal-directed learning in the human brain. J. Neurosci. **27:** 4019–4026.
49. Rushworth, M.F. *et al.* 2007. Functional organization of the medial frontal cortex. Curr. Opin. Neurobiol. **17:** 220–227.
50. Padoa-Schioppa, C. & J.A. Assad. 2006. Neurons in the orbitofrontal cortex encode economic value. Nature **441:** 223–226.
51. Thorpe, S.J., E.T. Rolls & S. Maddison. 1983. The orbitofrontal cortex: neuronal activity in the behaving monkey. Exp. Brain Res. **49:** 93–115.
52. Rescorla, R.A. & A.R. Wagner. 1972. A theory of Pavlovian conditioning: variations in the effectiveness of reinforcement and nonreinforcement. *In* Classical Conditioning II: Current Research and Theory. A.H. Black, & W.F. Prokasy, Eds.: 64–99. Appleton Crofts. New York.
53. Sutton, R.S. 1988. Learning to predict by the methods of temporal differences. Machine Learning **3:** 9–44.
54. Schultz, W. 1998. Predictive reward signal of dopamine neurons. J. Neurophysiol. **80:** 1–27.
55. Schultz, W., P. Dayan & P.R. Montague. 1997. A neural substrate of prediction and reward. Science **275:** 1593–1599.
56. Berns, G.S. *et al.* 2001. Predictability modulates human brain response to reward. J. Neurosci. **21:** 2793–2798.
57. O'Doherty, J. *et al.* 2003. Temporal difference models and reward-related learning in the human brain. Neuron **38:** 329–337.
58. Rolls, E.T. 2000. The orbitofrontal cortex and reward. Cereb. Cortex **10:** 284–294.
59. Hampton, A.N., P. Bossaerts & J.P. O'Doherty. 2006. The role of the ventromedial prefrontal cortex in abstract state-based inference during decision making in humans. J. Neurosci. **26:** 8360–8367.
60. O'Doherty, J.P., A. Hampton & H. Kim. 2007. Model-based fMRI and its application to reward learning and decision making. Ann. N. Y. Acad. Sci. **1104:** 35–53.
61. Hampton, A.N. & J.P. O'Doherty. 2007. Decoding the neural substrates of reward-related decision making with functional MRI. Proc. Natl. Acad. Sci. USA **104:** 1377–1382.
62. Montague, P.R. & G.S. Berns. 2002. Neural economics and the biological substrates of valuation. Neuron **36:** 265–284.
63. Carmichael, S.T. & J.L. Price. 1994. Architectonic subdivision of the orbital and medial prefrontal cortex in the macaque monkey. J. Comp. Neurol. **346:** 366–402.

64. SCHOENBAUM, G., A.A. CHIBA & M. GALLAGHER. 2000. Changes in functional connectivity in orbitofrontal cortex and basolateral amygdala during learning and reversal training. J. Neurosci. **20:** 5179–5189.
65. SCHOENBAUM, G. *et al.* 2003. Encoding predicted outcome and acquired value in orbitofrontal cortex during cue sampling depends upon input from basolateral amygdala. Neuron **39:** 855–867.
66. STALNAKER, T.A. *et al.* 2007. Basolateral amygdala lesions abolish orbitofrontal-dependent reversal impairments. Neuron **54:** 51–58.
67. OSTLUND, S.B. & B.W. BALLEINE. 2007. Orbitofrontal cortex mediates outcome encoding in Pavlovian but not instrumental conditioning. J. Neurosci. **27**(18): 4819–4825.

Orbitofrontal Cortex and Amygdala Contributions to Affect and Action in Primates

ELISABETH A. MURRAY[a] AND ALICIA IZQUIERDO[b]

[a]Section on the Neurobiology of Learning & Memory, Laboratory of Neuropsychology, National Institute of Mental Health, NIH, Bethesda, Maryland, USA

[b]Department of Psychology, California State University, Los Angeles, Los Angeles, California, USA

ABSTRACT: The amygdala and orbitofrontal cortex (OFC) work together as part of the neural circuitry guiding goal-directed behavior. This chapter explores the way in which the amygdala and OFC contribute to emotion and reward processing in macaque monkeys, taking into account recent methodological and conceptual advances. Although direct functional interaction of the amygdala and OFC is necessary for some types of stimulus–reward associations, it is not necessary for others. Both regions contribute to the expression of defensive responses to a potential predator. Contrary to the prevailing view, the amygdala and OFC make distinct contributions to emotional responses and reward processing.

KEYWORDS: reward; emotion; inferotemporal cortex; stimulus–reward association

INTRODUCTION

The ability to learn from experience—that is, to form memories—affords animals an astonishing adaptive advantage. Responding flexibly to the many changes in the environment would not be possible if it all had to be encoded into the genome. Yet memories *per se* provide no benefit; animals benefit from memories only to the extent that they exploit them to make advantageous actions.

So how, in the face of a bewildering array of behavioral options, do animals decide on advantageous actions? Of course, one answer is that they (and we)

Address for correspondence: Elisabeth A. Murray, Ph.D., Laboratory of Neuropsychology, National Institute of Mental Health, NIH, 49 Convent Drive, MSC 4415, Bethesda, MD 20892-4415. Voice: 301-496-5625, ext. 227; fax: 301-402-0046.
murraye@mail.nih.gov

Ann. N.Y. Acad. Sci. 1121: 273–296 (2007). © 2007 New York Academy of Sciences.
doi: 10.1196/annals.1401.021

do not always do so: maladaptive behavior and its causes are major topics in contemporary neuroscience. Yet, often enough, our ancestors succeeded in taking advantageous actions; we would not be here otherwise. This chapter explores the idea that affect mediates the relationship between memory and advantageous action. For the purposes of this chapter, "action" includes responses that are the product of visual choices of objects in addition to actions, *per se*.

In primates, three components of the telencephalon contribute to affect–action relations in a highly direct way: the amygdala, the orbitofrontal cortex (OFC), and the medial frontal cortex (MFC). This chapter concentrates on recent research regarding the contributions of OFC and amygdala to affect and action in primates. Monkeys with bilateral ablations of either the amygdala or OFC were assessed for their ability to assign value to stimuli based on reinforcement history, and for their emotional reactions to stimuli. After reviewing the findings, we argue that although the amygdala and OFC functionally interact in mediating some types of adaptive choices, contrary to the prevailing view, the amygdala and OFC make distinct contributions to emotional responses and reward processing. We close with speculation regarding the ways in which OFC and its neighbor MFC might provide complementary contributions to goal-directed behavior.

NEURAL SUBSTRATES OF AFFECTIVE PROCESSING

From the 1960s to the present, neuropsychological studies in nonhuman primates have employed the object reversal learning and "win-stay, lose-shift" tasks as assays for linking objects with reward. Both tasks require flexible associations of objects with food reward. For example, in the win-stay, lose-shift task, animals must return to an object that had led to food reward in the preceding acquisition phase and avoid one that did not. The implication was that animals were linking objects with the affective qualities of food reward. Because amygdala lesions produced severe impairment on these tasks, the amygdala emerged as a critical site of stimulus–reward association.[1-6] For decades these findings have been cited as evidence for a general role of the amygdala in stimulus–reward association, which pointed to a key role in affect–action relations. To anticipate the story outlined below, both methodological improvements and conceptual advances have reshaped the landscape in which these and related findings have been interpreted.

Two related developments have altered our view of amygdala contributions to stimulus–reward association as measured by object reversal learning and win-stay, lose-shift. First, we discovered that the effects of axon-sparing excitotoxic lesions of the amygdala in nonhuman primates differed dramatically from the traditional aspirative lesions.[7,8] The discrepant findings have been attributed to the fact that aspirative removals of the amygdala disrupt both inputs and outputs of inferotemporal visual cortex and perirhinal cortex.[9,10] Thus, damage to fibers passing near or through the amygdala, rather than loss of neurons in the amygdala, appears to account for many of the behavioral deficits observed after the aspirative removals. Improved methods for making selective lesions of deep structures together with the knowledge that the amygdala is not essential for recognition memory functions initially ascribed to it[11,12] opened the way to a more accurate understanding of amygdala function. Second, there has been a growing awareness that "reward" is not a unitary construct.[13,14] This has led to the development of new tasks to probe reward processing, including tasks that require the association of objects with either fixed or changing probabilities, magnitudes and values of rewards, as well as the application of traditional learning-theory models to begin to discern a more specific role for the amygdala.

Another substrate for affective processing is the OFC. Several neuropsychological studies in nonhuman primates have examined the role of the OFC in tasks such as object reversal learning, tests aimed at assessing behavioral inhibition, and other tasks that relate affect to action. But little of this research took into account the interactions between OFC and the amygdala. Accordingly, this chapter summarizes research comparing the contributions of the amygdala and OFC on a battery of tests of affective processing. All the experiments outlined here examined the effects of bilateral excitotoxic lesions of the amygdala or bilateral aspirative lesions of the OFC in primates. Where possible, tests of their interaction through crossed disconnections and unilateral lesions are discussed, as well.

Reinforcer Devaluation

As already indicated, earlier work in nonhuman primates used object reversal learning and win-stay, lose-shift tasks specifically to assess stimulus–reward associations. The underlying assumption was that "reward" in this context reflected the affective qualities of the food. This assumption, however, is without foundation; in these tasks and others, such as discrimination learning set, monkeys can improve their performance in at least two ways: via an object–outcome association (i.e., by choosing the object associated with the food of higher biological value) and via visually based performance rules (e.g., by choosing the object that is associated in memory with the appearance of a peanut). In the latter case, food provides information independent of its reinforcing value.[15] When monkeys acquire a visually based performance rule, it allows them to choose efficiently between two objects, only one of which is associated in memory with food. It has been hypothesized that this is instantiated in the form of a prospective memory, laid down at the time of trial x, for the object that should be chosen on the next trial, trial $x + 1$.[16] Although object choices in these circumstances can of course be defined as "stimulus–reward" association, this concept is at odds with what is conventionally meant by reward, namely, information about the biological value of the food.

Given the distinct possibility that previous tests[1-5] relied on visually-based performance rules rather than stimulus–reward value associations, my colleagues and I developed a different assessment of object–outcome associations more specifically: reinforcer devaluation. The task was adapted from work carried out by Hatfield et al.[17] In their experiment, rats learned about sensory cues that reliably predicted the delivery of food reward. Specifically, rats learned to make conditioned responses, in this case approaches to a food cup, in the presence of a light cue paired with food delivery. After experimental alterations of food value, rats' responses to the food-predicting cue were reassessed in the absence of food delivery. Control rats with central nucleus lesions, but not rats with basolateral amygdala lesions, responded to decreases in food value by reducing the amount of conditioned approaches to the food cup. By applying a similar method in monkeys we hoped to produce a more precise measure of stimulus–reward value association, with the intention of specifically probing the linkage of objects with food value. The test is carried out in two stages. First, monkeys are familiarized with a large number of objects, half of which are associated with one kind of food, designated Food 1, and half associated with a different food, designated Food 2. Second, the value of one food is decreased by feeding it to the monkey, and the effect of this selective satiety on choices between objects associated with Food 1 and Food 2 is compared with a baseline condition in which there was no such prefeeding.

In the experiments described here, each experimental group had surgical operations in two stages, with a behavioral test after each stage. In FIGURE 1, the scores for each group are reflected in a pair of bars: the left bars of each pair show the effects of the first stage surgery (after first lesion), and the right bars of each pair show the influence of the complete lesion (after second lesion). The control group was also tested twice, but received no surgery. This repeated test design was necessary for assessing the effect of the crossed surgical disconnection of amygdala and OFC (middle pair of bars), and we applied this design to all groups so that their data would be directly comparable.

Intact monkeys avoid choosing objects associated with a devalued food, as indicated by the high devaluation scores obtained by the unoperated control group (FIG. 1, left). On average, this group scored slightly better on the second test relative to the first. Scores on the second test (black bars) reveal that control monkeys shift their choices away from objects associated with the devalued (sated) food by about half, yielding a score of ~17 out of a possible 30. In contrast, monkeys with bilateral lesions of either OFC or the amygdala continue to choose much as they had before the selective satiation procedure. This deficit is reflected in the low devaluation scores obtained after the bilateral removal of either OFC or the amygdala (FIG. 1, right), findings recently confirmed by other investigators.[18] Likewise, monkeys with a surgical

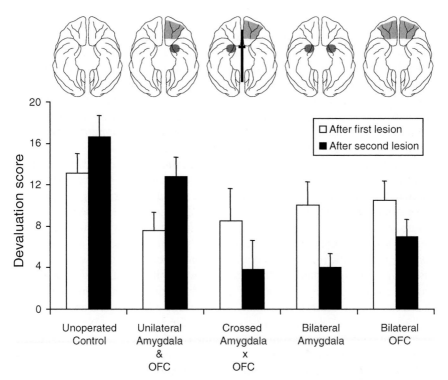

FIGURE 1. (Top) Ventral views of a standard rhesus monkey brain showing the location of the intended lesion for each operated group (shaded regions). Surgery was carried out in two stages. The group with the crossed disconnection lesion (crossed Amygdala x OFC) also received a section of the forebrain commissures (black line), which was carried out in the same stage as the OFC lesion. (Bottom) Group mean devaluation scores obtained on the reinforcer devaluation task. Error bars indicate ± SEM. The left bar of each pair shows scores obtained after the first stage surgery (either a unilateral amygdala lesion or unilateral OFC lesion). The right bar of each pair shows scores obtained after the second stage surgery. The site of the first surgery was counterbalanced for all operated groups. Each of the operated groups is significantly impaired relative to controls. Unoperated controls (N = 10); Unilateral amygdala & OFC lesion (N = 8); Crossed amygdala x OFC lesion (N = 4); Bilateral amygdala lesion (N = 5); Bilateral OFC lesion (N = 4).

disconnection that prevents the intrahemispheric interaction of the amygdala and OFC (Fig. 1, middle pair of bars) cannot efficiently link objects with the current value of a food reward. Finally, the effects of a unilateral removal of these two structures (Fig. 1, second pair of bars) gave an intermediate result. Monkeys with removal of the amygdala and OFC in one hemisphere—either left or right—scored roughly half way between the controls and the other experimental groups. This finding suggests that combined signals from the two hemispheres are summed to influence decisions about object choices.[19]

Control procedures have shown that changes in visual perceptual abilities, food preferences, level of motivation, and satiety mechanisms cannot account for the impairments. For example, monkeys with OFC lesions,[20] amygdala lesions,[21] and crossed disconnection of OFC and amygdala[22] have been found to perform just as much work as intact monkeys to earn food reward, suggesting that the motivation of the monkeys in these operated groups is intact. Nor can nonspecific effects of surgery account for the result; the performance of monkeys with bilateral damage to either the hippocampus or perirhinal cortex is indistinguishable from that of intact controls.[18,23]

An important feature of the task design was that in the second stage, when monkeys selected between objects after selective satiation, they received only a single trial per pair of objects. Thus, there was no opportunity to learn the association between the objects and the now devaluated food. The high devaluation scores of intact control monkeys therefore indicate that they were able to automatically integrate the updated food value into existing associations, and this is what the monkeys in operated groups could not achieve. In theory, given enough experience, all the monkeys would have eventually learned to choose objects yielding the food of higher biological value. Consistent with this idea, when monkeys with either OFC or amygdala lesions are given the opportunity to choose between two familiar foods with no objects covering them, like controls, they avoid choosing the sated food.[20,24,cf.18] Presumably, during the roughly 30-min selective satiation procedure, all monkeys, controls and operated alike, are able to acquire the association between the visual properties of the food and the updated value of the food, allowing them to make adaptive visual choices of the food items. That monkeys in the experimental groups are able to avoid choosing sated foods shows that their satiety mechanisms are intact, a finding that serves to further specify the nature of the impairment.

Still, the reinforcer devaluation test outlined above comprises several components: forming object representations, linking those representations with the incentive value of the associated food, registering and encoding a change in the reward value due to selective satiation, linking object representations with those updated values, and using these changed representations to choose between objects. Although, as mentioned earlier, we can rule out effects of the lesions on visual discrimination abilities, several possibilities remain.

Transient inactivation of the amygdala by focal infusion of the GABA agonist muscimol has clarified the mechanisms of stimulus valuation in primates. In these experiments, monkeys received infusions of either saline or muscimol, bilaterally, via cannulae lowered to the basolateral amygdala. The infusions were given either before or after selective satiation. As expected, when monkeys received saline infusions (either before or after selective satiation) they obtained robust devaluation scores. Similar scores were obtained when the basolateral amygdala was inactivated *after* the selective satiation procedure. By contrast, inactivation of the basolateral amygdala immediately *before and during* the satiation procedure prevented the shift in object choices that normally occurs with selective satiation.[25] Thus, the basolateral amygdala needs to be functionally intact for registration of a change in the incentive value of a food reward and the corresponding shift in the monkey's choices of objects based on food value. Apparently, once the value of the food reward has been updated, no further contribution of the basolateral amygdala is required. [We note this latter finding appears at odds with recent work in rats. Pickens *et al.*[26] found that after rats had learned stimulus–food associations, the amygdala was not necessary to register changes in the value of the food. Because there are several methodological differences in the test procedures used with rats and monkeys, additional studies will be required to determine the factors responsible for the apparent discrepancy.]

A possible mechanism for this updating function is suggested by neurophysiological studies of awake, behaving monkeys performing a task in which choices of visual stimuli lead to reward delivery. Typically, different visual stimuli are assigned to different types or quantities of juice rewards. Such studies have shown that the activity of OFC neurons discriminates between different rewards: the firing rates of OFC neurons reflect the value of expected rewards largely independently of the spatial and visual properties of the predicting stimuli and independently of motor-command signals that control the response.[27–29] Taste of the expected reward is also represented, though to a lesser degree. Importantly, OFC neurons appear to code the values of rewards independent of their type and amount, suggesting that the neurons represent value in a common mode.[29] On this basis, it has been suggested that OFC guides choice between "goods."

Another important finding from physiological studies is that the activity of OFC neurons reflects the value of expected outcomes while monkeys are viewing objects (or images), before reward is made available.[28] This type of object-elicited representation of expected outcomes is just what would be needed to guide monkeys' visual choices in the reinforcer devaluation task. Many neurons in the basolateral amygdala of monkeys likewise represent expected outcomes.[30] Interestingly, studies in rats have shown that this type of cue-elicited activity normally observed in OFC neurons is greatly reduced in rats with lesions of the basolateral amygdala. Thus, interaction of the amygdala and OFC underlies at least some aspects of the associative encoding normally observed in OFC neurons.[31]

Object Reversal Learning

Whereas reinforcer devaluation assesses monkeys' abilities to choose between positive objects ("goods") after changes in the value of the food associated with that object, object reversal learning assesses monkeys' abilities to choose between two objects when the reinforcement contingencies are

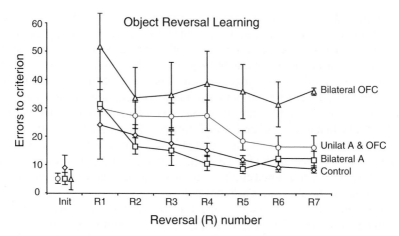

FIGURE 2. Group mean errors to criterion for initial learning of a single pair object discrimination problem (Init) and seven serial reversals (R) in the object discrimination reversal-learning task. Error bars indicate ± SEM. Unoperated controls (N = 10), diamonds; monkeys with bilateral OFC lesions (N = 3), triangles; monkeys with bilateral amygdala lesions (N = 5), squares; monkeys with unilateral amygdala and OFC lesions (N = 8), circles. A, amygdala.

reversed but food values remained unchanged. In this task there are two different objects, one arbitrarily designated the S+ (covering a baited food well) and the other the S− (covering an empty food well). On each trial, a monkey was allowed to choose one of the two objects and, if correct, to retrieve the food reward underneath it. After monkeys learned the original problem, as judged by their ability to consistently approach and displace the rewarded object, the reward contingencies were reversed (starting the next day), and each monkey was trained to the same criterion as before. This procedure was repeated until several serial reversals had been completed. During and after the first reversal, each of the objects available for choice had been associated with reward; hence, reinforcer devaluation and object reversal learning have in common the requirement to choose between two objects with a history of reward, at least as viewed over the long term.

FIGURE 2 illustrates the number of errors scored in acquisition of the initial discrimination and during the subsequent seven reversals. Although the groups did not differ in initial learning, some groups were impaired in acquiring the reversals. Specifically, monkeys with bilateral OFC lesions and those with unilateral OFC and amygdala lesions were significantly slower to learn the reversals than intact controls. By contrast, monkeys with bilateral amygdala lesions learned reversals as efficiently as the controls.

Reversals were also analyzed according to a stage of reversal learning (see Ref. 4). For each session, errors were assigned as follows: stage 1, 21 or more errors; stage 2, 10–20 errors; stage 3, 3–9 errors. Thus, stage 1 errors occur when the monkey is responding predominantly to the originally reinforced object, stage 2 errors occur when the monkey is near chance performance, and stage 3 errors happen as the monkey progresses from chance to criterion performance. Relative to controls, monkeys with bilateral OFC lesions made significantly more errors only in stage 2. This result contrasts with the earlier report of Jones and Mishkin.[4] They found that monkeys with OFC lesions made an inordinately large number of errors in stage 1, which they interpreted as response perseveration. Because the OFC lesion performed by Jones and Mishkin included the ventral convexity below the principal sulcus (area 12), in addition to the parts of orbital cortex traditionally identified as OFC, the greater deficit after OFC lesions in their report relative to ours probably reflects the larger lesion. When lesions are restricted to the orbital surface of the prefrontal cortex, and limited to the dysgranular and homotypical portions of areas 11, 13, and 14, the deficit is not perseverative, or at least not markedly so.[3,20,32] In future studies it may be profitable to use tasks with three or more choices, which are better able to identify perseverative errors,[33] or to employ other types of error analyses, ones that can tease apart the way in which monkeys benefit from incorrectly performed trials (i.e., errors) and correctly performed trials.[34]

There are at least two possible interpretations of the deficit that follows OFC lesions. First, the most parsimonious account is that a single mechanism underlies performance on both of the OFC-dependent tasks just reviewed: reinforcer devaluation and object reversal learning. On this view, OFC houses representations of expected outcomes, and visual cortical inputs to OFC (from inferotemporal and perirhinal cortex) are the route through which values of expected outcomes are accessed. After OFC lesions, in the absence of representations of expected outcomes, performance on both tasks is impaired. (Although amygdala−OFC interaction is essential for the reinforcer devaluation task, it is important only for updating the values of expected outcomes stored in OFC. Once that process has occurred, the amygdala is no longer necessary for guiding choices of objects based on the updated value.)

An alternative account posits that different mechanisms underlie performance on reinforcer devaluation and object reversal learning, with object reversal learning reflecting application of a visually guided rule. On this view, the role of food reward is informational rather than hedonic: to signal the current behavior-guiding rule. In our study, OFC lesions did not cause a significant deficit in the early reversals, only in later ones (FIG. 2). Indeed, our analysis revealed a significant group x reversal interaction; control monkeys, but not monkeys with OFC lesions, became more efficient at acquiring the reversals with increased experience. Thus, the deficit in the OFC group may be in acquiring a reversal learning set. As discussed earlier, learning set may depend on the ability to lay down a prospective memory about what stimulus should be selected next, when a similar choice arises in the future.[16] If so, then one effect of the OFC lesion—one underlying the deficit on object reversal learning—may be to disrupt either the acquisition or implementation of a prospective memory mechanism. This second interpretation is in line with the finding that activity of OFC neurons (as well as that of neurons in other frontal cortical regions) reflects behavior-guiding rules[35] and with preliminary data hinting that different subregions within OFC may be responsible for mediating reinforcer devaluation and object reversal learning.[36] This more cognitive interpretation of the results points away from accounts of OFC lesion effects invoking concepts such as perseveration, reward contingencies, and response inhibition, in the sense usually used in animal learning theory and in clinical practice.

Because few visual learning tasks are affected by unilateral lesions in nonhuman primates, it is of particular interest that combined lesions of the amygdala and OFC in one hemisphere were found to yield significant deficits on object reversal learning. To the extent that this signature can be linked to a particular neurotransmitter system or type of learning,[37,38] it may help elucidate the nature of the OFC contribution to object reversal learning.

Instrumental Extinction

We employed one additional test of reward processing: instrumental extinction. This task, like object reversal learning, measures monkeys' responses to changing reward contingencies. Unlike object reversal learning, however, there is no alternative response. There are two phases of the test: acquisition and extinction. During acquisition, monkeys were allowed to approach and to displace a single object to obtain the food reward hidden underneath. This behavior was allowed to become well established. During extinction, everything remained the same except food reward was no longer provided. The measure of interest was the number of unrewarded object displacements performed after the reward contingency changed from rewarded to nonrewarded (i.e., the number of responses made in extinction).

To our surprise, we found opposing effects of OFC and amygdala lesions on this task. Whereas monkeys with OFC lesions showed impaired instrumental extinction, monkeys with amygdala lesions displayed expedited extinction (data not shown).[39] The effect of OFC lesions can be considered an increase in impulsivity, although other, more cognitive interpretations remain possible. One interpretation of the deficit after OFC lesions is the same as that offered for object reversal learning: an inability to acquire or apply visually guided rules in which the appearance of food reward (or not) guides object choices. In addition, the opposing effects of OFC and amygdala lesions suggest that the two structures, under certain circumstances, work via a competitive interaction.[40] Although the nature of the interaction and the degree to which other regions are involved remain to be determined, one attractive possibility is that in the absence of the amygdala, OFC processing of (nonaffective) visual information is more efficient.

Reactions to an Artificial Snake

To examine the contributions of OFC and amygdala to emotion, we used a method adapted from Mineka and her colleagues to assess behavioral reactions to emotionally provocative stimuli, namely, an artificial snake.[41,42] In this task monkeys are presented with objects located inside a clear Plexiglas box. We used three classes of objects: rubber snake, rubber spider, and neutral objects. In addition, a food reward is placed on top of the far edge of the box. On each trial, the monkeys were allowed to reach for and to procure the food, which was always located at the edge of the top farthest from the monkey. Thus, this method pits approach responses elicited by food against defensive responses engendered by the snake.

As expected, intact monkeys showed robust emotional reactions to the rubber snake. Whereas intact monkeys quickly reached over neutral objects to obtain the food reward, they hesitated or failed to reach altogether when given the opportunity to reach over the rubber snake (FIG. 3). The facial expressions and movements made in the presence of the snake were mainly defensive, including moving to the back of the cage, eye and head aversion, freezing, and piloerection (FIG. 4). The intensity of the defensive behaviors matched closely the description of the snake-naïve monkeys studied by Nelson et al.,[43] in that the monkeys displayed a wide range of behaviors interpreted by human observers as orienting responses, wariness, and fear. These defensive behaviors are the same type of "disturbance behaviors" reported by Mineka and colleagues[41] in snake-naïve monkeys, fully consistent with the idea that snakes induce an innate fear response.

In contrast to the controls, the monkeys with either bilateral OFC or bilateral amygdala lesions displayed relatively shorter food-retrieval latencies on snake and spider trials (FIG. 3). In addition, when confronted with the snake, both operated groups displayed fewer defensive behaviors than did the controls (FIG. 4). Monkeys with unilateral OFC and amygdala lesions likewise exhibited reduced emotional responses to the rubber snake, and there was no difference in the effects of lesions in the left versus right hemisphere. These data are of interest because they are among the first to show that unilateral brain damage in monkeys is sufficient to disrupt emotional responses. Taken together, our data show that the monkeys with OFC and amygdala damage, unlike controls, had little or no fear of the snake. These data are consistent with the findings of Meunier et al.[44] and Kalin et al.,[45] who reported blunted emotional reactions to fake and real snakes in young adult macaque monkeys following selective bilateral amygdala lesions.

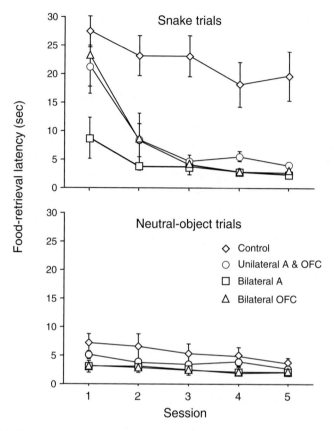

FIGURE 3. Group mean food-retrieval latency (sec) during exposure to an artificial snake (Snake trials) and neutral objects (Neutral-object trials) across five sessions. Error bars indicate ± SEM. Unoperated controls (N = 10), diamonds; monkeys with bilateral OFC lesions (N = 4), triangles; monkeys with bilateral amygdala lesions (N = 5), squares; monkeys with unilateral amygdala and OFC lesions (N = 8), circles. A, amygdala.

Reactions to Human Intruder

In response to the presence of an unfamiliar human—a "human intruder"—intact monkeys exhibit emotional behavior characterized by defensive, submissive, and aggressive behaviors,[46] many of them different from those elicited by a snake. We included this task to measure emotional responses to a social stimulus, which would complement our evaluation in the snake test of reactions to a potential predator. The behaviors elicited in response to an unfamiliar human, like those elicited by the snake, are held to be unconditioned responses; they are present early in life and reflect long-term emotional disposition or temperament.[47]

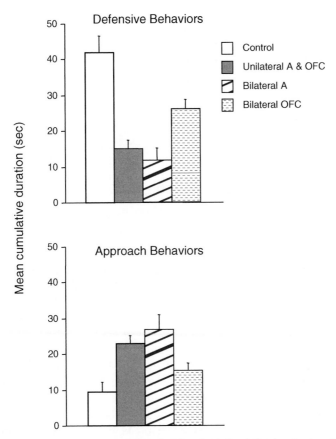

FIGURE 4. Group mean cumulative duration (sec) for defensive (top) and approach (bottom) behaviors during exposure to an artificial snake. Error bars indicate ± SEM. Unoperated controls (N = 10); monkeys with bilateral OFC lesions (N = 4); monkeys with bilateral amygdala lesions (N = 5); monkeys with unilateral amygdala and OFC lesions (N = 8). A, amygdala.

Monkeys were placed in a test cage, taken to a room they had never been in, and left alone for 5 min: the *alone* condition. A human male unfamiliar to the monkey then entered the room, sat approximately 2.5 m away from the cage, and presented his profile to the monkey for 5 min. The human never made eye contact with the monkey during this time: the *no eye contact* condition. After leaving the room for 3 min, the same human intruder returned to the room, sat 2.5 m away from the monkey, and proceeded to fixate the monkeys eyes for 5 min. The human remained motionless and projected a neutral face toward the monkey: the *stare* condition.

The hallmark responses include defensive freezing (especially in the no eye contact condition) and both submission and aggression (especially in

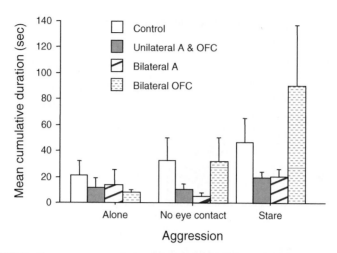

FIGURE 5. Group mean cumulative duration (sec) of aggressive behaviors in the three conditions of the human intruder task. Aggressive behaviors included both mild and high aggressive behaviors such as mouth threat, ears back, and cage shake. Error bars indicate ± SEM. Unoperated controls (N = 10); monkeys with bilateral OFC lesions (N = 4); monkeys with bilateral amygdala lesions (N = 5); monkeys with unilateral amygdala and OFC lesions (N = 8). A, amygdala.

the stare condition). Consistent with other published reports,[45] intact control monkeys showed more defensive behavior, especially freezing, in the no eye contact condition relative to the alone condition. In addition, they showed more defensive behavior in the stare condition relative to the alone condition, with a slight increase in aggressive behavior, as well. Relative to controls, the OFC group exhibited more mild aggression during the stare condition (FIG. 5). Consistent with the findings of Kalin *et al.*,[45] monkeys with amygdala lesions did not differ from controls.[cf.48]

Conclusions Concerning Neural Substrates of Affective Processing

In summary, both the OFC and amygdala are essential for linking objects with the current value of an outcome and for expression of snake fear. Presumably, the valuation process itself reflects an emotional bias gained through incentive learning.[49] Taken together, these data suggest that these structures necessarily interact in guiding choices of objects and foods based on value signals and danger (i.e., affective) signals. Indeed, in the case of linking objects with current food value, the crossed disconnection experiment indicates the amygdala and OFC directly interact to mediate the reinforcer devaluation effects. By contrast, OFC but not the amygdala is essential for object reversal learning, which, as we have argued elsewhere,[24] does not require processing changes in reward value, but, rather, requires the monkey to apply a visually guided rule based on the association between the same objects and the presentation of food (i.e., to learn a new reward contingency). Indeed, these data indicate a neurobiological distinction between stimulus–reward associations based on current reward value, as assessed by reinforcer devaluation, and stimulus–reward associations based on reward contingency, as assessed by object reversal learning.

Because we have studied the effects of aspirative lesions of OFC, the work is subject to the criticism that the lesions involve fibers of passage, and behavioral effects of the lesions might therefore be due to damage outside OFC, or in addition to OFC. For example, noradrenergic fibers course long distances within the cortical grey matter[50]; these and other projection fibers traveling in the grey matter would be disrupted by an aspirative lesion. We think it unlikely that damage to fibers of passage caused the behavioral effects in our monkeys with aspirative OFC lesions because selective lesions yield similar behavioral effects. For example, serotonergic depletions within OFC of marmoset monkeys, like aspirative lesions in macaque monkeys, produce a deficit in object reversal learning.[37] Nevertheless, future studies should make use of selective, excitotoxic lesions. In addition, the anatomical connections of different cytoarchitectonic fields within OFC differ, with areas 11 and 13 being preferentially connected with the amygdala and area 14 being preferentially connected with hippocampus.[51,52] Consequently, future studies should investigate the functions of subdivisions of primate OFC.

MODELS OF OFC–AMYGDALA INTERACTION

OFC versus Amygdala Function

The prevailing, textbook view holds that OFC and the amygdala have the same functions in reward processing and emotion. The idea that OFC and amygdala work together in affective processing, including both emotion and reward, arose from observations that the effects of bilateral amygdala lesions closely resembled those of bilateral OFC lesions. For example, damage to either structure disrupts emotional responses[6,44,45,53-56] and, until our results became available, damage to either structure was also thought to disrupt object reversal learning.[1,4,6,57] Consequently, several investigators have suggested a common circuitry for both emotional responses and reward processing, without distinguishing between the concepts of emotion and reward.[3,4,6,58] Indeed, it has been proposed that emotion is a by-product of received, omitted, and expected positive and negative reinforcements.[58] The present findings argue against the textbook view by showing that selective amygdala lesions have no effect on the kind of reward processing required by object reversal learning (FIG. 2), although the same lesions in the same monkeys have a clear effect on emotional responses.[56] Thus, OFC and the amygdala make distinct contributions to emotional responses and reward processing, which are distinctly different neuronal processes.

Our results may also inform models of the role of OFC in decision making. OFC is held to represent the value of expected outcomes of goal-directed behavior and to provide a common currency for the value of a goal, taking into account benefits (e.g., the biological value of food) and costs (e.g., the time required to obtain the food) thereby enabling organisms to make "good" selections among several possible choices.[29,59] On this view, the OFC is necessary only for representing the results of a cost–benefit analysis. The basic idea behind this model is that OFC operates downstream from the amygdala for the purpose of decisions and choices, based on predicted rewards. Put somewhat differently, this model holds that the amygdala provides the information needed for OFC to make value comparisons.

Although this idea is consistent with findings from the reinforcer devaluation task (FIG. 1), it does not accord with the results from the snake test, in which monkeys must reach over an artificial snake in order to obtain a food reward. If OFC neurons only compute and compare valuation signals, taking into account the positive biological value of the food (a benefit) with the negative biological value of the snake (a cost), we would have predicted that the emotional reactions to the snake, such as freezing or gaze aversion, would be intact after OFC lesions. After all, the amygdala was undamaged and could interact with the remainder of the brain, and the emotional reactions we measured do not depend on cost–benefit computations. This idea did not hold up, however. Instead, OFC lesions severely disrupted emotional responses such as freezing and gaze aversion (FIG. 4), as well as producing dramatic reductions in the latency to reach over the snake to obtain food (FIG. 3). Importantly, the disruption of emotional responses to snakes cannot be ascribed to an inability to produce these responses. Monkeys with damage to OFC expressed many of the same behaviors in response to the human intruder (FIG. 5) that they failed to show in response to the snake (FIGS. 3 and 4), in amounts equivalent to the controls. Because the amygdala is also essential for marshaling defensive responses to the fake snake, and because amygdala removal, unlike OFC damage, almost completely eliminates the emotional reactions to the snake, the effects of OFC lesions on emotional responses may well reflect an influence of OFC on the amygdala, although influences in the opposite direction cannot be ruled out. In fact, physiological studies in rodents suggest that OFC makes an essential contribution to the coding of expected outcomes in the amygdala.[31] This issue notwithstanding, the pattern of results argues against a simple model in which the OFC functions solely in cost–benefit analysis and operates downstream from the amygdala (FIG. 6A). So in order to understand the neural substrates of affective processing, we must look to a more realistic model of OFC–amygdala interactions.

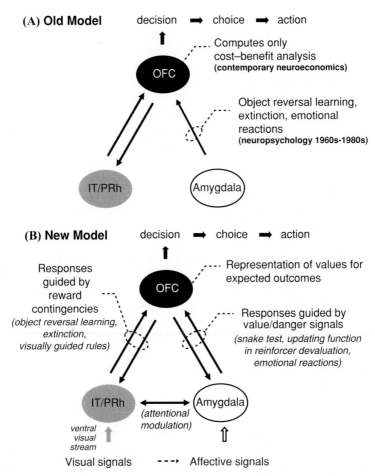

FIGURE 6. (**A**) The old model incorporates ideas derived from both neuropsychological findings from the 1960s–1980s as well as from contemporary neuroeconomics. The model indicates a joint role for the OFC and amygdala in stimulus–reward association and emotion, with no distinction between emotion and reward processing. Also according to this model, the sole function of the OFC is computation of a cost–benefit analysis that serves to guide decisions. Neither view can account for the data reviewed here (see text for explanation). (**B**) The new model suggests that both the amygdala and IT/PRh interact with OFC to guide decisions. In addition, each structure interacts with each of the others. For example, the amygdala can modulate activity in IT/PRh to enhance sensory processing of biologically significant stimuli and events. IT, inferotemporal cortex; PRh, perirhinal cortex.

A New View

The old model, illustrated in FIGURE 6A, implies that reward processing and emotion are more or less the same thing[58] and that the amygdala should therefore be necessary for both reward processing, as assessed by object re-versal performance, and emotion, as assessed by emotional reactions such as freezing or gaze aversion. The data discussed above show that view to be untenable. In addition, the old model encompasses the view that OFC, in representing values of expected outcomes, computes only a cost–benefit analysis. Our data indicate that this idea, too, is untenable. To accommodate the findings reviewed here, we propose a new model in which two routes to the OFC, one for visual information and the other for affective information, subserve both emotional responses and reward-driven response choices. On this view, interactions between OFC and both inferotemporal and perirhinal cortex (rather than interactions between OFC and amygdala) allow visual cues to elicit the predicted (long-term) values of food. Based on these and related findings,[60,61] we think that this network plays an analogous role in tasks in which high-order visual inputs determine the rules for future actions (FIG. 6B). By contrast, interactions between the OFC and amygdala would be important for updating the value of expected outcomes and generating appropriate emotional reactions to objects. If true, crossed surgical disconnections of OFC and the amygdala, on the one hand, and of OFC and inferotemporal cortex plus perirhinal cortex, on the other hand, would be expected to reveal a double dissociation. Crossed disconnection of OFC with inferotemporal cortex plus perirhinal cortex would be predicted to disrupt object reversal learning but not reinforcer devaluation, whereas crossed disconnection of OFC and amygdala would be predicted to disrupt reinforcer devaluation and emotional responses, but not object reversal learning.

The new view allows us to propose an answer to the question posed at the outset: "So how, in the face of a bewildering array of behavioral options, do animals decide on advantageous actions?" Put somewhat differently: How do animals employ their memories to make advantageous decisions? We propose that one aspect of affect—specifically, representations of the expected values of outcomes—provides the link between memory and action. Animals are armed with two mechanisms to realize this link: one dependent on the OFC, considered here, and the other on MFC, taken up in the next section. The first mechanism, the one mediated by amygdala–OFC interactions, allows monkeys to choose advantageously in the face of multiple competing cues, such as objects, assessed on the basis of their past experience and other factors, such as current drive states. Importantly, this mechanism allows animals to make good choices without having to experience the consequences of their actions in their current state. It does so through updating the value of expected food outcomes. Although most published work along these lines involves updating the values of positive outcomes such as food, it is likely that these principles apply equally to updating the value of negative outcomes.[62] This amygdala–OFC mechanism would provide an adaptive advantage by allowing organisms to maximize positive outcomes (e.g., food of high biological value, attainment of desirable sexual partners) and to minimize negative outcomes (e.g., distasteful or disgusting foods, pain-inducing stimuli) including those that might lead to injury.

AFFECT AND ACTION: THE BIG PICTURE

But how do the current, updated values of food outcomes and other affective signals provide a link between memories and advantageous action? To develop a more complete picture of how affect guides action we must consider two other sets of findings. First, accumulating evidence suggests that MFC, like OFC, represents expected outcomes, taking into account factors, such as the magnitude and probability of reward, as well as the effort required to obtain it.[63,64] The precise way in which expected outcomes in OFC and MFC are represented, and potential differences between these regions, is currently a subject of intensive investigation. Whereas OFC is thought to be important for guiding choices among objects or other stimuli, recent research suggests that major portions of MFC are important for guiding choices of actions *per se*.[34,63,65-69] If so, then the OFC and MFC collectively may guide goal-directed behavior, with OFC linking specific *cues* (including objects) with predicted outcomes and MFC linking particular *actions* with predicted outcomes (FIG. 7). On this account, OFC and MFC play complementary roles in using affect (especially the predicted value of outcomes) to guide biologically advantageous action. MFC may also play a role in processing feedback signals used to guide choices.[70] The complex web of interconnections between the lateral and medial parts of OFC, as well as between OFC and MFC,[71] likely reflects the interactions of these systems.

A second part of the "big picture" involves amygdala interactions with sensory cortex. As shown in FIGURE 6B, the amygdala interacts not only with OFC and MFC to promote adaptive responses, as described above, but also interacts with sensory cortical areas to influence perception. Functional imaging studies have shown that amygdala activity correlates with enhanced responses to emotionally charged stimuli in visual cortex, and there is greater functional connectivity between the amygdala and parts of visual cortex (e.g., fusiform cortex) when human subjects view fearful versus neutral faces. Because these effects depend on the integrity of the amygdala and nearby structures,[72] it has been suggested that amygdala-cortical pathways provide a route for increased perceptual processing of biologically significant stimuli. On this view, the amygdala is essential for a top-down influence of emotion on perceptual processing, a kind of "emotional attention." Additional support for this idea comes from a recent physiological study in cats, in which neuronal activity in the basolateral amygdala was found to correlate with increased transmission from the perirhinal cortex to entorhinal cortex.[73] As indicated at the outset, memories are only useful to the extent that animals can exploit them to make advantageous actions; as we have seen, the OFC and amygdala, likely together

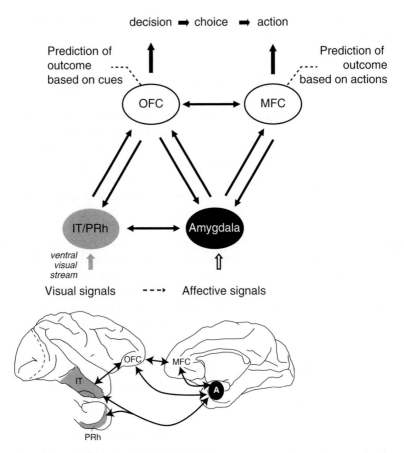

FIGURE 7. (Top) Neural circuits involved in goal-directed action based on visual sensory inputs. Neurons in OFC and MFC represent the values of expected outcomes, which can be updated via interaction with the amygdala. The OFC likely plays a major role in guiding choices of objects whereas the MFC likely plays a major role in guiding choices of actions. Both OFC and MFC make an essential contribution to making advantageous decisions. (Bottom) Lateral and medial views of a macaque brain showing the approximate locations of A, OFC, MFC, IT and PRh, as well as their interconnections. A, amygdala; IT, inferotemporal cortex; MFC, medial frontal cortex; PRh, perirhinal cortex.

with related cortical and thalamic networks, process affect to mediate the relationship between memory and advantageous actions.

ACKNOWLEDGMENTS

We thank P. H. Rudebeck and S. P. Wise for comments on an earlier version of the manuscript. This work was supported by the Intramural Research Program of the NIMH.

REFERENCES

1. SCHWARTZBAUM, J.S. & D.A. POULOS. 1965. Discrimination behavior after amygdalectomy in monkeys: learning set and discrimination reversals. J. Comp. Physiol. Psychol. **60:** 320–328.
2. BARRETT, T.W. 1969. Studies of the function of the amygdaloid complex in *Macaca mulatta*. Neuropsychologia **7:** 1–12.
3. BUTTER, C.M. 1969. Perseveration in extinction and in discrimination reversal tasks following selective frontal ablations in *Macaca mulatta*. Physiol. Behav. **4:** 163–171.
4. JONES, B. & M. MISHKIN. 1972. Limbic lesions and the problem of stimulus-reinforcement associations. Exp. Neurol. **36:** 362–377.
5. SPIEGLER, B.J. & M. MISHKIN. 1981. Evidence for the sequential participation of inferior temporal cortex and amygdala in the acquisition of stimulus-reward associations. Behav. Brain Res. **3:** 303–317.
6. AGGLETON, J.P. & R.E. PASSINGHAM. 1981. Syndrome produced by lesions of the amygdala in monkeys (*Macaca mulatta*). J. Comp. Physiol. Psychol. **95:** 961–977.
7. MURRAY, E.A. 1992. Medial temporal lobe structures contributing to recognition memory: the amygdaloid complex versus the rhinal cortex. *In* The Amygdala: neurobiological Aspects of Emotion, Memory, and Mental Dysfunction. J.P. Aggleton, Ed.: 453–470. Wiley-Liss. New York, NY.
8. BAXTER, M.G. & E.A. MURRAY. 2000. Reinterpreting the behavioural effects of amygdala lesions in nonhuman primates. *In* The Amygdala: a Functional Analysis. J.P. Aggleton, Ed.: 545–568. Oxford Univ. Press. Oxford.
9. GOULET, S., F.Y. DORE & E.A. MURRAY. 1998. Aspiration lesions of the amygdala disrupt the rhinal corticothalamic projection system in rhesus monkeys. Exp. Brain Res. **119:** 131–140.
10. EASTON, A. & D. GAFFAN. 2001. Crossed unilateral lesions of the medial forebrain bundle and either inferior temporal or frontal cortex impair object-reward association learning in Rhesus monkeys. Neuropsychologia **39:** 71–82.
11. MURRAY, E.A. 1996. What have ablation studies told us about the neural substrates of stimulus memory? Semin. Neurosci. **5:** 10–20.
12. ZOLA-MORGAN, S. *et al.* 1989. Lesions of perirhinal and parahippocampal cortex that spare the amygdala and hippocampal formation produce severe memory impairment. J. Neurosci. **9:** 4355–4370.
13. BALLEINE, B.W. 2005. Neural bases of food-seeking: affect, arousal and reward in corticostriatolimbic circuits. Physiol. Behav. **86:** 717–730.
14. BERRIDGE, K.C. & T.E. ROBINSON. 2003. Parsing reward. Trends Neurosci. **26:** 507–513.
15. GAFFAN, D. 1985. Hippocampus: memory, habit and voluntary movement. Philos. Trans. R. Soc. Lond. B Biol. Sci. **308:** 87–99.
16. MURRAY, E.A. & D. GAFFAN. 2006. Prospective memory in the formation of learning sets by rhesus monkeys (*Macaca mulatta*). J. Exp. Psychol. Anim. Behav. Process. **32:** 87–90.
17. HATFIELD, T. *et al.* 1996. Neurotoxic lesions of basolateral, but not central, amygdala interfere with Pavlovian second-order conditioning and reinforcer devaluation effects. J. Neurosci. **16:** 5256–5265.

18. MACHADO, C.J. & J. BACHEVALIER. 2007. The effects of selective amygdala, orbital frontal cortex or hippocampal formation lesions on reward assessment in nonhuman primates. Eur. J. Neurosci. **25:** 2885–2904.
19. IZQUIERDO, A. & E.A. MURRAY. 2004. Combined unilateral lesions of the amygdala and orbital prefrontal cortex impair affective processing in rhesus monkeys. J. Neurophysiol. **91:** 2023–2039.
20. IZQUIERDO, A., R.K. SUDA & E.A. MURRAY. 2004. Bilateral orbital prefrontal cortex lesions in rhesus monkeys disrupt choices guided by both reward value and reward contingency. J. Neurosci. **24:** 7540–7548.
21. AGGLETON, J.P. & R.E. PASSINGHAM. 1982. An assessment of the reinforcing properties of foods after amygdaloid lesions in rhesus monkeys. J. Comp. Physiol. Psychol. **96:** 71–77.
22. BAXTER, M.G. *et al.* 2000. Control of response selection by reinforcer value requires interaction of amygdala and orbital prefrontal cortex. J. Neurosci. **20:** 4311–4319.
23. CHUDASAMA, Y. & E.A. MURRAY. 2004. Hippocampal lesions in rhesus monkeys disrupt emotional responses but not reinforcer devaluation effects [abstract]. Society for Neuroscience Meeting Planner. Online. Program No. 84.4.
24. IZQUIERDO, A. & E.A. MURRAY. 2007. Selective bilateral amygdala lesions in rhesus monkeys fail to disrupt object reversal learning. J. Neurosci. **27:** 1054–1062.
25. WELLMAN, L.L., K. GALE & L. MALKOVA. 2005. $GABA_A$-mediated inhibition of basolateral amygdala blocks reward devaluation in macaques. J. Neurosci. **25:** 4577–4586.
26. PICKENS, C.L. *et al.* 2003. Different roles for orbitofrontal cortex and basolateral amygdala in a reinforcer devaluation task. J. Neurosci. **23:** 11078–11084.
27. TREMBLAY, L. & W. SCHULTZ. 1999. Relative reward preference in primate orbitofrontal cortex. Nature **398:** 704–708.
28. WALLIS, J.D. & E.K. MILLER. 2003. Neuronal activity in primate dorsolateral and orbital prefrontal cortex during performance of a reward preference task. Eur. J. Neurosci. **18:** 2069–2081.
29. PADOA-SCHIOPPA, C. & J.A. ASSAD. 2006. Neurons in the orbitofrontal cortex encode economic value. Nature **441:** 223–226.
30. PATON, J.J. *et al.* 2006. The primate amygdala represents the positive and negative value of visual stimuli during learning. Nature **439:** 865–870.
31. SCHOENBAUM, G. & M. ROESCH. 2005. Orbitofrontal cortex, associative learning, and expectancies. Neuron **47:** 633–636.
32. IVERSEN, S.D. & M. MISHKIN. 1970. Perseverative interference in monkeys following selective lesions of the inferior prefrontal convexity. Exp. Brain Res. **11:** 376–386.
33. BUSSEY, T.J., S.P. WISE & E.A. MURRAY. 2001. The role of ventral and orbital prefrontal cortex in conditional visuomotor learning and strategy use in rhesus monkeys (*Macaca mulatta*). Behav. Neurosci. **115:** 971–982.
34. KENNERLEY, S.W. *et al.* 2006. Optimal decision making and the anterior cingulate cortex. Nat. Neurosci. **9:** 940–947.
35. WALLIS, J.D., K.C. ANDERSON & E.K. MILLER. 2001. Single neurons in prefrontal cortex encode abstract rules. Nature **411:** 953–956.

36. KAZAMA, A.M. & J. BACHEVALIER. 2006. Selective aspiration or neurotoxic lesions of the orbital frontal areas 11 and 13 spared monkeys' performance on the object discrimination reversal task [abstract]. Society for Neuroscience Meeting Planner. Online. Program No. 670.25.

37. CLARKE, H.F. *et al.* 2007. Cognitive flexibility after prefrontal serotonin depletion is behaviorally and neurochemically specific. Cereb. Cortex **17:** 18–27.

38. IZQUIERDO, A. *et al.* 2007. Genetic modulation of cognitive flexibility in rhesus monkeys. Proc. Natl. Acad. Sci. USA **104:** 14128–14133.

39. IZQUIERDO, A. & E.A. MURRAY. 2005. Opposing effects of amygdala and orbital prefrontal cortex lesions on the extinction of instrumental responding in macaque monkeys. Eur. J. Neurosci. **22:** 2341–2346.

40. STALNAKER, T.A. *et al.* 2007. Basolateral amygdala lesions abolish orbitofrontal-dependent reversal impairments. Neuron **54:** 51–58.

41. MINEKA, S., R. KEIR & V. PRICE. 1980. Fear of snakes in wild- and laboratory-reared rhesus monkeys (*Macaca mulatta*). Anim. Learn. Behav. **8:** 653–663.

42. MINEKA, S. 1987. A primate model of phobic fears. *In* Theoretical Foundations of Behavior Therapy. H.J. Eysenck & I. Martin, Eds.: 81–111. Plenum Press. New York, NY.

43. NELSON, E.E., S.E. SHELTON & N.H. KALIN. 2003. Individual differences in the responses of naive rhesus monkeys to snakes. Emotion **3:** 3–11.

44. MEUNIER, M. *et al.* 1999. Effects of aspiration versus neurotoxic lesions of the amygdala on emotional responses in monkeys. Eur. J. Neurosci. **11:** 4403–4418.

45. KALIN, N.H. *et al.* 2001. The primate amygdala mediates acute fear but not the behavioral and physiological components of anxious temperament. J. Neurosci. **21:** 2067–2074.

46. KALIN, N.H. & S.E. SHELTON. 1989. Defensive behaviors in infant rhesus monkeys: environmental cues and neurochemical regulation. Science **243:** 1718–1721.

47. KALIN, N.H., S.E. SHELTON & L.K. TAKAHASHI. 1991. Defensive behaviors in infant rhesus monkeys: ontogeny and context-dependent selective expression. Child. Dev. **62:** 1175–1183.

48. KALIN, N.H., S.E. SHELTON & R.J. DAVIDSON. 2004. The role of the central nucleus of the amygdala in mediating fear and anxiety in the primate. J. Neurosci. **24:** 5506–5515.

49. BALLEINE, B.W. 2001. Incentive processes in instrumental conditioning. *In* Handbook of Contemporary Learning Theories. R.R. Mowrer & S.B. Klein, Eds.: 307–366. Lawrence Erlbaum Associates. Mahwah, NJ.

50. MORRISON, J.H. *et al.* 1982. Laminar, tangential and regional organization of the noradrenergic innervation of monkey cortex: dopamine-β-hydroxylase immunohistochemistry. Brain Res. Bull. **9:** 309–319.

51. CARMICHAEL, S.T. & J.L. PRICE. 1995. Limbic connections of the orbital and medial prefrontal cortex in macaque monkeys. J. Comp. Neurol. **363:** 615–641.

52. CAVADA, C. *et al.* 2000. The anatomical connections of the macaque monkey orbitofrontal cortex. A review. Cereb. Cortex **10:** 220–242.

53. WEISKRANTZ, L. 1956. Behavioral changes associated with ablation of the amygdaloid complex in monkeys. J. Comp. Physiol. Psychol. **49:** 381–391.

54. BUTTER, C.M. & D.R. SNYDER. 1972. Alterations in aversive and aggressive behaviors following orbital frontal lesions in rhesus monkeys. Acta Neurobiol. Exp. (Wars.) **32:** 525–565.

55. STEFANACCI, L., R.E. CLARK & S.M. ZOLA. 2003. Selective neurotoxic amygdala lesions in monkeys disrupt reactivity to food and object stimuli and have limited effects on memory. Behav. Neurosci. **117:** 1029–1043.
56. IZQUIERDO, A., R.K. SUDA & E.A. MURRAY. 2005. Comparison of the effects of bilateral orbital prefrontal cortex lesions and amygdala lesions on emotional responses in rhesus monkeys. J. Neurosci. **25:** 8534–8542.
57. BUTTER, C.M., D.R. SNYDER & J.A. MCDONALD. 1970. Effects of orbital frontal lesions on aversive and aggressive behaviors in rhesus monkeys. J. Comp. Physiol. Psychol. **72:** 132–144.
58. ROLLS, E.T. 1999. The Brain and Emotion. Oxford University Press. New York, NY.
59. MONTAGUE, P.R. & G.S. BERNS. 2002. Neural economics and the biological substrates of valuation. Neuron **36:** 265–284.
60. MURRAY, E.A., M.G. BAXTER & D. GAFFAN. 1998. Monkeys with rhinal cortex damage or neurotoxic hippocampal lesions are impaired on spatial scene learning and object reversals. Behav. Neurosci. **112:** 1291–1303.
61. BROWNING, P.G., A. EASTON & D. GAFFAN. 2007. Frontal-temporal disconnection abolishes object discrimination learning set in macaque monkeys. Cereb. Cortex **17:** 859–864.
62. FANSELOW, M.S. & G.D. GALE. 2003. The amygdala, fear, and memory. Ann. N. Y. Acad. Sci. **985:** 125–134.
63. PROCYK, E. *et al.* 2007. Modulations of prefrontal activity related to cognitive control and performance monitoring. *In* Sensorimotor Foundations of Higher Cognition. Y. Rossetti, Ed. Oxford University Press: in press.
64. KENNERLEY, S.W., A.H. LARA & J.D. WALLIS. 2005. Prefrontal neurons encode an abstract representation of value [abstract]. Society for Neuroscience Meeting Planner. Online. Program No. 194.16.
65. KILLCROSS, S. & E. COUTUREAU. 2003. Coordination of actions and habits in the medial prefrontal cortex of rats. Cereb. Cortex **13:** 400–408.
66. DE WIT, S. *et al.* 2006. Dorsomedial prefrontal cortex resolves response conflict in rats. J. Neurosci. **26:** 5224–5229.
67. RUSHWORTH, M.F. *et al.* 2007. Contrasting roles for cingulate and orbitofrontal cortex in decisions and social behaviour. Trends Cogn. Sci. **11:** 168–176.
68. MATSUMOTO, K. & K. TANAKA. 2004. The role of the medial prefrontal cortex in achieving goals. Curr. Opin. Neurobiol. **14:** 178–185.
69. SHIMA, K. & J. TANJI. 1998. Role for cingulate motor area cells in voluntary movement selection based on reward. Science **282:** 1335–1338.
70. AMIEZ, C., J.P. JOSEPH & E. PROCYK. 2005. Anterior cingulate error-related activity is modulated by predicted reward. Eur. J. Neurosci. **21:** 3447–3452.
71. CARMICHAEL, S.T. & J.L. PRICE. 1996. Connectional networks within the orbital and medial prefrontal cortex of macaque monkeys. J. Comp. Neurol. **371:** 179–207.
72. VUILLEUMIER, P. 2005. How brains beware: neural mechanisms of emotional attention. Trends Cogn. Sci. **9:** 585–594.
73. PAZ, R. *et al.* 2006. Emotional enhancement of memory via amygdala-driven facilitation of rhinal interactions. Nat. Neurosci. **9:** 1321–1329.

Synergistic and Regulatory Effects of Orbitofrontal Cortex on Amygdala-Dependent Appetitive Behavior

A. C. ROBERTS, Y. REEKIE, AND K. BRAESICKE

Department of Physiology, Development and Neuroscience, University of Cambridge, Cambridge, United Kingdom

Behavioural and Clinical Neuroscience Institute, University of Cambridge, Cambridge, United Kingdom

ABSTRACT: This paper will review two avenues of our research in marmosets that have focused on the role of the orbitofrontal cortex (OFC) in amygdala-dependent appetitive behavior. The first demonstrates the important contribution of both the OFC and the amygdala to conditioned reinforcement (CRF). The second reveals the regulatory effects of the OFC on amygdala-dependent autonomic and behavioral arousal in appetitive conditioning. The process of CRF is one way in which an environmental cue can guide emotional behavior. As a consequence of its previous relationship with reward, a cue can take on affective value and reinforce behavior. Lesion studies in marmosets are described that show that CRF is dependent upon both the amygdala and OFC. The synergistic interactions between these structures that have been shown to underlie other aspects of reward processing are then considered with respect to CRF. The results are contrasted with those that show the importance of the OFC in suppressing positive affective responses elicited by the amygdala in response to a conditioned stimulus (CS). Specifically, it will be shown that the OFC is involved in the rapid suppression of conditioned autonomic arousal upon CS withdrawal and in the co-ordination of conditioned autonomic and behavioral responses when adapting to changing reward contingencies. It will be argued that, overall, the OFC plays a critical role in the context-dependent regulation of positive affective responding governed by external cues, in keeping with a role in executive control.

Address for correspondence: A. C. Roberts, Department of Physiology, Development and Neuroscience, University of Cambridge, Downing Street, Cambridge, CB2 3DY, UK. Voice: 44 1223 333763/339015; fax: 44 1223 333786.
acr4@cam.ac.uk

Ann. N.Y. Acad. Sci. 1121: 297–319 (2007). © 2007 New York Academy of Sciences.
doi: 10.1196/annals.1401.019

KEYWORDS: positive emotion regulation; executive control; autonomic arousal; reversal learning; appetitive conditioning

INTRODUCTION

The amygdala and orbitofrontal cortex (OFC) are highly interconnected.[1,2] Not only do these two structures have direct reciprocal connections with one another,[3,4] but many of their inputs from, and outputs to, other forebrain and brain stem sites are overlapping. Their pattern of connectivity with structures, such as the anterior cingulate, ventral striatum, hypothalamus, insula, and brainstem as well as sensory association cortices,[1,5–8] suggests an involvement in emotional evaluation and expression, and indeed functional studies substantiate this view. Thus, both human functional neuroimaging[9–12] and electrophysiological studies in animals[13–16] have shown activity in the OFC and amygdala to be particularly sensitive to the incentive value of environmental stimuli, both negative and positive. Moreover, in all species studied so far, lesions of either structure disrupts various aspects of goal-directed behavior[17–21] and emotional and social behavior.[22–28] Together, these findings emphasize commonalities of function between the OFC and the amygdala but of themselves do not provide insight into the nature of any interaction. When studies have specifically investigated this interaction, they have provided evidence for a synergistic relationship, highlighting the inter-dependency of the two structures for certain of their reward-processing functions. Thus, disconnecting the OFC from the basolateral (BL) amygdala by lesioning the OFC on one side of the brain and the amygdala on the other[29] can produce as profound a deficit in choices guided by reward value as that seen following a bilateral lesion of either structure.[18] Such findings demonstrate that the contributions of each structure to the behavior under study are dependent upon their ability to interact with one another. Another illustration of interdependency between the OFC and BL amygdala has been provided by studies showing that specific aspects of neural encoding of reward-related information within each structure is disrupted in the absence of input from the other.[30,31]

Lesions of the amygdala and OFC do not always produce the same pattern of behavioral effects, and the marked differences that have been reported in a number of behavioral settings have provided important insight into the functional distinctions between the two.[32–34] In some cases these differences suggest antagonistic rather than synergistic interactions. Indeed, OFC termination patterns in the amygdala include the central nucleus as well as the intercalated cell masses, which in turn send inhibitory projections onto the central nucleus, providing anatomical evidence that the OFC may both enhance and suppress output from the central nucleus.[4] This chapter will consider two experimental preparations that have been used to study the role of the OFC and amygdala in reward processing that highlight both the synergistic and regulatory roles of the OFC in amygdala-dependent functioning.

CONTRIBUTIONS OF THE OFC TO AMYGDALA-DEPENDENT REWARD PROCESSING

OFC and the BL Nuclei of the Amygdala

A number of contexts have been identified in which behavior is dependent upon both the BL amygdala and OFC. For example, the ability of monkeys to select an object from an array of objects based upon the current incentive value of the rewards associated with those objects is disrupted not only by bilateral lesions of the amygdala[19] and OFC[18] but also by employing a unilateral lesion procedure that effectively disconnects the two structures.[35] For detailed discussion of these findings see Ref.36. Although in this particular context the deficit could be due either to an impairment in action-outcome learning or object-outcome learning, the latter is the more likely. Thus, the same deficit has been reported following OFC lesions in rats in an appetitive Pavlovian task.[17] In this task, conditioned approach behavior to the food hopper upon presentation of a stimulus associated with food, a behavior dependent upon the association between the stimulus and its outcome, is insensitive to changes in the value of the food following OFC lesions. In addition, behavior guided specifically by the knowledge of the incentive value of the outcome of an action, e.g., lever pressing, is not disrupted by OFC-lesions.[37]

However, the precise contribution of the amygdala and OFC to stimulus-outcome learning still remains to be determined. This is, in part, because the devaluation test used to determine knowledge about the incentive value of the outcome in amygdala and OFC- lesioned animals depends on changing the incentive value and accordingly, looking for a change in behavior.[19,38] Thus, any effect of a lesion may be due either to an inability to update incentive value and/or use that new value to change behavior, or alternatively, to a failure to learn the association between the stimulus and the incentive value of the outcome and/or use that information to guide behavior, in the first place. Whether the OFC impairs the latter remains to be determined.

Another context in which the OFC contributes to amygdala-dependent behavior is in responding for conditioned reinforcement (CRF). CRF is a process by which stimuli in the environment can control and maintain behavior in the absence of primary reinforcers such as food, sex, and warmth. Conditioned reinforcers acquire their motivational properties through direct Pavlovian association with primary reinforcers and subsequently act themselves as goals for actions. Thus, they can induce high rates of responding over protracted periods of time, helping to maintain behavior when rewards are not immediate. Moreover, they can act to reinforce new responding despite the new responding itself failing to result in primary reward. This reinforcing property of conditioned stimuli (CSs) may be dependent upon the CS evoking either a representation of the primary reward with which it is associated or generalized, non-specific affect.[39] Evidence for the latter was provided by

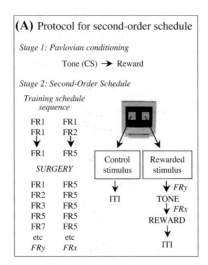

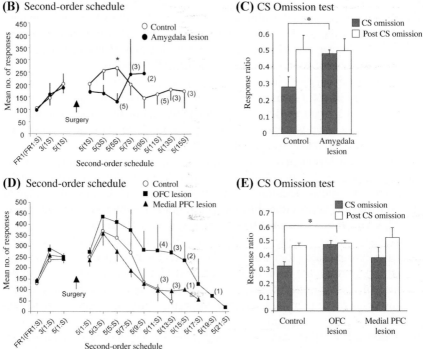

FIGURE 1. **(A)** For the second-order schedule study, animals first learned that a tone was associated with banana milkshake reward (Pavlovian conditioning). They then learned that a response to a stimulus presented on either the left or right of a touch-sensitive computer screen resulted in the presentation of the tone (CS) and access to the reward. Subsequently they had to make more and more responses to gain access to the reward (Fixed Ratio, $FRx = 1...5$) but each response resulted in the tone CS ($FRy = 1$). After

a recent study of lever pressing for CRF in rats,[40] but evidence for the former has been provided at this meeting.[41] Thus, both specific and general aspects of affect may underlie responding for CRF's, with the relative contribution of each varying as a consequence of task and stimulus parameters.

Typically two distinct behavioral procedures are used to study CRF in the laboratory: (1) second-order schedules (FIG. 1A) in which a CS maintains high rates of responding when there are only intermittent presentations of primary reward and (2) acquisition of a new response for CRF (FIG. 2A). Performance on both types of procedure is impaired in rats following amygdala lesions,[42-44] and although marmosets with amygdala lesions have not been tested with the latter procedure, their performance on second-order schedules is compromised as severely as that of amygdala-lesioned rats.[45] Thus, as the response requirements increased and the availability of primary reward became less frequent, amygdala-lesioned marmosets became progressively impaired at maintaining responding during periods when such behavior was reinforced primarily by the contingent presentation of the CS (FIG. 1B). Their insensitivity to the reinforcing efficacy of the CS was confirmed by their failure to show a decline in responding upon omission of the CS, in contrast to the marked decline in the performance of controls (FIG. 1C). This insensitivity to the reinforcing efficacy of a CS most likely underlies the enhanced rate of extinction in amygdala-lesioned monkeys following omission of reward for object displacement.[33]

Lesions of the OFC, but not the medial prefrontal cortex (PFC), in marmosets also disrupt the CRF process.[32] Animals with OFC lesions failed to

←——

surgery, 5 tone CS presentations always resulted in reward (FR$x = 5$), but the number of responses before receiving a tone presentation (S) was increased every fourth session from 1 to 3, 5 etc. (FR$y = 1...5$). Animals continued to progress up the schedule until they failed to gain a single reward on two consecutive sessions. **(B and D)** Mean number of responses performed by amygdala-lesioned and prefrontal-lesioned groups respectively, across the three sessions of each stage of the schedule. Numbers in brackets indicate the number of animals still performing at each stage. Amygdala-lesioned animals ($n = 6$) dropped out at earlier stages of the schedule compared to controls ($n = 6$). In contrast there were no differences between control ($n = 5$) and OFC- ($n = 5$) and medial PFC- ($n = 5$) lesioned groups. **(C and E)** Performance on the CS omission test is presented as the ratio of responses following omission of the CS (CS omission phase) relative to the two days immediately prior to CS omission (pre-CS omission phase), i.e., CS omission/(CS omission + pre-CS omission). A score of 0.5 indicates that responding was equivalent to the pre-CS omission phase, while a score below 0.5 indicates a decline in responding. For comparison purposes performance on the two days following the CS omission phase in which the CS was present (post-CS omission phase) is also shown. *indicates that the response ratio for the CS omission phase in the lesioned groups was significantly greater ($P < 0.05$), than their respective control groups. Adapted from Refs. 32, 45.

acquire a new discrimination based on the association of the discriminanda with one or other of a pair of auditory CSs, one of which had been previously associated with reward, the other not (FIG. 2A, B). The responding of OFC-lesioned marmosets was also insensitive to the omission of the CS on a second-order schedule (FIG. 1E). However, despite this insensitivity to the CS, and in contrast to amygdala-lesioned marmosets, their overall levels of responding on the second-order schedule remained equivalent to controls (FIG. 1D). Thus they were able to maintain their responding over lengthy periods when only a CS, but no unconditioned stimulus (US), was present. This finding suggests that additional effects of OFC lesions may have led to the persistent responding in the OFC-lesioned group on the second-order schedule. For example, lesions of the PFC have been shown to increase behavioral sensitivity to dopaminergic manipulations,[46–48] effects that may well depend upon the actions of dopamine (DA) at the level of the striatum. In addition, sensitization of dopaminergic systems with repeated amphetamine pretreatment leads to a rapid progression from goal-directed to habit-based responding,[49] the latter associated with the dorsal striatum.[50] Thus, despite being insensitive to the reinforcing properties of the CS, the responding of OFC-lesioned monkeys on the second-order schedule may have become habitual, prematurely, as a consequence of enhanced sensitivity to DA in the striatum.

In summary, the comparable deficits associated with lesions of the OFC and amygdala on CRF and outcome-devaluation tests highlight the critical role played by these two structures in processing the incentive value of reward-related stimuli; information that can be used to control goal-directed behavior. Although an interaction between the OFC and amygdala has only been shown to underlie performance on outcome-devaluation tests, it is likely that a similar interaction underlies responding for conditioned reinforcers. By lesioning the BL nuclei and recording from neurons in the OFC, it has been shown that such lesions disrupt the ability of OFC neurons to represent the value of expected outcomes. Based on these findings it has been proposed that the failure to represent expected outcomes in the OFC is due to the loss of specific information from the BL amygdala regarding the relationship between stimuli in the outside world and rewarding events,[51] leading to the observed deficits in goal-directed behavior.

It should be highlighted though that not all behavior dependent upon the BL amygdala is also dependent upon the OFC. For example, the ability of CSs to override satiety signals and stimulate eating in sated rats is dependent on the BL amygdala[52,53] and its connections with the lateral hypothalamus,[54] but not the OFC.[55] This suggests that it is specifically preparatory, and not consummatory, behaviors that are dependent upon an interaction between the BL nuclei and the OFC.

(A) Protocol

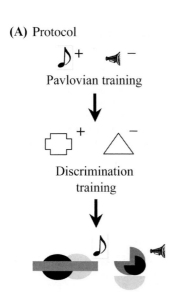

Pavlovian training

Discrimination
training

Responding for conditioned
reinforcement

(B) Acquisition of a new response
for conditioned reinforcement

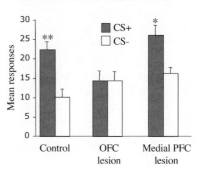

FIGURE 2. (A) For acquisition of a new response for conditioned reinforcement, animals were first trained on a Pavlovian schedule in which one of two noises, tone or white noise, predicted banana milkshake reward (CS^+). They then received training on a series of visual discriminations in which one of two visual patterns presented on a touch-sensitive computer screen was associated with reward. Subsequently they were presented with two novel visual patterns, one of which was associated with the auditory CS^+ and the other with the auditory CS^-. **(B)** Mean number of responses made to a visual stimulus associated with a CS^+ compared to a stimulus associated with a CS^- in control ($n = 5$), OFC-lesioned ($n = 5$), and medial PFC-lesioned ($n = 4$) groups. While the control-lesioned and medial PFC-lesioned groups showed differential responding to the stimulus associated with the CS^+ compared to that associated with the CS^-, OFC-lesioned animals responded equally to the two stimuli. ** and * indicate that the responding for the CS^+ was significantly greater than that for the CS^- in control and medial PFC-lesioned groups at $P < 0.01$ and 0.05, respectively. Adapted from Ref. 32.

OFC and the Central Nucleus of the Amygdala

The available evidence and thus the discussion so far, has emphasized the important contribution of the OFC to aspects of reward processing that are dependent upon the BL amygdala. Focus on the BL nuclei has been due, in part, to this region sending the greatest number of projections to the OFC compared to other regions of the amygdala, including central, cortical, and medial nuclei.[2,3] However, at least one behavior that is not dependent upon the BL nuclei, but is dependent instead upon the central nucleus of the amygdala,

(A) Apparatus

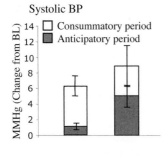

(B) Task protocol

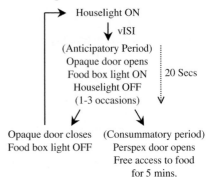

(C) Acquisition

Systolic BP

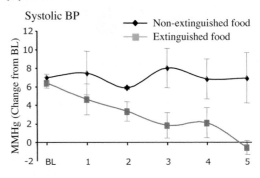

CS/US directed behavior

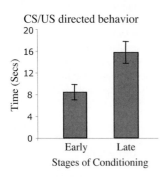

(D) Extinction

Systolic BP

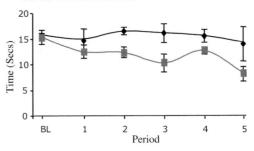

CS/US directed behavior

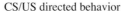

FIGURE 3. (A) A photograph of the apparatus used in the autonomic study. The task procedure for each session is summarized in **B.** During the anticipatory period an opaque door opened and the animal could view either high- (marshmallow, maltloaf) or low- (laboratory pellets) incentive food inside the box. Animals ($n = 4$) received between 1 and 3 such periods within a session, and at the end of the final anticipatory period, both the opaque and transparent doors opened and the animal gained access to the food (the consummatory period). **(C)** Early in acquisition, no changes in BP occurred during the anticipatory periods, but a rise in BP was seen during the consumption of the high-incentive food. In later stages of acquisition, all animals developed a rise in BP and directed their behavior toward the food box during the anticipatory period when they could "see" the high-incentive food

has also been found to be dependent upon the OFC. Thus, the conditioned approach response that develops to a CS as a consequence of pairings of the CS with food reward, is dependent upon the central, but not BL, nucleus of the amygdala for its acquisition,[56] although not its expression.[57] The acquisition, but not expression, of this conditioned approach response is also dependent upon the OFC.[58] This approach response to the CS in appetitive conditioning should not be confused with the approach response to the food cup itself during presentation of the CS. The latter is not affected by either BL or central nucleus lesions of the amygdala[38] and may be controlled by the discriminatory, and not the motivational properties of the CS. In contrast, approach to the CS itself has been proposed to reflect the CS's acquisition of positive incentive motivation[59] and is consistent with many other findings that implicate the central nucleus in the encoding of generalized motivation or affect that acts as a reinforcement signal to strengthen stimulus-response associations.[60,61] This therefore implicates the OFC too in generalized motivational or affective processes, at least during learning, but its precise role remains unclear, as does its interaction with the rest of the neural network that contributes to Pavlovian approach behavior, including the nucleus accumbens[62,63] and anterior cingulate cortex.[57]

REGULATORY EFFECTS OF THE OFC ON AMYGDALA-DEPENDENT REWARD PROCESSING

The involvement of the OFC in the control of Pavlovian appetitive responses is of particular relevance to our understanding of the role of the OFC in positive emotion regulation. Emotions are highly adaptive and complex states,[64,65] simultaneously involving psychological, behavioral, and physiological responses that are triggered by the cognitive appraisal of external stimuli. These responses enable the organism to fulfill goals, both internal and social, that preserve the individual and its reproductive success. They range from unlearned reflexes and fixed action patterns, through Pavlovian learning, in which novel stimuli come to elicit conditioned responses, to instrumental

---

through the window. (No such changes were seen during the anticipatory period when they could see low-incentive food.) **(D)** During the extinction stage, animals ($n = 2$) learned that they never got access to one particular type of high-incentive food (extinguished food, e.g., marshmallow; 20 sessions), but they did get access to the other (non-extinguished food, e.g. maltloaf; 20 sessions). These two types of session were intermingled with one another over the full 40-session extinction stage. Consequently, the anticipatory systolic BP rise to the sight of the "extinguished" food declined across sessions while the BP rise to the "non-extinguished food" was maintained. Behavior directed toward the sight of the "extinguished food" also declined across sessions. BL, baseline; 1–5, mean data from groups of 4 sessions across the 20 sessions; vISI, variable inter-stimulus interval.

behavior, whereby the organism takes active control of the environment in order to satisfy motivational and emotional needs. However, our immediate reactions to emotive stimuli are not always the most beneficial, and thus an important element of emotion is to appropriately adapt and rapidly modify emotional responses as contexts change. Recently there has been much emphasis on the importance of the ventromedial PFC in the regulation of Pavlovian conditioned negative emotional responses. Studies in humans have focused on the regulation of emotional experience and/or autonomic arousal elicited by the presentation of emotion-provoking stimuli, and in studies of rats, conditioned behavior, e.g., freezing, has frequently been the measure of emotion. Together, they have implicated the infralimbic cortex of rats[66,67] and the subgenual PFC of humans[68,69] in the suppression of negative emotion elicited by the amygdala to a currently extinguished, but previously aversive, CS. In addition, microstimulation studies of the medial PFC in rats have shown that the prelimbic and infralimbic regions up-regulate and down-regulate, respectively, the expression of conditioned fear responses.[70]

In contrast, there is a paucity of information regarding the regulation of such responses in the appetitive domain. Indeed, the majority of studies of the regulation of positive reinforcement have analyzed reward processing primarily from an economic perspective,[71] rather than in affective terms, and have focused mainly on how reward guides instrumental actions or choices.[18,72] Thus, there is a need to study concomitantly those physiological, behavioral, and, in humans, experiential responses evoked by appetitive stimuli that together define a positive emotional state. Very few studies though have investigated the autonomic correlates of appetitive conditioning[73-76] (unlike aversive conditioning), and in those that have, contrasting effects have been reported.[73,75] However, the OFC receives sensory information from the autonomic system and sends projections onto autonomic output centers.[77] In addition, the OFC has been shown to play a major role in appetitive tasks of behavioral flexibility including extinction,[33,78] discrimination reversal,[18,58,79,80] and reward devaluation.[17,18] Although, with the exception of one study,[17] these studies have investigated how the OFC contributes to the process by which discriminative stimuli guide instrumental actions, rather than how it contributes to the regulation of Pavlovian conditioned appetitive emotional responses, per se. Taken together though, these findings make it likely that the OFC is also involved in the regulation of Pavlovian conditioned appetitive emotional responses.

PAVLOVIAN CONDITIONED APPETITIVE RESPONSES AND THEIR REGULATION BY OFC

Recently, we have developed a primate model for studying the regulation of positive emotional responses that uses a telemetric device implanted into the descending aorta of marmosets, allowing for the remote measurement of cardiovascular responses in behaving animals. By measuring multiple behavioral and cardiovascular conditioned responses, it is possible to investigate the role of the OFC, not only in the regulation of positive appetitive responses but also in their coordination, the latter being an important element of executive control.

In our original studies[81] marmosets could view high-incentive or low-incentive food through a window for 20 s (anticipatory period) before gaining 5 min access to the food (consummatory period; FIG. 3A). In this case, the sight, i.e., shape and color, of the high-incentive food (marshmallow/maltloaf), acted as the CS^+. Cardiovascular responses, i.e., blood pressure (BP) and heart rate (HR), during this anticipatory period were compared with the same period during which the marmosets viewed low-incentive food (laboratory chow, CS^-). In any one session, marmosets were given the opportunity to view the food (either high-incentive or low-incentive) on 1–3 occasions (anticipatory periods), before they obtained access to the food (FIG. 3B). Repeated exposure to this contingency resulted in the marmosets developing anticipatory, conditioned autonomic and behavioral responses to the sight of the high-incentive food but not the low-incentive food. Since the physical properties of the food acted as the CS in this version of the task, it was not possible to separate out conditioned behavioral responses to the CS separately from that to the US. Thus the primary behavioral responses that developed during the CS period were "looking" and "scrabbling" at the window through which the food was clearly visible, responses that were both CS directed and US directed. Early on in acquisition, no changes in BP (and HR) were seen during this anticipatory period, although increases in BP did occur during the subsequent consummatory period when animals consumed the high-incentive food, but not the low-incentive food (FIG. 3C). However, in the later stages of acquisition, marked increases in BP (and HR) were seen during the anticipatory period when the animals viewed high-incentive food. This was accompanied by an increase in behavior directed toward the food box (FIG. 3C). If subsequently the sight of a particular high-incentive food, e.g., marshmallow, no longer led to access to that food, i.e., extinction, then the conditioned cardiovascular and behavioral responses to the sight of that food returned to base line (FIG. 3D). Conditioned cardiovascular and behavioral responses to the sight of food to which they still gained access remained high over this period.

Using this version of the task, it was shown that the expression of these CS-induced cardiovascular arousal responses were dependent upon the amygdala.[81] Excitotoxic lesions of the amygdala that targeted both the BL and central nucleus in the marmoset markedly attenuated the conditioned cardiovascular response to the sight of high-incentive food in animals that had been trained on the task prior to surgery (FIG. 4A). In contrast, there were no effects of the lesion on the cardiovascular arousal that occurred during consumption of the food (FIG. 4C). Neither was there any effect of the lesion on the expression

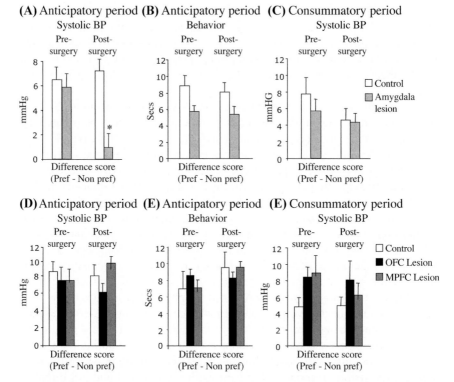

FIGURE 4. (A) Mean changes in systolic BP ($\pm$SEM) during the anticipatory period (20 s), compared to the preceding baseline period (20 s) are shown for both control ($n = 4$) and amygdala-lesioned ($n = 4$) groups. Mean durations of food box directed behavior ($\pm$SEM), including looking, approaching, and responding at the box during the anticipatory period, are shown in **B,** and mean changes in systolic BP ($\pm$SEM) during the first minute of the consummatory period, compared to the immediately preceding anticipatory period, are shown in **C**. These same measures are shown in **D–F**, respectively, for animals that received a lesion of either the OFC ($n = 6$), medial PFC ($n = 4$), or a sham operated control procedure ($n = 5$). Amygdala lesions disrupted the expression of the conditioned BP rise during the anticipatory period, but there were no other significant effects. *indicates a significant difference of $P = 0.005$ between the control and amygdala-lesioned groups, post surgery.

of the conditioned behavioral responses (FIG. 4B). The latter is consistent with the finding in rats that neither BL nor central nucleus lesions of the amygdala disrupt US-directed appetitive conditioned responses and that central nucleus lesions only disrupt the acquisition, but not expression, of CS-directed appetitive conditioned responses.[38] The latter also rules out the possibility that the conditioned cardiovascular arousal observed during the CS period merely reflected the accompanying increase in behavioral activity (e.g., scrabbling at the food box), given that these two measures were clearly dissociated by an amygdala lesion.

In a subsequent experiment, using protocols identical to those used for the study of the amygdala, we showed that excitotoxic lesions of neither the medial PFC nor OFC in marmosets had any effect on the expression of these conditioned cardiovascular or behavioral arousal responses or unconditioned arousal responses (FIG. 4D–F). Thus, it would appear that the amygdala is necessary for the expression of appetitive conditioned cardiovascular, but not CS/US directed, behavioral responses and neither the medial PFC nor OFC is critical for the expression of appetitive-conditioned cardiovascular or behavioral responses. Given that OFC lesions in rats disrupt the acquisition, but not expression, of conditioned behavioral approach responses to the CS, it will be interesting in a future study to investigate the role of the OFC in the acquisition of conditioned cardiovascular responses.

One aspect of peripheral autonomic arousal not considered so far is its role in regulating emotional processing. Evidence for such regulation has come from studies of long-term memory in humans[82] and animals[83] and emotional experience[84,85] in humans, although the extent to which peripheral feedback can influence the latter may depend upon an individual's level of interoceptive awareness.[86] In contrast, its role in biasing response selection[87] or increasing response vigor is less clear. Moreover, any contribution of autonomic arousal specifically in the context of responding on second-order schedules for CRF, as studied here, is unknown. However, it has been proposed that disjunctions between peripheral feedback and other emotional responses, including activity in emotion-related neural circuitry, may have a marked impact on emotional experience.[88,89] Such disjunctions have recently been highlighted in investigations of the role of the OFC in regulating autonomic and behavioral responses in reversal learning and are described below.

In order to determine the role of the OFC in the regulation of autonomic and behavioral responses, the effects of OFC lesions in marmosets on two distinct aspects of appetitive regulation have been studied. The first is the relatively automatic decline in cardiovascular arousal when the appetitive-eliciting stimulus is withdrawn from the environment. The second is the modification of appetitive responses following reversal of the reward contingencies. The former has already been investigated in studies of human negative emotion, and in one study prolonged autonomic arousal following the offset of an aversive stimulus was shown to be associated with low scores on a resilience questionnaire.[90] Such persistent negative affect has also been shown to correlate with greater relative right-sided anterior activation in scalp-recorded brain electric signals, although, in this study, the measure of affect was eyeblink startle magnitude, not autonomic arousal.[91] However, to date, no studies have investigated such regulation in the positive domain. The second aspect of regulation, namely reversal learning and its control by the OFC, is well documented in the context of the reversal of instrumental responses in appetitive conditioning.

However it has not been studied in the context of Pavlovian responses. More-over, traditionally, such reversal studies have only monitored a single response system across the reversal and that response has always been behavioral in nature. But, given that emotions or affective states are multifaceted with be-havioral, physiological, and experiential components, it is important, wherever possible, to monitor these separable components when studying emotion reg-ulation. As mentioned above, this may be of particular relevance to a number of neuropsychiatric disorders in which disjunctions between various measures of emotional processing have been reported.[88]

Instead of the sight of the food reward acting as the CS, one of two auditory stimuli (white noise or tone) acted as the CS. As before, one or other of the stimuli was presented for 20 s, after which the marmoset either gained 2 min access to a box full of high-incentive food or an empty box. As expected, marmosets developed anticipatory, conditioned cardiovascular and behavioral responses to the auditory stimulus when paired with the high-incentive food (CS$^+$) but not when paired with the empty food box (CS$^-$). In this ver-sion of the task, the most prominent conditioned behavioral responses were "head jerking" to the CS and "looking" at the food box, behaviors similar to those previously reported in rats and which have been described respec-tively as CS specific and US specific.[59,92,93] Preliminary findings replicate our previous results showing that lesions of the OFC do not affect the ex-pression of either conditioned autonomic or behavioral responses to an appet-itive CS that has been established prior to the lesion. However, OFC lesions do disrupt the *regulation* of those responses. Thus, compared with controls, OFC-lesioned animals showed prolonged cardiovascular arousal following the unexpected offset of the appetitive CS, and their performance was markedly disrupted following reversal of the reward contingencies.[94] Not only did OFC-lesioned animals take more sessions before their conditioned BP reflected the new contingencies compared with controls, but even when their BP did reverse, their CS-directed behavior remained non-discriminative. This is in marked contrast to the controls, all of which showed significantly elevated CS-directed responses to the new CS$^+$ compared with the CS$^-$ at the same stage in the reversal as their conditioned BP also reflected the new contingen-cies.

Together, these results demonstrate that the OFC plays an important role in the regulation of conditioned appetitive responses and, in particular, demon-strate the critical contribution of the OFC in the coordination of such responses when adapting to changes in the environment. Thus, in the absence of the OFC, autonomic and behavioral responses become uncoupled during reversal of the reward contingencies. The pathways through which the OFC normally coor-dinates these different outputs that make up the adaptive response remain to be determined, although it is likely that they include the projections from the OFC that directly innervate the amygdala. Indeed, it has been shown in rats performing a reversal of an odor go/no-go discrimination task that far fewer amygdala neurons reverse their odor preference following loss of OFC input,[31] highlighting the dependence of flexible neuronal firing in the amygdala upon the OFC. However, while the expression of conditioned cardiovascular arousal is dependent upon an intact amygdala,[81,95] the expression of various conditioned behaviors, including CS-elicited approach[56,57] and orienting responses,[96,97] are not, despite their dependence on the amygdala at acquisition. Thus, projections from the OFC onto other downstream structures involved in the expression of these conditioned responses, including the ventral and dorsal striatum, hypothalamus, and brain stem, may also contribute to a coordinated response output.

How the contribution of the OFC to affective regulation differs from that of the medial PFC is unclear. To date, studies of the latter have focused primarily on negative affect, while the example of regulation by the OFC provided here involves positive affect. Thus, distinct regions within the OFC and medial PFC could differentially regulate these affective valences. However, infralimbic lesions disrupt the memory of extinction for both conditioned fear[67] and appetitive responses,[98] suggesting that this region serves a more general, valence-independent function. For example, the infralimbic cortex has been proposed to play a specialized role in contextual processing,[98] consistent with its afferent input from the hippocampus[99] and the importance of contextual information in recalling the memory of extinction.[100,101] In contrast, the OFC may contribute to the acquisition of extinction by virtue of its ability to modify stimulus-reward associations in downstream structures.[31]

SUMMARY AND CONCLUSIONS

Data have been presented that highlight both the synergistic and regulatory effects of the OFC on amygdala-dependent appetitive behavior. Lesions of either the OFC[32] or amygdala[45] in marmosets disrupt the ability of reward-related stimuli to act as conditioned reinforcers, an impairment associated specifically with damage to the BL amygdala in rats.[42] Lesions of the OFC have also been shown to impair the ability of rats and monkeys to adjust their behavior to reward-related stimuli in response to changes in the incentive value of the reward.[17,18] This, too, is a deficit associated with damage to the BL amygdala[19] and one that is thought to reflect a loss of goal-directed behavior. In both cases, the findings are consistent with the proposal that the OFC encodes the incentive value of future outcomes, based upon the information it receives from the BL amygdala about the relationship between stimuli in the environment and reward.[17,35,102] However, while an intact OFC always appears necessary for this incentive information to guide responding whether in acquisition or performance,[32,103,104] there is some evidence to suggest that the role of the BL amygdala in this process is restricted to the initial learning of the stimulus-reward association.[103,105] These findings parallel those obtained from studies of the central nucleus in rats, in which the nucleus has been shown to play a role in the acquisition, but not expression, of CS-directed conditioned behavioral responses, i.e., approach[106] and orienting.[55,96] However, other findings do not concur with a role for these amygdala nuclei in reward processing that is restricted to acquisition.[42,45,81,107] Whether such discrepancies can be accounted for by differences in the nature of the responses between studies, e.g., Pavlovian versus instrumental[103,107] and behavioral versus autonomic,[81,97] remains to be determined.

In considering the interaction of the amygdala and OFC in goal-directed behavior, it should be emphasized that this network contributes specifically to behavior that is dependent upon the incentive value of the reward. However, in many tasks and contexts, including simple sensory discrimination tests in which the selection of a specific odor or visual stimulus leads to reward, response selection is not dependent upon knowledge of the relationship between a stimulus and the incentive value of that associated reward. Instead other, non-affective properties of the CS and its reward, i.e., physical properties, can enter into association and guide response selection (see Refs. 108–110 for detailed discussions). Thus, overall learning and performance on such tasks are not dependent upon either the amygdala or OFC.[78,80] However, recent findings would suggest that the particular neural network that is involved in the overall learning and performance of such discrimination tasks (including perhaps regions of temporal lobe[111] and striatum[112]) is nevertheless sensitive to incentive information and that activity in the network is disrupted when incentive information is incongruent with the current stimulus-reward contingencies.[113]

Data presented in this paper have also highlighted the regulatory role played by the OFC in amygdala functioning with respect to autonomic and behavioral arousal. Conditioned autonomic arousal that accompanies an appetitive CS was shown to be dependent upon the amygdala, but not the OFC or medial PFC, for its expression in marmosets. However, the relatively automatic decline in cardiovascular arousal when a CS is withdrawn from the environment was shown to be delayed following OFC lesions. In addition, following a reversal of the reward contingencies, OFC lesions not only impaired the rate at which conditioned autonomic arousal adapted to the reversed contingencies but also resulted in an uncoupling of conditioned autonomic and behavioral responses across the reversal. Together, these findings reveal the truly executive nature of this regulatory control, with the OFC acting to coordinate appetitive, conditioned responses when adapting to changes in the environment.

ACKNOWLEDGEMENTS

The research described here was funded by a Medical Research Council (MRC) Programme Grant awarded to ACR. The work was completed within the University of Cambridge Behavioural and Clinical Neuroscience Institute funded jointly by the MRC and the Wellcome Trust. We especially thank A. Newman for help preparing the figures and all my colleagues for their efforts in these studies.

REFERENCES

1. CARMICHAEL, S.T. & J.L. PRICE. 1995. Limbic connections of the orbital and medial prefrontal cortex in macaque monkeys. J. Comp. Neurol. **363:** 615–641.
2. AMARAL, D.G. *et al.* 1992. Anatomical organization of the primate amygdaloid complex. *In* The Amygdala: Neurobiological Aspects of Emotion, Memory, and Mental Dysfunction. J.P. Aggleton, Ed.: 1–66. Wiley-Liss. New York.
3. GHASHGHAEI, H.T. & H. BARBAS. 2002. Pathways for emotion: interactions of prefrontal and anterior temporal pathways in the amygdala of the rhesus monkey. Neuroscience **115:** 1261–1279.
4. GHASHGHAEI, H.T., C.C. HILGETAG & H. BARBAS. 2007. Sequence of information processing for emotions based on the anatomic dialogue between prefrontal cortex and amygdala. Neuroimage **34:** 905–923.
5. REMPEL-CLOWER, N.L. & H. BARBAS. 1998. Topographic organization of connections between the hypothalamus and prefrontal cortex in the rhesus monkey. J. Comp. Neurol. **398:** 393–419.
6. FERRY, A.T. *et al.* 2000. Prefrontal cortical projections to the striatum in macaque monkeys: evidence for an organization related to prefrontal networks. J. Comp. Neurol. **425:** 447–470.
7. ÖNGÜR, D., X. AN & J.L. PRICE. 1998. Prefrontal cortical projections to the hypothalamus in macaque monkeys. J. Comp. Neurol. **401:** 480–505.
8. FLOYD, N.S. *et al.* 2000. Orbitomedial prefrontal cortical projections to distinct longitudinal columns of the periaqueductal gray in the rat. J. Comp. Neurol. **422:** 556–578.
9. O'DOHERTY, J. *et al.* 2001. Abstract reward and punishment representations in the human orbitofrontal cortex. Nat. Neurosci. **4:** 95–102.
10. ARANA, F.S. *et al.* 2003. Dissociable contributions of the human amygdala and orbitofrontal cortex to incentive motivation and goal selection. J. Neurosci. **23:** 9632–9638.
11. GOTTFRIED, J.A., J. O'DOHERTY & R.J. DOLAN. 2003. Encoding predictive reward value in human amygdala and orbitofrontal cortex. Science **301:** 1104–1107.
12. BREITER, H.C. *et al.* 2001. Functional imaging of neural responses to expectancy and experience of monetary gains and losses. Neuron **30:** 619–639.
13. SCHOENBAUM, G., A.A. CHIBA & M. GALLAGHER. 1999. Neural encoding in orbitofrontal cortex and basolateral amygdala during olfactory discrimination learning. J. Neurosci. **19:** 1876–1884.
14. TREMBLAY, L. & W. SCHULTZ. 1999. Relative reward preference in primate orbitofrontal cortex. Nature **398:** 704–708.
15. PATON, J.J. *et al.* 2006. The primate amygdala represents the positive and negative value of visual stimuli during learning. Nature **439:** 865–870.
16. ROESCH, M.R. & C.R. OLSON. 2004. Neuronal activity related to reward value and motivation in primate frontal cortex. Science **304:** 307–310.

17. GALLAGHER, M., R.W. MCMAHAN & G. SCHOENBAUM. 1999. Orbitofrontal cortex and representation of incentive value in associative learning. J. Neurosci. **19:** 6610–6614.

18. IZQUIERDO, A., R.K. SUDA & E.A. MURRAY. 2004. Bilateral orbital prefrontal cortex lesions in rhesus monkeys disrupt choices guided by both reward value and reward contingency. J. Neurosci. **24:** 7540–7548.

19. MALKOVA, L., D. GAFFAN & E.A. MURRAY. 1997. Excitotoxic lesions of the amygdala fail to produce impairment in visual learning for auditory secondary reinforcement but interfere with reinforcer devaluation effects in rhesus monkeys. J. Neurosci **17:** 6011–6020.

20. BECHARA, A. *et al.* 1994. Insensitivity to future consequences following damage to human prefrontal cortex. Cognition **50:** 7–15.

21. BECHARA, A. *et al.* 1999. Different contributions of the human amygdala and ventromedial prefrontal cortex to decision-making. J. Neurosci. **19:** 5473–5481.

22. IZQUIERDO, A., R.K. SUDA & E.A. MURRAY. 2005. Comparison of the effects of bilateral orbital prefrontal cortex lesions and amygdala lesions on emotional responses in rhesus monkeys. J. Neurosci. **25:** 8534–8542.

23. MEUNIER, M. *et al.* 1999. Effects of aspiration versus neurotoxic lesions of the amygdala on emotional responses in monkeys. Eur. J. Neurosci. **11:** 4403–4418.

24. EMERY, N.J. *et al.* 2001. The effects of bilateral lesions of the amygdala on dyadic social interactions in rhesus monkeys (Macaca mulatta). Behav. Neurosci. **115:** 515–544.

25. BUTTER, C.M., D.R. SNYDER & J.A. MCDONALD. 1970. Effects of orbital frontal lesions on aversive and aggressive behaviors in rhesus monkeys. J. Comp. Physiol Psychol. **72:** 132–144.

26. KOLB, B. 1974. Social behavior of rats with chronic prefrontal lesions. J. Comp. Physiol. Psychol. **87:** 466–474.

27. SKUSE, D., J. MORRIS & K. LAWRENCE. 2003. The amygdala and development of the social brain. Ann. N. Y. Acad. Sci. **1008:** 91–101.

28. BLAIR, R.J. 2004. The roles of orbital frontal cortex in the modulation of antisocial behavior. Brain Cogn. **55:** 198–208.

29. BAXTER, M.G. *et al.* 2000. Control of response selection by reinforcer value requires interaction of amygdala and orbital prefrontal cortex. J. Neurosci. **20:** 4311–4319.

30. SCHOENBAUM, G. *et al.* 2003. Encoding predicted outcome and acquired value in orbitofrontal cortex during cue sampling depends upon input from basolateral amygdala. Neuron **39:** 855–867.

31. SADDORIS, M.P., M. GALLAGHER & G. SCHOENBAUM. 2005. Rapid associative encoding in basolateral amygdala depends on connections with orbitofrontal cortex. Neuron **46:** 321–331.

32. PEARS, A. *et al.* 2003. Lesions of the orbitofrontal, but not the medial prefrontal cortex, disrupt conditioned reinforcement in primates. J. Neurosci. **23:** 11189–11201.

33. IZQUIERDO, A. & E.A. MURRAY. 2005. Opposing effects of amygdala and orbital prefrontal cortex lesions on the extinction of instrumental responding in macaque monkeys. Eur. J. Neurosci. **22:** 2341–2346.

34. WINSTANLEY, C.A. *et al.* 2004. Contrasting roles of basolateral amygdala and orbitofrontal cortex in impulsive choice. J. Neurosci. **24:** 4718–4722.

35. BAXTER, M.G. *et al.* 2000. Control of response selection by reinforcer value requires interaction of amygdala and orbital prefrontal cortex. J. Neurosci. **20:** 4311–4319.
36. MURRAY, E.A. & A. IZQUIERDO. 2007. Orbitofrontal cortex and amygdala contributions to affect and action in primates. Ann. N. Y. Acad. Sci. in press.
37. OSTLUND, S. & B. BALLEINE. 2007. Linking affect to action: critical contributions of orbitofrontal cortex. Ann. N. Y. Acad. Sci. in press.
38. HATFIELD, T. *et al.* 1996. Neurotoxic lesions of basolateral, but not central, amygdala interfere with Pavlovian second-order conditioning and reinforcer devaluation effects. J. Neurosci. **16:** 5256–5265.
39. DICKINSON, A. & M.F. DEARING. 1979. Appetitive-aversive interactions and inhibitory processes. *In* Mechanisms of Learning and Motivation. A. Dickinson & R.A. Boakes, Eds.: 203–231. Erlbaum. Hillsdale, New Jersey.
40. PARKINSON, J.A. *et al.* 2005. Acquisition of instrumental conditioned reinforcement is resistant to the devaluation of the unconditioned stimulus. Q. J. Exp. Psychol. B. **58:** 19–30.
41. BURKE, A.K. *et al.* 2007. Orbitofrontal cortex lesions abolish conditioned reinforcement mediated by a representation of the expected outcome. Ann. N. Y. Acad. Sci. abstract 3: in press.
42. CADOR, M., T.W. ROBBINS & B.J. EVERITT. 1989. Involvement of the amygdala in stimulus-reward associations: interaction with the ventral striatum. Neuroscience **30:** 77–86.
43. BURNS, L.H., T.W. ROBBINS & B.J. EVERITT. 1993. Differential effects of excitotoxic lesions of the basolateral amygdala, ventral subiculum and medial prefrontal cortex on responding with conditioned reinforcement and locomotor activity potentiated by intra-accumbens infusions of D-amphetamine. Behav. Brain Res. **55:** 167–183.
44. WHITELAW, R.B. *et al.* 1996. Excitotoxic lesions of the basolateral amygdala impair the acquisition of cocaine-seeking behaviour under a second-order schedule of reinforcement. Psychopharmacology **127:** 213–224.
45. PARKINSON, J.A. *et al.* 2001. The role of the primate amygdala in conditioned reinforcement. J. Neurosci. **21:** 7770–7780.
46. LIPSKA, B.K. *et al.* 1995. Prefrontal cortical and hippocampal modulation of haloperidol-induced catalepsy and apomorphine-induced stereotypic behaviors in the rat. Biol. Psychiatry **38:** 255–262.
47. BRAUN, A.R. *et al.* 1993. Effects of ibotenic acid lesion of the medial prefrontal cortex on dopamine agonist-related behaviors in the rat. Pharmacol. Biochem. Behav. **46:** 51–60.
48. WILKINSON, L.S. *et al.* 1997. Contrasting effects of excitotoxic lesions of the prefrontal cortex on the behavioural response to D-amphetamine and presynaptic and postsynaptic measures of striatal dopamine function in monkeys. Neuroscience **80:** 717–730.
49. NELSON, A. & S. KILLCROSS. 2006. Amphetamine exposure enhances habit formation. J. Neurosci. **26:** 3805–3812.
50. YIN, H.H., B.J. KNOWLTON & B.W. BALLEINE. 2004. Lesions of dorsolateral striatum preserve outcome expectancy but disrupt habit formation in instrumental learning. Eur. J. Neurosci. **19:** 181–189.
51. ROESCH, M. & G. SCHOENBAUM. 2006. From associations to expectancies:orbitofrontal cortex as gateway tbetween limbic system and representa-

tional memory. *In* The Orbitofrontal Cortex. D.H. Zald & S.L. Rauch, Eds.: 199–236. Oxford University Press. Oxford, UK.

52. HOLLAND, P.C. & M. GALLAGHER. 2003. Double dissociation of the effects of lesions of basolateral and central amygdala on conditioned stimulus-potentiated feeding and Pavlovian-instrumental transfer. Eur. J. Neurosci. **17:** 1680–1694.

53. HOLLAND, P.C., G.D. PETROVICH & M. GALLAGHER. 2002. The effects of amygdala lesions on conditioned stimulus-potentiated eating in rats. Physiol. Behav. **76:** 117–129.

54. PETROVICH, G.D. *et al.* 2002. Amygdalo-hypothalamic circuit allows learned cues to override satiety and promote eating. J. Neurosci. **22:** 8748–8753.

55. McDANNALD, M.A. *et al.* 2005. Lesions of orbitofrontal cortex impair rats' differential outcome expectancy learning but not conditioned stimulus-potentiated feeding. J. Neurosci. **25:** 4626–4632.

56. PARKINSON, J.A., T.W. ROBBINS & B.J. EVERITT. 2000. Dissociable roles of the central and basolateral amygdala in appetitive emotional learning. Eur. J. Neurosci. **12:** 405–413.

57. CARDINAL, R.N. *et al.* 2002. Effects of lesions of the nucleus accumbens core, anterior cingulate cortex, and central nucleus of the amygdala on autoshaping performance in rats. Behav. Neurosci. **116:** 553–567.

58. CHUDASAMA, Y. & T.W. ROBBINS. 2003. Dissociable contributions of the orbitofrontal and infralimbic cortex to pavlovian autoshaping and discrimination reversal learning: further evidence for the functional heterogeneity of the rodent frontal cortex. J. Neurosci. **23:** 8771–8780.

59. HOLLAND, P.C. 1977. Conditioned stimulus as a determinant of the form of the Pavlovian conditioned response. J. Exp. Psychol. Anim. Behav. Process **3:** 77–104.

60. BALLEINE, B.W. & S. KILLCROSS. 2006. Parallel incentive processing: an integrated view of amygdala function. Trends Neurosci. **29:** 272–279.

61. EVERITT, B.J. *et al.* 2000. Differential involvement of amygdala subsystems in appetitive conditioning and drug addiction. *In* The Amygdala: a Functional Analysis. J.P. Aggleton, Ed.: 353–390. Oxford University Press. New York.

62. PARKINSON, J.A. *et al.* 2002. Nucleus accumbens dopamine depletion impairs both acquisition and performance of appetitive Pavlovian approach behaviour: implications for mesoaccumbens dopamine function. Behav. Brain Res. **137:** 149–163.

63. PARKINSON, J.A. *et al.* 2000. Disconnection of the anterior cingulate cortex and nucleus accumbens core impairs Pavlovian approach behavior: further evidence for limbic cortical-ventral striatopallidal systems. Behav. Neurosci. **114:** 42–63.

64. PANKSEPP, J. 1994. Evolution constructed the potential for subjective experience within the neurodynamics of the mammalian brain. *In* The Nature of Emotion: fundamental Questions. P. Ekman & R. Davidson, Eds.: 396–399. Oxford University Press. Oxford.

65. ROLLS, E.T. 1999. The Brain and Emotion. Oxford University Press. Oxford.

66. MORGAN, M.A. & J.E. LEDOUX. 1995. Differential contribution of dorsal and ventral medial prefrontal cortex to the acquisition and extinction of conditioned fear in rats. Behav. Neurosci. **109:** 681–688.

67. QUIRK, G.J. *et al.* 2000. The role of ventromedial prefrontal cortex in the recovery of extinguished fear. J. Neurosci. **20:** 6225–6231.

68. MILAD, M.R. *et al.* 2007. Recall of fear extinction in humans activates the ventromedial prefrontal cortex and hippocampus in concert. Biol. Psychiatry **62:** 446–454.

69. PHELPS, E.A. *et al.* 2004. Extinction learning in humans: role of the amygdala and vmPFC. Neuron **43:** 897–905.

70. VIDAL-GONZALEZ, I. *et al.* 2006. Microstimulation reveals opposing influences of prelimbic and infralimbic cortex on the expression of conditioned fear. Learn Mem. **13:** 728–733.

71. SANFEY, A.G. *et al.* 2006. Neuroeconomics: cross-currents in research on decision-making. Trends Cogn. Sci. **10:** 108–116.

72. O'DOHERTY, J.P. 2004. Reward representations and reward-related learning in the human brain: insights from neuroimaging. Curr. Opin. Neurobiol. **14:** 769–776.

73. POWELL, D.A. *et al.* 2002. Heart rate changes accompanying jaw movement Pavlovian conditioning in rabbits: concomitant blood pressure adjustments and effects of peripheral autonomic blockade. Integr. Physiol. Behav. Sci. **37:** 215–227.

74. BILLMAN, G.E., D.M. HASSON & D.C. RANDALL. 1978. Acquisition and discrimination of appetitively and aversively conditioned heart rate responses in rhesus monkeys. Pavlov J. Biol. Sci. **13:** 145–150.

75. RANDALL, D.C., J.V. BRADY & K.H. MARTIN. 1975. Cardiovascular dynamics during classical appetitive and aversive conditioning in laboratory primates. Pavlov J. Biol. Sci. **10:** 66–75.

76. HUNT, P.S. & B.A. CAMPBELL. 1997. Autonomic and behavioral correlates of appetitive conditioning in rats. Behav. Neurosci. **111:** 494–502.

77. BARBAS, H. 1995. Anatomic basis of cognitive-emotional interactions in the primate prefrontal cortex. Neurosci. Biobehav. Rev. **19:** 499–510.

78. BUTTER, C.M. 1969. Perseveration in extinction and in discrimination reversal tasks following selective frontal ablations in macaca mulatta. Physiol. Behav. **4:** 163–171.

79. DIAS, R., T.W. ROBBINS & A.C. ROBERTS. 1996. Dissociation in prefrontal cortex of affective and attentional shifts. Nature **380:** 69–72.

80. IVERSEN, S.D. & M. MISHKIN. 1970. Perseverative interference in monkeys following selective lesions of the inferior prefrontal convexity. Exp. Brain Res. **11:** 376–386.

81. BRAESICKE, K. *et al.* 2005. Autonomic arousal in an appetitive context in primates: a behavioural and neural analysis. Eur. J. Neurosci. **21:** 1733–1740.

82. CAHILL, L. 2000. Modulation of long-term memory storage in humans by emotional arousal: adrenergic activation and the amygdala. *In* The Amygdala: a Functional Analysis. J.P. Aggleton, Ed.: 425–445. Oxford University Press. New York.

83. MCGAUGH, J.L. *et al.* 2000. Amygdala: role in modulation of memory storage. *In* The Amygdala: a Functional Analysis. J.P. Aggleton, Ed.: 391–423. Oxford University Press. New York.

84. NICOTRA, A. *et al.* 2006. Emotional and autonomic consequences of spinal cord injury explored using functional brain imaging. Brain **129:** 718–728.

85. CRITCHLEY, H.D. *et al.* 2007. Vagus nerve stimulation for treatment-resistant depression: behavioral and neural effects on encoding negative material. Psychosom. Med. **69:** 17–22.

86. CRITCHLEY, H.D. *et al.* 2004. Neural systems supporting interoceptive awareness. Nat. Neurosci. **7:** 189–195.
87. DAMASIO, A.R. 1996. The somatic marker hypothesis and the possible functions of the prefrontal cortex. Philos. Trans. R. Soc. Lond. B Biol. Sci. **351:** 1413–1420.
88. WILLIAMS, L.M. *et al.* 2007. Fronto-limbic and autonomic disjunctions to negative emotion distinguish schizophrenia subtypes. Psychiatry Res. **155:** 29–44.
89. HIRSTEIN, W., P. IVERSEN & V.S. RAMACHANDRAN. 2001. Autonomic responses of autistic children to people and objects. Proc. Biol. Sci. **268:** 1883–1888.
90. TUGADE, M.M. & B.L. FREDRICKSON. 2004. Resilient individuals use positive emotions to bounce back from negative emotional experiences. J. Pers. Soc. Psychol. **86:** 320–333.
91. JACKSON, D.C. *et al.* 2003. Now you feel it, now you don't: frontal brain electrical asymmetry and individual differences in emotion regulation. Psychol. Sci. **14:** 612–617.
92. HOLLAND, P.C. 1980. CS-US interval as a determinant of the form of Pavlovian appetitive conditioned responses. J. Exp. Psychol. Anim. Behav. Process **6:** 155–174.
93. HOLLAND, P.C. 1979. Differential effects of omission contingencies on various components of Pavlovian appetitive conditioned responding in rats. J. Exp. Psychol. Anim. Behav. Process **5:** 178–193.
94. REEKIE, Y. *et al.* 2006. The role of the primate orbitofrontal cortex in emotional regulation: A behavioural and autonomic analysis of positive affect. Soc. Neurosci. abstracts. 370.30.
95. IWATA, J. *et al.* 1986. Intrinsic neurons in the amygdaloid field projected to by the medial geniculate body mediate emotional responses conditioned to acoustic stimuli. Brain Res. **383:** 195–214.
96. GROSHEK, F. *et al.* 2005. Amygdala central nucleus function is necessary for learning, but not expression, of conditioned auditory orienting. Behav. Neurosci. **119:** 202–212.
97. MCDANNALD, M. *et al.* 2004. Amygdala central nucleus function is necessary for learning but not expression of conditioned visual orienting. Eur. J. Neurosci. **20:** 240–248.
98. RHODES, S.E. & S. KILLCROSS. 2004. Lesions of rat infralimbic cortex enhance recovery and reinstatement of an appetitive Pavlovian response. Learn. Mem. **11:** 611–616.
99. JAY, T.M. & M.P. WITTER. 1991. Distribution of hippocampal CA1 and subicular efferents in the prefrontal cortex of the rat studied by means of anterograde transport of Phaseolus vulgaris-leucoagglutinin. J. Comp. Neurol. **313:** 574–586.
100. BOUTON, M.E. 1988. Context and ambiguity in the extinction of emotional learning: implications for exposure therapy. Behav. Res. Ther. **26:** 137–149.
101. RESCORLA, R.A. 2001. Experimental extinction. *In* Handbook of Contemporary Learning Theories. R.R. Mowrer & S.B. Klein, Eds.: 119–154. Lawrence Erlbaum Associates. Mahwah.
102. SCHOENBAUM, G. & M. ROESCH. 2005. Orbitofrontal cortex, associative learning, and expectancies. Neuron **47:** 633–636.
103. PICKENS, C.L. *et al.* 2003. Different roles for orbitofrontal cortex and basolateral amygdala in a reinforcer devaluation task. J. Neurosci. **23:** 11078–11084.

104. PICKENS, C.L. *et al.* 2005. Orbitofrontal lesions impair use of cue-outcome associations in a devaluation task. Behav. Neurosci. **119:** 317–322.
105. SETLOW, B., M. GALLAGHER & P.C. HOLLAND. 2002. The basolateral complex of the amygdala is necessary for acquisition but not expression of CS motivational value in appetitive Pavlovian second-order conditioning. Eur. J. Neurosci. **15:** 1841–1853.
106. CARDINAL, R.N. *et al.* 2002. Effects of selective excitotoxic lesions of the nucleus accumbens core, anterior cingulate cortex, and central nucleus of the amygdala on autoshaping performance in rats. Behav. Neurosci. **116:** 553–567.
107. WELLMAN, L.L., K. GALE & L. MALKOVA. 2005. GABAA-mediated inhibition of basolateral amygdala blocks reward devaluation in macaques. J. Neurosci. **25:** 4577–4586.
108. ROBERTS, A.C. 2006. A componential analysis of the functions of primate orbitofrontal cortex. *In* The Orbitofrontal Cortex. D.H. Zald & S.L. Rauch, Eds.: 237–264. Oxford University Press. Oxford, UK.
109. GAFFAN, D. 1979. Acquisition and forgetting in mokeys' memory of informational object-reward associations. Learn. Motiv. **10:** 419–444.
110. MEDIN, D. 1977. Information processing and discrimination learning set. *In* Behavioral Primatology. A.M. Schier, Ed.: 33–69. Erlbaum. Mahwah.
111. MURRAY, E.A. & B.J. RICHMOND. 2001. Role of perirhinal cortex in object perception, memory, and associations. Curr. Opin. Neurobiol. **11:** 188–193.
112. FERNANDEZ-RUIZ, J. *et al.* 2001. Visual habit formation in monkeys with neurotoxic lesions of the ventrocaudal neostriatum. Proc. Natl. Acad. Sci. USA **98:** 4196–4201.
113. STALNAKER, T.A. *et al.* 2007. Basolateral amygdala lesions abolish orbitofrontal-dependent reversal impairments. Neuron **54:** 51–58.

Reconciling the Roles of Orbitofrontal Cortex in Reversal Learning and the Encoding of Outcome Expectancies

GEOFFREY SCHOENBAUM,[a,b] MICHAEL P. SADDORIS,[c]
AND THOMAS A. STALNAKER[a]

[a]Departments of Anatomy and Neurobiology and Psychiatry, University of Maryland School of Medicine, Baltimore, Maryland 21201, USA

[b]Department of Psychology, University of Maryland Baltimore County, Baltimore, Maryland 21228, USA

[c]Department of Psychological and Brain Sciences, Johns Hopkins University, Baltimore, Maryland 21218, USA

ABSTRACT: Damage to orbitofrontal cortex (OFC) has long been associated with decision-making deficits. Such deficits are epitomized by impairments in reversal learning. Historically, reversal learning deficits have been linked to a response inhibition function or to the rapid reversal of associative encoding in OFC neurons. However here we will suggest that OFC supports reversal learning not because its encoding is particularly flexible—indeed it actually is not—but rather because output from OFC is critical for flexible associative encoding downstream in basolateral amygdala (ABL). Consistent with this argument, we will show that reversal performance is actually inversely related to the flexibility of associative encoding in OFC (i.e., the better the reversal performance, the less flexible the encoding). Further, we will demonstrate that associative correlates in ABL are more flexible during reversal learning than in OFC, become less flexible after damage to OFC, and are required for the expression of the reversal deficit caused by OFC lesions. We will propose that OFC facilitates associative flexibility in downstream regions, such as ABL, for the same reason that it is critical for outcome-guided behavior in a variety of setting—namely that processing in OFC signals the value of expected outcomes. In addition to their role in guiding behavior, these outcome expectancies permit the rapid recognition of unexpected outcomes, thereby driving new learning.

KEYWORDS: orbitofrontal cortex; basolateral amygdala; reversal; associative learning; expectancies

Address for correspondence: Geoffrey Schoenbaum, M.D., Ph.D., 20 Penn Street HSF-2, Rm S251, Baltimore, MD 21201. Voice: 410-706-3814; fax: 410-706-2512.
schoenbg@schoenbaumlab.org

Ann. N.Y. Acad. Sci. 1121: 320–335 (2007). © 2007 New York Academy of Sciences.
doi: 10.1196/annals.1401.001

Orbitofrontal cortex (OFC) has long been implicated in cognitive flexibility.[1,2] The loss of this ability is evident in impairments in rapid reversal learning that are observed after OFC damage in a variety of species.[1,3–13] In these settings, animals are first taught to respond to one cue to receive reward and to withhold or inhibit a similar response to avoid punishment or non-reward. After animals are responding correctly based on these contingencies, the meaning of the cues is reversed, such that animals must respond to the cue to which they had previously withheld responding and withhold responding to the cue to which they had previously responded. Animals with OFC damage typically acquire the initial discrimination normally but require many more trials than controls to relearn the discrimination after the cue-outcome associations are reversed. This deficit has been taken as evidence that OFC promotes flexible responding. Yet why is OFC important for this function?

THE ORBITOFRONTAL CORTEX
AND RESPONSE INHIBITION

The role of OFC in promoting reversal learning has been explained historically as a result of the involvement of OFC in inhibiting responses.[1,2] While this has been proposed to be a general prefrontal function, reports often identify disinhibited, perseverative, or impulsive responding as hallmarks of the "orbitofrontal syndrome." Thus, much of the behavior of orbitofrontal damaged humans has been conceptualized as an inability to inhibit so-called "prepotent" responses. To the extent that this is more than just a restatement of the deficit, this proposal suggests that output from OFC somehow directly inhibits expression of the response, as illustrated in FIGURE 1A. Unfortunately this account is contradicted by the observation that, in most of the discrimination reversal studies in which OFC lesions impair reversal, lesioned animals are fully capable, before reversal, of withholding a response that is identical to the one that they are unable to withhold after reversal. This is particularly true in go, no-go tasks, in which this initial response is often highly ingrained. For example, in our studies the rats are shaped for many hundreds of trials to respond for reward on every trial. Yet rats with OFC lesions learn to inhibit this response at the same rate as controls when presented with a series of discrimination problems, both on the initial and subsequent problems. Only after reversal are these rats unable to withhold responding.

Moreover, animals with OFC lesions are also able to inhibit responses normally in many other settings. For example, although OFC-lesioned monkeys and rats fail to suppress cue-evoked conditioned responses after reinforcer devaluation, they do inhibit consummatory responses like controls.[8,14,15] In these tasks, the animals are trained to associate cues with rewards. If the rewards are devalued by overfeeding or pairing with illness, normal animals exhibit reduced responding to the cues that predict those rewards. OFC-lesioned

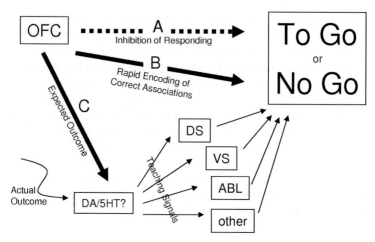

FIGURE 1. Schematic summarizing proposed roles for the OFC in reversal learning. **(A)** Historical proposal that output from OFC directly inhibits "prepotent" responses and thus is critical for reversal learning. **(B)** More recent idea that OFC acts as a highly flexible associative look-up table to guide correct responding and thus is critical for reversal learning. **(C)** Our proposal that OFC is critical for reversal learning because it facilitates associative learning in other structures, by facilitating the generation of teaching signals when actual outcomes do not match OFC signals of expected outcomes. DS, dorsal striatum; VS, ventral striatum; DA, dopamine; 5-HT, serotonin.

animals fail to show this decline in conditioned responding. However, they are able to suppress actual consumption of the devalued food item after this critical probe test. Further, during the probe test, which is conducted under extinction conditions, lesioned rats show normal extinction of conditioned responding. Thus while OFC-lesioned rats fail to suppress conditioned responding as a result of prior devaluation of the outcome, they are able to suppress conditioned responding as a result of non-reward. In fact, it has recently been reported that rats with OFC lesions can even suppress instrumental responses normally after reinforcer devaluation.[16]

Furthermore, it has recently been shown that OFC-lesioned monkeys are able to inhibit prepotent responses normally in the so-called reversed reward contingency task.[17] In this task, the monkeys were asked to select the smaller of two available food quantities in order to obtain presentation of the larger quantity. Thus monkeys were presented with a choice between one half peanut or four half peanuts. In order to obtain the four half peanuts, the monkeys had to select the one half peanut. This requires the monkeys to suppress their natural tendency to select the thing that they want to receive, which is the larger of the two rewards. OFC-lesioned monkeys learned to do this at the same rate as controls.

These studies show that there are circumstances in which OFC is not required for response inhibition. Thus while there may be situations in which OFC

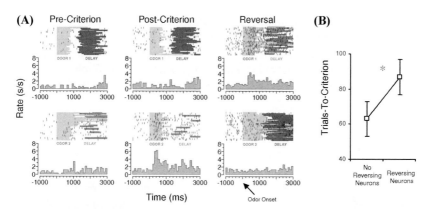

FIGURE 2. Flexibility of associative encoding in OFC is inversely related to speed of reversal learning. **(A)** Example of associative encoding in a rat OFC neuron recorded during acquisition and reversal of a two-odor discrimination problem. Neural activity is shown synchronized to odor onset on each trial, in both raster and peri-event time histograms, for trials before learning (pre-criterion), after learning (post-criterion), and after reversal (reversal). Before reversal, odor 1 predicts sucrose, and odor 2 predicts quinine. The neuron exhibits a phasic response during odor sampling that develops with learning and tracks the predicted outcome (quinine) across reversal. **(B)** Average trials required to attain criterion on the reversal in sessions in which reversing cue-selective neurons were recorded versus sessions in which cue-selective neurons were recorded that did not reverse. Rats performed significantly worse in sessions with reversing neurons. (Data adapted from Stalnaker *et al.*[22]) (In color in *Annals* online.)

promotes response inhibition, response inhibition per se is not the underlying function of this area. In other words, disinhibited and impulsive responding after OFC lesions is a symptom, rather than an explanation.

THE ORBITOFRONTAL CORTEX AS AN ASSOCIATIVE LOOK-UP TABLE

More recently, the role of OFC in promoting reversal learning has been linked to the finding that cue-selective neurons in OFC reverse firing selectivity for cues during reversal learning.[18–20] Reversal of cue-selective activity in OFC neurons presumably reflects acquisition of the reversed associations. An example of such flexible associative encoding is given in FIGURE 2A, which shows a single neuron recorded in OFC in a rat learning and reversing a novel odor discrimination problem. During initial learning, the neuron becomes selective to odor two, which predicts quinine, then after reversal, the same neuron switches to fire to odor one now that this odor predicts quinine. Similar correlates are also observed for the positive odor cue. When these neurons were first reported by Rolls and colleagues in great numbers in OFC,[19] flexible associative encoding had not been prominently demonstrated

in other brain areas. The apparent uniqueness of these correlates, in combination with the close correspondence between their apparent function and the
effects of OFC damage, led to the readily accepted proposal that the critical
contribution of OFC to behavior was to be a rapidly modifiable associative
look-up table of sorts. By this account, illustrated in FIGURE 1B, the reversed

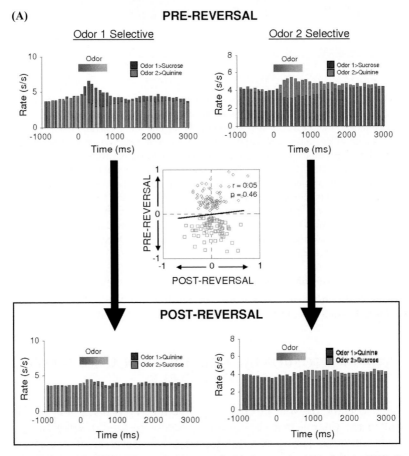

FIGURE 3. Flexibility of associative encoding is greater in ABL than in OFC. Population response of neurons in OFC **(A)** and ABL **(B)** identified as cue-selective during
learning. Average activity per neuron is shown, synchronized to odor onset, during and after
reversal. The population response reverses cue-selectivity in ABL but not in OFC. Inset
scatterplot compares the cue-selectivity indices before (X-axis) and after reversal (Y-axis)
for all the cue-selective neurons used to construct the population histogram. *Blue* and *red*
symbols show data for "Odor One Selective" neurons and "Odor Two Selective" neurons,
respectively. The cue-selectivity indices are inversely correlated in ABL, consistent the
reversal of cue-selectivity, whereas they show no correlation in OFC. (Data adapted from
Stalnaker *et al.*.[22,36]) (In color in *Annals* online.)

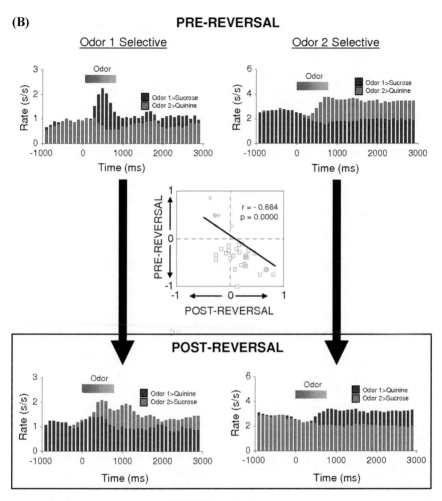

FIGURE 3. *Continued.*

associations would be learned most rapidly in OFC and then employed to drive the behavioral reversal.

However more recent neurophysiological findings are inconsistent with this hypothesis. Specifically, though single-unit recording studies in rats and primates have shown that about a quarter of cue-selective OFC neurons reverse their stimulus selectivity after reversal of the stimulus-outcome associations,[18,20,21] the population of cue-selective neurons actually becomes nonselective after reversal and is, in effect, replaced by the emergence of a new cue-selective population. This is illustrated in FIGURE 3A, which shows the effect of reversal of a two-odor discrimination problem on the firing of OFC neurons selective for each odor cue during learning. Both populations fire selectively during sampling of their respective cue before reversal but not after reversal. Loss of selectivity is also shown graphically for each neuron in the two populations by the inset scatter plot in FIGURE 3A. This figure plots a cue-selectivity index for each neuron before and after reversal. This calculation consisted of the difference in firing rate to the odor cues divided by the sum of those rates. If a population of neurons maintained the same cue-selectivity before and after reversal, one would expect a regression with a positive correlation. On the other hand, if a population of neurons reversed cue-selectivity, one would expect a regression with a negative correlation. However, this plot shows that cue-selective neurons in OFC are actually equally likely to fire to either odor cue after reversal. As a result, there is no correlation between the cue-selectivity indices of these OFC neurons before and after reversal. This encoding pattern is at odds with the proposal that OFC rapidly encodes reversals of cue-outcome associations.

Furthermore, we have recently reported that the probability of observing reversal of cue-selectivity in OFC neurons is actually inversely related to the rate of reversal learning.[22] This relationship, illustrated in FIGURE 2B, is inconsistent with the notion that flexible encoding in OFC drives behavioral reversal, since if it did one would expect the opposite relationship (i.e., better performance when reversing neurons are plentiful). Instead, this relationship suggests that reversal of cue-selectivity in OFC reflects feedback regarding discrepancies between expected and actual outcomes. Such feedback would be greatest when reversal performance is poor. Indeed, OFC BOLD response is sensitive to violations of expected outcomes, and a small number of neurons in OFC respond strongly when errors are detected.[23–25]

Finally, recent work shows that associative encoding in other brain regions can be more flexible than that in OFC. The best example of this is activity in basolateral amygdala (ABL), a region that receives strong projections from OFC.[26–28] ABL is critical for associative learning,[29–32] and neurons in ABL rapidly become selective to cues that predict biologically relevant appetitive or aversive outcomes.[18,33–35] An analysis of the effect of reversal on cue-selectivity in ABL[18,34,36] is presented in FIGURE 3B. This figure, which parallels the analysis of OFC neurons in FIGURE 3A, shows the effect of reversal of a two-odor discrimination problem on the firing of ABL neurons selective for each odor cue during learning. Both populations switch their cue-selectivity across reversal, thereby rapidly encoding the reversed cue-outcome associations. This pattern is also evident in the inset scatterplot, which plots the cue-selectivity index for each neuron before and after reversal. These values were inversely correlated across the population, consistent with a reversal of cue-selectivity. Comparison of data in FIGURE 3A and B is particularly revealing, showing that though OFC has received the greatest attention for the flexibility of its neural correlates, encoding in ABL neurons actually appears to provide a more rapidly flexible associative look-up table. Importantly this impression has been confirmed in primates in the past year in an elegant study by Salzman and colleagues showing that primate amygdala neurons reverse cue-selectivity in large proportions during reversal learning.[37]

THE ORBITOFRONTAL CORTEX AND ENCODING OF OUTCOME-EXPECTANCIES

So what then is the contribution of OFC to flexible responding in situations such as reversal learning? An alternative explanation for the role of OFC in promoting flexible responding is found in the neural activity in OFC that anticipates expected outcomes.[25,38–45] This is evident across different species and tasks; neural activity or BOLD changes in OFC are often triggered by cues and events that convey information about the value of impending outcomes.[25,38,40,43,44,46–51] (Note that this is different from prediction error signaling thought to characterize dopaminergic activity.[52]) The importance of OFC for signaling such information is evident in lesion studies in which damage to OFC causes selective deficits in the ability of animals to use information about the value of expected outcomes to guide existing or established behavior. For example, as described earlier OFC-lesioned animals fail to modify responding to cues after reinforcer devaluation.[8,14,15] Deficits in these settings, which do not involve new learning, likely reflect a critical function for OFC in modulating the expression of previously acquired associative information, perhaps in downstream areas such as the basal ganglia or amygdala.[53]

We have proposed that neural encoding of expected outcomes by OFC might also provide a signal that could be compared to actual outcomes to drive new learning.[54] When an actual outcome fails to match expectations, this comparison could promote changes in old associative representations and the acquisition of new ones. Presumably this function would be helpful even in initial learning, but it might be particularly critical during reversals, in which the discrepancy between actual and expected outcomes is maximal. By this account, illustrated in FIGURE 1C, OFC would support reversal learning not directly due to its role in rapid encoding new associations but rather indirectly, by facilitating changes in associative encoding in other brain regions. Such old or persistent memories might otherwise slow or impede behavioral reversal. Perhaps the best candidate region for showing this effect is ABL; as outlined above, ABL is critically involved in associative learning, and associative encoding in ABL normally changes rapidly after reversal. This proposal makes at least two testable predictions:

1. The flexibility of associative correlates in ABL should depend on input from OFC.
2. Expression of the reversal deficit caused by OFC lesions should be mediated through ABL.

We will describe these predictions—and the data that addresses them—in the remaining sections of this chapter.

Flexibility of Associative Encoding in Basolateral Amygdala Depends on Input from Orbitofrontal Cortex

The first prediction of our hypothesis is that associative encoding in amygdala should depend on OFC. Consistent with this proposal, we have recently reported that cue-selective firing in ABL neurons fails to reverse in rats with unilateral OFC lesions.[34] These data are illustrated in FIGURE 4, which shows the effects of reversal of a two-odor discrimination on the firing of cue-selective ABL neurons recorded in rats with ipsilateral neurotoxic lesions of OFC. Because the connections between OFC and ABL are largely (though not completely) ipsilateral, this lesion would have substantially diminished the influence of OFC on ABL in the lesioned hemisphere while leaving processing in the intact hemisphere largely unaffected. This manipulation caused associative correlates in ABL to become both less prevalent and, when followed across reversal, significantly less flexible. This is evident in the population histograms, in which neither population of cue-selective neurons shows any selectivity to the odor cues after reversal, and in the scatterplot, where there was no correlation between cue-selectivity before and after reversal in the cue-selective neurons. Thus removal of OFC dramatically reduced the flexibility of encoding in ABL.

Of course associative encoding (and flexibility of that encoding) was not completely eliminated by OFC lesions. Obviously such preserved encoding could reflect input from the intact contralateral hemisphere or compensatory mechanisms in the lesioned brain. However the partially preserved encoding is also consistent with recent studies showing that some outcome-guided behaviors depend on ABL but not OFC. For example, ABL lesions cause deficits in fear conditioning,[30,55–57] but OFC lesions typically do not.[58] ABL lesions also abolish conditioned stimulus-potentiated feeding,[59,60] while OFC lesions do not.[61] Thus ABL neurons may be able to encode associative information, albeit at a slower rate, even in the absence of signaling from OFC. This would be consistent with the idea that other brain areas may signal aspects of impending outcomes independent of contributions from OFC.

Reversal Deficits Caused by Orbitofrontal Lesions Are Mediated through Basolateral Amygdala

The second prediction of our hypothesis is that the reversal deficits caused by OFC lesions should be mediated by the inflexible correlates in ABL. In other words, if OFC normally promotes reversal by facilitating changes in associative

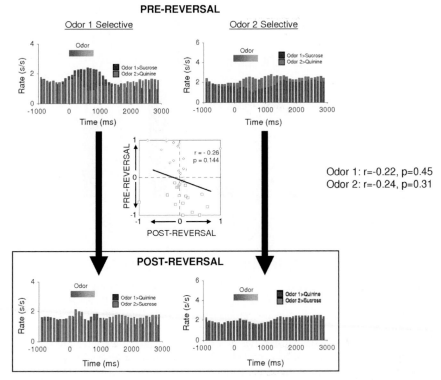

FIGURE 4. Flexibility of associative encoding in ABL depends on input from OFC. Population response of cue-selective neurons in ABL in rats with ipsilateral lesions of OFC. Average activity per neuron is shown, synchronized to odor onset, during and after reversal. Unlink the populations recorded in intact rats, illustrated in FIGURE 3B, the population response recorded in OFC-lesioned rats does not reverse cue-selectivity. Inset scatterplot compares the cue-selectivity indices before (X-axis) and after reversal (Y-axis) for all the cue-selective neurons used to construct the population histograms. *Blue* and *red symbols* show data for "Odor One Selective" neurons and "Odor Two Selective" neurons, respectively. Again in contrast to the inverse correlation in intact rats, illustrated in FIGURE 3B, the cue-selectivity indices in OFC-lesioned rats showed no correlation, indication that ABL neurons in OFC-lesioned rats had lost their tendency to reverse. (Data adapted from Saddoris *et al.*[34]) (In color in *Annals* online.)

encoding in ABL, then damage to ABL in OFC-lesioned animals should mitigate or even abolish the reversal impairment. Note that this prediction contrasts with the prediction that other ideas regarding OFC function would make. For example, if OFC normally promotes reversal directly either by inhibiting responding or by rapidly acquiring the reversed associations, then damage to these downstream areas should either worsen or have no effect on the OFC-dependent reversal deficit. To test this, we assessed reversal learning in rats with bilateral neurotoxic lesions of either OFC or ABL and rats with

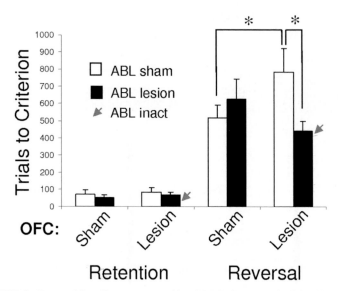

FIGURE 5. Reversal impairments caused by OFC lesions are abolished by lesions or inactivation of ABL. Bars show the average number of trials ($\pm$SEM) required to retain and reverse a two-odor discrimination problem for controls, rats with OFC lesions, and rats with OFC lesions combined with bilateral ABL lesions or unilateral ABL lesions and inactivation of contralateral ABL via infusions of muscimol + baclofen immediately prior to reversal (*red arrows*). As expected, OFC lesions impaired reversal learning. This impairment was abolished by pre-training lesions of ABL or by inactivation at the time of reversal. ABL lesions alone had no effect. *Significant difference with $P < 0.05$. (Data adapted from Stalnaker et al.,[62]) (In color in *Annals* online.)

bilateral OFC lesions combined with bilateral ABL lesions or unilateral ABL lesions plus inactivation of contralateral ABL during reversal.[62] The results are shown in FIGURE 5. Consistent with our hypothesis, we found that removal or inactivation of ABL completely abolished the reversal deficit caused by OFC lesions.

Importantly, lesions of ABL in otherwise intact rats did not facilitate reversal learning, and neither did ABL lesions have any effect on the acquisition of the initial discriminations. This argues against an account by which ABL lesions corrected the reversal impairment by an effect on initial acquisition of the discriminations or by independently improving cognitive flexibility. The absence of effects of ABL lesions on reversal learning is consistent with our own prior work and other reports that have used fiber-sparing lesion techniques to examine the role of amygdala in reversal learning.[6,8,61,63] In these studies, damage to amygdala did not facilitate or impair reversal learning performance, although ABL damage did affect differential changes in response latencies, consistent with a role in encoding the associative information acquired with learning. (Note that OFC + ABL lesions do not fix the latency effects observed with either lesion in isolation—see supplemental material in Ref. 62.) The simplest explanation of these results is that changes in such associative encoding in ABL during reversal learning normally occur more rapidly than those in other regions (at least in paradigms similar to ours). As a result, removing ABL has little effect in otherwise intact rats. However, OFC lesions impair reversal of associative encoding in ABL, rendering it slow enough to retard the rate of behavioral reversal.

CONCLUSIONS

Damage to OFC has long been associated with deficits in adaptive decision making. Such deficits are epitomized by impairments in reversal learning. Here we have shown that reversal performance is actually inversely related to the flexibility of associative encoding in OFC. Further, we have demonstrated that associative correlates in ABL are more flexible than those in OFC during reversal learning, become less flexible after damage to OFC, and are required for the expression of the reversal deficit caused by OFC lesions. This is consistent with the proposal that OFC supports rapid reversal learning by facilitating associative flexibility in downstream regions, such as ABL, rather than due to any role in directly driving reversals either through a role in response inhibition or in rapidly encoding the reversed associations. This proposal is consistent with the idea that OFC is critical for signaling the value of expected outcomes. In addition to guiding behavior, these outcome expectancies permit the rapid recognition of unexpected outcomes, thereby driving new learning.

ACKNOWLEDGMENTS

This work was supported by grants from the NIDA (R01-DA015718, GS).

REFERENCES

1. JONES, B. & M. MISHKIN. 1972. Limbic lesions and the problem of stimulus-reinforcement associations. Exp. Neurol. **36:** 362–377.
2. MISHKIN, M. 1964. Perseveration of central sets after frontal lesions in monkeys. *In* The Frontal Granular Cortex and Behavior. J.M. Warren & K. Akert, Eds.: 219–241. McGraw-Hill. New York.
3. SCHOENBAUM, G. *et al.* 2002. Orbitofrontal lesions in rats impair reversal but not acquisition of go, no-go odor discriminations. Neuroreport **13:** 885–890.
4. BOHN, I., C. GIERTLER & W. HAUBER. 2003. Orbital prefrontal cortex and guidance of instrumental behavior in rats under reversal conditions. Behav. Brain Res. **143:** 49–56.
5. DIAS, R., T.W. ROBBINS & A.C. ROBERTS. 1996. Dissociation in prefrontal cortex of affective and attentional shifts. Nature **380:** 69–72.

6. SCHOENBAUM, G. *et al.* 2003. Lesions of orbitofrontal cortex and basolateral amyg-
    dala complex disrupt acquisition of odor-guided discriminations and reversals.
    Learn. Mem. **10:** 129–140.
7. ROLLS, E.T. *et al.* 1994. Emotion-related learning in patients with social and
    emotional changes associated with frontal lobe damage. J. Neurol. Neurosurg.
    Psychiatry **57:** 1518–1524.
8. IZQUIERDO, A.D., R.K. SUDA & E.A. MURRAY. 2004. Bilateral orbital prefrontal
    cortex lesions in rhesus monkeys disrupt choices guided by both reward value
    and reward contingency. J. Neurosci. **24:** 7540–7548.
9. MEUNIER, M., J. BACHEVALIER & M. MISHKIN. 1997. Effects of orbital frontal
    and anterior cingulate lesions on object and spatial memory in rhesus monkeys.
    Neuropsychologia **35:** 999–1015.
10. CHUDASAMA, Y. & T.W. ROBBINS. 2003. Dissociable contributions of the or-
    bitofrontal and infralimbic cortex to pavlovian autoshaping and discrimination
    reversal learning: further evidence for the functional heterogeneity of the rodent
    frontal cortex. J. Neurosci. **23:** 8771–8780.
11. KIM, J. & K.E. RAGOZZINO. 2005. The involvement of the orbitofrontal cortex
    in learning under changing task contingencies. Neurobiol. Learn. Mem. **83:**
    125–133.
12. BROWN, V.J. & K. MCALONAN. 2003. Orbital prefrontal cortex mediates reversal
    learning and not attentional set shifting in the rat. Behav. Brain Res. **146:** 97–
    130.
13. TEITELBAUM, H. 1964. A comparison of effects of orbitofrontal and hippocampal
    lesions upon discrimination learning and reversal in the cat. Exp. Neurol. **9:**
    452–462.
14. GALLAGHER, M., R.W. MCMAHAN & G. SCHOENBAUM. 1999. Orbitofrontal cortex
    and representation of incentive value in associative learning. J. Neurosci. **19:**
    6610–6614.
15. PICKENS, C.L. *et al.* 2003. Different roles for orbitofrontal cortex and basolateral
    amygdala in a reinforcer devaluation task. J. Neurosci. **23:** 11078–11084.
16. OSTLUND, S.B. & B.W. BALLEINE. 2007. Orbitofrontal cortex mediates outcome
    encoding in Pavlovian but not instrumental learning. J. Neurosci. **27:** 4819–
    4825.
17. CHUDASAMA, Y., J.D. KRALIK & E.A. MURRAY. 2006. Rhesus monkeys with orbital
    prefrontal cortex lesions can learn to inhibit prepotent responses in the reversed
    reward contingency task. Cereb. Cortex **17:** 1154–1159.
18. SCHOENBAUM, G., A.A. CHIBA & M. GALLAGHER. 1999. Neural encoding in
    orbitofrontal cortex and basolateral amygdala during olfactory discrimination
    learning. J. Neurosci. **19:** 1876–1884.
19. THORPE, S.J., E.T. ROLLS & S. MADDISON. 1983. The orbitofrontal cor-
    tex: neuronal activity in the behaving monkey. Exp. Brain Res. **49:** 93–
    115.
20. ROLLS, E.T. *et al.* 1996. Orbitofrontal cortex neurons: role in olfactory and visual
    association learning. J. Neurophysiol. **75:** 1970–1981.
21. CRITCHLEY, H.D. & E.T. ROLLS. 1996. Olfactory neuronal responses in the primate
    orbitofrontal cortex: analysis in an olfactory discrimination task. J. Neurophysiol.
    75: 1659–1672.
22. STALNAKER, T.A. *et al.* 2006. Abnormal associative encoding in orbitofrontal
    neurons in cocaine-experienced rats during decision-making. Euro. J. Neurosci.
    24: 2643–2653.

23. NOBRE, A.C. *et al.* 1999. Orbitofrontal cortex is activated during breaches of expectation in tasks of visual attention. Nat. Neurosci. **2:** 11–12.
24. TOBLER, P.N. *et al.* 2006. Human neural learning depends on reward prediction errors in the blocking paradigm. J. Neurophysiol. **95:** 301–310.
25. FEIERSTEIN, C.E. *et al.* 2006. Representation of spatial goals in rat orbitofrontal cortex. Neuron **51:** 495–507.
26. KRETTEK, J.E. & J.L. PRICE. 1977. Projections from the amygdaloid complex to the cerebral cortex and thalamus in the rat and cat. J. Comp. Neurol. **172:** 225–254.
27. KITA, H. & S.T. KITAI. 1990. Amygdaloid projections to the frontal cortex and the striatum in the rat. J. Comp. Neurol. **298:** 40–49.
28. SHI, C.J. & M.D. CASSELL. 1998. Cortical, thalamic, and amygdaloid connections of the anterior and posterior insular cortices. J. Comp. Neurol. **399:** 440–468.
29. WEISKRANTZ, L. 1956. Behavioral changes associated with ablations of the amygdaloid complex in monkeys. J. Comp. Physiol. Psychology **9:** 381–391.
30. DAVIS, M. 2000. The role of the amygdala in conditioned and unconditioned fear and anxiety. *In* The Amygdala: a Functional Analysis. J.P. Aggleton, Ed.: 213–287. Oxford University Press. Oxford.
31. GALLAGHER, M. 2000. The amygdala and associative learning. *In* The Amygdala: a Functional Analysis. J.P. Aggleton, Ed.: 311–330. Oxford University Press. Oxford.
32. EVERITT, B.J. *et al.* 2000. Differential involvement of amygdala subsystems in appetitive conditioning and drug addiction. *In* The Amygdala: a Functional Analysis. J.P. Aggleton, Ed.: 353–390. Oxford University Press. New York.
33. QUIRK, G.J., J.L. ARMONY & J.E. LEDOUX. 1997. Fear conditioning enhances different temporal components of tone-evoked spike trains in auditory cortex and lateral amygdala. Neuron **19:** 613–624.
34. SADDORIS, M.P., M. GALLAGHER & G. SCHOENBAUM. 2005. Rapid associative encoding in basolateral amygdala depends on connections with orbitofrontal cortex. Neuron **46:** 321–331.
35. QUIRK, G.J., J.C. REPA & J.E. LEDOUX. 1995. Fear conditioning enhances short-latency auditory responses of lateral amygdala neurons: parallel recordings in the freely behaving rat. Neuron **15:** 1029–1039.
36. STALNAKER, T.A. *et al.* 2007. Cocaine-induced decision-making deficits are mediated by miscoding in basolateral amygdala. Nat. Neurosci. **10:** 949–951.
37. PATTON, J.J. *et al.* 2006. The primate amygdala represents the positive and negative value of visual stimuli during learning. Nature **439:** 865–870.
38. SCHOENBAUM, G., A.A. CHIBA & M. GALLAGHER. 1998. Orbitofrontal cortex and basolateral amygdala encode expected outcomes during learning. Nat. Neurosci. **1:** 155–159.
39. PADOA-SCHIOPPA, C. & J.A. ASSAD. 2006. Neurons in orbitofrontal cortex encode economic value. Nature **441:** 223–226.
40. SCHOENBAUM, G. *et al.* 2003. Encoding predicted outcome and acquired value in orbitofrontal cortex during cue sampling depends upon input from basolateral amygdala. Neuron **39:** 855–867.
41. SCHOENBAUM, G. *et al.* 2006. Encoding changes in orbitofrontal cortex in reversal-impaired aged rats. J. Neurophysiol. **95:** 1509–1517.

42. HIKOSAKA, K. & M. WATANABE. 2000. Delay activity of orbital and lateral prefrontal neurons of the monkey varying with different rewards. Cereb. Cortex **10:** 263–271.
43. ROESCH, M.R., A.R. TAYLOR & G. SCHOENBAUM. 2006. Encoding of time-discounted rewards in orbitofrontal cortex is independent of value representation. Neuron **51:** 509–520.
44. HIKOSAKA, K. & M. WATANABE. 2004. Long- and short-range reward expectancy in the primate orbitofrontal cortex. Eur. J. Neurosci. **19:** 1046–1054.
45. TREMBLAY, L. & W. SCHULTZ. 2000. Reward-related neuronal activity during go-no go task performance in primate orbitofrontal cortex. J. Neurophysiol. **83:** 1864–1876.
46. ROESCH, M.R. & C.R. OLSON. 2004. Neuronal activity related to reward value and motivation in primate frontal cortex. Science **304:** 307–310.
47. O'DOHERTY, J. *et al.* 2002. Neural responses during anticipation of a primary taste reward. Neuron **33:** 815–826.
48. GOTTFRIED, J.A., J. O'DOHERTY & R.J. DOLAN. 2003. Encoding predictive reward value in human amygdala and orbitofrontal cortex. Science **301:** 1104–1107.
49. ROESCH, M.R. & C.R. OLSON. 2005. Neuronal activity in primate orbitofrontal cortex reflects the value of time. J. Neurophysiol. **94:** 2457–2471.
50. TREMBLAY, L. & W. SCHULTZ. 1999. Relative reward preference in primate orbitofrontal cortex. Nature **398:** 704–708.
51. BLAIR, K. *et al.* 2006. Choosing the lesser of two evils, the better of two goods: specifying the roles of ventromedial prefrontal cortex and dorsal anterior cingulate in object choice. J. Neurosci. **26:** 11379–11386.
52. CALU, D.J., M.R. ROESCH & G. SCHOENBAUM. 2007. Orbitofrontal cortex does not signal reward prediction errors. Society for Neuroscience Abstracts. 749.16.
53. FRANK, M.J. & E.D. CLAUS. 2006. Anatomy of a decision: striato-orbitofrontal interactions in reinforcement learning, decision making, and reversal. Psychol. Rev. **113:** 300–326.
54. SCHOENBAUM, G., M.R. ROESCH & T.A. STALNAKER. 2006. Orbitofrontal cortex, decision-making, and drug addiction. Trends Neurosci. **29:** 116–124.
55. MAREN, S. & K.A. GOOSENS. 2001. Contextual and auditory fear conditioning are mediated by the lateral, basal, and central amygdaloid nuclei in rats. Learn. Mem. **8:** 148–155.
56. AMORAPANTH, P., J.E. LEDOUX & M.A. NADER. 2000. Different lateral amygdala outputs mediate reactions and actions elicited by a fear-arousing stimulus. Nat. Neurosci. **3:** 74–79.
57. LEDOUX, J.E. *et al.* 1990. The lateral amygdaloid nucleus: sensory interface of the amygdala in fear conditioning. J. Neurosci. **10:** 1062–1069.
58. MORGAN, M.M. & J.E. LEDOUX. 1999. Contribution of ventrolateral prefrontal cortex to the acquisition and extinction of conditioned fear in rats. Neurobiol. Learn. Mem. **72:** 244–251.
59. PETROVICH, G.D. *et al.* 2002. Amygdalo-hypothalamic circuit allows learned cues to override satiety and promote eating. J. Neurosci. **22:** 8748–8753.
60. HOLLAND, P.C. & M. GALLAGHER. 2003. Double dissociation of the effects of lesions of basolateral and central amygdala on conditioned stimulus-potentiated feeding and Pavlovian-instrumental transfer. E. J. Neurosci. **17:** 1680–1694.

61. McDannald, M.A. *et al.* 2005. Lesions of orbitofrontal cortex impair rats' differential outcome expectancy learning but not conditioned stimulus-potentiated feeding. J. Neurosci. **25:** 4626–4632.
62. Stalnaker, T.A. *et al.* 2007. Basolateral amygdala lesions abolish orbitofrontal-dependent reversal impairments. Neuron **54:** 51–58.
63. Baxter, M.G. & E.A. Murray. 2002. The amygdala and reward. Nat. Rev. Neurosci. **3:** 563–573.

Flexible Neural Representations of Value in the Primate Brain

C. DANIEL SALZMAN, JOSEPH J. PATON, MARINA A. BELOVA, AND SARA E. MORRISON

Departments of Neuroscience and Psychiatry, Columbia University, New York State Psychiatric Institute, New York, New York 10032, USA

ABSTRACT: The amygdala and orbitofrontal cortex (OFC) are often thought of as components of a neural circuit that assigns affective significance—or value—to sensory stimuli so as to anticipate future events and adjust behavioral and physiological responses. Much recent work has been aimed at understanding the distinct contributions of the amygdala and OFC to these processes, but a detailed understanding of the physiological mechanisms underlying learning about value remains lacking. To gain insight into these processes, we have focused initially on characterizing the neural signals of the primate amygdala, and more recently of the primate OFC, during appetitive and aversive reinforcement learning procedures. We have employed a classical conditioning procedure whereby monkeys form associations between visual stimuli and rewards or aversive stimuli. After learning these initial associations, we reverse the stimulus-reinforcement contingencies, and monkeys learn these new associations. We have discovered that separate populations of neurons in the amygdala represent the positive and negative value of conditioned visual stimuli. This representation of value updates rapidly upon image value reversal, as fast as monkeys learn, often within a single trial. We suggest that representations of value in the amygdala may change through multiple interrelated mechanisms: some that arise from fairly simple Hebbian processes, and others that may involve gated inputs from other brain areas, such as the OFC.

KEYWORDS: amygdala; OFC; orbitofrontal cortex; reinforcement learning; conditioning; learning; reward; aversive; value; monkey

EMOTION, VALUATION, AND REINFORCEMENT LEARNING

In humans, the regulation of emotion is extremely flexible, adapting to different sensory cues, social situations, and cognitive operations, such as the application of rules. How does the brain mediate these different aspects of

Address for correspondence: C. Daniel Salzman, Departments of Neuroscience and Psychiatry, Columbia University, New York State Psychiatric Institute, 1051 Riverside Drive, Unit 87, NY, NY 10032. Voice: 212-543-6931; fax: 212-543-5816.

cds2005@columbia.edu

Ann. N.Y. Acad. Sci. 1121: 336–354 (2007). © 2007 New York Academy of Sciences.
doi: 10.1196/annals.1401.034

emotional processing? Most prior efforts to understand emotion at the neural level have employed rodents, often using fear-conditioning and related behavioral paradigms. In human and non-human primates, however, a more flexible control of emotion is thought to be conferred by interactions between the amygdala and prefrontal cortex (PFC).[1] Indeed, in primates, as compared to non-primates, there is an extensive elaboration of the PFC and its connections with the amygdala.[2] In addition, because the visual system is a dominant sensory modality in primates, there are dense connections among the amygdala, PFC, and visual system. Thus, although many aspects of the function and organization of the amygdala and interconnected structures are conserved across species, amygdala function in primates likely expands upon and differs from processing in rodents in significant ways. For these reasons, it is important to elucidate the complex neural circuitry that regulates emotion in the rhesus monkey. Their rich behavioral and cognitive repertoire makes rhesus monkeys ideal for helping to fill a critical gap between studies in rodents and humans.

One way to approach these questions is to exploit different conditioning procedures developed by experimental psychologists to investigate the neural basis of appetitive and aversive reinforcement learning. During reinforcement learning, subjects learn that particular sensory stimuli are associated with rewards and punishments. Emotional responses, such as excitement or fear, commonly occur upon exposure to sensory stimuli that have been endowed with affective value through reinforcement learning.

Associative learning, such as that which links a sensory stimulus with punishment or reward, is frequently assumed to arise gradually via changing synaptic weights; computational models of reinforcement learning have often worked from this assumption.[3] The seminal Rescorla–Wagner model posits that the value representation should be updated on a trial-by-trial basis by "error signals"—that is, signals reflecting the difference between expected and received reinforcement—and recent theories (e.g., temporal difference [TD] models), have extended this model so that reinforcement learning may be described quantitatively in real time.[4-6] TD models require a neural representation of value as a function of time, with error signals being computed continuously by taking the difference in the value of situations or "states" at successive time steps. However, more complex forms of conditioning that often occur in nature—such as conditioning in which the value of stimuli changes depending upon context—require representations of value that can be flexibly activated depending on contextual cues or other information. Consider the game of blackjack, whereby being dealt the same card, such as a king, can be rewarding (if it makes a total of 21) or punishing (if it makes a total greater than 21) depending upon the cards dealt earlier in the hand, which define a context that dictates whether receiving the king would be good or bad. TD and other reinforcement learning models, in their simplest form and on their own, may not be able to explain this kind of flexible control of neural activity reflecting value. Instead, such models would need to be extended to incorporate information, such as rules, so that a potentially infinite number of contexts can be interpreted appropriately; furthermore, describing these processes may require mechanisms that operate on a short timescale to gate, or regulate, neural representations of value. Finally, beyond model development, we still need to understand how the brain actually represents value in a flexible manner.

As a first step to understand how value may be represented flexibly, and building upon the theoretical framework of reinforcement learning,[4,5,7] we have targeted two brain areas, the amygdala and orbitofrontal cortex (OFC). We focused on these brain areas because of their known anatomic connectivity and because of a long history of research linking them to reinforcement learning and emotional processes.[8-10] The amygdala is a structurally and functionally heterogeneous collection of nuclei lying in the anterior medial portion of each temporal lobe.[11,12] Sensory information is provided to the amygdala from advanced levels of sensory cortices, the olfactory system, and polysensory brain areas such as perirhinal cortex.[11] This information enters the amygdala primarily, but not exclusively, in the lateral nucleus, and then flows—either directly or through multiple synapses—to the basal, accessory basal, central, and other more medial nuclei. Output from the amygdala is directed to a wide range of target structures, including PFC, sensory cortices, the hippocampus, perirhinal cortex, entorhinal cortex, the striatum, and the basal forebrain; and also to subcortical structures responsible for physiological responses related to emotion, such as autonomic responses, hormonal responses, and startle. In general, subcortical projections originate from the central nucleus, and projections to cortex and the striatum originate from the basal, accessory basal and in some cases the lateral nuclei.

Modulation of intrinsic processing in the amygdala can occur via multiple pathways. In particular, OFC projects to numerous amygdala nuclei, including the basal, accessory basal, intercalated masses, and lateral nuclei.[13] Other inputs, such as dopaminergic input from the ventral tegmental area and the substantia nigra and serotonergic input from the raphe nuclei, also probably modulate intrinsic amygdala processing, though this has primarily been studied in the rodent.[11] Each of these processing streams, as well as others not mentioned, may modulate amygdala processing substantially, potentially helping induce plastic changes important to learning and memory formation, as well as facilitating the expression of physiological and behavioral responses. Thus the amygdala can receive information from all sensory modalities about conditioned and unconditioned stimuli (CSs and USs), and also from structures that might transmit instructive or supervisory signals to the amygdala, such as midbrain dopamine neurons or PFC, especially the OFC.[13,14]

THE ROLE OF OFC AND THE AMYGDALA

Prior neurophysiological studies in rodent amygdala have suggested that the amygdala supplies neural signals involved in associative learning.[15-25] Most of these studies have been conducted in the context of fear conditioning or related tasks, and they have revealed that amygdala neural activity changes during fear conditioning. Compared with investigations in rodents, only a few studies have investigated amygdala neurophysiology in primates,[26–32] and results were often conflicting. Prior to our recent paper,[33] there had been no systematic study of the neurophysiological properties of primate amygdala neurons during classical conditioning with a well-controlled experimental design.

The OFC, which comprises much of the ventral surface of the frontal lobe, is an area that also has frequently been implicated in the control of emotional behavior. It receives extensive innervation from the amygdala, hippocampus, striatum, and hypothalamus, as well as from many other cortical areas.[34,35] The amygdala sends projections throughout OFC, but most densely to the caudal areas (e.g., area 13).[36] Similarly, OFC (mainly area 13, but also areas 12o, 14 and 11) sends projections to several nuclei of the amygdala, including the basal and lateral nuclei, which partially overlaps with input from temporal cortices.[13,14,37] OFC may therefore modulate the processing of sensory information in the amygdala.

The OFC, together with other parts of the PFC, the striatum and amygdala, is thought to assign values to stimuli, which in turn can contribute to emotional responses and decision making.[38,39] Human patients with lesions of the OFC have abnormal emotional and social behavior (including disinhibition), are impaired on decision-making tasks, and have an inability to generate normal physiological reactions to negatively CSs.[38,40,41] Lesion studies in non-human primates have been consistent with these findings; for example, monkeys with OFC lesions, or even an effective "disconnection" of OFC and amygdala, are impaired on a reinforcer-devaluation paradigm.[42,43] Functional imaging studies have revealed OFC involvement in anticipating and acting upon positive and negative outcomes.[44–46]

Studies of OFC neurophysiology in rats and monkeys have suggested a role for the OFC in associative learning.[16,47–51] Nearly all of these studies have used instrumental tasks, that is, tasks in which the subject must perform (or actively refrain from performing) an action in order to obtain reward or avoid punishment. In these types of tasks, aversive stimuli do not occur after learning occurs; therefore, one cannot conclude that neural activity recorded during task performance represents the anticipation of aversive stimuli. Conclusions about the encoding of negative value are best supported by tasks in which aversive stimuli always occur, even after learning. However, the responses of OFC neurons have not been examined using classical aversive conditioning, in which the CS is consistently predictive of punishment.

Recent primate studies have largely focused on operant forms of appetitive conditioning. Many OFC neurons develop responses to visual cues that predict reward, as well as anticipatory responses to uncued predictable rewards, which are often modulated by the type and amount of reward anticipated.[52–56] These signals have often been interpreted as reflecting expectation of the value of the anticipated reward, although two new studies have called into question whether all aspects of value are integrated in the OFC.[57,58] Furthermore, one recent study suggests that OFC in rodents is involved in updating value representations during procedures containing Pavlovian features, but not during procedures containing only instrumental procedures.[59] Interestingly, several studies have suggested that reward signals in OFC are context dependent—that is, some OFC neurons respond differentially to a stimulus predicting a particular reward depending upon the available alternatives.[52,55,56] Overall, OFC carries information about the identity and value of rewards that are available, rewards that are expected, and rewards that are actually received. Considered together with the OFC's anatomic connectivity, this makes OFC a prime candidate for the flexible modulation of value representations for stimuli associated with reward or punishment.

In the studies described here, we have employed both appetitive and aversive classical conditioning procedures to ask two fundamental questions: (1) What information is represented by neurons in the amygdala and OFC during reinforcement learning? and (2) How are these response properties related to behavioral learning?

HOW IS VALUE REPRESENTED IN THE AMYGDALA?

Our initial studies have been aimed at describing neural signals in the amygdala during the learning and reversal of affective associations. Monkeys performed a trace-conditioning task in which novel, abstract visual stimuli were followed by USs: either a liquid reward, nothing, or an aversive air-puff directed at the face (FIG. 1A). Trace conditioning is a version of classical conditioning in which a brief temporal gap is inserted between CS offset and US onset.[60,61] It is possible that differential responses to CSs associated with rewards and punishments could be attributed to the sensory properties of the CSs themselves, rather than to their reinforcement contingencies; therefore, after initial learning occurred, without warning, and at a variable trial number across experiments, we reversed the contingencies of the images initially associated with rewards and air-puffs, and the monkeys learned the new associations. The monkeys demonstrated their learning by licking a spout in anticipation of a liquid reward, or closing their eyes—a defensive behavior—in anticipation of an air-puff. Note that in our task, CSs predicted USs with 100% certainty, so aversive stimuli could not be avoided.

While monkeys performed the trace-conditioning task, we recorded the activity of individual amygdala neurons. We hypothesized that neurons encoding value would change their response profile to the same CSs once the US associated with them switched. Furthermore, we hypothesized that separate populations of neurons would preferentially respond to positive and negative values, respectively, and that these neurons would rapidly update their responses to CSs during learning. We defined "value" operationally, with positive and negative "CS value-coding neurons" referring to neurons whose activity was higher in

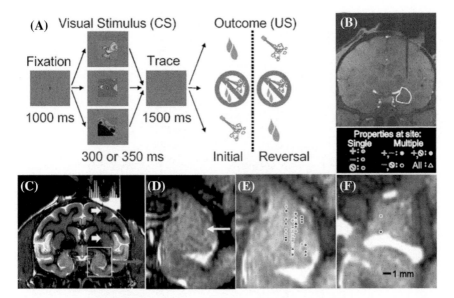

FIGURE 1. The trace-conditioning task and localization of recording sites in the amygdala. (**A**) Sequence of events in the three trial types during trace-conditioning. *Top and bottom squares:* images that reverse values from positive to negative or vice-versa. *Middle square:* image does not reverse and was always non-reinforced. (**B**) Coronal MRI acquired with a two-dimensional (2D) spoiled gradient recalled acquisition (SPGR) sequence in monkey V. The susceptibility artifact from a tungsten microelectrode dorsal to the amygdala (*circled*) is visible. (**C–F**) Coronal MRI with 2D inversion recovery (IR) sequence (**C**, *arrows* point to the electrode artifact, which is less evident). Magnified images show the recording site locations (slice in **F** is immediately posterior to **E**). The *arrow* in **D** corresponds to a possible border of the lateral nucleus, which contains a fiber tract. Recording sites spanning 2 mm in the anterior–posterior dimension were collapsed onto each image slice. In many cases, this resulted in the superposition of multiple cells with different properties (the key above **F** gives the properties denoted by symbols: "+" denotes positive value-coding, "−" denotes negative value-coding, and "no" symbol indicates no value-coding). Recording sites from monkey P occurred in an overlapping region of the amygdala. (From Paton et al.[33] Reproduced by permission.) (In color in *Annals* online.)

response to a CS paired with rewards or a CS paired with aversive air-puffs, respectively.

We found that some amygdala neurons encoded positive value, whereas other amygdala neurons encoded negative value. FIGURE 2 shows an experiment in which we recorded a neuron encoding positive value. Anticipatory licking and blinking behavior (FIG. 2A,B) demonstrated that the monkey learned about the value of the images. We scored every trial according to whether the monkey licked or blinked during the last 500 ms of the trace interval. For both images, licking response rates were greater, and blinking response rates lower, when an image was positive than when the same image was negative. In this

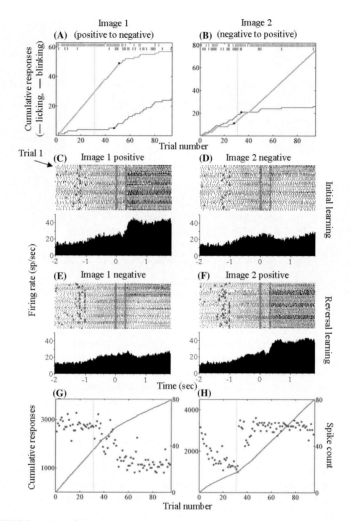

FIGURE 2. Neural activity from a single amygdalar neuron that encoded positive value during learning, in relation to behavioral learning. (**A,B**) Behavioral performance. Cumulative (*curves*) and trial-by-trial (*tick marks*) licking (red) and blinking (blue) responses, plotted as a function of trial number for images 1 and 2; *black dots* represent change points. Value reversals occurred at the vertical green lines. (**C–F**) Rasters and peri-stimulus time histograms (PSTHs) for the amygdala cell recorded during the same experiment. The plots are truncated at US delivery. Each *dot* represents one action potential, and each *row of dots* represents the timing of action potentials during one trial. PSTHs sum and average activity across trials, smoothing with a 10-ms moving average of activity. *Blue ticks* indicate fixation point onset; *red ticks* indicate visual stimulus onset/offset. (**G,H**) Spike count and cumulative spike count during the trace interval for the cell depicted in **C–F**, plotted as a function of trial number separately for images 1 and 2. *Red dots* show change points that demarcate the onset of a significant change in neural firing rate. (From Paton et al.[33] Reproduced by permission.) (In color in *Annals* online.)

experiment, activity in the neuron under study was higher during the trace interval when images had a positive value compared to when the same images had a negative value (FIG. 2C–F), typical of a positive value-coding neuron. FIGURE 3 shows the results from another experiment, in which we recorded the activity of a neuron encoding negative value, predominantly during the visual stimulus interval. Neurons encoding positive and negative value were dispersed throughout our recording sites in the amygdala, which largely spanned the lateral, basal, accessory basal, and central nuclei, as estimated by reconstructing recording sites with MRI (FIG. 1B–F). These recording sites overlapped those used in prior monkey neurophysiology studies of the amygdala.[26–32]

The activity of neurons encoding positive and negative values was not related to motor responses. When neural activity was aligned on licking and blinking onset, no amygdala neurons had neural responses that were related to either motor action.[33] Thus value-related response properties are not well described as representing the link between a CS and a particular response. Moreover, many neurons responded to both rewards and air-puff, suggesting that these cells do not simply represent a link between CS and the sensory modality of the US it is associated with. Finally, it is difficult to account for the value-related signals as simply being related to autonomic reactivity. In general, arousing stimuli of both positive and negative valences can trigger autonomic responses.[62]

To understand how neural activity in the amygdala might relate to activity in other brain areas, such as the OFC, it is critical to characterize the response dynamics of amygdala neurons during learning so that these dynamics can be compared across areas. In particular, it is important to know how rapidly amygdala neurons learn in relation to changes in reinforcement contingencies, and how rapidly amygdala neurons can encode value after the onset of a CS. Therefore, to examine how individual neurons changed their response level when a CS reversed its value, we applied a change-point test[63] to neural responses that reflected value during either the trace (FIG. 2) or visual stimulus (FIG. 3) time epochs. The change-point test identifies the onset of a significant change in response rate in relation to the reversal of image value ($P < 0.05$), represented graphically by a change in slope of the cumulative record of responses.[63] Inspection of the data for the neuron depicted in FIGURE 2 reveals that neural activity changed over the course of a number of trials after the change point for Image 1, but activity changed in a single trial for Image 2. We used the same change-point test to detect the onset of changes in behavioral responses in this experiment (FIG. 2A,B). For the experiments depicted in FIGURES 2 AND 3, changes in neural activity and in behavioral responses indicative of learning occurred at about the same time.

Across experiments, behavioral learning of image value reversals was correlated with changes in neural activity. FIGURE 4A,B shows the change points of neural activity plotted against the corresponding change points for the behavioral data. Each data point compares a neural activity change point with either a blinking or licking change point. The distributions of licking and

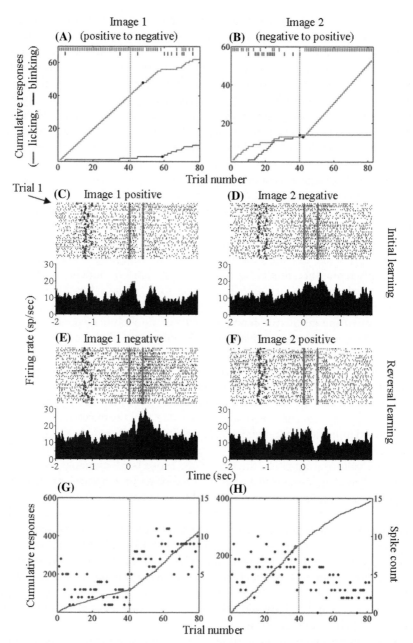

FIGURE 3. Neural activity from an amygdala neuron encoding negative value in relation to behavioral learning. (**A,B**) Behavioral performance. (**C–F**) Rasters and peristimulus time histograms (PSTHs) for the neuron recorded during the same experiment as the behavior shown in **A,B**. (**Gs,H**) Change-point analysis of neural responses during the visual stimulus epoch. All labeling conventions in this figure follow those shown in FIGURE 2. (In color in *Annals* online.)

blinking change points were not significantly different from one another, so they were combined here ($P > 0.25$, t-test). For both monkeys tested, and in both the visual stimulus and trace intervals, behavioral learning was significantly correlated with changes in neural activity (visual stimulus interval: monkey V, $P = 0.02$, $r = 0.24$; monkey P, $P < 10^{-5}$, $r = 0.66$; trace interval: monkey V, $P < 10^{-5}$, $r = 0.63$; monkey P, $P < 10^{-5}$, $r = 0.57$). Moreover, there was not a significant difference between neural and behavioral change points in all cases (paired t-test, $P > 0.05$). Finally, change points during the visual stimulus and trace intervals were not significantly different from each other ($P > 0.1$, t-test).

The tight correlation between the onset of changes in behavior and neural activity suggested that the time course of behavioral and neural learning was similar. We confirmed this by comparing, across neurons encoding image value, the time course of average neural responses with the time course of average behavioral responses. FIGURE 4C shows the normalized and then averaged neural activity and behavior from the 20 trials before and after the value reversal of each image. The data were fit with sigmoidal functions to construct "neural" and "behavioral" learning curves. The time courses of these curves were quite similar and statistically indistinguishable. Moreover, the changing activity and behavior was specific for the images that changed image value, as demonstrated by the same analysis applied to the same cells from the trials with non-reinforced images (FIG. 4D). Thus, the dynamics of behavioral learning could be accounted for if monkeys based their decisions to lick or blink on the evolving representation of value in the amygdala.

It is also worth emphasizing that both neural activity and behavior changed very rapidly after image value reversal, becoming asymptotic within 4–10 trials, on average. These data imply that amygdala neurons update their response profile on a short timescale, since changes in their activity occur within very few trials of a change in image value. Amygdala neurons may update their representation of value rapidly by virtue of receiving information about reinforcement that does not match expectations; indeed, amygdala responses to reinforcement are often stronger when rewards or aversive stimuli occur unexpectedly, such as immediately after a reversal.[64] Neural signals representing reinforcement in relation to expectation could come to the amygdala from a variety of subcortical and cortical pathways. In particular, OFC is a candidate for providing rapid, flexible regulation of amygdala neural activity, consistent with a proposed role for OFC in helping account for amygdala response flexibility during reversal learning.[65]

In addition to rapidly updating its representation during learning of reversed CS-US contingencies, amygdala neurons provide a temporally extended representation of value that appears shortly after visual CS onset and spans until the time of reinforcement. To quantify this, we used a receiver operating characteristic (ROC) analysis[66] to estimate the extent to which activity was different before and after an identified change point (FIG. 5). By convention, ROC values

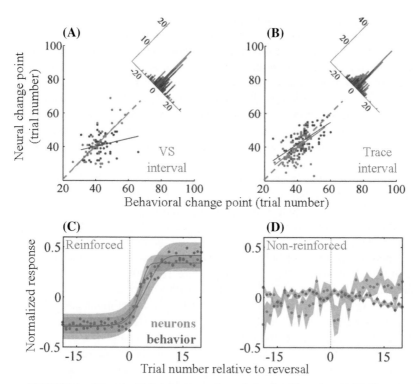

FIGURE 4. Neural activity changes as fast as behavioral learning. (**A,B**) Change points from neural data in the visual stimulus and trace intervals plotted against the change points found for licking or blinking responses reflecting learning. Histograms show that on average there is no difference between neural and behavioral change points. Data and regression lines for monkey V are shown in *blue*; data and regression lines for monkey P are shown in *red*. (**C**) Average normalized neural activity and behavioral responses plotted as a function of trial number relative to the reversal in image value. *Shaded regions* indicate 95% prediction intervals for best-fit Weibull functions. Behavioral and neural learning curves overlap. (**D**) Neural responses do not change to the non-reinforced image, as shown by applying the same analysis done for **C** to the trials containing non-reinforced images. *Shaded regions* show SEM of data points. (From Paton et al.[33] Reproduced by permission.) (In color in *Annals* online.)

> 0.5 indicated activity that was greater when an image was associated with reward, and values < 0.5 indicated activity that was greater when an image was associated with air-puff. Using this approach, we characterized how neurons represent value across time during a trial by repeating the ROC analysis in consecutive overlapping time-windows of 100 ms (advanced in steps of 20 ms). FIGURE 5 shows how each value-coding cell represented the value of images as a function of time within trials (each row corresponds to how a single cell represented the value of a single image, as quantified by the ROC analysis). On average, for positive-coding cells, the first bin significantly greater than

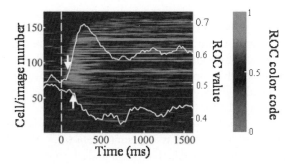

FIGURE 5. The temporally extended representation of value in the amygdala. Value signals in the amygdala plotted as a function of time, with positive and negative value-coding neurons represented by different colors. Each row in the color map shows how value was represented by a neuron during the presentation of a single image. Positive and negative cell rows are sorted in opposite order according to the latency of the first post-visual-stimulus data point significantly different from 0.5 ($P < 0.05$, permutation test). The *white curves* depict the mean ROC values across the populations of neurons encoding positive and negative value. Time 0 corresponds to the start of the bin spanning from 0–99 ms after visual stimulus onset. *White arrows* indicate the first bins significantly different from 0.5 for the mean ROC values ($P < 0.05$, *t*-test). (Adapted from FIG. 3D in Paton *et al.*[33]) (In color in *Annals* online.)

0.5 occurred 80–180 ms after visual stimulus onset; all subsequent bins were also significantly greater than 0.5 (downward white arrow, $P < 0.05$, *t*-test). The first significant bin for neurons encoding negative value was 120–220 ms after visual stimulus onset (upward white arrow). This representation of value over time could correspond to the sort of representation posited by models of reinforcement learning to be required for computations of prediction error signals.[6] However, the temporal dynamics of amygdala neurons have not been compared quantitatively during learning with neurons encoding prediction errors, such as dopamine neurons.[6]

HOW IS VALUE REPRESENTED IN PRIMATE OFC?

Given the anatomic interconnections between the amygdala and OFC, a significant challenge for neuroscientists is to understand how neural activity in the two brain areas is interrelated during appetitive and aversive reinforcement conditioning. We have therefore been interested in comparing neural signals in the OFC and amygdala during learning induced by classical conditioning. How and when might signals representing value develop during learning in each area, and what is the timing of these signals relative to each other? OFC is frequently thought of as being critical for reversal learning, but are the response dynamics of OFC neurons appropriate for regulating amygdala responses during our task?

To address these questions, we have been recording simultaneously from individual neurons in the OFC (primarily area 13) and amygdala while monkeys performed a trace-conditioning task similar to the one described above. We find that the responses of neurons in the OFC, like those in the amygdala, can be modulated by image value during one or more periods of the task.[67] Value-related signals in the amygdala and OFC develop with a range of overlapping latencies after CS onset. Furthermore, both OFC and amygdala neurons can rapidly change their activity during reversal learning, with the time course appearing to be similar in a small data set.[67] Both OFC and the amygdala therefore contain signals that could underlie appetitive and aversive learning during classical conditioning. On the basis of these preliminary data, amygdala and OFC may be seen to represent closely connected and interrelated components of a neural circuit that assigns affective significance to sensory stimuli, and the two areas may largely act in unison during learning.

SUMMARY AND REFLECTIONS ON THE REGULATION OF VALUE REPRESENTATIONS IN THE BRAIN

Both the amygdala and OFC have long been hypothesized to play a role in aspects of emotional learning and behavior. We are investigating the neurophysiology of the amygdala and OFC during learning induced by appetitive and aversive classical conditioning, and during the reversal of learned reinforcement contingencies. We have discovered that the amygdala contains different populations of neurons, some that respond more strongly to a CS associated with a reward, and others that respond more strongly to a CS associated with an aversive stimulus. This representation of CS "value" is rapidly updated during reversal of contingencies. In some cells, and for some CSs, it occurs within a single trial, and on average it occurs within 4–10 trials, at the same time as changes in behavior indicative of learning. In addition, the representation of value appears rapidly after CS onset. Similar signals appear to be present in OFC. We are in the process of characterizing the rates of learning in OFC neurons compared to amygdala neurons, and the relative latency and duration of value-related signaling in the two brain areas. If one brain area is driving the other, then learning rates should be faster, and latencies shorter, in that brain area. In general we are interested in determining the different roles of OFC and amygdala during learning induced by classical conditioning. Does the amygdala or OFC drive learning in the other brain area, or do the two brain areas function in a parallel fashion? Do distinct response properties in each area depend upon input from the other brain area? What mechanisms are responsible for the flexible representation of value in these brain areas?

The data presented here and in our recent paper,[33] characterize the neurophysiological properties of primate amygdala neurons during appetitive and aversive classical conditioning. Prior work provided conflicting data about whether primate amygdala neurons rapidly changed their response properties upon reversal of reinforcement contingencies using instrumental tasks,[28,29,68] but analogous instrumental tasks in rodents had shown that amygdala neurons were sensitive to reversals in contingencies.[16,48] Our use of classical conditioning procedures (rather than avoidance tasks, where the aversive stimuli do not occur after learning), our use of novel CSs in every experiment, and our tighter requirements for visual fixation all may have contributed to our identification of a flexible representation of value in primate amygdala.

Several lines of experiments have suggested that the OFC is itself a critical structure for reversal learning. In monkeys, lesions of OFC disrupt performance on an operant task involving stimulus-reward reversal learning.[42] Similar findings have been reported in human clinical populations.[69] Moreover, selective lesions in primate amygdala, in contrast to OFC, do not appear to impair performance on a similar operant task.[70] Overall, these results mirror the effects of OFC lesions reported in rodents on a different operant task in which animals learned to use cues to acquire rewards and to avoid aversive stimuli.[71] Interestingly, rat OFC lesions decreased the proportion of amygdala neurons that reversed cue-related responses during this task. The extent of homology between the parts of rat OFC that were lesioned in these studies, and those which we are studying physiologically in monkeys, needs to be determined. Nonetheless, these studies raise the possibility that the flexible representation of value in the amygdala may depend, directly or indirectly, on OFC input. If this is the case, however, the regulation must be sufficiently rapid to account for the largely overlapping temporal dynamics of amygdala and OFC neural activity during learning. Furthermore, it is worth noting that the tasks establishing that OFC is required for reversal learning have all been operant tasks, and it remains unclear how amygdala and OFC lesions would affect performance on a classical conditioning task that includes a reversal of contingencies, such as the one we have employed.

Our experiments have revealed that the primate amygdala provides a flexible representation of the positive and negative value of visual CSs. The rate of learning exhibited by cells, however, was variable. Even the same cell could learn at different rates for different CSs (see, for example, the cell in FIG. 2). This raises the possibility that combinations of different types of mechanisms may be employed in regulating the representation of value in the amygdala. At one extreme, synaptic weights may gradually change during learning through a Hebbian mechanism; this is possible because the amygdala is anatomically well-situated to receive the required coincident input from sensory stimuli and reinforcers. At the other extreme, gated inputs might dictate the response level of amygdala neurons, perhaps explaining how single-trial reversal learning could occur. For a model of this type of flexible learning, we might look to supervised response modulation.[72,73] In this scheme, a neural network is set up to perform a certain function (e.g., compute expected reinforcement); based on the result of the network's performance, a supervising neural circuit will make direct adjustments to the response properties of the neurons in the network. By interacting with Hebbian plasticity in the synapses of the main network, this kind of supervising circuit can result in efficient learning, even when multiple outputs are required. Thus, gradually changing synaptic weights are not the only physiologically plausible mechanisms for modulating the output of amygdala neurons. OFC could constitute a part of the supervising circuit that may help control representations of value in the amygdala.

ACKNOWLEDGMENTS

We thank S. Dashnaw and J. Hirsch for MRI support. This work was supported by the Keck Foundation, grants from the NIMH, and the Klingenstein, Sloan, James S. McDonnell, Gatsby and NARSAD Foundations, and by a Charles E. Culpeper Scholarship award from Goldman Philanthropic Partnerships to C.D.S. J.J.P. received support from NICHD and NEI institutional training grants. S.E.M. received support from an NSF graduate research fellowship.

REFERENCES

1. OCHSNER, K.N. & J.J. GROSS. 2005. The cognitive control of emotion. Trends Cogn. Sci. **9:** 242–249.
2. MURRAY, E.A. 2008. Neuropsychology of primate reward processes. *In* New Encyclopedia of Neuroscience. L.R. Squire Ed. Elsevier. In press.
3. PENNARTZ, C.M. 1997. Reinforcement learning by Hebbian synapses with adaptive thresholds. Neuroscience **81:** 303–319.
4. RESCORLA, R.A. & A.R. WAGNER. 1972. A theory of Pavlovian conditioning: variations in the effectiveness of reinforcement and non-reinforcement. *In* Classical Conditioning II: Current Research and Theory. A.H. Black & W.F. Prokasy Eds.: 64–99. Appleton Century Crofts. New York.
5. SUTTON, R. & A. BARTO. 1998. Reinforcement Learning. MIT Press. Cambridge, MA.
6. SCHULTZ, W., P. DAYAN & P.R. MONTAGUE. 1997. A neural substrate of prediction and reward. Science **275:** 1593–1599.
7. PEARCE, J. & G. HALL. 1980. A model for Pavlovian conditioning: variations in the effectiveness of conditioned but not unconditioned stimuli. Psychol. Rev. **87:** 532–552.
8. LEDOUX, J.E. 2000. Emotion circuits in the brain. Annu. Rev. Neurosci. **23:** 155–184.
9. EVERITT, B.J., R.N. CARDINAL, J.A. PARKINSON & T.W. ROBBINS. 2003. Appetitive behavior: impact of amygdala-dependent mechanisms of emotional learning. Ann. N. Y. Acad. Sci. **985:** 233–250.
10. BAXTER, M. & MURRAY, EA. 2002. The amygdala and reward. Nat. Rev. Neurosci. **3:** 563–573.

11. AMARAL, D., J. PRICE, A. PITKANEN & S. CARMICHAEL. 1992. Anatomical organi-
    zation of the primate amygdaloid complex. *In* The Amygdala: Neurobiological
    Aspects of Emotion, Memory, and Mental Dysfunction. J. Aggleton Ed.: 1–66.
    Wiley–Liss. New York.

12. SWANSON, L.W. & G.D. PETROVICH. 1998. What is the amygdala? Trends Neurosci.
    21: 323–331.

13. GHASHGHAEI, H.T. & H. BARBAS. 2002. Pathways for emotion: interactions of
    prefrontal and anterior temporal pathways in the amygdala of the rhesus monkey.
    Neuroscience **115:** 1261–1279.

14. STEFANACCI, L. & D.G. AMARAL. 2002. Some observations on cortical inputs to
    the macaque monkey amygdala: an anterograde tracing study. J. Comp. Neurol.
    451: 301–323.

15. REPA, J.C. *et al.* 2001. Two different lateral amygdala cell populations contribute
    to the initiation and storage of memory. Nat. Neurosci. **4:** 724–731.

16. SCHOENBAUM, G., A.A. CHIBA & M. GALLAGHER. 1999. Neural encoding in
    orbitofrontal cortex and basolateral amygdala during olfactory discrimination
    learning. J. Neurosci. **19:** 1876–1884.

17. PASCOE, J.P. & B.S. KAPP. 1985. Electrophysiological characteristics of amygdaloid
    central nucleus neurons during Pavlovian fear conditioning in the rabbit. Behav.
    Brain Res. **16:** 117–133.

18. QUIRK, G.J., C. REPA & LEDOUX, J.E. 1995. Fear conditioning enhances short-
    latency auditory responses of lateral amygdala neurons: parallel recordings in
    the freely behaving rat. Neuron **15:** 1029–1039.

19. APPLEGATE, C.D., R.C. FRYSINGER, B.S. KAPP & M. GALLAGHER. 1982. Multiple
    unit activity recorded from amygdala central nucleus during Pavlovian heart rate
    conditioning in rabbit. Brain Res. **238:** 457–462.

20. GOOSENS, K.A., J.A. HOBIN & S. MAREN. 2003. Auditory-evoked spike firing in
    the lateral amygdala and Pavlovian fear conditioning: mnemonic code or fear
    bias? Neuron **40:** 1013–1022.

21. COLLINS, D.R. & D. PARE. 2000. Differential fear conditioning induces reciprocal
    changes in the sensory responses of lateral amygdala neurons to the CS(+) and
    CS(-). Learn. Mem. **7:** 97–103.

22. MAREN, S. & G.J. QUIRK. 2004. Neuronal signaling of fear memory. Nat. Rev.
    Neurosci. **5:** 844–852.

23. SCHOENBAUM, G., A.A. CHIBA & M. GALLAGHER. 1998. Orbitofrontal cortex and
    basolateral amygdala encode expected outcomes during learning. Nat. Neurosci.
    1: 155–159.

24. MAREN, S. 2000. Auditory fear conditioning increases CS-elicited spike firing in
    lateral amygdala neurons even after extensive overtraining. Eur. J. Neurosci. **12:**
    4047–4054.

25. RORICK-KEHN, L.M. & J.E. STEINMETZ. 2005. Amygdalar unit activity during three
    learning tasks: eyeblink classical conditioning, Pavlovian fear conditioning, and
    signaled avoidance conditioning. Behav. Neurosci. **119:** 1254–1276.

26. SUGASE-MIYAMOTO, Y. & B.J. RICHMOND. 2005. Neuronal signals in the monkey
    basolateral amygdala during reward schedules. J. Neurosci. **25:** 11071–11083.

27. DEHAENE, S. & J.P. CHANGEUX. 2000. Reward-dependent learning in neuronal
    networks for planning and decision making. Prog. Brain Res. **126:** 217–
    229.

28. SANGHERA, M.K., E.T. ROLLS & A. ROPER-HALL. 1979. Visual responses of neurons
    in the dorsolateral amygdala of the alert monkey. Exp. Neurol. **63:** 610–626.

29. NISHIJO, H., T. ONO & H. NISHINO. 1988. Single neuron responses in amygdala of alert monkey during complex sensory stimulation with affective significance. J. Neurosci. **8:** 3570–3583.

30. NAKAMURA, K., A. MIKAMI & K. KUBOTA. 1992. Activity of single neurons in the monkey amygdala during performance of a visual discrimination task. J. Neurophysiol. **67:** 1447–1663.

31. WILSON, F.A. & E.T. ROLLS. 2005. The primate amygdala and reinforcement: a dissociation between rule-based and associatively-mediated memory revealed in neuronal activity. Neuroscience **133:** 1061–1072.

32. ROLLS, E. 1992. Neurophysiology and functions of the primate amygdala. *In* The Amygdala: Neurobiological Aspects of Emotion, Memory, and Mental Dysfunction. J. Aggleton, Ed.: 143–166. Wiley–Liss. New York.

33. PATON, J., M. BELOVA, S. MORRISON & C. SALZMAN. 2006. The primate amygdala represents the positive and negative value of visual stimuli during learning. Nature **439:** 865–870.

34. HABER, S.N., K. KUNISHIO, M. MIZOBUCHI & E. LYND-BALTA. 1995. The orbital and medial prefrontal circuit through the primate basal ganglia. J. Neurosci. **15:** 4851–4867.

35. CAVADA, C., T. COMPANY, J. TEJEDOR, *et al.* 2000. The anatomical connections of the macaque monkey orbitofrontal cortex: a review. Cereb. Cortex **10:** 220–242.

36. CARMICHAEL, S.T. & J.L. PRICE. 1995. Limbic connections of the orbital and medial prefrontal cortex in macaque monkeys. J. Comp. Neurol. **363:** 615–641.

37. STEFANACCI, L. & D.G. AMARAL. 2000. Topographic organization of cortical inputs to the lateral nucleus of the macaque monkey amygdala: a retrograde tracing study. J. Comp. Neurol. **421:** 52–79.

38. BECHARA, A., H. DAMASIO & A.R. DAMASIO. 2000. Emotion, decision making and the orbitofrontal cortex. Cereb. Cortex **10:** 295–307.

39. BECHARA, A., H. DAMASIO & A.R. DAMASIO. 2003. Role of the amygdala in decision-making. Ann. N.Y. Acad. Sci. **985:** 356–369.

40. BECHARA, A., D. TRANEL, H. DAMASIO & A.R. DAMASIO. 1996. Failure to respond autonomically to anticipated future outcomes following damage to prefrontal cortex. Cereb. Cortex **6:** 215–225.

41. CHOW, T.W. 2000. Personality in frontal lobe disorders. Curr. Psychiatry Rep. **2:** 446–451.

42. IZQUIERDO, A., R.K. SUDA & E.A. MURRAY. 2004. Bilateral orbital prefrontal cortex lesions in rhesus monkeys disrupt choices guided by both reward value and reward contingency. J. Neurosci. **24:** 7540–7548.

43. BAXTER, M., A. PARKER, C.C. LINDNER, *et al.* 2000. Control of response selection by reinforcer value requires interaction of amygdala and orbital prefrontal cortex. J. Neurosci. **20:** 4311–4319.

44. COX, S.M., A. ANDRADE & I.S. JOHNSRUDE. 2005. Learning to like: a role for human orbitofrontal cortex in conditioned reward. J. Neurosci. **25:** 2733–2740.

45. URSU, S. & C.S. CARTER. 2005. Outcome representations, counterfactual comparisons and the human orbitofrontal cortex: implications for neuroimaging studies of decision-making. Cogn. Brain Res. **23:** 51–60.

46. O'DOHERTY, J., M.L. KRINGELBACH, E.T. ROLLS, *et al.* 2001. Abstract reward and punishment representations in the human orbitofrontal cortex. Nature Neurosci. **4:** 95–102.

47. THORPE, S.J., E.T. ROLLS & S. MADDISON. 1983. The orbitofrontal cortex: neuronal activity in the behaving monkey. Exp. Brain Res. **49:** 93–115.

48. SCHOENBAUM, G., A. CHIBA & M. GALLAGHER. 1998. Orbitalfrontal cortex and basolateral amygdala encode expected outcomes during learning. Nature Neurosci. **1:** 155–159.
49. SCHOENBAUM, G., A.A. CHIBA & M. GALLAGHER. 1999. Neural encoding in orbitofrontal cortex and basolateral amygdala during olfactory discrimination learning. J. Neurosci. **19:** 1876–1884.
50. SCHOENBAUM, G., B. SETLOW, M.P. SADDORIS & M. GALLAGHER. 2003. Encoding predicted outcome and acquired value in orbitofrontal cortex during cue sampling depends upon input from basolateral amygdala. Neuron **39:** 855–867.
51. ROLLS, E.T., H.D. CRITCHLEY, R. MASON & E.A. WAKEMAN. 1996. Orbitofrontal cortex neurons: role in olfactory and visual association learning. J. Neurophysiol. **75:** 1970–1981.
52. TREMBLAY, L. & W. SCHULTZ. 1999. Relative reward preference in primate orbitofrontal cortex. Nature **398:** 704–708.
53. WALLIS, J.D. & E.K. MILLER. 2003. Neuronal activity in primate dorsolateral and orbital prefrontal cortex during performance of a reward preference task. Eur. J. Neurosci. **18:** 2069–2081.
54. TREMBLAY, L. & W. SCHULTZ. 2000. Modifications of reward expectation-related neuronal activity during learning in primate orbitofrontal cortex. J. Neurophysiol. **83:** 1877–1885.
55. ROESCH, M.R. & C.R. OLSON. 2004. Neuronal activity related to reward value and motivation in primate frontal cortex. Science **304:** 307–310.
56. PADOA-SCHIOPPA, C. & J.A. ASSAD. 2006. Neurons in the orbitofrontal cortex encode economic value. Nature **441:** 223–226.
57. FEIERSTEIN, C.E., M.C. QUIRK, N. UCHIDA, *et al.* 2006. Representation of spatial goals in rat orbitofrontal cortex. Neuron **51:** 495–507.
58. ROESCH, M.R., A.R. TAYLOR & G. SCHOENBAUM. 2006. Encoding of time-discounted rewards in orbitofrontal cortex is independent of value representation. Neuron **51:** 509–520.
59. OSTLUND, S.B. & B.W. BALLEINE. 2007. Orbitofrontal cortex mediates outcome encoding in Pavlovian but not instrumental conditioning. J. Neurosci. **27:** 4819–4825.
60. MAZUR, J.E. 2006. Learning and Behavior. Prentice Hall. Upper Saddle River, NJ.
61. PAVLOV, I.P. 1927. Conditioned Reflexes. Oxford University Press. London.
62. LANG, P.J., M.M. BRADLEY & B.N. CUTHBERT. 1990. Emotion, attention, and the startle reflex. Psychol. Rev. **97:** 377–395.
63. GALLISTEL, C.R., S. FAIRHURST & P. BALSAM. 2004. The learning curve: implications of a quantitative analysis. Proc. Natl. Acad. Sci. USA **101:** 13124–13131.
64. BELOVA, M.A., J.J. PATON, S.E. MORRISON & C.D. SALZMAN. 2007. Expectation modulates neural responses to pleasant and aversive stimuli in primate amygdala. Neuron. **55(6):** 970–984.
65. SADDORIS, M.P., M. GALLAGHER & G. SCHOENBAUM. 2005. Rapid associative encoding in basolateral amygdala depends on connections with orbitofrontal cortex. Neuron **46:** 321–331.
66. GREEN, D.M. & J.A. SWETS. 1966. Signal Detection Theory and Psychophysics. Wiley. New York.
67. MORRISON, S.E. & C.D. SALZMAN. 2007. Primate orbitofrontal cortex and amygdala encode stimulus value with a similar time course during reinforcement learning. Soc. Neurosci. Abstr. 934.4.

68. ROLLS, E. 2000. Neurophysiology and functions of the primate amygdala, and the neural basis of emotion. *In* The Amygdala: a Functional Analysis. J. Aggleton, Ed.: 447–478. Oxford University Press. New York.
69. FELLOWS, L.K. & M.J. FARAH. 2003. Ventromedial frontal cortex mediates affective shifting in humans: evidence from a reversal learning paradigm. Brain **126:** 1830–1837.
70. IZQUIERDO, A. & E.A. MURRAY. 2007. Selective bilateral amygdala lesions in rhesus monkeys fail to disrupt object reversal learning. J. Neurosci. **27:** 1054–1062.
71. SCHOENBAUM, G., B. SETLOW, S.L. NUGENT, M.P. SADDORIS & M. GALLAGHER. 2003. Lesions of orbitofrontal cortex and basolateral amygdala complex disrupt acquisition of odor-guided discriminations and reversals. Learn. Mem. **10:** 129–140.
72. SWINEHART, C.D. & L.F. ABBOTT. 2005. Supervised learning through neuronal response modulation. Neural Comput. **17:** 609–631.
73. SWINEHART, C.D., K. BOUCHARD, P. PARTENSKY & L.F. ABBOTT. 2004. Control of network activity through neuronal response modulation. Neurocomputing **58–60:** 327–335.

The Contribution of the Medial Prefrontal Cortex, Orbitofrontal Cortex, and Dorsomedial Striatum to Behavioral Flexibility

MICHAEL E. RAGOZZINO

Department of Psychology, University of Illinois at Chicago, Chicago, Illinois 60607, USA

ABSTRACT: Behavioral flexibility refers to the ability to shift strategies or response patterns with a change in environmental contingencies. The frontal lobe and basal ganglia are two brain regions implicated in various components for successfully adapting to changed environmental contingencies. This paper discusses a series of experiments that investigate the contributions of the rat prelimbic area, infralimbic area, orbitofrontal cortex, and dorsomedial striatum to behavioral flexibility. Orbitofrontal cortex inactivation did not impair initial learning of discrimination tests, but it impaired reversal learning due to perseverance in the previously learned choice pattern. Inactivation of the prelimbic area did not affect acquisition or reversal learning of different discrimination tests, but it selectively impaired learning when rats had to inhibit one strategy and shift to using a new strategy. However, comparable to orbitofrontal cortex inactivation, strategy-switching deficits following prelimbic inactivation resulted from a perseverance of the previously relevant strategy. Fewer studies have examined the infralimbic region, but there is some evidence suggesting that this region supports reversal learning by maintaining the reliable execution of a new choice pattern. Dorsomedial striatal inactivation impaired both reversal learning and strategy switching. The behavioral flexibility deficits following dorsomedial striatal inactivation resulted from the inability to maintain a new choice pattern once selected. Taken together, the results suggest that orbitofrontal and prelimbic subregions differentially contribute to behavioral flexibility, but they are both critical for the initial inhibition of a previously learned strategy, while the dorsomedial striatum plays a broader role in behavioral flexibility and supports a process that allows the reliable execution of a new strategy once selected.

KEYWORDS: orbitofrontal cortex; prelimbic; infralimbic; striatum; learning

Address for correspondence: Michael E. Ragozzino, Department of Psychology, University of Illinois at Chicago, 1007 West Harrison Street, Chicago, IL 60607. Voice: 312-413-2630; fax: 312-413-4122.

mrago@uic.edu

Ann. N.Y. Acad. Sci. 1121: 355–375 (2007). © 2007 New York Academy of Sciences.
doi: 10.1196/annals.1401.013

INTRODUCTION

In an ever-changing environment, the ability to adapt new choice patterns is essential for daily living and often survival. Considerable evidence indicates that the frontal cortex supports learning when conditions require inhibition of a previously relevant strategy and acquiring a new strategy.[1–5] The frontal cortex, however, consists of several subregions, which raises the important issue of whether these separate subareas support distinct behavioral flexibility functions. The frontal cortex is also known to project heavily to the basal ganglia in a highly organized manner in which there are distinct cortico-basal ganglia loops.[6] This raises a further issue of whether and how distinct cortico-striatal circuits in this highly organized network may differentially support a shift in strategy.

A model put forth by Wise and colleagues to explain the functional organization of the primate frontal cortex proposes that different conditions require different types of cognitive/behavioral processes to facilitate behavioral flexibility, and these processes are mediated by separate primate prefrontal cortex areas.[7] Specifically, the model proposes that there is a lower-order process for the shifting of specific choices within a dimension. This process allows the approach to and avoidance of a particular stimulus or scene as required in discrimination tasks that involve reversal learning. The model also states that there is a higher-order process when conditions demand learning about stimulus attributes as opposed to a stimulus as a whole. In these cases, learning must go beyond simply attaching a positive or negative valence to stimuli within a particular dimension and instead require attention to components of an object or scene or abstract rules about component objects or scenes. This may involve learning the relationship between different stimulus components—e.g., paired associate learning—or complete response inhibition to stimuli in one dimension while learning what stimulus in a different dimension is correct. For example, one may use street signs to reach a location during the day but use directional information, such as memory for turn sequences and distance, to reach the same location at night. Thus, higher-order processing enables a subject to reconceptualize his or her approach to a task and attend to a new type of information. This type of flexibility is required during extradimensional shifts. Reversal learning is representative of lower-order processing because it involves a change only in exemplar, not in category. The extradimensional shift is representative of higher-order processing because it requires taking a fundamentally new approach to solving a task that entails using a new strategy. Although the terms *lower-order* and *higher-order* might suggest a serial hierarchical organization, the model explicitly hypothesizes that different operations are subserved by different prefrontal subregions that function independently of each other.

To explore the model proposed by Wise and colleagues[7] related to rodent prefrontal cortex functioning, we conducted a series of experiments that

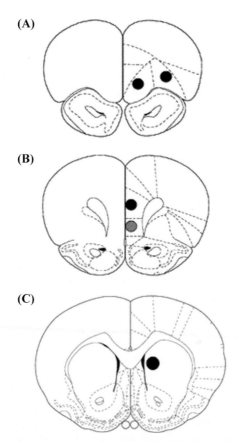

FIGURE 1. Highlight of prelimbic area with black circle and infralimbic area with grey circle **(A)**; ventral and lateral orbitofrontal cortex **(B)** and dorsomedial striatum **(C)**. The rat brain sections were modified from the atlas of Paxinos and Watson.[43]

investigated whether temporarily inactivating the prelimbic cortex or the orbitofrontal cortex affected separate processes that enabled behavioral flexibility (see FIG. 1). The experiments were conducted using a variety of discrimination tasks that tested the effects of inactivation on initial learning, reversal learning, and times when conditions required a shift in strategy. Because the orbitofrontal cortex and the prelimbic area both project to the dorsomedial striatum,[8] the effects of dorsomedial striatal inactivation were also on examined on various discrimination tests.

PRELIMBIC INVOLVEMENT IN BEHAVIORAL FLEXIBILITY

In initial experiments, the role of the medial prefrontal cortex in switching strategies was examined. In particular, the contribution of the prelimbic subregion was investigated on tasks that involved learning a discrimination based on one type of strategy and then being required to learn a new strategy in the same context, e.g., to make a choice based on visuospatial information first and then base a choice on odor information.[9–11] In one set of studies, rats were permanently implanted with guide cannula aimed toward the prelimbic subregion (see FIG. 1A). Subsequently, rats were trained to dig in a sand cup to receive a cereal reinforcement using a procedure similar to that of Bunsey and Eichenbaum.[12] The sands cups contained a spice, such as cinnamon or nutmeg, mixed in with the sand to provide a distinct odor to the sand cups. The two odor cups were randomly switched between two different spatial locations across trials. In this task, rats first learned to base their choice on either odor information or visuospatial information (location of the sand cup). After learning to discriminate based on one of these strategies in one session, rats had to switch their choice pattern based on the other strategy in the following session; e.g., odor information could be relevant on acquisition and spatial information could be relevant on the shift phase. Five minutes prior to each test session, a rat received an intracranial infusion of either saline or the local anesthetic, bupivacaine, into the prelimbic area. The learning criterion for each session was ten consecutive correct trials. The finding revealed that prelimbic inactivation did not impair the initial learning of either odor or spatial discrimination.[11] In contrast, prelimbic inactivation did impair learning when rats had to shift between an odor and spatial discrimination (see FIG. 2A). This was the case whether rats first learned an odor discrimination or first learned a spatial discrimination. The pattern of results suggests that the prelimbic area supports behavioral flexibility when conditions require a shift in strategy.

The contribution of the prelimbic area to extradimensional shifts does not appear to be limited to specific attribute information. For example, the prelimbic area does not facilitate extradimensional shifts that only involve the flexible use of spatial or visual cue information. This is because neurotoxic lesions of the prelimbic and infralimbic areas impair a shift between the use of odor information and the use of texture information.[13] Furthermore, dopamine receptor blockade or N-methyl-D-aspartate (NMDA) receptor blockade in the prelimbic area impairs a shift between egocentric response and visual cue strategies.[14–16] Together, these findings suggest that the prelimbic area enables a shift in strategy across a variety of stimulus dimensions.

Several studies have explored what process or processes are disrupted following prelimbic inactivation that produces a deficit in shifting strategies. One possibility is that the prelimbic region facilitates the ability to *initially* inhibit a previously relevant strategy and/or to generate a new strategy. In this case, prelimbic inactivation should produce a predominance of errors during the initial trials in the shift phase. These errors are commonly referred to as perseverative errors. Another possibility is that the prelimbic area supports a process that allows an individual to reliably execute or learn a new strategy once the new strategy is selected. This process would prevent or minimize regressions to

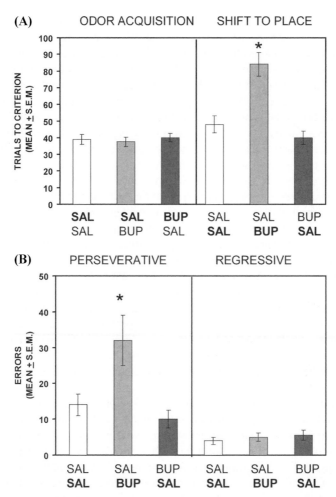

FIGURE 2. (A) Mean (± s.e.m.) trials to criterion in odor acquisition and shift to a spatial discrimination following bilateral infusions of saline or bupivacaine into the prelimbic area. Prelimbic inactivation did not affect acquisition, but did impair a shift to a spatial strategy. The treatment received in each phase of testing is in bold. SAL = saline; BUP = bupivacaine. *$P < 0.05$ versus controls. **(B)** Mean (± s.e.m.) number of perseverative and regressive errors in reversal learning after bilateral infusions of saline or bupivacaine into the prelimbic area. There was a significant increase in perseverative, but not regressive errors following prelimbic inactivation. SAL = saline; BUP = bupivacaine. *$P < 0.05$ versus controls.

the previously relevant strategy once the new, presently relevant strategy is selected. In this case, prelimbic inactivation should not produce a significant increase in errors during the initial trials of the shift phase, but rather should lead to a greater number of errors once a rat has selected the new, presently relevant strategy. We have referred to these errors as regressive errors because a subject has chosen the new correct choice and has been reinforced for it, but regresses to the previous strategy that is no longer reinforced. There have been different operational definitions used to define perseverative and regressive errors but the patterns of results have remained the same whatever definition was used. More specifically, in some studies perseveration was defined as making the previously correct choice three or four times in consecutive blocks of four trials. Once a rat made less than three previously correct choices in a block the errors were no longer counted as perseverative errors, but rather were counted as regressive errors. With this definition, a rat was considered to be perseverating when it was choosing the previously correct choice on the majority of trials. Once it was just as likely to make the new correct choice as the previous correct choice, the errors were considered regressive. We have also defined perseveration as the number of trials a rat continued to make the previously correct choice after making an initial error until it made the new correct choice. Subsequently, every error after making the first correct choice was counted as a regressive error. In multiple experiments in which manipulations of the prelimbic area impaired a shift in strategy, the deficit resulted from an increase in perseverative errors but not regressive errors.[9–11,15] This includes the study described above in which prelimbic inactivation impaired a shift from an odor to a spatial strategy (see FIG. 2B). The pattern of results suggests that the prelimbic area enables a shift in strategy by facilitating the initial inhibition of a previously learned strategy and/or the generation of a new strategy.

The findings described above suggest that the prelimbic area contributes to behavioral flexibility, at least in part, by supporting a shift in strategy. A number of other experiments have also investigated whether the prelimbic area plays a role in other types of behavioral flexibility, such as reversal learning. In one study using the sand-digging test, rats were trained on acquisition and reversal learning of a two-choice odor discrimination.[11] Prelimbic inactivation did not impair acquisition or reversal learning of a two-choice odor discrimination (see FIG. 3A). This lack of effect on reversal learning has also been reported with prelimbic inactivation or lesions on other types of reversal-learning tests, such as spatial, egocentric response, and texture.[9,13] Thus, based on multiple behavioral-flexibility tests, the findings might suggest that the prelimbic area supports a higher-order process that involves a shift in strategy, but not a lower-order process as assessed by reversal learning.

One issue that arises when examining a brain region on extradimensional shifts versus reversal-learning tests is that extradimensional shifts are often more difficult than reversal-learning tests.[11,13] Because of the difference in level of difficulty between reversal-learning tests and extradimensional shifts, it is unknown whether a differential effect of prefrontal subregion inactivation in these tasks is related to the behavioral operation necessary to learn the task or due to the level of difficulty. To address this issue, a two-choice odor

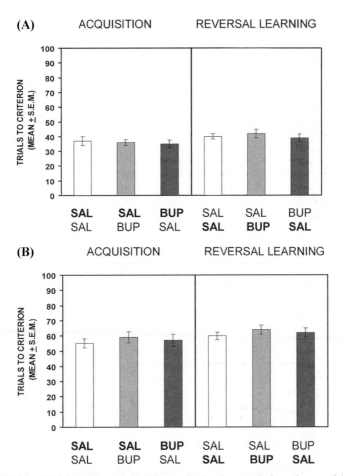

FIGURE 3. (A) Mean (± s.e.m.) trials to criterion in two-choice odor acquisition and reversal learning following bilateral infusions of saline or bupivacaine into the prelimbic area. Prelimbic inactivation did not affect acquisition or reversal learning. The treatment received in each phase of testing is in bold. SAL = saline; BUP = bupivacaine. (B) Mean (± s.e.m.) trials to criterion in four-choice odor acquisition and reversal learning following bilateral infusions of saline or bupivacaine into the prelimbic area. Prelimbic inactivation did not affect acquisition or reversal learning. The treatment received in each phase of testing is in bold. SAL = saline; BUP = bupivacaine.

reversal-learning test was changed to a four-choice odor reversal-learning test. A four-choice discrimination test required significantly more trials to acquire and reverse than a two-choice discrimination, but it was comparable to an extradimensional shift. Thus, the same behavioral operation was required in the four-choice reversal-learning test as in the two-choice reversal-learning test, but the four-choice test required a greater number of trials to learn. Even in the four-choice odor discrimination test, prelimbic inactivation did not impair reversal learning (see FIG. 3B). This suggests that the prelimbic area supports a higher-order process that enables a shift in strategy but is not involved in a lower-order process in which the same general strategy remains the same, but a shift in specific choices is reversed.

A possible alternative interpretation of prelimbic inactivation's affecting extradimensional shifts, but not reversal-learning tests, is not related to the behavioral operation required but rather is due to different reinforcement contingencies in the shift phase. In particular, in a reversal-learning task the previously reinforced choice is never reinforced during the reversal phase (e.g., the cinnamon odor would be reinforced in 100% of the trials on acquisition and in 0% of the trials on reversal). In an extradimensional shift, the previously reinforced choice or strategy is reinforced in 50% of the trials during the shift phase. For example, in acquisition a rat first learns to choose the cinnamon odor cue and to avoid the nutmeg odor cue, as well as to disregard the spatial location of the cup. During the shift, a rat learns to choose spatial location A and to avoid spatial location B while ignoring odor information. However, the different odor cues and spatial locations are pseudorandomly combined such that for half the trials the previously relevant cinnamon odor cue is in spatial location A and therefore is still reinforced in 50% of the trials. Thus, manipulation of the prelimbic area may lead to a deficit in an extradimensional shift, but not in reversal-learning, because of a difficulty abandoning a previously relevant strategy a or choice that is still being partially reinforced.

To investigate this possibility, we examined the effects of prelimbic inactivation on a test that has the same reinforcement contingencies as an extradimensional shift, but involves reversal learning. Specifically, prelimbic inactivation on spatial reversal learning was examined. To inactivate the prelimbic area, the gamma aminobutryic acid (GABA)-A agonist muscimol was infused into the prelimbic area. The same learning criterion of ten consecutive correct trials was used as in past experiments. Acquisition of the spatial discrimination was the same as past studies such that a rat learned to choose the sand cup in spatial location A and to avoid the sand cup in spatial location B. In reversal learning, the previously correct spatial location A was still reinforced in 50% of the trials when chosen, while location B was reinforced in 100% of the trials when chosen. This mimics the reinforcement contingencies in the extradimensional shift in which the stimulus choice that was reinforced on acquisition is still reinforced in 50% of the trials when chosen. However, in this test, the relevant stimulus information remained the same in the switch. Prelimbic inactivation did not impair spatial reversal learning using a 50%/100% reinforcement contingency. These findings suggest that the prelimbic inactivation–induced deficit in an extradimensional shift, but not a reversal-learning task, cannot be due to a difference in reinforcement contingencies, but rather is due to a difference in the strategic requirements of the two tasks. Therefore, the findings suggest that the prelimbic areas support particular types of behavioral flexibility based on the behavioral operation required.

As stated above, a lower-order process allows the approach to and avoidance of a particular stimulus or scene. A lower-order process treats a stimulus or scene as a whole by applying a positive or negative valence. A higher-order process is required when conditions demand learning about stimulus attributes as opposed to a stimulus as a whole. In these cases, learning must go beyond simply attaching a positive or negative valence to stimuli within a particular dimension and instead requires attention to components of an object or scene—or abstract rules about component objects or scenes. Based on this idea of a higher-order process, there should be other conditions besides extradimensional shifts that would require a higher-order process. In one experiment, Dias and Aggleton[17] studied learning in a spatial-delayed match-to-sample test and nonmatch-to-sample test. Rats have a natural tendency to alternate[18] and thus can readily acquire a nonmatch-to-sample task that requires a subject to alternate choices between the sample and the test phase. This tendency to alternate has been commonly shown in spontaneous alternation tests in which a rat tends to choose the least-recently visited arm of a maze.[19] If rats are first trained to acquire a match-to-sample rule and therefore must switch away from their natural bias of using a nonmatch-to-sample strategy, prelimbic lesions impair acquisition.[17] Furthermore, if rats are first trained on a match-to-sample task and then switched to the nonmatch-to-sample version, prelimbic lesions still impair the shift. Thus, based on a situation where a valence could not simply be applied to either spatial location, but a more abstract rule applied, the prelimbic area appears critical for behavioral flexibility.

Paired-associate learning represents another way to examine whether a prefrontal cortex subregion supports a higher-order process. In paired-associate learning, a subject must learn to make a choice when two specific stimuli are associated together, but avoid choosing either stimulus when associated with other stimuli. Under these conditions a valence cannot be simply attributed to a particular stimulus. To examine whether the prelimbic area is critical for paired-associate learning, rats were trained on an object-spatial location paired-associate test using a go/no-go procedure.[20] Two objects, black and white blocks, were each placed in two different spatial locations. An object in one spatial location was associated with reinforcement, while in the other spatial location the object was never associated with reinforcement. The two objects had opposite pairings of spatial locations associated with reinforcement or no reinforcement. Therefore, in this task a rat must learn the association between spatial and visual object pairs and flexibly adapt responding. Prelimbic lesions impaired the learning of this paired-associate test. However, prelimbic lesions do not impair learning of either a visual object discrimination or a spatial discrimination.[10]

In summary, the prelimbic areas support behavioral flexibility in a number of conditions that include extradimensional shifts, switching between match-to-sample and nonmatch-to-sample rules, and paired-associate learning. In contrast, the prelimbic area does not appear critical for behavioral flexibility when conditions require the use of the same general strategy, but a shift in specific choices is required in reversal learning. Furthermore, when conditions require a shift in strategies, the prelimbic area may support the initial inhibition of the previously learned strategy and/or the ability to generate a new strategy.

INFRALIMBIC INVOLVEMENT IN BEHAVIORAL FLEXIBILITY

In several of the experiments described above, inactivation or lesions of the prelimbic area also partly encompassed the infralimbic area, which is found ventral to the prelimbic cortex. Thus, the deficits observed on certain set-shifting tests may have arisen because of damage to the infralimbic area or to a combination of the prelimbic and infralimbic subregions. A few experiments have specifically studied the infralimbic cortex in behavioral flexibility. Taken together, the experiments have not led to a clear understanding of how the infralimbic cortex may contribute to behavioral flexibility. For example, a couple of experiments have found that infralimbic lesions do not impair initial acquisition of a visual cue discrimination, but do impair visual cue reversal learning.[21,22] Interestingly, one study found that the reversal-learning deficit was not due to perseveration of the previously relevant choice pattern, but was due to the inability to reliably execute the new choice pattern once selected.[21] However, other studies reported that infralimbic lesions do not impair extinction of tone-shock pairings,[23] spatial reversal learning,[24] or latent inhibition.[25] Thus, infralimbic lesions impair learning when conditions require a shift in choice patterns in certain studies but not in others.

Killcross and Coutureau have investigated the effects of infralimbic lesions on the formation of habits with instrumental conditioning.[26] The study follows from the idea that in the early stage of instrumental conditioning a response is based on acquiring an action–outcome association, and the goal-directed outcome must be actively maintained for accurate responding.[27,28] With more extensive training, a stimulus–response habit is formed in which the goal-directed outcome no longer is actively maintained. This idea of the formation of actions and habits has received empirical support using instrumental devaluation procedures.[29] In particular, with limited instrumental training of a bar-press response for a food reward, instrumental performance reduces when the food reward or outcome is devalued either by pairing the food with lithium chloride or by satiating the rat with the food prior to the test session. In contrast, with extensive training, devaluing the outcome does not reduce instrumental performance. Lesions or temporary inactivation of the infralimbic area prevented the insensitivity to the instrumental devaluation observed with extensive training such that infralimbic lesions now showed a decreased instrumental performance.[26] These findings suggest that the infralimbic area may be important for the development of a stimulus–response habit or a more routed choice pattern. These results may be comparable to the reversal-learning deficit observed by Chudasama and Robbins following infralimbic lesions.[21] In this case, a reversal-learning deficit did not cause an increase in perseverative errors, but it did cause an increase in regressive errors. More specifically, if the infralimbic region is critical for the formation and maintenance of a habit or routine choice pattern, then lesions of the infralimbic area will not lead to perseverance of the learned choice pattern when conditions are reversed and a subject must inhibit the expression of the previously relevant choice pattern. That is, a subject will be more likely to initially give up the previously relevant choice pattern, but will have difficulty forming the new relevant choice pattern because the infralimbic region is critical for habit formation. In reversal-learning, this would not lead to an increase in perseveration, but it would lead to an increase in reliably executing the new choice pattern once selected. This is the pattern observed with infralimbic lesions in a visual cue reversal-learning task.[21]

One limitation of the interpretation provided above is that the findings from Killcross and Coutureau suggest that the infralimbic area is critical for the development of a habit formation, and thus in the acquisition phase of these discrimination tests infralimbic lesions should impair this initial learning.[26] However, different studies have reported that infralimbic lesions do not impair acquisition.[21,23,24] One possibility is that in these tasks a subject is still operating in an action–outcome mode even at the end of the acquisition phase, and thus the infralimbic area is not engaged. An alternative possibility is that in many of the discrimination tests there is extensive pretraining before acquisition testing begins, and this pretraining influences the initial learning process. Clearly, there is a need for a more systematic examination of experiments of the infralimbic area to better understand how this area may contribute to behavioral flexibility.

ORBITOFRONTAL CORTEX INVOLVEMENT IN BEHAVIORAL FLEXIBILITY

The rat orbitofrontal cortex is located predominantly in the lateral portion of the frontal cortex. Comparable to the medial frontal cortex in rats, it contains different subdivisions.[8] The majority of experiments that have investigated the role of the rat orbitofrontal cortex in behavioral flexibility have focused on the lateral orbital, ventral orbital, and/or agranular insular regions. The findings described below come from studies that involve manipulations of the lateral areas of the orbitofrontal cortex.

Studies investigating the contribution of the orbitofrontal cortex to behavioral flexibility have predominantly used reversal-learning tests. Studies involving lesions centered in the orbitofrontal cortex have commonly found that orbitofrontal damage does not impair acquisition of different discrimination tests, but does impair reversal-learning.[21,24,30–33] This occurred in a number of different types of reversal-learning tests that involved the flexible use of odor, visual cue, tactile, or spatial information. In a comparable manner, we found that infusion of muscimol into the lateral orbital or ventral orbital frontal cortex did not impair acquisition of a two-choice odor discrimination, but did impair reversal-learning (see FIG. 4A).[34] The reversal-learning impairment observed with orbitofrontal cortex inactivation was comparable whether muscimol injections were centered in the lateral or the ventral regions of the orbitofrontal cortex. Similar to that observed with prelimbic inactivation in extradimensional shifts, orbitofrontal cortex inactivation impaired reversal learning by selectively increasing perseverative errors (see FIG. 4B). This selective increase in perseverative errors has also been observed in other studies in which neurotoxic lesions of the orbitofrontal cortex impaired reversal learning.[21,24] These findings suggest that the orbitofrontal cortex supports learning when conditions require a switch in choice patterns as required in reversal learning and facilitates the ability to initially inhibit a previously relevant choice pattern and/or to generate a new choice pattern.

Orbitofrontal cortex lesions or inactivation producing perseveration during reversal learning has been reported for two-choice reversal-learning tests.[21,24,30–34] We explored whether a similar deficit would occur with orbitofrontal cortex inactivation during a four-choice odor discrimination. One advantage of using a four-choice discrimination is that two of the stimuli are never reinforced during acquisition or reversal learning. Therefore, this can provide information about whether the orbitofrontal cortex is important in reducing interference to irrelevant stimuli. In this study, irrelevant errors during the reversal-learning phase were counted as the number of trials in which a rat chose the never-reinforced stimuli after an initial choice. Comparable to the two-choice discrimination, orbitofrontal cortex inactivation did not impair initial learning, but did impair reversal learning (see FIG. 5A). However, the error pattern that emerged was unique. Specifically, orbitofrontal cortex inactivation increased perseverative, regressive, and irrelevant errors (see FIG. 5B). This pattern of results suggests that under these conditions the orbitofrontal cortex is not only critical for initial inhibition of a previously relevant choice pattern, but also critical for maintaining a choice pattern once selected, as well as reducing interference to irrelevant stimuli. With the increased number of stimuli to discriminate among, orbitofrontal cortex inactivation may lead to this broader range of errors in reversal learning because the orbitofrontal cortex is critical for a lower-order process that applies a valence to particular stimuli. Therefore, increasing the number of stimuli that must be inhibited from choosing requires an increased elimination process that manifests itself following orbitofrontal cortex inactivation as an increase in perseverative, regressive, and irrelevant errors.

There are findings from devaluation paradigms that also suggest that the orbitofrontal cortex is critical for flexible responding when a valence can

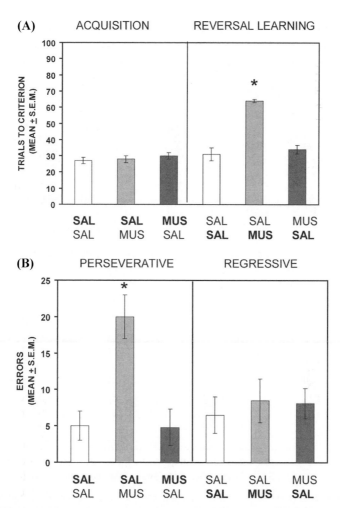

FIGURE 4. (A) Mean (± s.e.m.) trials to criterion in two-choice odor acquisition and reversal learning following bilateral infusions of saline or muscimol into the orbitofrontal cortex. Orbitofrontal cortex inactivation did not affect acquisition but impaired reversal learning. The treatment received in each phase of testing is in bold. SAL = saline; MUS = muscimol. *$P < 0.05$ versus controls. **(B)** Mean (± s.e.m.) number of perseverative and regressive errors in two-choice odor reversal learning after bilateral infusions of saline or muscimol into the orbitofrontal cortex. There was a significant increase in perseverative, but not regressive errors following orbitofrontal cortex inactivation. SAL = saline; MUS = muscimol. *$P < 0.05$ versus controls.

be applied to a stimulus. More specifically, orbitofrontal cortex lesions fail to decrease responding to a conditioned stimulus following devaluation of a reinforcer.[35,36] In devaluation paradigms a subject must first learn to respond to a cue that is associated with presentation of a food reinforcer. After the

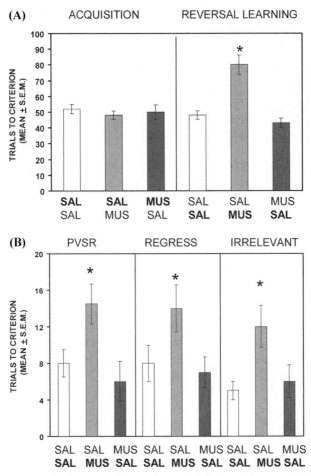

FIGURE 5. (A) Mean (± s.e.m.) trials to criterion in four-choice odor acquisition and reversal learning following bilateral infusions of saline or muscimol into the orbitofrontal cortex. Orbitofrontal cortex inactivation did not affect acquisition but impaired reversal learning. The treatment received in each phase of testing is in bold. SAL = saline; MUS = muscimol. *$P < 0.05$ versus controls. **(B)** Mean (± s.e.m.) number of perseverative, regressive, and irrelevant errors in four-choice odor reversal learning after bilateral infusions of saline or muscimol into the orbitofrontal cortex. There was a significant increase in perseverative, regressive, and irrelevant errors following orbitofrontal cortex inactivation. SAL = saline; PVSR = perseverative; MUS = muscimol. *$P < 0.05$ versus controls.

reinforcer is devalued by pairing the food with illness, this new association leads a normal rat to decrease responding to the previously associated cue, but orbitofrontal cortex lesions prevent rats from adjusting their responding to the cue.

Although there is convincing evidence that the rat orbitofrontal cortex is involved in learning when contingencies are reversed, few studies have examined the rat orbitofrontal cortex in other tests that require behavioral flexibility. One investigation studied whether orbitofrontal cortex lesions affect an extradimensional shift involving the use of odor and tactile information.[32] The study found that orbitofrontal cortex lesions do not impair performance in an extradimensional shift, but the same lesions do impair reversal learning. Taken together with the findings from prelimbic inactivation, these findings suggest that the prelimbic and orbitofrontal cortex support different behavioral operations to enable behavioral flexibility. This double dissociation observed between the orbitofrontal cortex and the prelimbic cortex on reversal-learning tests and extradimensional shifts cannot be explained by differences in the level of difficulty because orbitofrontal cortex inactivation also leads to impairments on a four-choice reversal-learning test, but prelimbic inactivation does not impair four-choice reversal learning. Instead, the pattern of results suggests that these separate prefrontal cortex regions differentially contribute to behavioral flexibility.

DORSOMEDIAL STRIATAL INVOLVEMENT IN BEHAVIORAL FLEXIBILITY

There is evidence that the orbitofrontal cortex and the prelimbic cortex differentially contribute to behavioral flexibility related to the behavioral operation required to flexibly adapt. Both the orbitofrontal cortex and the prelimbic area project to the dorsomedial striatum.[8] Because the dorsomedial striatum receives input from both of these prefrontal cortex areas, this brain area may also contribute to behavioral flexibility. Using a similar approach to investigate the contributions of the prefrontal cortex subregions to behavioral flexibility, a series of experiments have examined the effects of dorsomedial striatal inactivation on acquisition, reversal learning, and extradimensional shifts of different discrimination tests.

In the initial experiment, the effects of tetracaine injections into the dorsomedial striatum were investigated on the acquisition of either a visual cue or an egocentric response discrimination, then a shift to the other strategy.[37] In the egocentric response discrimination, a rat was required to make the same turn relative to its body (left or right) in order to receive a cereal reinforcement. In an egocentric response discrimination, the idea is that a rat learns to use proprioceptive and vestibular information to guide its response. Dorsomedial striatal inactivation did not impair acquisition of either a visual cue or an egocentric response strategy. Dorsomedial striatal inactivation did impair a shift between a visual cue and an egocentric response strategy. These results are comparable to those observed with manipulations of the prelimbic area. However, an examination of the error pattern revealed that dorsomedial striatal inactivation did not increase perseveration, but rather led to an increase in regressive errors. This was the opposite pattern to that observed with prelimbic inactivation, suggesting that these two areas both enable a shift in strategy, but they support different processes to facilitate an adaptation in strategy.

The dorsomedial striatum also plays a role in reversal learning. While inactivation of dorsomedial striatum did not impair acquisition of different discrimination tests, inactivation did impair reversal learning.[38,39] This was the case for spatial reversal learning as well as egocentric response reversal learning (see FIG. 6A). These findings are comparable to previous studies demonstrating that dorsomedial striatal lesions impair reversal learning.[40–42] In our experiments, an examination of the error pattern revealed that dorsomedial striatal inactivation also led to a selective increase in regressive errors during reversal learning comparable to that observed during the extradimensional shift (see FIG. 6B). Again, this is the opposite pattern to that observed in two-choice reversal-learning tests following orbitofrontal cortex inactivation.

The findings from studying the effects of dorsomedial striatal inactivation suggest that this striatal region plays a broader role in behavioral flexibility then either the prelimbic area or the orbitofrontal cortex alone. This may not be surprising because both regions project to the dorsomedial striatum. Furthermore, the dorsomedial striatum appears critical for the maintenance or reliable execution of a strategy once selected, but it is not critical for the initial inhibition of the previously relevant strategy or the generation of a new strategy. These results suggest that the dorsomedial striatum may dynamically interact with multiple prefrontal cortex subregions to facilitate behavioral flexibility in a distinct but complementary manner. More specifically, prefrontal cortex subregions may be critical for the generation of a new strategy. This allows the initial inhibition of the previously relevant strategy. However, once a new strategy is generated, it must be executed into the appropriate response pattern. The striatum, in coordination with different prefrontal cortex areas, may facilitate the execution of the appropriate response pattern for a particular strategy that is generated. Thus, the striatum in linking a particular response pattern with a specific strategy allows the reliable execution of a strategy once generated, as well as continual inhibition of previously relevant strategies.

SUMMARY AND CONCLUSIONS

The findings from a series of experiments indicate that the prelimbic cortex and the orbitofrontal cortex differentially contribute to behavioral flexibility. The prelimbic area supports behavioral flexibility when conditions require a shift in strategies or rules. This is observed in conditions in which an individual must inhibit responding based on one stimulus dimension and instead respond based on a different dimension. Under these conditions, the prelimbic area facilitates the ability to initially shift away from a previously relevant strategy, but once a new strategy is selected the prelimbic area is not critical for the reliable execution of that strategy. The prelimbic area is also involved in adaptive

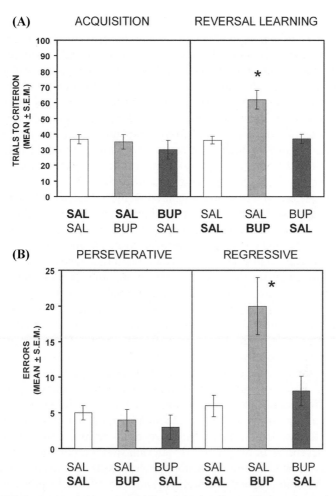

FIGURE 6. (A) Mean ($\pm$ s.e.m.) trials to criterion in two-choice egocentric response acquisition and reversal learning following bilateral infusions of saline or bupivacaine into the dorsomedial striatum. Dorsomedial striatal inactivation did not affect acquisition but impaired reversal learning. The treatment received in each phase of testing is in bold. SAL = saline; BUP = bupivacaine. *$P < 0.05$ versus controls. **(B)** Mean ($\pm$ s.e.m.) number of perseverative and regressive errors in two-choice egocentric response reversal learning after bilateral infusions of saline or bupivacaine into the dorsomedial striatum. There was a significant increase in regressive, but not perseverative, errors following dorsomedial striatal inactivation. SAL = saline; BUP = bupivacaine. *$P < 0.05$ versus controls.

responses when more abstract rules must be used in a context, e.g., switching between match-to-sample and nonmatch-to-sample rule. Furthermore, the prelimbic area supports learning when different stimuli must be integrated and the relationship between different stimuli learned as in paired-associate tasks. In contrast, the prelimbic area does not appear critical for flexibly adapting when conditions require a reversal in choice patterns or exemplars. Taken together, the pattern of findings suggests that the prelimbic area supports a higher-order process for flexibly adapting to a change in environmental conditions.

Several studies indicate that the orbitofrontal cortex supports learning when the general strategy remains the same but a shift in specific choices is required. This is commonly observed in reversal-learning tasks. Comparable to the prelimbic area, the orbitofrontal cortex supports a process that enables the ability to initially shift away from a previously relevant choice. However, as the level of difficulty is increased with more stimuli to discriminate among, the orbitofrontal cortex may support multiple processes for facilitating a switch in choice patterns. One study examined the effects of rat orbitofrontal cortex lesions on an extradimensional shift and revealed that there was no deficit. These results suggest that the orbitofrontal cortex and the prelimbic cortex support different behavioral operations to enable behavioral flexibility. However, future studies are clearly needed to better understand how the orbitofrontal cortex contributes to behavioral flexibility. One issue is that within the orbitofrontal cortex there are different subregions. It is unknown whether the separate orbitofrontal subregions differentially contribute to behavioral flexibility. Related to this point, it should be noted that at the rostral pole in the ventromedial frontal cortex the rat contains a medial orbital subregion that makes up part of the larger orbitofrontal cortex. There is a paucity of experiments that have investigated the medial orbital region.

There is some evidence that the infralimbic subregion contributes to behavioral flexibility. A role for the infralimbic region in behavioral flexibility has come from studies that have demonstrated that infralimbic lesions impair reversal learning but do not impair the initial acquisition of a discrimination. One study further demonstrated that the reversal-learning impairment was not due to perseverance of the previously relevant strategy, but once a new choice pattern was selected infralimbic lesions prevented the maintenance of that new strategy. This contrasts with the prelimbic and orbitofrontal regions, which are important for the initial inhibition of a previously relevant strategy. Although there is some evidence that the infralimbic region supports behavioral flexibility, not all studies have demonstrated this. Furthermore, the range of tests to examine infralimbic involvement in behavioral flexibility has been limited. A more comprehensive examination of possible infralimbic contributions to behavioral flexibility is needed. Future studies should utilize a wider range of behavioral paradigms.

The dorsomedial striatum, which receives input from both the orbitofrontal cortex and the prelimbic area, plays a broader role in behavioral flexibility in that this region supports both reversal-learning and extradimensional shifts. In contrast to prefrontal cortex subregions, the dorsomedial striatum does not facilitate the initial shift away from a previous strategy, but it is critical for the maintenance of a new strategy once selected. These results indicate that the dorsomedial striatum, in conjunction with prefrontal cortex subregions, can enable behavioral flexibility by supporting distinct but complementary functions. Thus, these areas together are part of a larger neural system that allows one to adapt successfully in an ever-changing environment.

REFERENCES

1. DIAS, R., T.W. ROBBINS & A.C. ROBERTS. 1997. Dissociable forms of inhibitory control within prefrontal cortex with an analog of the Wisconsin Card Sort Test: Restriction to novel situations and independence from "on-line" processing. J. Neurosci. **17:** 9285–9287.
2. JONES, B. & M. MISHKIN. 1972. Limbic lesions and the problem of stimulus-reinforcement associations. Exp. Neurol. **36:** 362–377.
3. MILNER, B. 1963. Effects of different brain lesions of card sorting. Arch. Neurol. **9:** 90–100.
4. MONCHI, O., M. PETRIDES, V. PETRE, *et al.* 2001. Wisconsin card sorting revisited: distinct neural circuits participating in different stages of the task identified by event-related functional magnetic resonance imaging. J. Neurosci. **21:** 7733–7741.
5. NONNEMAN, A.J., J. VOIGT & B.E. KOLB. 1974. Comparisons of behavioral effects of hippocampal and prefrontal cortex lesions in the rat. J. Comp. Physiol. Psychol. **87:** 249–260.
6. ALEXANDER, G.E., M.R. DELONG & P.L. STRICK. 1986. Parallel organization of functionally segregated circuits linking basal ganglia and cortex. Ann. Rev. Neurosci. **9:** 357–381.
7. WISE, S.P., E.A. MURRAY & C.R. GERFEN. 1996. The frontal cortex—basal ganglia system in primates. Crit. Rev. Neurobiol. **10:** 317–356.
8. BERENDSE, H.W., Y. GALIS-DE GRAAF & H.J. GROENEWEGEN. 1992. Topographical organization and relationship with ventral striatal compartments of prefrontal corticostriatal projections in the rat. J. Comp. Neurol. **316:** 314–347.
9. RAGOZZINO, M.E., S. DETRICK & R.P. KESNER. 1999. Involvement of the prelimbic-infralimbic areas of the rodent prefrontal cortex in behavioral flexibility for place and response learning. J. Neurosci. **19:** 4585–4594.
10. RAGOZZINO, M.E., C. WILCOX, M. RASO & R.P. KESNER. 1999. Involvement of rodent prefrontal cortex subregions in strategy switching. Behav. Neurosci. **113:** 32–41.
11. RAGOZZINO, M.E., J. KIM, D. HASSERT, *et al.* 2003. The contribution of the rat prelimbic-infralimbic areas to different forms of task switching. Behav. Neurosci. **117:** 1054–1065.
12. BUNSEY, M. & H. EICHENBAUM. 1996. Selective damage to the hippocampal region blocks long-term retention of a natural and nonspatial stimulus-stimulus association. Nature **379:** 255–257.
13. BIRRELL, J.M. & V.J. BROWN. 2000. Medial frontal cortex mediates perceptual attentional set-shifting in the rat. J. Neurosci. **20:** 4320–4324.
14. FLORESCO, S.B., O. MAGYAR, S. GHODS-SHARIFI, *et al.* 2006. Multiple dopamine receptor subtypes in the medial prefrontal cortex of the rat regulate set-shifting. Neuropsychopharmacology **31:** 297–309.
15. RAGOZZINO, M.E. 2002. The effects of dopamine D1 receptor blockade in the prelimbic-infralimbic areas on behavioral flexibility. Learn. Mem. **9:** 18–28.

16. STEFANI, M.R., K. GROTH & B. MOGHADDAM. 2003. Glutamate receptors in the rat medial prefrontal cortex regulate set-shifting ability. Behav. Neurosci. **117:** 728–737.

17. DIAS, R. & J.P. AGGLETON. 2000. Effects of selective excitotoxic prefrontal lesions on acquisition of nonmatching- and matching-to-place in the T-maze in the rat: differential involvement of the prelimbic-infralimbic and anterior cingulate cortices in providing behavioural flexibility. Eur. J. Neurosci. **12:** 4457–4466.

18. DEMBER, W.N. & H. FOWLER. 1958. Spontaneous alternation behavior. Psychol. Bull. **55:** 412–428.

19. RAGOZZINO, M.E., K. UNICK & P.E. GOLD. 1996. Hippocampal acetylcholine release during memory testing: Augmentation by glucose. Proc. Nat. Acad. Sci. USA **93:** 4693–4698.

20. KESNER, R.P. & M.E. RAGOZZINO. 2003. The role of the prefrontal cortex object-place learning: a test of the attribute specificity model. Behav. Brain Res. **146:** 159–165.

21. CHUDASAMA, Y. & T.W. ROBBINS. 2003. Dissociable contributions of the orbitofrontal and infralimbic cortex to Pavlovian autoshaping and discrimination reversal learning: further evidence for the functional heterogeneity of the rodent frontal cortex. J. Neurosci. **23:** 8771–8780.

22. LI, L. & J. SHAO. 1998. Restricted lesions to ventral prefrontal subareas block reversal learning but not visual discrimination learning in rats. Physiol. Behav. **65:** 371–379.

23. QUIRK, G.J., G.K. RUSSO, J.L. BARRON & K. LEBRON. 2000. The role of ventromedial prefrontal cortex in the recovery of extinguished fear. J. Neurosci. **20:** 6225–6231.

24. BOULOUGOURIS, V., J.W. DALLEY & T.W. ROBBINS. 2007. Effects of orbitofrontal, infralimbic and prelimbic cortical lesions on serial spatial reversal learning in the rat. Behav. Brain Res. **179:** 219–228.

25. JOEL, D., I. WEINER & J. FELDON. 1997. Electrolytic lesions of the medial prefrontal cortex in rats disrupt performance on an analog of the Wisconsin Card Sorting Test, but do not disrupt latent inhibition: implications for animal models of schizophrenia. Behav. Brain Res. **85:** 187–201.

26. KILLCROSS A.S. & E. COUTUREAU. 2003. Coordination of actions and habits in the medial prefrontal cortex of rats. Cereb. Cortex. **13:** 400–408.

27. BALLEINE, B.W. 1992. The role of incentive learning in instrumental performance following shifts in primary motivation. J. Exp. Psychol. Anim. Behav. Process. **18:** 236–250.

28. DICKINSON, A. 1985. Actions and habits: the development of behavioural autonomy. Phil. Trans. R. Soc. Lond. **308:** 67–78.

29. BALLEINE, B.W. & A. DICKINSON. 1998. Goal-directed instrumental action: contingency and incentive learning and their cortical substrates. Neuropharmacology **37:** 407–419.

30. BOHN, I., C. GIERTLER & W. HAUBER. 2003. Orbital prefrontal cortex and guidance of instrumental behaviour in rats under reversal conditions. Behav. Brain Res. **143:** 49–56.

31. FERRY, A.T., X.C.M. LU & J.L. PRICE. 2000. Effects of excitotoxic lesions in the ventral striatopallidal-thalamocortical pathway on odor reversal learning: inability to extinguish an incorrect response. Exp. Brain Res. **131:** 320–335.

32. MCALONAN, K. & V.J. BROWN. 2003. Orbital prefrontal cortex mediates reversal learning and not attentional set-shifting in the rat. Behav. Brain Res. **146:** 97–103.

33. SCHOENBAUM, G., S.L. NUGENT, M.L. SADDORIS & B. SETLOW. 2002. Orbitofrontal lesions in rats impair reversal but not acquisition of go, no-go odor discriminations. Neuroreport **13:** 885–890.
34. KIM, J. & M.E. RAGOZZINO. 2005. The involvement of the orbitofrontal cortex in learning under changing task contingencies. Neurobiol. of Learn. Mem. **83:** 125–133.
35. GALLAGHER, M., R.W. MCMAHAN & G. SCHOENBAUM. 1999. Orbitofrontal cortex and representation of incentive value in associative learning. J. Neurosci. **19:** 6610–6614.
36. PICKENS, C.L., M.P. SADDORIS, B. SETLOW, *et al.* 2003. Different roles for orbitofrontal cortex and basolateral amygdala in a reinforcer devaluation task. J. Neurosci. **23:** 11078–11084.
37. RAGOZZINO, M.E., K.E. RAGOZZINO, S.J. MIZUMORI & R.P. KESNER. 2002. Role of the dorsomedial striatum in behavioral flexibility for response and visual cue discrimination learning. Behav. Neurosci. **116:** 105–115.
38. RAGOZZINO, M.E., J. JIH & A. TZAVOS. 2002. Involvement of the dorsomedial striatum in behavioral flexibility: role of muscarinic cholinergic receptors. Brain Res. **953:** 205–214.
39. RAGOZZINO, M.E. & D. CHOI. 2004. Dynamic changes in acetylcholine output in the medial striatum during place reversal learning. Learn. Mem. **11:** 70–77.
40. KIRKBY, R.J. 1969. Caudate nucleus lesions and perseverative behavior. Physiol. Behav. **4:** 451–454.
41. KOLB, B. 1977. Studies on the caudate-putamen and the dorsomedialthalamic nucleus of the rat: implications for mammalian frontal-lobe functions. Physiol. Behav. **18:** 237–244.
42. PISA, M. & J. CYR. 1990. Regionally selective roles of the rat's striatum in modality specific discrimination learning and forelimb reaching. Behav. Brain Res. **37:** 281–292.
43. PAXINOS, G. & C. WATSON. 1996. The rat brain in stereotaxic coordinates. 3rd Edition. Academic Press.

A Comparison of Reward-Contingent Neuronal Activity in Monkey Orbitofrontal Cortex and Ventral Striatum

Guiding Actions toward Rewards

JANINE M. SIMMONS,[a] SABRINA RAVEL,[a] MUNETAKA SHIDARA,[b] AND BARRY J. RICHMOND[a]

[a]Laboratory of Neuropsychology, National Institute of Mental Health, Bethesda, Maryland, USA

[b]Graduate School of Comprehensive Human Sciences, University of Tsukuba, Tsukuba, Japan

ABSTRACT: We have investigated how neuronal activity in the orbitofrontal-ventral striatal circuit is related to reward-directed behavior by comparing activity in these two regions during a visually guided reward schedule task. When a set of visual cues provides information about reward contingency, that is, about whether or not a trial will be rewarded, significant subpopulations of neurons in both orbitofrontal cortex and ventral striatum encode this information. Orbitofrontal and ventral striatal neurons also differentiate between rewarding and non-rewarding trial outcomes, whether or not those outcomes were predicted. The size of the neuronal subpopulation encoding reward contingency is twice as large in orbitofrontal cortex (50% of neurons) as in ventral striatum (26%). Reward-contingency-dependent activity also appears earlier during a trial in orbitofrontal cortex than in ventral striatum. The peak reward-contingency representation in orbitofrontal cortex (31% of neurons), occurs during the wait period, a period of high anticipation prior to any action. The peak ventral striatal representation of reward contingency (18%) occurs during the go period, a time of action. We speculate that signals from orbitofrontal cortex bias ventral striatal activity, and that a flow of reward-contingency information from orbitofrontal cortex to ventral striatum serves to guide actions toward rewards.

KEYWORDS: motivation; limbic system; basal ganglia; electrophysiology

Address for correspondence: Janine M. Simmons, M.D., Ph.D., Room 1B80, Building 49, Laboratory of Neuropsychology, National Institute of Mental Health, Bethesda, MD 20892. Voice: 301-402-4599; fax: 301-402-0046.

simmonsj@mail.nih.gov

Ann. N.Y. Acad. Sci. 1121: 376–394 (2007). © 2007 New York Academy of Sciences.
doi: 10.1196/annals.1401.028

INTRODUCTION

The neural processes underlying complex reward-directed behaviors must include the integration of signals from many brain regions. To study how coordinated activity across brain regions is related to these behaviors, we have recorded responses from neurons in a series of closely and heavily connected regions while monkeys perform a reward schedule task. Here, we compare activity in the orbitofrontal cortex and ventral striatum. Both orbitofrontal cortex and ventral striatum play important roles in encoding reward-related information, and the orbitofrontal-ventral striatal circuit has been proposed as one pathway by which emotional and motivational signals from the limbic system influence action signals in striatum.[1,2]

Physiological responses in orbitofrontal cortex and ventral striatum show relatively similar activation patterns to rewards and to stimuli that predict rewards. In animals and humans, differential activations occur in both regions during anticipation and/or delivery of primary rewards.[3–14,36] In humans, orbitofrontal and striatal areas also respond to the direct experience of winning money and in anticipation of an upcoming financial payoff.[15–17] Additional studies have shown that orbitofrontal cortex and striatum specifically encode the values of anticipated and delivered rewards.[18–31]

Below, we directly compare the activity of orbitofrontal and ventral striatal neurons during a visually guided reward schedule task and determine the extent to which reward information modulates activity during different time periods in this task. We find that orbitofrontal neurons are more likely to encode information about reward contingency before any action is performed, whereas ventral striatal neurons encode this information at the time of the needed action. Taking into account the known neuroanatomic projections from orbitofrontal cortex to ventral striatum, we suggest that signals from the orbitofrontal cortex serve to bias ventral striatal activity, and in so doing, to guide actions toward rewards.

BEHAVIOR IN THE REWARD SCHEDULE TASK

In the reward schedule task, monkeys perform schedules of trials, in which each trial consists of a sequential red–green color discrimination (FIG. 1A). Monkeys must complete each trial correctly before progressing to the next trial in a schedule (FIG. 1B). If an error is made on a given trial, no explicit penalty is imposed, but that trial is presented again until it is completed correctly. Early trials in the multi-trial schedules are unrewarded. A liquid reward is delivered after successful completion of the final trial in each schedule. Schedules of 1, 2, or 3 trials are randomly inter-mixed during a session.

The visual cues presented at the beginning of each trial provide two different contexts. In the Valid cue context, the brightness of each visual cue and schedulestate are paired (as in FIG. 1B), so each cue provides information about

(A)

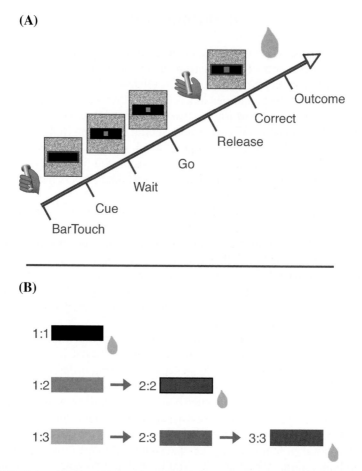

(B)

FIGURE 1. **(A)** Events occurring in each trial of the reward schedule task. Trials begin when the monkey touches a bar mounted at the front of the chair. A visual cue then appears alone for a time period between 0.4 and 2.5 s. The visual cue remains on for the duration of the trial. The wait signal (a red spot) appears for 0.4–1.5 s, and the monkey must hold the bar until the red spot turns green (the go signal). A trial is performed correctly when the monkey releases the bar between 0.2 and 1.0 s after the go signal. Correct trials are signaled by the green spot turning blue. Trial outcome follows the correct signal. In rewarded trials (as illustrated) a liquid reward is delivered. **(B)** Cue sequences within each schedule. Schedules contain sequences of 1, 2, or 3 trials. The schedule state (e.g., 1:1, 1:2, 2:2, 1:3, 2:3, and 3:3) indicates the trial and schedule length. In the Valid cue context, schedule states are differentiated by the brightness of the visual cue (as illustrated). In the Random cue context, the visual cue on each trial is randomly chosen from the four possible brightnesses ($P = 0.25$/cue) and has no relation to the underlying schedule state. After correct performance on each trial, the monkey progresses to the next trial in the schedule (*arrows*), receiving a reward at the end of a complete schedule (liquid drop). If an error is made, the monkey must repeat that trial, but is not required to return to the beginning of the schedule. After successful completion of the current schedule, a new schedule is picked at random. (In color in *Annals* online.)

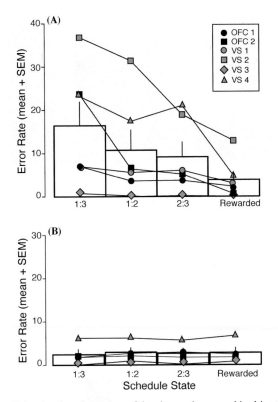

FIGURE 2. Behavioral performance of the six monkeys used in this study. Behavioral sessions consist of blocks of Valid and Random cue trials. Monkeys are not specifically trained to use cue-related information to perform the task. Monkeys must release a touch bar after detection of the red–green color change in every trial, regardless of the cue or context. Error rate serves as a behavioral measure of the monkey's motivational level during each trial. **(A)** Valid cue context: As a group, monkeys had the lowest error rates in the rewarded schedule states, and progressively higher error rates as a function of the number of trials remaining in the schedule (group chi-square tests for linear trend in 2- and 3-trial schedules, $P < 0.001$). Schedule states are indicated on the abscissa (1:3, 1:2, 2:3; rewarded schedule states include 1:1, 2:2, 3:3). The error rate is plotted on the ordinate (mean % errors across 6 monkeys + SEM). Note that individual monkeys had widely differing sensitivities to the schedules in this context, but the behavioral trend remained the same in each monkey. Data points from individual monkeys (OFC1-OFC 2 [black symbols], VS1-VS 4 [gray symbols]) are superimposed and connected with line segments to show the decreasing trend in error rates (individual chi-square tests for linear trend in 2-trial schedules, $P < 0.001$ for all monkeys except VS3; individual chi-square tests for linear trend in 3-trial schedules, $P < 0.001$ for all monkeys). **(B)** Random cue context: Cues were randomly selected on each trial; across a block of Random cue trials, each schedule state included cues of every brightness. Monkeys responded with low and indistinguishable error rates across all schedule states (group chi-square tests for linear trend in 2- and 3-trial schedules, $P = 0.6$ and 0.35, respectively). Data were analyzed from four monkeys in the Random context (OFC 1-OFC 2 [black symbols], VS 3- VS 4 [gray symbols]), and individual data points are superimposed and connected with line segments.

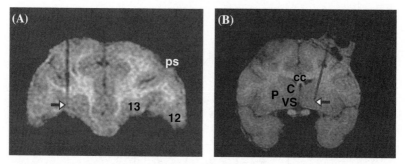

FIGURE 3. MRIs showing recording electrodes in **(A)** area 13 of orbitofrontal cortex (approximately 32.7 mm rostral to the interaural line in monkey OFC 1; ps: principal sulcus) and **(B)** ventral striatum (approximately 22.35 mm rostral to the interaural line in monkey VS3; cc: corpus callosum; C: caudate; P: Putamen; VS: ventral striatum). *Dark lines* indicate MR artifacts caused by the electrodes themselves. *Arrowheads* placed to mark electrode tips and highlight recording sites. MRIs were obtained on a 1.5 T GE Signa unit, using a 5-inch GP surface coil and a 3D volume SPGR pulse sequence (TE 6, TR 25, flip angle 30, FOV of 11 cm, slice thickness of 1 mm).

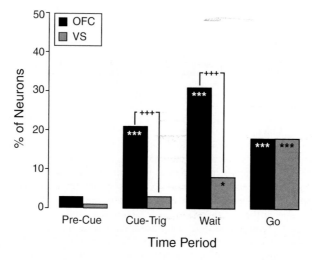

FIGURE 4. Percentages of OFC (*black*) and VS (*gray*) neurons with reward-contingency-dependent activity modulations in the pre-cue, cue-triggered, wait, and go time periods during the Valid cue context. Neither OFC nor VS neurons encoded reward contingency prior to cue onset. Significant proportions of OFC neurons encoded reward contingency in all other periods (1-sided binomial tests, ***$P < 0.001$); this OFC subpopulation reached its peak size during the wait period. The proportion of VS neurons encoding reward contingency increased as each trial progressed, reaching a size statistically greater than chance in the wait period (1-sided binomial test, *$P < 0.05$) and peaking during the go period (1-sided binomial test, ***$P < 0.001$). In the cue-triggered and wait periods, the proportion of neurons with reward-contingency-dependent activity was significantly larger in the OFC than the VS context (2-sided proportions tests, +++$P < 0.001$).

whether or not a trial will be rewarded. In the Random cue context, the cue on any given trial is chosen randomly from the set of cues, so the cue provides no information about reward contingency.

During the Valid cue context, monkeys' error rates are directly related to the number of trials remaining before the reward: the largest number of errors occurs in the first trial of the three trial schedules, and the fewest errors occur in the rewarded trials (FIG. 2A).[7,9,32,34–36] In the Random cue context, error rates are low and indistinguishable across all schedule states (FIG. 2B). From their performance in the Random cue context, we know that monkeys are capable of performing well in every trial. We therefore interpret the behavior in the Valid cue context as showing that monkeys are most highly motivated when the current trial will be rewarded and become progressively less motivated to perform as the number of remaining trials increases.[7,9,32–36]

NEURONAL ENCODING OF REWARD-RELATED INFORMATION

In our study of orbitofrontal cortex, we observed that neurons appear to have changes in activity over the course of each trial, and our analyses of orbitofrontal recordings were designed to characterize these activity modulations. Rather than identifying and counting the number of neurons with phasic changes in firing rate to each event, we identified neurons with differences in neuronal activity between groups of schedule states during a series of event-related time periods. We found that orbitofrontal neurons encode information about preceding as well as upcoming rewards.[36]

In the reward schedule task, ventral striatal neurons respond phasically at cue onset, near bar release and near reward delivery, and carry information about reward contingency primarily at the time of bar release and reward delivery.[9,37] To compare directly the timing of activity modulations in ventral striatum with those seen in orbitofrontal cortex, we have now carried out the same analysis as was done for orbitofrontal cortex. We have included Valid cue data from the earlier study of ventral striatum[9] as well as data from another ventral striatal experiment (Ravel and Richmond, unpublished data) in which the cue-randomization procedure was the same as that used in the orbitofrontal study.[36]

Different monkeys were used in the orbitofrontal and each of the two ventral striatal experiments. Single neurons were recorded after behavior on the reward schedule task had stabilized. Data were analyzed from every well-isolated neuron recorded for at least 100 trials. Neuronal activity was quantified by counting spikes during five 300-ms time periods in each trial: (1) prior to cue appearance (precue period), (2) after cue appearance (cue-triggered period), (3) during the wait period, (4) after the go signal (go period), and (5) after trial outcome (outcome period).

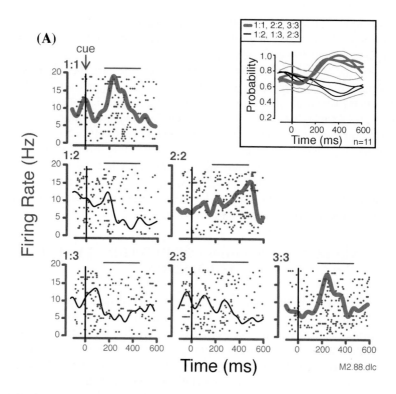

FIGURE 5. Reward-contingency-dependent activity of orbitofrontal neurons during the cue-triggered and wait periods in the Valid cue context. Individual rasters are shown for each of the six schedule states. Each row of *dots* represents an individual trial in the task. The ordinate shows firing rate per trial (in spikes/s). Spike density function curves (bandwidth = 25 ms) are superimposed on each raster. *Thick gray lines* indicate the rewarded schedule states; *thin black lines*, the unrewarded schedule states. For this study, a 2-level ANOVA was used to quantify differences in firing rates between the rewarded and unrewarded schedule states. **(A)** Cue-triggered period: In this example, activity levels in the rewarded trials (1:1, 2:2, 3:3, *thick gray lines*) were significantly higher than in the unrewarded trials (1:2, 1:3, 2:3, *thin black lines*; 2-level, 1-way ANOVA, $F_{1,201} = 28.7$, $P < .001$). Rasters are aligned on cue onset (0 ms, vertical line), and the cue-triggered period extended from 150 to 450 ms (*horizontal lines* above rasters). *Inset:* Normalized population spike density functions for the 11 cells with higher firing rates in rewarded trials. Six additional cells had higher firing rates in unrewarded trials. Each *thick gray line* represents one of the three rewarded schedule states. Each *thin black line* represents one of the three unrewarded schedule states. *Thin light gray lines* represent the outer bounds of the standard errors for each set of curves. **(B)** Wait period: In this example, activity levels in the rewarded trials were significantly higher than in the unrewarded trials (2-level, 1-way ANOVA, $F_{1,125} = 33.5$, $P < 0.001$). Rasters are aligned on the time at which the red spot appeared (0 ms, vertical line), and the wait period extended from 300 to 600 ms after the appearance of the red spot (*horizontal lines* above rasters). *Inset:* Normalized population spike density functions for the 17 cells with higher firing rates in rewarded trials. Eight additional cells had higher firing rates in unrewarded trials.

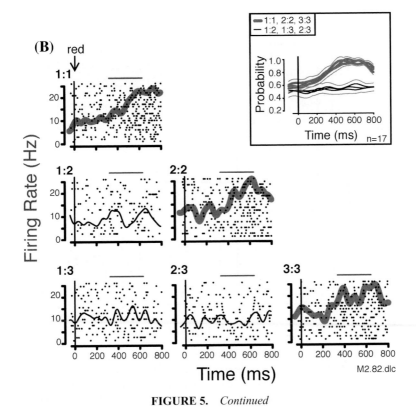

FIGURE 5. *Continued*

We have focused our analyses on the relationships between neuronal activity and reward contingency, and neuronal activity and trial outcome. We categorized neurons as encoding information about reward contingency when the spike counts in rewarded versus unrewarded trials were significantly different during one or more of the first four time periods (2-level, 1-way ANOVA, $P < 0.01$). The same analysis was applied during the outcome period: we categorized neurons as encoding trial outcome information when the spike counts during this last period were significantly different between rewarded and unrewarded trials (2-level, 1-way ANOVA, $P < 0.01$).

Eighty neurons were recorded in two monkeys from areas 11/13 of orbitofrontal cortex (FIG. 3A) during the Valid cue context; 58 of these were also recorded during the Random cue context.[36] In the ventral striatum (FIG. 3B), 267 neurons were recorded from four monkeys during the Valid cue context, with 46 neurons from two monkeys recorded during the Random cue context(Ravel and Richmond, unpublished data).[9]

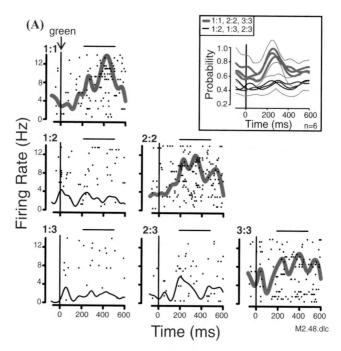

FIGURE 6.   Reward-contingency-dependent activity in the Valid Cue context during the go period. **(A)** Orbitofrontal neurons: In this example, activity levels in the rewarded trials (1:1, 2:2, 3:3, *thick gray lines*) were significantly higher than in the unrewarded trials (1:2, 1:3, 2:3, *thin black lines*; 2-level, 1-way ANOVA, $F_{1,166} = 71.6$, $P < 0.001$). Rasters are aligned on the time at which the red spot turned green (0 ms, vertical line), and the go period extended from 200 to 500 ms after the spot turned green (*horizontal lines* above rasters). *Inset:* Normalized population spike density functions for the 6 cells with higher firing rates in rewarded trials. Eight additional cells had higher firing rates in unrewarded trials. **(B)** Ventral striatal neurons: In this example, activity levels in the rewarded trials were significantly higher than in the unrewarded trials (2-level, 1-way ANOVA, $F_{1,164} = 33.9$, $P < 0.001$). Rasters are aligned on the time at which the red spot turned green (0 ms, vertical line), and the go period extended from 150 to 450 ms after the spot turned green (*horizontal lines* above rasters). *Inset:* Normalized population spike density functions for the 33 cells with higher firing rates in rewarded trials. Fourteen additional cells had higher firing rates in unrewarded trials. The proportion of ventral striatal neurons with higher firing rates in rewarded trials (33/267) was indistinguishable from that in orbitofrontal cortex (6/80) (2-sided proportions test, $P = 0.31$). Plotting conventions as in FIGURE 5.

Activity Modulations across Time Periods

In the Valid cue context, activity was modulated in relation to reward contingency in both orbitofrontal cortex and ventral striatum. The proportion of neurons encoding reward contingency was significantly larger in orbitofrontal cortex (40/80; 50%) than in ventral striatum (70/267; 26%; 2-sided propor-

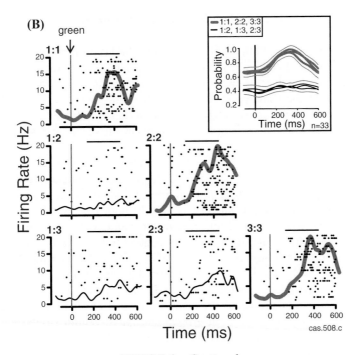

FIGURE 6. *Continued*

tions test, $\chi^2 = 15.0$, df $= 1$, $P < 0.001$). The proportion of neurons with reward-contingency-dependent activity modulations in more than one time period was also significantly larger in orbitofrontal cortex (22/80; 28%) than in ventral striatum (30/267; 11%; 2-sided proportions test, $\chi^2 = 11.5$, df $= 1$, $P < 0.001$).

Reward-contingency-dependent activity modulations began and peaked earlier in orbitofrontal cortex than in ventral striatum (FIG. 4). Prior to cue onset, neither orbitofrontal nor ventral striatal neurons encoded reward-contingency information (1-sided binomial tests; OFC $P = 0.9$; VS $P = 0.99$). In orbitofrontal cortex, a significant proportion of neurons (21%) began to differentiate between to-be-rewarded and unrewarded trials during the cue-triggered period (example in FIG. 5A). This proportion increased to reach a peak of 31% during the wait period (example in FIG. 5B), and then decreased to 18% during the go period (example in FIG. 6A). In contrast, the proportion of ventral striatal neurons encoding reward contingency increased steadily across time in a trial, peaking at 18% during the go period (example in FIG. 6B).

Activity Modulations between Contexts

Neuronal activity in both orbitofrontal cortex and ventral striatum depended upon task context. In the Valid cue context, where the visual cues provide information about reward, neuronal firing rates depended upon reward contingency (see above). In the Random cue context, where the visual cues provided no information about reward contingency, neuronal activity did not differ significantly between rewarded and unrewarded trials in any of the time periods prior to trial outcome (FIG. 7).

At the time of the trial outcome, the monkeys know whether or not they received a reward in both the Valid and Random cue contexts. As has been shown before, neuronal activity in both orbitofrontal cortex and ventral striatum depends upon reward delivery.[5,7,10,11] In both regions, the proportion of neurons encoding the trial outcome in the Valid context was not significantly different from that in the Random context (OFC: Valid 35%, Random 23%, 2-sided proportions test: $\chi^2 = 1.8$, df $= 1$, $P = 0.2$; VS: Valid 26% Random 26%, $\chi^2 = 0$, df $= 1$, $P = 1$). However, the time of onset of the activity modulations depended on context (FIG. 8). In the Valid cue context, where the trial outcome can be predicted, the neuronal activity changed before the time of reward delivery in 13/28 orbitofrontal and 26/70 ventral striatal neurons. In the Random context, the activity differences did not occur until after the time of possible reward onset, when the monkey would know whether or not a reward had been delivered.

DISCUSSION

An overarching goal of ours is to understand how the functions of interconnected brain regions are related to reward-directed behavior. Here, we have focused on the orbitofrontal cortex and ventral striatum. Neurons in both orbitofrontal cortex and ventral striatum encode information about reward contingency and trial outcome. We have found that the population of neurons encoding reward contingency is larger in orbitofrontal cortex than in ventral striatum. Neuronal activity differences due to reward contingency also appear earlier in orbitofrontal cortex than in ventral striatum. Representations of trial outcome are similar in orbitofrontal cortex and ventral striatum, with significant reward-dependent activity in both the Valid and Random cue contexts.

Reward-Contingency Encoding

Orbitofrontal neurons have responses related to stimulus-reinforcer associations and expected reward value.[4,10,11,19,20,26,27,29,38] Ventral striatal neurons also anticipate and respond to rewards.[5-7,9,39,40] By directly comparing unit

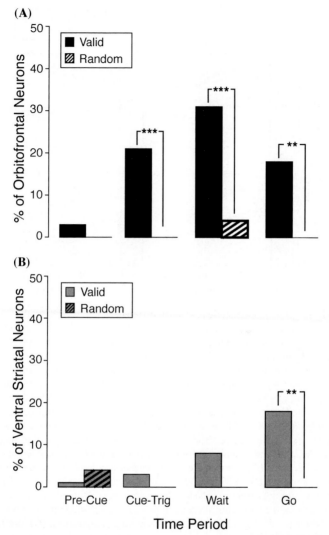

FIGURE 7. Percentages of orbitofrontal and ventral striatal neurons with reward-contingency-dependent activity in the pre-cue, cue-triggered, wait, and go time periods during the Valid cue (*solid bars*) and Random cue (*hatched bars*) contexts. **(A)** Orbitofrontal neurons: Significantly more orbitofrontal neurons showed reward-contingency-dependent activity in the Valid (*solid black bars*) than the Random (*hatched bars*) context during the cue-triggered, wait and go periods (2-sided proportions tests; **$P < 0.01$, ***$P < 0.001$). **(B)** Ventral striatal neurons: Significantly more ventral striatal neurons showed reward-contingency-dependent activity in the Valid (*solid gray bars*) than the Random (*hatched bars*) context during the go period (2-sided proportions test; **$P < 0.01$). The difference between the proportion of ventral striatal neurons encoding reward contingency in the Valid and Random cue contexts during the wait period did not reach statistical significance (2-sided proportions test; $P = 0.09$).

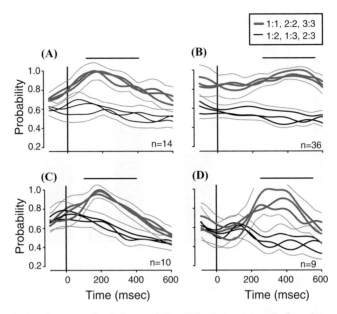

FIGURE 8. Outcome-dependent activity differences appear before the outcome in the Valid cue context and after the outcome in the Random context in both orbitofrontal cortex and ventral striatum. **(A)** Orbitofrontal neurons in the Valid cue context: Normalized population spike density functions for the 14 orbitofrontal neurons with higher firing rates in rewarded trials (*thick gray lines*) than unrewarded trials (*thin black lines*). Fourteen additional cells had higher firing rates in unrewarded trials. Spike density functions are aligned on the time at which the reward was delivered or the time at which the reward would have been delivered in the unrewarded trials (0 ms, *vertical line*). In orbitofrontal cortex, this period extended from 100 to 400 ms after the trial outcome (*horizontal lines above plots*). **(B)** Ventral striatal neurons in the Valid cue context: Normalized population spike density functions for the 36 ventral striatal neurons with higher firing rates in rewarded trials. Thirty-four additional cells had higher firing rates in unrewarded trials. In ventral striatum, the outcome period extended from 250 to 550 ms after the trial outcome (*horizontal lines above plots*). **(C)** Orbitofrontal neurons in the Random cue context: Normalized population spike density functions for the ten orbitofrontal neurons with higher firing rates in rewarded trials. Thirteen additional cells had higher firing rates in unrewarded trials. **(D)** Ventral striatal neurons in the Random cue context: Normalized population spike density functions for the eight ventral striatal neurons with higher firing rates in rewarded trials. Four additional cells had higher firing rates in unrewarded trials. The proportions of ventral striatal neurons with higher firing rates in rewarded trials were indistinguishable from that in orbitofrontal cortex (2-sided proportions tests, Valid (36/267 versus 14/80) $P = 0.47$; Random (9/46 versus 10/80) $P = 0.42$).

data from orbitofrontal cortex and ventral striatum using a single task, we now have shown that the overall size of the neuronal population encoding reward contingency is larger in the orbitofrontal cortex (50%) than in ventral striatum (26%). The combined data from two other studies using a go–no go task also show approximately twice as many task-related neurons in orbitofrontal cortex as in striatum.[12,40]

Orbitofrontal neurons begin to encode information about reward contingency early in a trial. The early phases of each trial are a time of reward anticipation prior to action. Previous work has shown that reaction times decrease as the duration of the wait period increases, indicating an increase in anticipation as each trial progresses.[7] The increase in reward-contingency-dependent activity in orbitofrontal cortex during the wait period may reflect this increasing anticipation.

Ventral striatal neurons frequently show phasic responses at the time of the cue onset in other tasks.[22,23,28,40,43,44] In these tasks, the cue determined not only the trial outcome, but also the action required by the subject. Therefore, the extent to which cue-triggered ventral striatal responses depended on action selection versus reward contingency could not be determined. In human imaging studies that show BOLD activations in ventral striatum during reward anticipation, the anticipation phase also involved both action selection and outcome expectation.[16,45,46] When cue-elicited BOLD activations have been examined in the absence of action, reward-predicting cues elicited orbitofrontal activity only.[47]

In the Reward Schedule Task, the cue predicts trial outcome, but does not instruct the monkey to perform one action versus another. The type of action performed in each correct trial is identical and independent of trial outcome. In this situation, ventral striatal activity during the cue-triggered period is seldom modulated by reward contingency (3/150 [2%] neurons in our previous study[9] and 9/267 [3%] in the analysis presented here).

Reward-contingency-dependent activity in ventral striatum peaks in the go period, after an event that triggers the action leading to the trial outcome itself. Similar peri-trigger responses have been seen previously in several different striatal sub-regions.[6,7,23,40–42] Differences in timing between ventral striatal and orbitofrontal responses have also been observed, and the greater dependence of ventral striatal responses on movement and orbitofrontal responses on reward has been recognized.[11] Together, these findings suggest that ventral striatal neurons encode the value of an action when it occurs and support the idea that the striatum acts as a limbic–motor interface.[1,2,43]

Stimulus-Outcome versus Action-Outcome Encoding

Although this study was not designed to study learning, two types of learning seem to occur in the reward schedule task. Monkeys learn to release a bar at the go signal, thereby mastering a simple instrumental task. Although not required to do so, monkeys also learn to associate visual cues with trial outcome in the Valid cue context. These are Pavlovian associations in that the monkeys have no control over the cue-outcome contingencies. Activity modulations in orbitofrontal cortex during the cue-triggered period may reflect these action-independent, stimulus-outcome associations. The peak ventral striatal activity modulations during the go period appear to reflect action-outcome associations. Therefore, orbitofrontal cortex may be more critically involved in Pavlovian conditioning and ventral striatum more so in instrumental conditioning.[48]

Information Flow

Orbitofrontal neurons appear to encode reward-contingency information earlier in a trial than ventral striatal neurons. There are at least three possible explanations for this finding. In one scenario, orbitofrontal cortex and ventral striatum would receive separate inputs from amygdala and the midbrain dopaminergic nuclei,[49–53] integrate information from these regions separately, and reflect the resulting reward-contingency information at different time periods.

In a second scenario, representations of reward value might flow from orbitofrontal cortex to dorsolateral prefrontal cortex[26] to striatum, or inputs from both orbitofrontal and dorsolateral prefrontal cortex might converge in the striatum. Although orbitofrontal and dorsolateral projections to striatum have classically been seen as segregated, recent anatomic work has shown overlap of diffuse terminals from orbital and dorsolateral prefrontal cortex within the rostral striatum.[54–57] In this way, the rostral striatum provides a potential region for integration of reward-value information and action plans. Our ventral striatal recordings provide another piece of evidence for just this type of integration.

In a third scenario, orbitofrontal cortex could integrate multi-modal sensory information with other limbic inputs to calculate the expected reward value in each trial[10,58]; orbitofrontal cortex could then transmit this information to the ventral striatum.[59] In this model, visual information provided by the cue has direct access to the orbitofrontal cortex, leading to reward-contingency-dependent activity during the cue-triggered period. The ramping up of activity in orbitofrontal cortex and the increase in the reward-contingency-dependent population size during the wait period could lead to sub-threshold changes in membrane potential in ventral striatal neurons. The green spot then could serve as a trigger to release ventral striatal responses (perhaps through a separate cortical striatal pathway), and ventral striatal responses would reflect the conjunction of the action trigger and the anticipated reward contingency.

The orbitofrontal-ventral striatal-thalamic loop has been proposed as one of the fundamental units of corticostriatal processing, dedicated to processing reward-related information critical for incentive learning and decision-making.[54,55,57,59–61] Here, we use a common analysis of recordings from the orbitofrontal cortex and ventral striatum during the reward schedule task to propose a conceptual model for how this circuit might function.

Neuronal activity in orbitofrontal cortex reflects reward-contingency information during anticipation. Neuronal activity in ventral striatum reflects reward-contingency information during action. We suggest that the signals from orbitofrontal cortex serve to bias ventral striatal activity, and in so doing, to guide actions toward rewards. We argue that this bias leads monkeys to perform the same action more quickly and accurately in rewarded trials in the Valid cue context of the Reward Schedule Task. We predict that this same bias could lead monkeys to perform different actions during different trials in a decision-making task, ensuring that choices are consistently directed toward the most likely source of a reward.

ACKNOWLEDGEMENTS

This work was funded by a NARSAD Young Investigator Award and by the NIMH/DIRP.

REFERENCES

1. MOGENSON, G.J., D.L. JONES & C.Y. YIM. 1980. From motivation to action: functional interface between the limbic system and the motor system. Prog. Neurobiol. **14:** 69–97.
2. NAUTA, W.J. & V.B. DOMESICK. 1984. Afferent and efferent relationships of the basal ganglia. Ciba Found. Symp. **107:** 3–29.
3. ROSENKILDE, C.E., R.H. BAUER & J.M. FUSTER. 1981. Single cell activity in ventral prefrontal cortex of behaving monkeys. Brain Res. **209:** 375–394.
4. THORPE, S.J., E.T. ROLLS & S. MADDISON. 1983. The orbitofrontal cortex: neuronal activity in the behaving monkey. Exp. Brain Res. **49:** 93–115.
5. APICELLA, P. *et al.* 1991. Responses to reward in monkey dorsal and ventral striatum. Exp. Brain Res. **85:** 491–500.
6. SCHULTZ, W. *et al.* 1992. Neuronal activity in monkey ventral striatum related to the expectation of reward. J. Neurosci. **12:** 4595–4610.
7. BOWMAN, E.M., T.G. AIGNER & B.J. RICHMOND. 1996. Neural signals in the monkey ventral striatum related to motivation for juice and cocaine rewards. J. Neurophysiol. **75:** 1061–1073.
8. SCHOENBAUM, G., A.A. CHIBA & M. GALLAGHER. 1998. Orbitofrontal cortex and basolateral amygdala encode expected outcomes during learning. Nat. Neurosci. **1:** 155–159.
9. SHIDARA, M., T.G. AIGNER & B.J. RICHMOND. 1998. Neuronal signals in the monkey ventral striatum related to progress through a predictable series of trials. J. Neurosci. **18:** 2613–2625.
10. ROLLS, E.T. 2000. The orbitofrontal cortex and reward. Cereb. Cortex **10:** 284–294.
11. SCHULTZ, W., L. TREMBLAY & J.R. HOLLERMAN. 2000. Reward processing in primate orbitofrontal cortex and basal ganglia. Cereb. Cortex **10:** 272–284.
12. TREMBLAY, L. & W. SCHULTZ. 2000. Reward-related neuronal activity during go-nogo task performance in primate orbitofrontal cortex. J. Neurophysiol. **83:** 1864–1876.

13. O'DOHERTY, J.P. *et al.* 2002. Neural responses during anticipation of a primary taste reward. Neuron **33**: 815–826.
14. HOSOKAWA, T. *et al.* 2005. Correspondence of cue activity to reward activity in the macaque orbitofrontal cortex. Neurosci. Lett. **389**: 146–151.
15. THUT, G. *et al.* 1997. Activation of the human brain by monetary reward. Neuroreport **8**: 1225–1228.
16. KNUTSON, B. & J. TAYLOR. 2001. Dissociation of reward anticipation and outcome with event-related fMRI. Neuroreport **12**: 3683–3687.
17. ELLIOTT, R. *et al.* 2003. Differential response patterns in the striatum and orbitofrontal cortex to financial reward in humans: a parametric functional magnetic resonance imaging study. J. Neurosci. **23**: 303–307.
18. CRITCHLEY, H.D. & E.T. ROLLS. 1996. Hunger and satiety modify the responses of olfactory and visual neurons in the primate orbitofrontal cortex. J. Neurophysiol. **75**: 1673–1686.
19. TREMBLAY, L. & W. SCHULTZ. 1999. Relative reward preference in primate orbitofrontal cortex. Nature **398**: 704–708.
20. HIKOSAKA, K. & M. WATANABE. 2000. Delay activity of orbital and lateral prefrontal neurons of the monkey varying with different rewards. Cereb. Cortex **10**: 263–271.
21. BREITER, H.C. *et al.* 2001. Functional imaging of neural responses to expectancy and experience of monetary gains and losses. Neuron **30**: 619–639.
22. HASSANI, O.K., H.C. CROMWELL & W. SCHULTZ. 2001. Influence of expectation of different rewards on behavior-related neuronal activity in the striatum. J. Neurophysiol. **85**: 2477–2489.
23. CROMWELL, H.C. & W. SCHULTZ. 2003. Effects of expectations for different reward magnitudes on neuronal activity in primate striatum. J. Neurophysiol. **89**: 2823–2838.
24. GOTTFRIED, J.A., J. O'DOHERTY & R.J. DOLAN. 2003. Encoding predictive reward value in human amygdala and orbitofrontal cortex. Science **301**: 1104–1107.
25. KRINGELBACH, M.L. *et al.* 2003. Activation of the human orbitofrontal cortex to a liquid food stimulus is correlated with its subjective pleasantness. Cereb. Cortex **13**: 1064–1071.
26. WALLIS, J.D. & E.K. MILLER. 2003. Neuronal activity in primate dorsolateral and orbital prefrontal cortex during performance of a reward preference task. Eur. J. Neurosci. **18**: 2069–2081.
27. ROESCH, M.R. & C.R. OLSON. 2004. Neuronal activity related to reward value and motivation in primate frontal cortex. Science **304**: 307–310.
28. GALVAN, A. *et al.* 2005. The role of ventral frontostriatal circuitry in reward-based learning in humans. J. Neurosci. **25**: 8650–8656.
29. PADOA-SCHIOPPA, C. & J.A. ASSAD. 2006. Neurons in the orbitofrontal cortex encode economic value. Nature **441**: 223–226.
30. KNUTSON, B. *et al.* 2001. Anticipation of increasing monetary reward selectively recruits nucleus accumbens. J. Neurosci. **21**: RC159.
31. KNUTSON, B. *et al.* 2005. Distributed neural representation of expected value. J. Neurosci. **25**: 4806–4812.
32. LIU, Z., E.A. MURRAY & B.J. RICHMOND. 2000. Learning motivational significance of visual cues for reward schedules requires rhinal cortex. Nat. Neurosci. **3**: 1307–1315.
33. SHIDARA, M. & B.J. RICHMOND. 2002. Anterior cingulate: single neuronal signals related to degree of reward expectancy. Science **296**: 1709–1711.

34. SUGASE-MIYAMOTO, Y. & B.J. RICHMOND. 2005. Neuronal signals in the monkey basolateral amygdala during reward schedules. J. Neurosci. **25:** 11071–11083.
35. RAVEL, S. & B.J. RICHMOND. 2006. Dopamine neuronal responses in monkeys performing visually cued reward schedules. Eur. J. Neurosci. **24:** 277–290.
36. SIMMONS, J.M. & B.J. RICHMOND. 2007. Dynamic changes in representations of preceding and upcoming reward in monkey orbitofrontal cortex. Cereb. Cortex. doi:10.1093/cercor/bhm034.
37. SHIDARA, M. & B.J. RICHMOND. 2004. Differential encoding of information about progress through multi-trial reward schedules by three groups of ventral striatal neurons. Neurosci. Res. **49:** 307–314.
38. SCHOENBAUM, G. & B. SETLOW. 2001. Integrating orbitofrontal cortex into prefrontal theory: common processing themes across species and subdivisions. Learn. Mem. **8:** 134–147.
39. WILLIAMS, G.V. *et al.* 1993. Neuronal responses in the ventral striatum of the behaving macaque. Behav. Brain Res. **55:** 243–252.
40. HOLLERMAN, J.R., L. TREMBLAY & W. SCHULTZ. 1998. Influence of reward expectation on behavior-related neuronal activity in primate striatum. J. Neurophysiol. **80:** 947–963.
41. APICELLA, P. *et al.* 1992. Neuronal activity in monkey striatum related to the expectation of predictable environmental events. J. Neurophysiol. **68:** 945–960.
42. WATANABE, K., J. LAUWEREYNS & O. HIKOSAKA. 2003. Neural correlates of rewarded and unrewarded eye movements in the primate caudate nucleus. J. Neurosci. **23:** 10052–10057.
43. NICOLA, S.M. *et al.* 2004. Cue-evoked firing of nucleus accumbens neurons encodes motivational significance during a discriminative stimulus task. J. Neurophysiol. **91:** 1840–1865.
44. SETLOW, B., G. SCHOENBAUM & M. GALLAGHER. 2003. Neural encoding in ventral striatum during olfactory discrimination learning. Neuron **38:** 625–636.
45. KIRSCH, P. *et al.* 2003. Anticipation of reward in a nonaversive differential conditioning paradigm and the brain reward system: an event-related fMRI study. Neuroimage **20:** 1086–1095.
46. ERNST, M. *et al.* 2003. Choice selection and reward anticipation: an fMRI study. Neuropsychologia **42:** 1585–1597.
47. COX, S.M., A. ANDRADE & I.S. JOHNSRUDE. 2005. Learning to like: a role for human orbitofrontal cortex in conditioned reward. J. Neurosci. **25:** 2733–2740.
48. OSTLUND, S.B. & B.W. BALLEINE. 2007. Orbitofrontal cortex mediates outcome encoding in Pavlovian but not instrumental conditioning. J. Neurosci. **27:** 4819–4825.
49. KITA, H. & S.T. KITAI. 1990. Amygdaloid projections to the frontal cortex and the striatum in the rat. J. Comp. Neurol. **298:** 40–49.
50. HABER, S.N., J.L. FUDGE & N.R. MCFARLAND. 2000. Striatonigrostriatal pathways in primates form an ascending spiral from the shell to the dorsolateral striatum. J. Neurosci. **20:** 2369–2382.
51. FUDGE, J.L. *et al.* 2002. Amygdaloid projections to ventromedial striatal subterritories in the primate. Neuroscience **110:** 257–275.
52. AMARAL, D.G. & J.L. PRICE. 1984. Amygdalo-cortical projections in the monkey (*Macaca fascicularis*). J. Comp. Neurol. **230:** 465–496.
53. OADES, R.D. & G.M. HALLIDAY. 1987. Ventral tegmental (A10) system: neurobiology. 1. Anatomy and connectivity. Brain Res. **434:** 117–165.

54. ALEXANDER, G.E., M.R. DELONG & P.L. STRICK. 1986. Parallel organization of functionally segregated circuits linking basal ganglia and cortex. Annu. Rev. Neurosci. **9:** 357–381.
55. EBLEN, F. & A.M. GRAYBIEL. 1995. Highly restricted origin of prefrontal cortical inputs to striosomes in the macaque monkey. J. Neurosci. **15:** 5999–6013.
56. SELEMON, L.D. & P.S. GOLDMAN-RAKIC. 1985. Longitudinal topography and interdigitation of corticostriatal projections in the rhesus monkey. J. Neurosci. **5:** 776–794.
57. HABER, S.N. et al. 2006. Reward-related cortical inputs define a large striatal region in primates that interface with associative cortical connections, providing a substrate for incentive-based learning. J. Neurosci. **26:** 8368–8376.
58. ONGUR, D. & J.L. PRICE. 2000. The organization of networks within the orbital and medial prefrontal cortex of rats, monkeys and humans. Cereb. Cortex **10:** 206–219.
59. HABER, S.N. et al. 1995. The orbital and medial prefrontal circuit through the primate basal ganglia. J. Neurosci. **15:** 4851–4867.
60. MIDDLETON, F.A. & P.L. STRICK. 2000. A revised neuroanatomy of frontal subcortical circuits. In Frontal-Subcortical Circuits in Psychiatry and Neurology. D.G. Licter & J.L. Cummings, Eds.: 44–58. Guilford Press. New York.
61. FERRY, A.T. et al. 2000. Prefrontal cortical projections to the striatum in macaque monkeys: evidence for an organization related to prefrontal networks. J. Comp. Neurol. **425:** 447–470.

Orbital Versus Dorsolateral Prefrontal Cortex

Anatomical Insights into Content Versus Process Differentiation Models of the Prefrontal Cortex

DAVID H. ZALD

Department of Psychology, Vanderbilt University, Nashville, Tennessee 37203, USA

ABSTRACT: Content differentiation models posit that different areas of the prefrontal cortex perform similar operations but differ in terms of the content that is operated on. For example, it has been suggested that the orbitofrontal cortex (OFC) and the dorsolateral prefrontal cortex (DLPFC) perform similar working memory or inhibitory operations, but on different types of content (e.g., reward versus spatial or feature-based versus abstract). In contrast to the above models, process differentiation models posit that different areas of the prefrontal cortex perform fundamentally different operations. Surprisingly, discussions of these dueling models rarely incorporate information about anatomy. The only exception is that advocates of content differentiation models appropriately note that different parts of the prefrontal cortex receive different afferents. Yet, an examination of the anatomy of the OFC and the DLPFC reveal numerous differences in cortical structure and interneuron composition. These structural differences necessitate that the OFC and the DLPFC will have strikingly different computational features. Given such computational differences, strong versions of content differentiation models are untenable. While overarching themes may help explain the operations in both the OFC and the DLPFC, the specific operations performed in the two regions are likely to be both quantitatively and qualitatively different in nature.

KEYWORDS: cytoarchitecture; decision making; interneuron; orbitofrontal; working memory

As its name implies, the orbitofrontal cortex (OFC) is part of the frontal lobe. While that simple anatomical conclusion is unavoidable, theoretical models

Address for correspondence: David H. Zald, Ph.D., Department of Psychology, Vanderbilt University, 301 Wilson Hall, 111 21ˢᵗ Avenue South, Nashville, TN 37203. Voice: 615-343-6076; fax: 615-343-8449.

david.zald@vanderbilt.edu

Ann. N.Y. Acad. Sci. 1121: 395–406 (2007). © 2007 New York Academy of Sciences.
doi: 10.1196/annals.1401.012

of frontal-lobe functions have often stumbled in their attempts to integrate the OFC with other aspects of prefrontal processing. Even in the latter half of the 20th century, it was not unusual for researchers to describe the OFC as an enigma. Indeed, the most significant predecessor to the present conference was a 1998 symposium entitled The Mysterious Orbitofrontal Cortex. This mysteriousness was particularly apparent when comparing what was known about the OFC relative to other prefrontal regions. When more dorsolateral prefrontal cortex (DLPFC) regions came to be associated with classic frontal measures, such as the Wisconsin Card Sorting Task,[1] lesions of the OFC rudely failed to produce typical perseverative errors.[2] Similarly, as studies in monkeys implicated the area around the principal sulcus in delayed spatial response tasks, animals with OFC lesions failed to show such deficits.[3]

OFC lesions not only failed to produce deficits on standard frontal measures, but also produced deficits on other measures that were not affected by DLPFC lesions.[4–7] This posed a major problem for early models of prefrontal functions, which emphasized the idea that the prefrontal cortex has a relatively unitary function. The observation of double dissociations between OFC and DLPFC lesions made such unitary models relatively untenable, and by the 1970s such models had given way to models that posit functional heterogeneity.[8,9]

Nevertheless, the idea that there is a unitary theme relating different frontal areas has remained popular. For instance, in her classic monograph on the prefrontal cortex, Goldman-Rakic[10] proposed a *content differentiation* model of prefrontal regions. Content differentiation models hold that all prefrontal areas perform similar processes (i.e., operations or computations) but differ in terms of the input (type of representation) on which they act. In line with this conceptualization, Goldman-Rakic[10] put forth that different areas of the prefrontal cortex perform similar working memory operations but operate on different types of representations. Whereas the DLPFC operated on spatial information, a more ventrolateral region operated on object information, and orbital areas operated on emotional information. In support of such a conceptualization, delay period activity has been found during single cell recordings of nonhuman primate OFC.[11–13] This activity appears critically linked to the current reinforcement value of the expected reward, as opposed to simply representing the identity of the reinforcer.[12] Importantly, this delay period activity qualitatively differs from that typically seen in the DLPFC. Whereas DLPFC activity is characterized by sustained tonic elevations during delay periods, only a minority of OFC cells shows this type of sustained activity.[13] In contrast, the majority of delay period activity in the OFC follows an ascending or descending firing pattern in advance of the expected reward delivery time. Taken together, these findings suggest that a substantial portion of the OFC's delay activity reflects a reward expectancy. These expectancies may be updated and brought forth on a trial-by-trial basis, but they are not an exact parallel to the persistent activity associated with working memory in more dorsal regions. It is also notable that conceptualizations of working memory, especially in humans, include a manipulation component.[14] This allows us to manipulate the order of different pieces of information, such as numbers, letters, or spatial locations. While it is possible that we might select an order of rewards (for instance, choosing the order in which we wish to eat items), the parallel to the online reordering of information in other modalities seems limited. Just ask yourself: when is the last time you had a need to do an online manipulation of the order of expected rewards?

The beauty of Goldman-Rakic's[10] content differentiation model is that it provided an organizing principle for understanding the operations of different prefrontal regions. However, this model has been vigorously opposed by researchers who have instead argued for a *process differentiation* model for understanding frontal involvement in working memory.[15] Process differentiation models hold that different areas of the frontal lobe perform fundamentally different operations or computations. For instance, it has been proposed that specific prefrontal regions can be dissociated based on whether they are involved in the process of holding information online or in the operations necessary for the manipulation of internal representations.[15] The human neuroimaging data has proven difficult to reconcile with Goldman-Rakic's[10] original content differentiation model, as the process being performed has often appeared more important than the specific stimulus modality.[16,17]

An alternative content differentiation model of prefrontal involvement in working memory focuses on level of abstraction. Ranganath states, "all prefrontal cortex subregions play a role in selecting (i.e., accentuating or inhibiting the activation of) memory representations. . . . but that different subregions may be selecting information at different levels of analysis" (p. 280).[18] In contrast to Goldman-Rakic's[10] original model, Ranganath[18] proposes that rostral and dorsal prefrontal regions select representations of abstract relations between currently active items, whereas caudal and ventral regions select representations of relevant items. Overall, this model helps to explain the distributions of functional neuroimaging activations in many lateral areas, including ventrolateral regions along the inferior frontal gyrus. However, specific reference to areas along the orbital surface are absent from this model, and the neuroimaging data cited in support of the model focuses exclusively on lateral prefrontal regions. Thus, although all prefrontal regions are argued to play a role in a common process, the specific role of the OFC in working memory is left unspecified.

Content differentiation models have also been applied to decision-making tasks. In a pioneering study, Dias et al.[19,20] used an intradimensional/extradimensional shift task to isolate responses to changes within a dimension (stimulus reward reversal) and across dimensions (abstract rule changes). Marmosets with OFC lesions showed impairments only on the intradimensional shifts, while marmosets with DLPFC lesions showed impairments only on extradimensional shifts. The question naturally arises whether this reflects two different operations or similar operations being performed on different types of representations. Dias et al.[19,20] proposed a content differentiation model in which both the dorsal and the orbital areas are involved in inhibition, with the orbital area involved in inhibition of affective information (relating to previous rewarded stimuli) and the dorsal region involved in inhibition of attention (to the previously relevant dimension). Their 1997 paper states this model in the abstract: "These findings suggest that inhibitory control is a general process that operates across functionally distinct regions within the prefrontal cortex. Although damage to lateral prefrontal cortex causes a loss of inhibitory control in attentional selection, damage to orbitofrontal cortex causes a loss of inhibitory control in affective processing" (p. 9285).[20] Based on some other passages in the Dias et al.[19,20] papers, O'Reilly and colleagues[21] assert that Dias et al.'s[19,20] arguments actually conform to a process differentiation model in which the OFC is involved in affective inhibition, while the DLPFC is involved in attention selection. This distinction is not just semantic: in the original framework presented by Dias,[19,20] the DLPFC and the OFC are both argued to work through similar inhibitory operations, whereas O'Reilly's[21] presentation of the Dias model suggests that the attention selection mechanisms of the DLPFC work through other types of operations. Regardless of the accuracy of their characterization, O'Reilly et al.[21] themselves propose an alternative content differentiation model, which focuses on an abstract versus stimulus-specific gradient similar to that described above for working memory. Specifically, they propose that the DLPFC processes more abstract information, whereas the OFC processes more specific stimulus feature information. They argue that both areas use a dynamic gating mechanism to implement changes when contingencies change; the OFC implements changes when stimulus-reinforcer contingencies change, and the DLPFC implements changes when abstract (extra-) dimensional shifts occur. The feasibility of this model is supported by computational modeling that reproduces the double dissociation observed by Dias et al.[19,20]

In summary, while unitary hypotheses of prefrontal function have proven untenable, the extent to which the different prefrontal regions are engaged in similar or different types of operations remains a matter of debate. Both content differentiation and process differentiation models attempt to explain how different regions may be necessary for specific tasks, but these models stand in opposition in their characterization of the operations subserved by the different regions of the prefrontal cortex.

Anatomical Insights

In assessing the process differentiation versus content differentiation debate, it is helpful to consider the anatomical characteristics of the OFC and the DLPFC. At the most basic level, it is quickly apparent that different parts of the prefrontal cortex receive afferents from different regions.[22] Because of this, there are certainly some differences in the content of what is processed in different prefrontal regions. However, anatomical differences do not stop here. There are several fundamental anatomical factors that show that the computational characteristics of the OFC will be quite different from more lateral prefrontal regions. Whereas the DLPFC is composed of well-defined, six-layered, granular cortex (eulaminate II),[23] the OFC does not reach this level of definition. The most posterior aspects of the OFC are agranular, followed by dysgranular cortex (area 13, caudal area 14), and modestly to moderately defined granular (eulaminate I) areas in the more rostral and lateral aspects of the OFC (areas 11 and 12, rostral area 14).[23-25] In addition to differences in the extent of granularity, prefrontal areas differ in terms of neuronal density, relative amounts of neurons in superficial or deep layers of cortex, the ratio of neurons to glia, the ratio of feedback to feedforward afferents and efferents, and levels of parvalbumin and calbindin.[23,26] These neuroanatomical differences have substantial functional implications, including the degree of tonic activity, the extent of local circuit processing, the balance of excitatory to inhibitory processing, and the nature of input and output from the region.[23,26-28]

A full characterization of the anatomical differences between the OFC and the DLPFC is beyond the scope of this review, but several specific features warrant mention. The superficial layers of the DLPFC possess high neuronal density (FIG. 1). Importantly, the pyramidal cells in the superficial layers of the DLPFC possess widespread horizontal intrinsic axon projections, which have been proposed to form a critical substrate for recurrent lateral projections that produce persistent activity following a response to a preferred cue.[29-33] Such persistent activity forms the basis of working memory. In contrast to the DLPFC, the superficial layers of the agranular and dysgranular OFC possess far fewer pyramidal neurons.[23] Lacking dense lateral connections between pyramidal neurons, the dysgranular and agranular regions of the OFC probably do not possess the ability to maintain the sort of tuned persistent firing that is seen in the DLFPC.

Increasing data indicates that the types of interneurons in a region markedly influence the region's computational features.[32,34,35] Parvalbumin and calbindin are found in separate types of interneurons.[36,37] Critically, the densities of these different types of interneurons differs dramatically across prefrontal regions.[23] Parvalbumin levels double as one moves from agranular and dysgranular OFC to the DLPFC. In contrast, calbindin levels are approximately threefold greater in dysgranular OFC than in the DLPFC. Based on observed differences in the characteristics of interneurons, Wang et al.[32] argue that these parvalbumin and calbindin interneurons serve different functions in the prefrontal cortex. They note that within the DLPFC, parvalbumin-containing interneurons, presumably of the large basket-cell type, have fast firing characteristics and target the perisomal region of pyramidal cells. Based on computational modeling, Wang et al.[32] propose that the

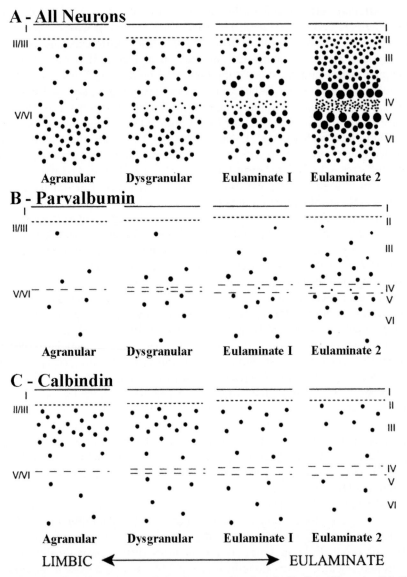

FIGURE 1. Differences in cell density (**A**), parvalbumin binding (**B**), and calbindin binding (**C**) in agranular, dysgranular, and granular prefrontal regions. The posteriormost aspects of the OFC are agranular, followed by dysgranular areas (such as area 13), and modestly to moderately defined eulaminate I cortex in the rostral and lateral OFC. The DLPFC is composed of eulaminate II cortex. The OFC has not only fewer cells but also very different ratio of calbindin to parvalbumin interneurons. (Figure adapted from Dombrowski, S.M., C.C. Hilgetag & H. Barbas. 2001. Quantitative architecture distinguishes prefrontal cortical systems in the rhesus monkey. Cereb. Cortex 11: 975–988,[23] with permission from Oxford University Press.)

parvalbumin-containing interneurons provide widespread perisomatic inhibition, which allows for stimulus (spatial) tuning of persistent activity during working memory. In contrast, calbindin-containing interneurons fire at a slower rate and target dendrites. Within their model, the calbindin-containing interneurons play a particular role in inhibiting interference from extraneous stimuli. Similarly elegant models are lacking for the OFC, but if we extend Wang et al.'s[32] reasoning, we would predict that the high levels of calbindin-containing interneurons in the OFC would lead to a network in which the inhibiting of extraneous information is robust. In contrast, the low levels of parvalbumin in the OFC would deprive it of the widespread inhibition necessary for tuning persistent activity.

Finally, the DLPFC and the OFC possess different levels of feedback and feedforward connections.[26,38] Feedforward projections can be defined structurally, in that they start from superficial layers and project to deep layers of cortex (FIG. 2).[39] In sensory systems, early stages of the processing stream provide information to subsequent stages through this type of feedforward projection. By contrast, feedback projections start in deep layers of cortex and project to superficial layers of cortex. Feedback projections act to modify or to bias the computations being performed in the earlier processing stages. For instance, feedback projections act to help accentuate the responses of cells coding attended objects or locations, while attenuating or suppressing responses to unattended objects.[40,41] Such feedback aids in basic perceptual processes such as figure-ground discrimination,[42] as well as allowing top-down control of what is processed in the information stream.

Based on analyses of the laminar patterns of axon projections, the agranular and dysgranular areas of the OFC are characterized by strong feedback

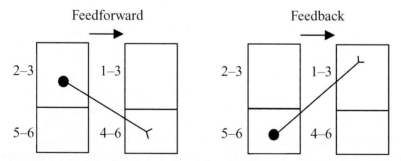

FIGURE 2. Feedforward versus feedback connections based on the laminar distribution of projections. Feedforward projections arise from superficial layers of cortex and project to deep layers of cortex. The projections carry information forward to later stages of the processing pathway. In contrast, feedback projections arise from deep layers and project to superficial layers of cortex. These projections allow modulation or biasing of early processing stages. The OFC efferents are more frequently of the feedback variety, whereas the DLPFC has a high percentage of feedforward projections.

features in their connections with other regions.[26,38] By analogy to sensory systems, this would mean that the OFC projections are geared toward biasing or modifying computations in earlier stages of information flow. By contrast, the eulaminate DLPFC has substantially higher levels of feedforward projections, which allow it to feed the results or output of its computations to subsequent brain regions. Thus, it appears the OFC and the DLPFC act upon other regions quite differently.

Taken together, the large number of anatomical differences between the orbital and dorsal prefrontal regions make evident that the orbital cortex has very different computational features than the DLPFC. Rather than simply performing similar operations on different types of input, these anatomical constraints indicate that the OFC's computational characteristics are both quantitatively and qualitatively different from the dorsal prefrontal regions. Thus, even if they are performing a similar type of operation on different content, the ways in which those operations are implemented are likely to be quite different. Such a conclusion is incompatible with a strong form of the content differentiation model, in which the computations or operations are considered to be equivalent.

CAVEATS AND CONCLUSIONS

I have argued that the anatomical differences between the OFC and more dorsal prefrontal areas make it unlikely that these two regions could perform equivalent computations. This conclusion runs counter to a strong content differentiation model that holds that the OFC and other prefrontal areas perform the same operations, but on separate input. In contrast, the anatomical differences would be fully compatible with a process differentiation model in which the two regions are held to perform fundamentally different operations. Such fundamental differences would be expected to lead to significant double dissociations in the effects of OFC lesions, which would extend beyond simple differences in content.

Before declaring a process differentiation model victorious, it is worth noting that a weaker content differentiation model is still viable. In a weak version of the content differentiation model, the OFC may be argued to perform operations similar to dorsal prefrontal regions, but with different computational properties. For instance, both the DLPFC and the OFC regions could perform operations necessary for inhibitory control, but using operations that differ due to the varied computational properties of the different regions. Indeed, it seems likely that different contents (such as abstract rules versus stimulus features) necessitate some computational differences in order to accomplish similar results. Ideally, such weaker versions of content differentiation models should specify the nature of these computational differences. Similarly, process differentiation models could afford to articulate the computational features that would be necessary to carry out different operations. At present, this remains difficult, as our knowledge of the precise computational features of various prefrontal regions remains quite coarse, but we can anticipate that our ability to specify these differences will increase dramatically in the coming years.

While I have focused on the anatomical arguments against strong content differentiation models, a similar line of reasoning could be used to target a strong process differentiation model that totally disregards differences in content. While some aspects of prefrontal processing appear quite multimodal in nature (allowing an area's operations to be performed on multiple types of stimulus representations),[43] differential inputs place constraints on the range of representations that can be processed in any given area. These constraints make a pure process differentiation model, in which all prefrontal regions are considered to operate on identical content, untenable. However, because knowledge regarding differential connections preceded the recent era of process differentiation models, it has generally been assumed (if not always stated explicitly) that inputs are not identical. In other words, while process differentiation models focus primarily on differences in operations, they are typically not predicated on the idea that the content itself is identical.

Perhaps a similar argument can be made that most proponents of content differentiation models also believe there are some differences in the operations being performed across regions. As such, it could be argued that the type of strong content differentiation model articulated in this article is really a "straw man" argument. Do theorists really believe that different areas of the prefrontal cortex are performing identical operations? O'Reilly et al.[21] state that different regions in their model perform a "common processing" function (p. 246). The word common leaves open the possibility of some computational differences among regions. Indeed, their model itself provides computational differences in the OFC and the lateral prefrontal areas (the OFC has more units in order to represent detailed features, and the lateral prefrontal has only enough units to represent the relevant dimensions). So it seems safe to assume that the authors did not intend to imply that the processes were identical in their computational properties. Thus, the model can absorb some degree of computational differences, as long as it can be shown that the basic architecture necessary to accomplish the common operations is present in both regions. The degree to which other content differentiation models accept computational differences is less clear. The sorts of qualifications that would indicate that the theorists intended a weak version of the model are rarely explicitly stated. If the theorists intended a weaker version of the content differentiation model, they do not state it. It seems safe to assume that many readers do not consider these unstated qualifications, and thus interpret the models in their strong form.

The argument put forth in this paper stands or falls on the degree to which the OFC and the DLPFC differ in their anatomical features. A quick glance at FIGURE 1 makes evident the strong contrast between the agranular/dysgranular OFC and the well-defined eulaminate II cortex that defines the DLPFC.

However, the degree of difference is weaker when one compares the eulaminate I cortex in the rostral and lateral OFC to the DLPFC. Does this mean that the arguments in this paper only apply to agranular/dysgranular OFC? No, but the argument is certainly strongest when contrasting more posterior and medial OFC regions to the DLPFC. Because transitions between different types of cortex occur gradually, computational features are also likely to vary gradually. Indeed, while maps of cortical areas often include sharp boundaries, in truth these boundaries are often gradual. The same is likely true for computational features. Neighboring regions may have computational features that differ in only mild quantitative rather than qualitative ways. However, as one moves through successive stages, the computational features and the operations they are capable of serving are likely to become progressively more differentiated. The difficulty in such a situation is determining at what point the anatomy or the operations that they serve has changed enough to consider them distinct.

This issue of boundaries is particularly tricky in regards to the ventrolateral prefrontal cortex. One could argue that while the content differentiation models have often been extended to the OFC, in the working memory literature, the greatest focus of debate has been on comparing the DLPFC with the ventrolateral prefrontal cortex rather than the OFC. Given the greater degree of similarity between the dorsolateral and ventrolateral prefrontal cortex, such areas are more likely to be able to perform similar operations. Even here, I maintain that care needs to be taken to look at the anatomical and resultant computational differences between these more proximal regions. Nevertheless, a content differentiation model is certainly more viable when comparing two areas of granular isocortex than when trying to extend such models to agranular and dysgranular regions of the OFC.

REFERENCES

1. MILNER, B. 1963. Effects of different brain lesions on card sorting. Arch. Neurol. **9:** 90–100.
2. STUSS, D.T. *et al.* 2000. Wisconsin Card Sorting Test performance in patients with focal frontal and posterior brain damage: effects of lesion location and test structure on separable cognitive processes. Neuropsychologia **38:** 388–402.
3. BRUTKOWSKI, S., M. MISHKIN & H.E. ROSVOLD. 1963. Positive and inhibitory motor conditioned reflexes in monkeys after ablation of orbital or dorso-lateral surface of the frontal cortex. *In* Central and Peripheral Mechanisms of Motor Functions. E. Gutman & P. Hnik, Eds.: 133–141. Czechoslovak Academy of Sciences. Prague, CZ.
4. MISHKIN, M.M. 1964. Preservation of central sets after frontal lesions in monkeys. *In* The Frontal Granular Cortex and Behavior. J.M. Warren & K. Akert, Eds.: 219–241. McGraw-Hill. New York.
5. PRIBRAM, K.H. & M. MISHKIN. 1956. Analysis of the effects of frontal lesions in monkey: III. Object alternation. J. Comp. Physiol. Psychol. **49:** 41–45.

6. IVERSEN, S. & M. MISHKIN. 1970. Perseverative interference in monkeys following selective lesions of the inferior prefrontal convexity. Exp. Brain Res. **11:** 376–386.

7. ZALD, D.H. 2006. Neuropsychological assessment of the orbitofrontal cortex. *In* The Orbitofrontal Cortex. D.H. Zald & S.L. Rauch, Eds.: 449–480. Oxford University Press. Oxford, UK.

8. ROSENKILDE, C.E. 1979. Functional heterogeneity of the prefrontal cortex in the monkey: a review. Beh. Neural. Biol. **25:** 301–345.

9. FUSTER, J.M. 1989. The Prefrontal Cortex. Raven Press. New York.

10. GOLDMAN-RAKIC, P.S. 1987. Circuitry of primate prefrontal cortex and regulation of behavior by representational memory. *In* Handbook of Physiology, **5:** 373–417. Yale University School of Medicine. New Haven.

11. ROSENKILDE, C.E., R.H. BAUER & J.M. FUSTER. 1981. Single cell activity in ventral prefrontal cortex of behaving monkeys. Brain Res. **209:** 375–394.

12. HIKOSAKA, K. & M. WATANABE. 2000. Delay activity of orbital and lateral prefrontal neurons of the monkey varying with different rewards. Cereb. Cortex **10:** 263–271.

13. ICHIHARA-TAKEDA, S. & S. FUNAHASHI. 2007. Activity of primate orbitofrontal and dorsolateral prefrontal neurons: task-related activity during an oculomotor delayed-response task Exp. Brain Res. **181:** 409–425.

14. BADDELEY, A. 1992. Working memory: the interface between memory and cognition. J. Cogn. Neurosci. **4:** 281–288.

15. PETRIDES, M. 1994. Frontal lobes and behaviour. Curr. Opin. Neurobiol. **4:** 207–211.

16. CURTIS, C.E., D.H. ZALD & J.V. PARDO. 2000. Organization of working memory within the human prefrontal cortex: a PET study of self-ordered object working memory. Neuropsychologia **38:** 1503–1510.

17. D'ESPOSITO, M. *et al.* 1998. Functional MRI studies of spatial and nonspatial working memory. Brain Res. Cogn. Brain Res. **7:** 1–13.

18. RANGANATH, C. 2006. Working memory for visual objects: complementary roles of inferior temporal, medial temporal, and prefrontal cortex. Neuroscience **139:** 277–289.

19. DIAS, R., T.W. ROBBINS & A.C. ROBERTS. 1996. Dissociation in prefrontal cortex of affective and attentional shifts. Nature **380:** 69–72.

20. DIAS, R., T.W. ROBBINS & A.C. ROBERTS. 1997. Dissociable forms of inhibitory control within prefrontal cortex with an analog of the Wisconsin Card Sort Test: restriction to novel situations and independence from "on-line" processing. J. Neurosci. **17:** 9285–9297.

21. O'REILLY, R.C. *et al.* 2002. Prefrontal cortex and dynamic categorization tasks: representational organization and neuromodulatory control. Cereb. Cortex **12:** 246–257.

22. BARBAS, H. 2000. Connections underlying the synthesis of cognition, memory, and emotion in primate prefrontal cortices. Brain Res. Bull. **52:** 319–330.

23. DOMBROWSKI, S.M., C.C. HILGETAG & H. BARBAS. 2001. Quantitative architecture distinguishes prefrontal cortical systems in the rhesus monkey. Cereb. Cortex **11:** 975–988.

24. PETRIDES, M. & S. MACKEY. 2006. Topography of the human OFC. *In* The Orbitofrontal Cortex. D.H. Zald & S.L. Rauch, Eds.: 19–38. Oxford University Press. Oxford, UK.

25. PRICE, J.L. 2006. Architectonic structure of the orbital and medial prefrontal cortex. *In* The Orbitofrontal Cortex. D.H. Zald & S.L. Rauch, Eds.: 3–18. Oxford University Press. Oxford, UK.

26. BARBAS, H. & N. REMPEL-CLOWER. 1997. Cortical structure predicts the pattern of corticocortical connections. Cereb. Cortex **7**: 635–646.

27. MONTAGNINI, A. & A. TREVES. 2003. The evolution of mammalian cortex, from lamination to arealization. Brain Res. Bull. **60**: 387–393.

28. ELSTON, G.N. *et al.* 2006. Specializations of the granular prefrontal cortex of primates: implications for cognitive processing. Anat. Rec. A Discov. Mol. Cell Evol. Biol. **288**: 26–35.

29. PUCAK, M.L. *et al.* 1996. Patterns of intrinsic and associational circuitry in monkey prefrontal cortex. J. Comp. Neurol. **376**: 614–630.

30. GONZALEZ-BURGOS, G., G. BARRIONUEVO & D.A. LEWIS. 2000. Horizontal synaptic connections in monkey prefrontal cortex: an in vitro electrophysiological study. Cereb. Cortex **10**: 82–92.

31. MELCHITZKY, D.S. *et al.* 2001. Synaptic targets of the intrinsic axon collaterals of supragranular pyramidal neurons in monkey prefrontal cortex. J. Comp. Neurol. **430**: 209–221.

32. WANG, X.J. *et al.* 2004. Division of labor among distinct subtypes of inhibitory neurons in a cortical microcircuit of working memory. Proc. Natl. Acad. Sci. USA **101**: 1368–1373.

33. COMPTE, A. *et al.* 2000. Synaptic mechanisms and network dynamics underlying spatial working memory in a cortical network model. Cereb. Cortex **10**: 910–923.

34. GUPTA, A., Y. WANG & H. MARKRAM. 2000. Organizing principles for a diversity of GABAergic interneurons and synapses in the neocortex. Science **287**: 273–278.

35. BUZSAKI, G. *et al.* 2004. Interneuron diversity series: circuit complexity and axon wiring economy of cortical interneurons. Trends Neurosci. **27**: 186–193.

36. ELSTON, G.N. & M.C. GONZALEZ-ALBO. 2003. Parvalbumin-, calbindin-, and calretinin-immunoreactive neurons in the prefrontal cortex of the owl monkey (Aotus trivirgatus): a standardized quantitative comparison with sensory and motor areas. Brain Behav. Evol. **62**: 19–30.

37. DEFELIPE, J. 2002. Cortical interneurons: from Cajal to 2001. Prog. Brain Res. **136**: 215–238.

38. REMPEL-CLOWER, N.L. & H. BARBAS. 2000. The laminar pattern of connections between prefrontal and anterior temporal cortices in the Rhesus monkey is related to cortical structure and function. Cereb. Cortex **10**: 851–865.

39. ROCKLAND, K.S. & D.N. PANDYA. 1979. Laminar origins and terminations of cortical connections of the occipital lobe in the rhesus monkey. Brain Res. **179**: 3–20.

40. MEHTA, A.D., I. ULBERT & C.E. SCHROEDER. 2000. Intermodal selective attention in monkeys. II: physiological mechanisms of modulation. Cereb. Cortex **10**: 359–370.

41. SAALMANN, Y.B., I.N. PIGAREV & T.R. VIDYASAGAR. 2007. Neural mechanisms of visual attention: how top-down feedback highlights relevant locations. Science **316**: 1612–1615.

42. ROLAND, P.E. *et al.* 2006. Cortical feedback depolarization waves: a mechanism of top-down influence on early visual areas. Proc. Natl. Acad. Sci. USA **103**: 12586–12591.

43. RAINER, G., W.F. ASAAD & E.K. MILLER. 1998. Memory fields of neurons in the primate prefrontal cortex. Proc. Natl. Acad. Sci. USA **95**: 15008–15013.

Difficulty Overcoming Learned Non-reward during Reversal Learning in Rats with Ibotenic Acid Lesions of Orbital Prefrontal Cortex

DAVID SCOTT TAIT AND VERITY J. BROWN

School of Psychology, The University of St Andrews, St Mary's College, St Andrews, Fife, KY16 9JP, United Kingdom

ABSTRACT: Behavioral flexibility is a concept often invoked when describing the function of the prefrontal cortex. However, the psychological substrate of behavioral flexibility is complex. Its key components are allocation of attention, goal-directedness, planning, working memory, and response selection. Furthermore, there is evidence that different regions of the prefrontal cortex might be implicated in these different components. In rule-switching tasks, a distinction is made between errors that are perseverative (difficulty switching from a previously rewarded strategy) and errors due to learned-irrelevance (difficulty switching to a strategy previously uncorrelated with reward). A similar distinction might be made for reversal learning, which involves inhibition of a previously rewarded response and activation of a previously unrewarded response. Damage to the orbital prefrontal cortex (OPFC) results in a deficit in reversal learning. The present study was designed to examine whether one or both of either perseveration or learned non-reward might account for the deficit. Rats with bilateral ibotenic acid-induced lesions of the OPFC were not impaired in acquisition of discriminations. They were impaired, relative to controls, only when they had to overcome learned non-reward. They did not show enhanced perseveration. We conclude that an inability to overcome learned non-reward significantly contributes to OPFC lesion-induced deficits in behavioral flexibility.

KEYWORDS: orbital prefrontal cortex; attentional set-shifting; ibotenic acid; reversal learning; perseveration; rat

INTRODUCTION

Lesions of both the orbital prefrontal cortex (OPFC)[1,2] and the basal forebrain[3,4] impair reversal learning in rats and monkeys during attentional

Address for correspondence: Prof. Verity J. Brown, School of Psychology, The University of St Andrews, St Mary's College, South Street, St Andrews, Fife, KY16 9JP, UK. Voice: +441334 462050; fax: +441334 463042.
vjb@st-andrews.ac.uk

Ann. N.Y. Acad. Sci. 1121: 407–420 (2007). © 2007 New York Academy of Sciences.
doi: 10.1196/annals.1401.010

set-shifting tasks[5,6] without affecting acquisition of discriminations or the ability to shift attentional set. Increases in the number of errors during reversal learning are often referred to as perseverative because subjects continue to respond to a previously reinforced stimulus.[7–9] However, in a typical test of reversal learning, the subject must both inhibit responding to the previously correct stimulus and start responding to the previously unrewarded stimulus. Thus, impairment could arise either because of perseverative responding or because of a process akin to latent inhibition or learned irrelevance, in which prior exposure to a stimulus uncorrelated with reward retards subsequent learning about that stimulus. From the nature of errors that are made in the ID/ED test of attentional set-shifting, it is possible to infer that both perseveration and learned irrelevance contribute to the increased frequency of errors with shifts of attentional set.[10–13] In reversal learning, rather than being uncorrelated with reward, the previously rewarded stimulus is now negatively correlated. Thus, although similar to learned irrelevance, a more accurate term is *learned non-reward*. We also favor this term over *learned avoidance* (which has been used previously),[14] which might be understood to imply that responding is punished, which is not the case here.

This study was designed to examine the relative contribution of perseveration and learned non-reward in both normal reversal learning and the impaired reversal learning following cell-body lesions of the OPFC. Although it is widely accepted that deficits in reversal learning are a feature of OPFC lesions, it is also known that not all aspects of reversal learning are impaired following OPFC lesions. For example, using the observation that rats respond with greater vigor when they expect rewards of greater value, and that they are sensitive to cues or signals that indicate the value of reward, it has been shown that rats with OFPC lesions can learn that cues have "reversed" in the reward-values they signal.[15,16] Thus, an OFPC lesion–induced reversal impairment would appear not to arise from insensitivity to cues predicting reward, but rather is specific to conditions in which the rat must inhibit a previously rewarded response and/or make a previously unrewarded response. To examine the extent to which these processes might contribute differentially to the reversal-learning impairment, a two-choice discrimination task was used. Rats learned to find food-bait hidden in small bowls filled with various scented digging media. In a procedure similar to that used with monkeys,[14] rats were required to overcome perseverative tendencies and learn that bait was no longer in a previously rewarded bowl or, in a separate condition, to overcome learned non-reward and learn to dig in a previously unbaited bowl.

MATERIALS AND METHODS

Twenty-eight male Lister hooded rats (Harlan, Bicester, UK) were used. The rats were pair-housed until surgery and maintained on a 12 hour light–dark schedule (lights on at 7 am), with a diet of 15–20 g of standard laboratory chow each day with water available *ad libitum*. The initial weight range was 280–330 g. At completion of the procedure, weight range was 370–420 g. All procedures were carried out in accordance with the UK Animals (Scientific Procedures) Act 1986.

Equipment

The set-shifting box was constructed from a large, opaque plastic housing cage (69.5 cm long × 40.5 cm wide × 18.5 cm deep), with internal wooden runners fitted to permit Perspex panels to be lowered to divide the cage into compartments. The cage was divided into three areas: a large waiting area, taking up the width and two-thirds of the length of the cage, and two equal areas large enough to accommodate a ceramic digging bowl. Two panels, which could be lowered independently of each other, were used to prevent access to either or both of the digging bowls. To prevent escape, there was a hinged lid over the waiting area. There were independent hinged lids over the two stimulus compartments, to enable the experimenter to reposition and/or to rebait the digging bowls between trials. The set-shifting apparatus and bowls are described in detail in Birrell and Brown.[6]

Bilateral OPFC Lesions with Ibotenic Acid

Sixteen rats were anesthetized with an isoflurane (4% and reduced to 2% to maintain anesthesia) and oxygen mix. Ibotenic acid (0.06M (n = 16)) or sterile phosphate buffer (n = 12) was administered bilaterally using a 0.5 μL Hamilton syringe with a 30-gauge needle attached, at stereotaxic coordinates[17]; level skull −3.3 mm, AP +4.0 mm, ML ±2.0 mm, DV −4.5 mm (from skull surface) (0.2 μL per site) over 2 mins. The needle was left *in situ* for 3 mins after administration. Rats were administered a 0.05 mL injection (s.c.) of the anti-inflammatory drug carprofen (Rimadyl; Pfizer, Kent, UK) and a 0.25 mL injection (i.p.) of the sedative diazepam (Hameln Pharmaceuticals, Gloucester, UK). Behavioral testing was carried out a minimum of one week and no more than three weeks after surgery.

Behavioral Testing

The day before testing, ceramic bowls (of the size used for the test) were placed in the home-cage and filled with sawdust and a quantity of Honey Loops® (Kellogg Company, Manchester, UK). By the following morning, the food was always eaten. On the first testing day, rats were placed in the larger compartment of the testing cage. Sawdust-filled bowls, with food bait (half of a Honey Loop) buried in each, were placed in the two smaller compartments, and the partitions were removed, allowing rats to approach the bowls and to uncover and eat both of the cereal pieces. This was repeated for a total of six trials. If the rat did not uncover the rewards from both bowls within 10 mins of being given access to them, then the partitions were lowered, both bowls were rebaited, and the trial was repeated. Then the rat learned two simple discriminations (SD), in which the bowls had different odors (the sawdust was scented with mint or oregano) or were filled with different digging media (paper confetti or small Styrofoam beads), and the rat had to learn which bowl was baited.

The side on which the baited bowl was placed was determined pseudo-randomly for each trial, with the constraint that there were no more than three consecutive trials with the reward on the same side. If the rat dug in the correct bowl, the latency to dig was recorded and that trial was recorded as correct. The trial terminated when the rat returned to the waiting area of the box, at which point the barrier was lowered and the bowls rebaited. If the rat dug in the incorrect bowl, the latency to dig was recorded and the trial was marked as incorrect, but the rat was still permitted to continue to explore the bowl; the trial was terminated only when the rat returned to the waiting area, at which point the barrier was lowered. For the initial four trials at each stage of the test, the rat was allowed subsequently to dig in the correct bowl to recover the reward; after four trials, however, an incorrect response terminated the trial. Whether the rat initiated digging in the first bowl he encountered or whether he explored both bowls prior to initiating digging was also recorded. The rat was given up to 10 mins to uncover the reward from the baited bowl, after which time the partitions were lowered and the experimenter waited until the rat showed interest again.

Criterion performance was six consecutive correct trials (the probability of making a correct choice six times consecutively by chance is 0.015), which could include the first four trials.

The following day, in a single session, the rat performed five discriminations:

- SD of odors or digging media
- compound discrimination (CD) in which novel, but irrelevant, stimuli were introduced so that the bowls differed according to both their smell and the digging media, but the correct and incorrect stimulus exemplars remained the same
- reversal (perseveration condition (R_P) or learned non-reward condition (R_{LNR}))
- new compound discrimination (NCD), with a novel stimulus, but the bowls were still discriminated according to the same sensory feature as previously (in other words, there was no requirement to shift attentional set)
- reversal (R_{LNR} or R_P)

TABLE 1. Stimulus sets[a]

Dimension	Training Pairs	Set 1	Set 2
Odor	Mint	Thyme	Nutmeg
	Oregano	Paprika	Cloves
		Coriander	Ginger
Medium	Polystyrene	Gravel	Coarse Sawdust
	Confetti	Pebbles	Fine Sawdust
		Sand	Woodchip

[a]To facilitate counterbalancing, exemplars were used in sets, and presentation of those sets was counterbalanced so that equal numbers of rats were exposed to the different stimuli for each learning and reversal condition.

All rats performed both of two reversal conditions. In the perseveration reversal condition (R_P), the previously baited bowl was now unbaited, and a novel stimulus was introduced as the baited bowl. The previously unrewarded stimulus was removed. In the learned non-reward reversal condition (R_{LNR}), the previously unbaited bowl was now baited. A novel stimulus replaced the previously baited bowl, which was removed. The order of presentation of the two reversal conditions was counterbalanced.

Protocol, discrimination learning criteria, and data recording methods were the same for all stages of testing (see description above).

Counterbalancing of Task

The large number of possible exemplar combinations meant that full counterbalancing of stimuli could not be achieved. Exemplars were therefore used in sets, with all animals receiving the same training pairs, and equal numbers of rats performing odor and media discriminations. The exemplars used are shown in TABLE 1. The order of exposure to the stimulus sets was counterbalanced between the SD/CD/R_P and NCD/R_{LNR} discriminations, as was relevance of the particular stimulus (odor or digging medium).

Histology

Operated rats were perfused with 4% paraformaldehyde in 0.1M phosphate buffer after anesthesia with 0.8 ml Dolethal (Univet, Bicester, Oxfordshire, UK). Brains were stored overnight at 4°C in 20% sucrose solution, washed in distilled water, dried, set in egg yolk in a 40% formaldehyde bath for 2 days, then removed and cut to 50-μm sections into 0.1M phosphate buffer saline (0.9%) (PBS). Three sets of sections were stained: one for vesicular acetylcholine transporter protein (VAChT; incubated in anti-VAChT (Phoenix Pharmaceuticals, Inc., CA) (1:4000) in antibody diluting solution (ADS)); one for acetylcholinesterase; and one set double-stained for neuronal nuclei (NeuN; incubated in anti-NeuN (Chemicon International, Temecula, CA) (1:4000)

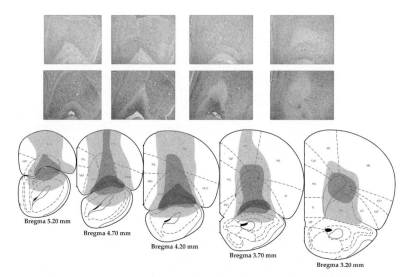

FIGURE 1. Photomicrographs (magnification X2.5) and schematic of the rat brain in coronal section (AP stereotaxic coordinates Bregma +5.20 to +3.20 left to right). Sections show NeuN/cresyl violet-stained tissue from control (top) and lesioned (middle) prefrontal cortex. The schematics on the bottom show greatest extent of lesion (light grey), typical lesion (middle grey), and smallest lesion (dark grey).

overnight in ADS) and with cresyl violet and mounted on gel-coated glass slides. Sections were analyzed under light microscope at magnifications X10 and X40. NeuN/cresyl violet–stained sections were used to visualize the extent of the lesion in the OPFC. VAChT- and acetylcholinesterase-stained sections were used to investigate the effect of the lesion on cholinergic function, specifically the basal forebrain cholinergic projections to the cortex.

Data Analysis

Trials to criterion and errors by type (incorrect digs and non-digs) were analyzed by ANOVA (SPSS v 12.0 for Windows; SPSS, Surrey, UK), with restricted ANOVA conducted to assess the origin of significant interactions following the procedure described in Winer.[18]

RESULTS

Histology

Lesion placement was visualized in the NeuN/cresyl violet–stained sections (FIG. 1). Two subjects were dropped from behavioral analyses due to small

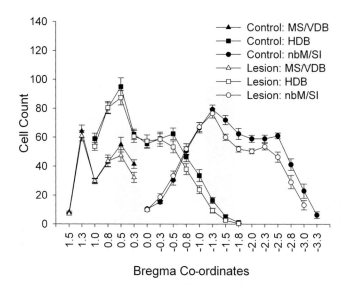

Bregma Co-ordinates

FIGURE 2. Mean ± SEM basal forebrain cell counts (VAChT) for control rats (n = 12) and ibotenic acid lesioned rats (n = 16). Injection point was Bregma +4.0. There is a reduction in cholinergic neurons in the nucleus basalis magnocellularis (nbM)/substantia innominata (SI), but not the medial septum (MS)/vertical (VDB) or horizontal limb of the diagonal band of Broca (HDB).

lesions and extensive, atypical prefrontal acetylcholinesterase loss. All other lesioned subjects showed reduction of acetylcholinesterase staining around the lesion site only. Lesioned rats had cell loss and gliosis in the ventral OPFC, extending to lateral OPFC (Bregma level +5.20 – +3.00). There was also a reduction of VAChT-positive neurons in the nucleus basalis magnocellularis/substantia innominata (mean $10.5\% \pm 2.5$, lesion n = 14) (FIG. 2), indicating a distal effect of the lesion on neurons either projecting to, or receiving projections from, the target area of the lesion. This reduction in cholinergic neurons in the basal forebrain is unlikely to be sufficient to affect performance in the task, however.[4]

Trials to Criterion

As the analysis of the number of trials to criterion (correct plus incorrect digs) and the analysis of the number of errors to criterion gave the same result, for the sake of clarity, only the former analysis is presented.

The performance of the rats with lesions was not different from that of controls for any of the acquisition phases (SD, CD, NCD), but performance was different from controls at both of the reversals (R_P and R_{LNR}) (interaction of Condition and Group: $(F(4,88) = 44.83, P < 0.01)$.

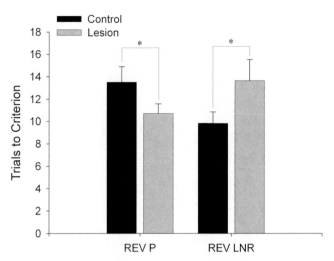

FIGURE 3. Mean ± SEM of the number of trials to criterion for each reversal condition. Control rats required fewer trials to reach criterion in the R_{LNR} condition than in the R_P condition. The lesioned rats performed significantly better than controls in the R_P condition and significantly worse than controls in the R_{LNR} condition. Statistically significant differences are marked with an "*".

An analysis restricted to the acquisition stages confirmed that, for both lesion and control groups, all three acquisitions were achieved in a similar number of trials (main effect of condition, $F(2,88) = 1.7$, ns) and there was no effect of the lesion (main effect of Group, $F(1,22) = 2.4$, ns; interaction of Condition and Group, $F(2,88) = 0.31$, ns).

The lesion and control group were different from each other in both conditions (interaction of Condition and Group: $F(1,88) = 8.4$, $P < 0.01$) (FIG. 3). Specifically, the lesioned animals required fewer trials than controls to reach criterion in the R_P condition (where the previously rewarded exemplar becomes unrewarded, and a novel rewarded exemplar replaces the previously unrewarded exemplar) ($t(24) = 1.8$, $P < 0.05$), while the opposite pattern (lesioned animals requiring more trials than control animals) occurred in the R_{LNR} condition (where the previously unrewarded exemplar becomes rewarded, and a novel exemplar replaces the previously rewarded exemplar) ($t(24) = -1.7$, $P < 0.05$).

In addition, the control rats required more trials to reach criterion in the R_P compared to the R_{LNR} ($t(11) = 2.2$, $P < 0.05$), whereas the lesioned group did not; if anything the lesioned group required fewer trials to reach criterion in the R_P condition, compared to the R_{LNR} condition, although this difference was not statistically significant ($t(11) = -1.5$, ns).

There was no effect of the order in which each reversal was performed; neither did condition order interact with other variables.

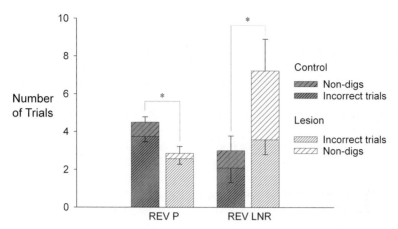

FIGURE 4. Mean ± SEM incorrect and "non-digs" trial to criterion. Lesioned rats make more error overall (i.e., incorrect + non-digs combined) than control in the R_{LNR} condition and fewer in the R_P condition.There was no statistical difference between the group when either type of error was considered alone. Statistically significant differences are marked with an "*".

Analysis of Errors

Rats learn to discriminate baited bowls by their odor or the digging medium very readily, and overall there are few errors. For this reason, it is not possible to consider errors according to whether they were made before or after a correct response (see Roberts et al.[3]).

However, in this modification of the task, rats were more likely to make "refusals to dig"—that is to say, they failed to dig in either bowl within 10 mins of being given access to the bowls. Under these circumstances, an error is not recorded (thus, these trials do not feature in the analysis of trials to criterion). Rather, they are considered suspended trials; the dividers are lowered and not raised until the rat appears to be engaged in the task again.

In the R_P condition, it was usual to see incorrect responses but almost no suspended trials, whereas suspended trials were more likely in the R_{LNR} condition (interaction of Condition and Error type, $F(1,24) = 5.66$, $P < 0.03$) (FIG. 4).

The lesioned rats were not more likely than the controls to make either kind of error (interaction of Group by Error type, ns), but (confirming the pattern seen in the analysis of Trials to criterion, see above) control rats made more errors in the R_P condition and lesioned animals made more errors in the R_{LNR} condition (interaction of Condition and Group, $F(1,24) = 7.84$, $P < 0.01$), although there was no interaction by Error type.

DISCUSSION

Confirming previous demonstrations,[1] OPFC lesions did not affect rats' abilities to learn simple (SD) or complex (NCD) discriminations of novel stimuli. Nor did the lesions impact performance when an additional, irrelevant, stimulus attribute was introduced (CD)—the lesioned rats were not disrupted or distracted by the novel aspects of the bowls and continued to respond to the relevant feature.

Rats with OPFC lesions were impaired relative to controls when they had to overcome learned non-reward (R_{LNR}) to form a new reward–stimulus association; they made both more errors and more non-dig responses than controls. By contrast, and somewhat surprisingly, when they had to inhibit responding to a previously rewarded stimulus (R_P), they made fewer perseverative errors than did controls.

The significant improvement, relative to controls, in performance in the R_P condition in the OPFC-lesioned group was unexpected. It is possible that both the improved performance in the R_P condition and the impaired performance in the R_{LNR} condition are due to an enhanced preference for novelty in the lesioned rats (see FIG. 4 of Ref. 14). We consider this unlikely for several reasons. First, we included an additional stage (CD) in which a novel stimulus aspect was introduced after a SD had been acquired, and we observed no disruption of behavior resulting from this—in particular, the lesioned animals were not distracted by (or attracted by, such that they directed reponses toward) the new stimulus features. That said, it was nevertheless the case that the new stimulus features were introduced after the rats had learned to discriminate between two stimuli, and they were additional to, and not replacing, any stimulus. Thus it is possible that their introduction was insufficiently salient to disrupt ongoing behavior even if the lesions do increase a preference for novelty. However, although a novelty bias would lead to an increase in errors in the R_{LNR} condition (by definition, errors in this condition are digging in the novel bowl), it is not apparent how a novelty bias alone would account for the difficulty in acquiring this stage. In particular, there was also a significant increase in "refusals to dig" in the R_{LNR} condition, a result that was independent of the increase in Trials to Criterion (which includes only correct trials and error digs). We consider reluctance to dig as indicative of learned non-reward as it is a passive reluctance to initiate a dig in the previously unrewarded bowl, rather than an approach to the novel bowl.

In terms of the R_P condition, an improvement in performance might indeed be due to some form of novelty bias, but further consideration of what is meant by this is warranted. We have previously reported that similar lesions to those made here resulted in a very large—on average almost 100%—increase in trials to criterion in a test of classic reversal learning where the correct and incorrect stimuli were simply exchanged.[1] The improvement in the R_P condition that we report here might be considered as suggesting that perseveration does not contribute to the previous reversal deficit. However, even in the R_{LNR} condition, in which the lesioned animals were impaired relative to controls, they still made fewer errors than might have been expected given the magnitude of the deficit in the classic reversal. Thus it is not possible to conclude that learned non-reward provides a complete account of the reversal deficit. In a typical reversal experiment, lesioned rats perseverate in the context of having to overcome learned non-reward: in the present experiment, the previously correct stimulus was competing with an entirely novel stimulus. It is therefore likely that the reduced perseverative tendency seen here might only be evident when the rat is given the option of responding to novelty and that under standard reversal conditions, perseveration and learned non-reward interact to produce greater deficits overall.

Clarke et al.,[14] using a procedure in essence the same as the one employed here, recently reported that serotonergic OPFC lesions in monkeys increased perseveration and did not increase learned avoidance. As this is in direct contrast to the effect reported here, an explanation is required. There is a growing body of evidence from many laboratories using similar procedures to suggest that rats and monkeys behave quite similarly in tests of set-shifting and in reversal learning. Therefore we think it is unlikely that the difference is species-specific, and it would be premature to dismiss it thus. Apart from the species, the next most obvious difference between the studies is that the lesions are different: we used excitotoxic cell-body lesions, while they used neurochemically specific lesions. Whereas depletion of serotonin increased perseveration relative to controls, depletion of dopamine was without effect. It is therefore quite possible that whereas serotonin is required for effective inhibition of learned responding, the intrinsic circuits of the OFPC, compromised by the excitotoxic lesions, are required to overcome learned non-reward. Having said that, we have not observed impairment in reversal learning in the context of the ID/ED task in rats with depletion of serotonin effected by intracerebroventricular infusion of 5,7-DHT (Tait, Laidlaw and Brown, unpublished observations). In addition, the improvement in reversal-learning performance following 5-HT$_6$ antagonism[19] has been interpreted as due not necessarily to the effects of manipulation of serotonergic transmission but rather to the effects on other transmitter systems, particularly acetylcholine. Thus, there might be other differences between the studies that also require consideration.

One procedural difference between the test as applied to rats and the test as applied to monkeys is based on the nature of the sampling of the stimuli and the availability of reward. When a rat approaches and digs in a bowl without having first explored the other bowl, regardless of whether or not it recovers a reward, its learning can be based only on the bowl sampled; the characteristics of an unsampled bowl are unknown. But when a monkey or a human views adjacent visual stimuli on a computer screen, both the responded-to and the not-responded-to stimuli can be seen, compared, and processed, and if the responded-to stimulus is not rewarded, it may be inferred that the other stimulus would have been. For this reason, for the initial four trials, if the rat makes an incorrect choice, our standard procedure is to allow the rat to sample and recover the bait from the other bowl. This was intended to enable the rat to learn as much about the other stimulus as the monkey might be learning. However, this procedural difference might give the rat more information than that available to the monkey: from the very first trial of a reversal, the rat has the opportunity to discover not only that the previously baited bowl is now not baited, but also where the bait is now located. On the other hand, the monkey, although seeing the stimulus, does not have the opportunity to learn that it is now associated with reward: the first trial of a reversal is always unrewarded, and the animal will not know that the other stimulus is rewarded until it overcomes perseveration. This additional information available to the rat might have aided in overcoming perseveration.

By contrast, in the R_{LNR} condition, the information available to the rat will be limited if the rat fails to dig in the other bowl after an unrewarded dig in the novel bowl. Although given the opportunity, rats sometimes do not explore and recover the reward from the other bowl after first digging in an unbaited bowl, and this was seen particularly in the R_{LNR} condition. These trials were not recorded as non-dig responses (because the rat had dug in the unbaited, incorrect, bowl); instead they were terminated when the rat showed no interest in exploring or digging further. Given that the rat cannot be forced to explore or to dig, if it chooses not to do so and avoids sampling the stimulus, this would retard learning. On the other hand, one might imagine that the monkey cannot help but "see" the alternative stimulus to which it did not respond so that in the condition of learned non-reward the monkey will still visually sample the stimulus. This difference in the way stimuli are sampled and how much can be learned in each trial might account for some of the behavior that is different for monkeys and rats. In particular, we would highlight the fact that normal rats solve the R_{LNR} more rapidly than the R_P, and a classic reversal (although not directly compared here) is generally solved with an intermediate number of errors. Monkeys, on the other hand, make fewer errors in both of the modified reversal conditions, compared to a classic reversal, and the modified reversals do not differ from each other.

In summary, in the two reversal conditions explored in this study, rats with OPFC lesions were only impaired when they had to overcome learned non-reward. To conclude from this that learned non-reward accounts for the deficit in reversal learning, however, would be premature. The limitations of the use of subtractive logic in the design of behavioral experiments have been acknowledged in the psychology literature for many years, but of most relevance here is that the subtraction of one factor rarely can have a fundamental impact on— so changing the nature of the effects of—the remaining factors. Furthermore, in both conditions a novel stimulus was introduced, and this also changes the nature of the response conflict. Neither of the conditions tested here is a full reversal: perseveration and learned non-reward may interact when the animal is lesioned and together produce failure to reverse responding. Nevertheless, it is clear that, as a single mechanism, perseveration alone cannot account for all aspects of the reversal-learning impairment following cell-body lesions of ventral OPFC. Learned non-reward also contributes to these deficits.

REFERENCES

1. MCALONAN, K. & V.J. BROWN. 2003. Orbital prefrontal cortex mediates reversal learning and not attentional set shifting in the rat. Behav. Brain Res. **146:** 97–103.
2. DIAS, R., T.W. ROBBINS & A.C. ROBERTS. 1996. Dissociation in prefrontal cortex of affective and attentional shifts. Nature **380:** 69–72.
3. ROBERTS, A.C. et al. 1992. A specific form of cognitive rigidity following excitotoxic lesions of the basal forebrain in marmosets. Neuroscience **47:** 251–264.
4. TAIT, D.S. & V.J. BROWN. 2007. Lesions of the basal forebrain impair reversal learning but not shifting of attentional set in rats. Behav. Brain Res. doi: 10.1016/j.bbr.2007.08.035.
5. ROBERTS, A.C., T.W. ROBBINS & B.J. EVERITT. 1988. The effects of intradimensional and extradimensional shifts on visual discrimination learning in humans and non-human primates. Q. J. Exp. Psychol. B. **40:** 321–341.
6. BIRRELL, J.M. & V.J. BROWN. 2000. Medial frontal cortex mediates perceptual attentional set shifting in the rat. J. Neurosci. **20:** 4320–4324.
7. CHUDASAMA, Y. & T.W. ROBBINS. 2003. Dissociable contributions of the orbitofrontal and infralimbic cortex to pavlovian autoshaping and discrimination reversal learning: further evidence for the functional heterogeneity of the rodent frontal cortex. J. Neurosci. **23:** 8771–8780.
8. CLARKE, H.F. et al. 2004. Cognitive inflexibility after prefrontal serotonin depletion. Science **304:** 878–880.
9. CLARKE, H.F. et al. 2005. Prefrontal serotonin depletion affects reversal learning but not attentional set shifting. J. Neurosci. **25:** 532–538.
10. GAUNTLETT-GILBERT, J., R.C. ROBERTS & V.J. BROWN. 1999. Mechanisms underlying attentional set-shifting in Parkinson's disease. Neuropsychologia **37:** 605–616.
11. MAES, J.H., M.D. DAMEN & P.A. ELING. 2004. More learned irrelevance than perseveration errors in rule shifting in healthy subjects. Brain Cogn. **54:** 201–211.
12. OWEN, A.M. et al. 1993. Contrasting mechanisms of impaired attentional setshifting in patients with frontal lobe damage or Parkinson's disease. Brain **116**(Pt 5): 1159–1175.
13. BARCELO, F. & R.T. KNIGHT. 2002. Both random and perseverative errors underlie WCST deficits in prefrontal patients. Neuropsychologia **40:** 349–356.
14. CLARKE, H.F. et al. 2007. Cognitive inflexibility after prefrontal serotonin depletion is behaviorally and neurochemically specific. Cereb. Cortex **17:** 18–27.
15. BOHN, I., C. GIERTLER & W. HAUBER. 2003. Orbital prefrontal cortex and guidance of instrumental behavior of rats by visuospatial stimuli predicting reward magnitude. Learn Mem. **10:** 177–186.
16. WARD, N.M. et al. 1998. Simple and choice reaction-time performance following occlusion of the anterior cerebral arteries in the rat. Exp. Brain Res. **123:** 269–281.

17. PAXINOS, G. & C. WATSON. 1998. The Rat Brain in Stereotaxic Coordinates. Academic Press. San Diego.
18. WINER, B.J. 1971. Statistical Principles in Experimental Design. McGraw-Hill. New York.
19. HATCHER, P.D. et al. 2005. 5-HT6 receptor antagonists improve performance in an attentional set shifting task in rats. Psychopharmacology (Berl.) **181**: 253–259.

The Role of Orbitofrontal Cortex in Decision Making

A Component Process Account

LESLEY K. FELLOWS

Montreal Neurological Institute, McGill University, Montréal, Québec, Canada

ABSTRACT: Clinical accounts of the effects of damage to orbitofrontal cortex (OFC) have provided important clues about the functions of this region in humans. Patients with OFC injury can demonstrate relatively isolated difficulties with decision making, and the development of laboratory tasks that captured these difficulties was an important advance. However, much of the work to date has been limited by the use of a single, complex decision-making task and by a narrow focus on risky decisions. A fuller understanding of the neural basis of decision making requires identification of the simpler components that underlie this complex behavior. Here, I review evidence that OFC lesions disrupt reversal learning in humans, as in animals, and show that this deficit in reversal learning is an important mechanism underlying the difficulties of such patients in the Iowa gambling task. Reversal learning, in turn, can be decomposed into simpler processes: a failure to rapidly learn from negative feedback may be the critical difficulty for OFC patients. OFC damage can also affect forms of decision making that do not require trial-by-trial learning. Preference judgment is a simple form of decision making that requires comparing the relative value of options. Humans with OFC lesions are more inconsistent in their choices, even in very simple preference judgment tasks. These results are broadly consistent with the view that OFC is critically involved in representing the relative value of stimuli, but also raise the possibility that this region plays distinct roles in reinforcement learning and value-based judgment.

KEYWORDS: reversal learning; neuroeconomics; executive function; prefrontal cortex; human; lesion

Clinical descriptions of patients with ventral frontal lobe damage have heavily influenced current thinking about the functions of orbitofrontal cortex (OFC) in humans. However, despite vivid anecdotal accounts of social, emotional, and personality changes following OFC injury stretching back many

Address for correspondence: Lesley K. Fellows, M.D., C.M., DPhil, Montreal Neurological Institute, 3801 University St., Rm 276, Montréal, QC H3A 2B4, Canada. Voice: (514) 398 8980; fax: (514) 398 1338.
lesley.fellows@mcgill.ca

Ann. N.Y. Acad. Sci. 1121: 421–430 (2007). © 2007 New York Academy of Sciences.
doi: 10.1196/annals.1401.023

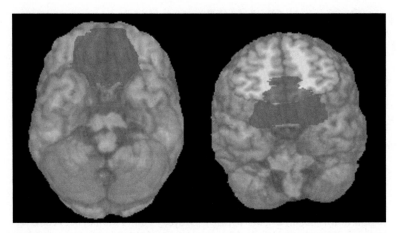

FIGURE 1. Schematic representation of the region of the frontal lobes referred to as ventromedial frontal (VMF) in the text. This includes medial OFC (shown in dark grey in the base of the brain view in the left panel) and the adjacent ventral region of medial PFC (shown in oblique view, with the anterior portion of the frontal lobe cut away, in the right panel). The common causes of focal injury to these areas in humans typically affect both sectors, often bilaterally, albeit to varying degree.

decades,[1-4] a principled understanding of the basis of these deficits has been slow to emerge. As with many disorders of complex behavior, the sticking point has been how best to frame these clinical observations: One influential model proposes that a fundamental impairment in decision making is at the heart of the real-life difficulties of OFC-damaged patients.[5] Experimental evidence for this claim came from the observation that those patients with OFC damage who displayed clinical evidence of impaired decision making were also impaired on a laboratory decision task now known as the Iowa gambling task (IGT).[6] Prompted in part by these findings, other investigators began asking more general questions about how economic information important to decision making, such as expectancies, risk, and uncertainty, might be represented in the brain.[7-10] This line of research, sometimes called "neuroeconomics," has provided evidence that activity within OFC (and the anatomically closely related ventral aspect of medial prefrontal cortex [PFC]; FIG. 1) reflects the relative value of potential choices (see Padoa-Schioppa *et al.*—this volume).

Although it was developed to study decision making, the IGT could equally be viewed as a reinforcement learning task: Good performance requires learning the reward and punishment contingencies associated with the different decks of cards and integrating these varying contingencies over multiple trials. Could the poor performance of OFC-damaged patients reflect a basic difficulty in some aspect of reinforcement learning? This formulation of the problem brings to bear a different literature. There is abundant evidence for a role for OFC in specific forms of reinforcement learning, primarily from animal studies. In particular, OFC lesions in several species lead to a characteristic deficit in reversal learning (reviewed in Ref. 11 and elsewhere in this volume). Two features of the initial IGT work in patients with frontal damage raise the possibility that reversal learning might be playing a role in this task. First, the task itself involves a reversal of initial reward and punishment contingencies. Second, at least in the initial IGT study, patients with ventromedial frontal (VMF) damage failed to learn to avoid the disadvantageous decks,[6,12] a behavior that echoes the tendency of animals with OFC damage to perseverate on the initially rewarded stimulus after reinforcement contingencies change in reversal-learning tasks.

The IGT requires participants to choose among four decks of cards. On each trial, a card is drawn, which either provides a win, or a win and a loss. Overall, two of the decks are associated with large wins, but even larger losses. The other two ('advantageous') decks provide smaller wins, but even smaller losses. Crucially, the order of the cards in each deck is fixed. The large losses associated with the disadvantageous decks only begin to accrue after several trials in which only large wins are experienced.[13] Unsurprisingly, healthy controls and patients alike show a preference for these (eventually) disadvantageous decks in the first block of 20 trials, because the reinforcement contingencies that have been experienced up to that point indicate that these decks are "the best bet." As the task proceeds, and the large losses begin to accrue, healthy subjects gradually shift their choices to the two advantageous decks. In contrast, those with VMF damage persist in choosing more often from the initially attractive, but overall disadvantageous decks. We hypothesized that the specific pattern of reinforcement in the IGT required reversal learning, and that the persistently disadvantageous choices of VMF patients reflected a fundamental impairment in reversal learning similar to that seen in other species after OFC damage.

This hypothesis was tested in work I carried out with Martha Farah. We first asked whether VMF damage in humans impaired simple reversal learning, following up an earlier lesion study which suggested as much.[14] Eight subjects with fixed focal damage to VMF due to stroke or aneurysm rupture were compared to 12 subjects with damage to other areas of the frontal lobes, and to 12 healthy, demographically matched control subjects. The reversal-learning task was a simple, two deck card game. Choosing from one deck led to a $50 play-money win, from the other a $50 loss. Once subjects had chosen from the winning deck eight trials in a row, the contingencies were switched without warning. The task continued for a further 50 trials, allowing up to five reversals. All subjects were quick to learn the initial associations in this simple task. However, those with VMF damage made substantially more errors in the reversal phase[15] (FIG. 2).

Having confirmed that VMF damage specifically impaired reversal learning, we went on to ask whether this explained the characteristic difficulties with the IGT experienced by patients with VMF damage. To that end, we designed

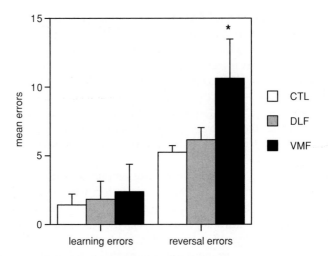

FIGURE 2. Initial stimulus–reinforcer association learning and reversal-learning performance in subjects with fixed damage of VMF lobes (VMF), compared to subjects with damage to the frontal lobes outside VMF (DLF) and healthy control subjects (CTL). Initial learning performance is expressed as the mean number of errors made before the learning criterion was met and reversal learning as the mean number of errors in the reversal phase of the experiment. Error bars show the upper bound of the 95% confidence intervals. The asterisk indicates a significant group X error type interaction, $P < 0.05$. From Fellows, L.K. & M.J. Farah. Ventromedial frontal cortex mediates affective shifting in humans: evidence from a reversal learning paradigm. *Brain* 2003; 126: 1830–1837, by permission of Oxford University Press.[15]

a "shuffled" variant of this task. By changing the order of the cards in each deck so that the large losses associated with the disadvantageous decks were experienced early, we attempted to eliminate the reversal-learning requirement of the original task. All other features of the task were identical to the original. Ten subjects with VMF damage (again compared to subjects with non-VMF frontal damage [N = 12] and healthy control subjects) completed both the original and "shuffled" versions of the IGT. As in previous reports, those with VMF damage chose from the disadvantageous decks more often than did the healthy control group. However, when the reversal requirement was eliminated in the shuffled task, the performance of VMF subjects was indistinguishable from that of healthy controls (FIG. 3).[16] Interestingly, the subjects with non-VMF frontal damage were also impaired on the standard IGT, consistent with other work.[17] However, their performance did not improve in the shuffled version, indicating that deficits in processes other than reversal learning (perhaps working memory[18] or attention[19]) contribute to their impairment.

   Taken together, these two studies argue that a fundamental deficit in reversal learning underlies the aberrant performance on the IGT of patients with VMF damage. This work also suggests that it may be more useful to characterize

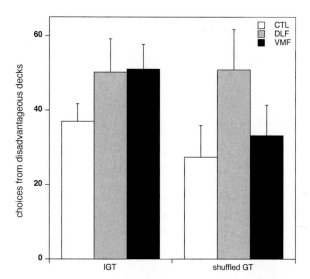

FIGURE 3. Total number of cards chosen from the two disadvantageous decks (over 100 trials) in the original IGT (*left*), and a "shuffled" version of the same task (*right*) designed to eliminate the requirement for reversal learning. Those with VMF damage made poor choices in the original IGT, but performed as well as healthy control subjects in the shuffled version. Those with non-VMF damage (DLF) were equally impaired on the two tasks. Error bars show the upper bound of the 95% confidence intervals. Data from Ref. 16.

the difficulties of such patients as deficits in flexible reinforcement learning, rather than impaired decision making. In a similar vein, others have argued that the particular form of "affective" perseveration captured by reversal learning may also be the basis for the real-life socially inappropriate behavior that can follow VMF damage.[14] This formulation raises other potential avenues of research. For example, while reversal learning is simpler than the IGT, it might be decomposed into still simpler underlying processes. Can the particular process or processes for which VMF is critical be specified in more detail? Finally, can links be made between this learning-based account of VMF function and the neuroeconomics-influenced view that this area is representing value?

Successful reversal learning requires a shift in behavior in response to unexpected negative feedback—either non-reward, or outright punishment, depending on the paradigm. Failure to shift away from punishment in this task also prevents the subject from experiencing (and so learning from) the rewards now available with the alternative choice, even if the ability to learn from reward is intact. One parsimonious explanation of the reversal-learning findings is that VMF is critically involved in adjusting behavior in response to negative outcomes. We found preliminary support for this hypothesis in a study of the effects of VMF damage on the ability to learn from positive and negative feedback, tested with a probabilistic learning paradigm developed by Frank and colleagues.[20]

Subjects chose between three pairs of arbitrary visual stimuli on the basis of probabilistic positive or negative feedback. Once they met a learning criterion for each pair, they moved to a test phase in which they chose between all possible combinations of the six stimuli, without feedback. Their tendency to choose the stimulus that had been most highly associated with positive reinforcement, and to avoid the stimulus that had been most highly associated with negative reinforcement separately probed their ability to learn from positive and negative feedback. Only five of the 11 VMF subjects (compared with 22 of 24 age-matched control subjects) learned the task to criterion. Consistent with previous work, controls who proceeded to the test phase learned about equally from positive and negative reinforcement. In contrast, those with VMF damage who completed the test phase were markedly and selectively impaired at learning from negative feedback (Wheele and Fellows, manuscript submitted for publication).

Instrumental avoidance learning differs from reward-driven learning in interesting ways: successful learning leads to reduced experience of the negative feedback, which in principle should lead to extinction of the no-longer-reinforced avoidance response. In practice, of course, avoidance learning is not easily extinguished. Various mechanisms have been proposed to explain this phenomenon.[21] Although it is debatable whether probabilistically delivered negative feedback is strictly comparable to outright punishment,[22] the finding that VMF damage disrupted learning from such feedback, while leaving positive feedback-driven learning intact suggests that there are differences in the neural substrates that support the two. It may be that dopaminergic-striatal mechanisms are sufficient for effectively learning from positive feedback, at least in a probabilistic context (and over a few hundred trials), with VMF additionally required for optimally learning from negative feedback over the same time scale.

The links between this reinforcement learning perspective on VMF function, with its emphasis on reversal learning and negative feedback, and neuroeconomic models of VMF as important in representing relative (and typically positively valenced) value are not self-evident. While the work just reviewed argues that VMF is not *necessary* for simple, incremental forms of probabilistic reward-driven learning, it nevertheless may still be involved, perhaps in more subtle or context-sensitive ways (see, e.g., Refs. 23, 24). It may also be that the role played by this region in reinforcement learning paradigms is different from its role (or roles) in other decision contexts. Indeed, even whether the VMF mechanisms important in simple reversal learning are the same as those tapped by probabilistic learning tasks remains to be directly established. Finally, different sub-regions within this relatively large area of the brain may be differentially involved in learning and decision making.

"Relative value" (and the closely related concept of subjective utility) is a powerful construct because it provides a parsimonious mechanism to solve a variety of decision problems. Value is not a fixed feature of a stimulus: it varies according to intrinsic factors, such as satiety, and extrinsic factors, such as the value of other available options. Value can be adjusted for uncertainty or delay and provides a common currency for comparing very different kinds of options and for calculating the total worth of options that have multiple attributes. Determining whether relative value is represented, as such, in the brain is obviously a central problem in understanding the neural basis of decision making. This question has been addressed by functional imaging studies in humans and by electrophysiological work in non-human primates. Both methods have provided evidence that activity in OFC and/or medial PFC reflects relative value, providing an "accounting" that can incorporate many of the factors described above.

This work, reviewed in detail elsewhere in this volume (Padoa-Schioppa, O'Doherty, Wallis), leaves open whether the information about value that seems to be represented in VMF is *necessary* for decision making. This question is most directly answered by loss-of-function methods, such as lesion studies. If we accept that the IGT is detecting the role of VMF in learning, rather than decision making, then the evidence that VMF plays a critical role in decision making is relatively limited. A handful of studies using other gambling or risk paradigms have shown that VMF or orbitofrontal damage can affect decision making in the absence of the need for new learning.[25–27] However, it is not clear whether this effect is specific to risky decision making, or reflects a more fundamental difficulty in determining relative value.

In order to explore these issues further, we examined the effects of VMF damage on a simple form of decision making that involves comparing the relative value of choices in the absence of risk, ambiguity, or trial-by-trial learning. Adapting a paradigm first used in non-human primates,[28] we asked whether VMF damage in humans would disrupt pair-wise preference judgments. Subjects were asked to indicate which of two stimuli they preferred, or "liked better." Categories included colors, foods, and famous people. Within each category, all possible pairs of stimuli were presented. Since subjective preferences are idiosyncratic, there is no right or wrong answer in such a task. Instead, we examined how internally consistent the choices were for each subject. If a given subject preferred food A over food B, and B over C, that subject should prefer A over C. The choice of C over A would be considered inconsistent. We reasoned that if VMF played a critical role in calculating or representing relative value, then damage there should degrade the ability to make these value-based preference judgments, resulting in an increase in inconsistent choices. As predicted, patients with VMF damage (N = 10) made significantly more inconsistent choices than either a healthy control group or a group with damage to the frontal lobes sparing VMF.[29]

This result is consistent with a role for VMF in representing relative value, with this region apparently necessary for even this very simple form of decision making. A deficit in this basic process may also explain the changes observed in more complex, multi-attribute decision making after VMF damage.[30] It seems reasonable to suppose that the additional complexity of risky or ambiguous decisions would magnify any deficit in determining relative value in such patients, although this is a claim that remains to be tested directly. Thus, the poor choices made by VMF-damaged patients in many contexts may derive from a degraded ability to compare the value of decision options. This impairment may result in a higher frequency of poor choices, choices that are less consistently risk-averse than those made by healthy subjects, or at least choices that are less consistent than those the patient might have made prior to his or her brain injury.

Could a deficit in comparing relative value also be at the root of reversal-learning impairments that follow VMF damage? After all, reversal-learning tasks require a series of choices between options with changing values. If VMF supports a common component process underlying both reversal learning and preference judgment, then performance on these two tasks should not be dissociable in patients with VMF damage. In fact, in the 10 patients we studied who completed both tasks, overall reversal learning and preference judgment performance were not correlated.[29] At the individual level, three of 10 subjects with VMF damage were clearly normal in their ability to make preference judgments, and two of these three were either moderately or severely impaired at reversal learning. Of the three subjects with the worst preference-task performance, one had only slight difficulty with reversal learning. These findings provide preliminary evidence that reversal learning and judging relative value can be dissociated in some patients with VMF damage, arguing that they are distinct processes with separable neural substrates (although there was no clear relationship between these dissociable behaviors and lesion location in this small sample). These data require further validation, however, not least because the preference task appears to be less sensitive than the reversal learning paradigm.

The series of studies reviewed here illustrates a component process approach to understanding the role played by VMF in human decision making. Candidate component processes were identified based on studies of OFC function in animals and on economic and psychologic models of decision making. This fundamental work has followed separate streams. The first has focused on the role of OFC in reinforcement learning and implicated the region specifically in particular forms of learning, notably reversal learning. The second, less-developed stream is consistent with a role for OFC in representing the relative, subjective value of potential choices. The work described here argues that OFC plays a necessary role in reversal learning in humans, just as it does in animals. Furthermore, this basic process seems to explain the deficits of patients with VMF damage in the more complex IGT. At an even more basic level, the reversal-learning deficit that follows VMF damage may rest, in turn, on a specific difficulty learning from negative feedback. However, VMF damage also disrupts preference judgments, simple decisions that isolate the comparison of relative value from other aspects of decision making. This supports the hypothesis that this region of the brain is involved in representing or comparing the relative value of options, thereby playing a critical role in human decision making. More generally, these studies underline that work on basic aspects of behavior in animal models can be a powerful starting point for understanding the neural basis of complex human behavior.

ACKNOWLEDGMENTS

I thank Martha Farah and Elizabeth Wheeler for their substantial contributions to the work reviewed here. Funding was provided by NIH R21NS045074, CIHR MOP-77583, and by a CIHR Clinician-Scientist award.

REFERENCES

1. ACKERLY, S. 2000. Prefrontal lobes and social development. 1950. Yale J. Biol. Med. **73:** 211–219.
2. DAMASIO, A.R. 1994. Descartes' Error: Emotion, Reason, and the Human Brain. Avon Books.
3. LOEWENSTEIN, G.F. *et al.* 2001. Risk as feelings. Psychol. Bull. **127:** 267–286.
4. ESLINGER, P.J. & A.R. DAMASIO. 1985. Severe disturbance of higher cognition after bilateral frontal lobe ablation: patient EVR. Neurology **35:** 1731–1741.
5. BECHARA, A., H. DAMASIO, & A.R. DAMASIO. 2000. Emotion, decision making and the orbitofrontal cortex. Cereb. Cortex **10:** 295–307.
6. BECHARA, A. *et al.* 1997. Deciding advantageously before knowing the advantageous strategy. Science **275:** 1293–1295.
7. FELLOWS, L.K. 2007. Advances in understanding ventromedial prefrontal function: the accountant joins the executive. Neurology **68:** 991–995.
8. MONTAGUE, P.R., B. KING-CASAS, & J.D. COHEN. 2006. Imaging valuation models in human choice. Annu. Rev. Neurosci. **29:** 417–448.
9. O'DOHERTY, J.P. 2004. Reward representations and reward-related learning in the human brain: insights from neuroimaging. Curr. Opin. Neurobiol. **14:** 769–776.
10. SUGRUE, L.P., G.S. CORRADO, & W.T. NEWSOME. 2005. Choosing the greater of two goods: neural currencies for valuation and decision making. Nat. Rev. Neurosci. **6:** 363–375.
11. ROBERTS, A.C. 2006. Primate orbitofrontal cortex and adaptive behaviour. Trends Cogn. Sci. **10:** 83–90.
12. BECHARA, A. *et al.* 1994. Insensitivity to future consequences following damage to human prefrontal cortex. Cognition **50:** 7–15.
13. BECHARA, A., D. TRANEL, & H. DAMASIO. 2000. Characterization of the decision-making deficit of patients with ventromedial prefrontal cortex lesions. Brain **123**(Pt 11): 2189–2202.

14. ROLLS, E.T. *et al.* 1994. Emotion-related learning in patients with social and emotional changes associated with frontal lobe damage. J. Neurol. Neurosurg. Psychiatry **57:** 1518–1524.
15. FELLOWS, L.K. & M.J. FARAH. 2003. Ventromedial frontal cortex mediates affective shifting in humans: evidence from a reversal learning paradigm. Brain **126:** 1830–1837.
16. FELLOWS, L.K. & M.J. FARAH. 2005. Different underlying impairments in decision-making following ventromedial and dorsolateral frontal lobe damage in humans. Cereb. Cortex **15:** 58–63.
17. MANES, F. *et al.* 2002. Decision-making processes following damage to the prefrontal cortex. Brain **125:** 624–639.
18. BECHARA, A. *et al.* 1998. Dissociation of working memory from decision making within the human prefrontal cortex. J. Neurosci. **18:** 428–437.
19. HORNAK, J. *et al.* 2004. Reward-related reversal learning after surgical excisions in orbito-frontal or dorsolateral prefrontal cortex in humans. J. Cogn. Neurosci. **16:** 463–478.
20. FRANK, M.J., L.C. SEEBERGER, & C. O'REILLY R. 2004. By carrot or by stick: cognitive reinforcement learning in parkinsonism. Science **306:** 1940–1943.
21. KIM, H., S. SHIMOJO, & J.P. O'DOHERTY. 2006. Is avoiding an aversive outcome rewarding? Neural substrates of avoidance learning in the human brain. PLoS Biol. **4:** e233.
22. SEYMOUR, B. *et al.* 2007. Differential encoding of losses and gains in the human striatum. J. Neurosci. **27:** 4826–4831.
23. FRANK, M.J. & E.D. CLAUS. 2006. Anatomy of a decision: striato-orbitofrontal interactions in reinforcement learning, decision making, and reversal. Psychol. Rev. **113:** 300–326.
24. SCHOENBAUM, G. & M. ROESCH. 2005. Orbitofrontal cortex, associative learning, and expectancies. Neuron **47:** 633–636.
25. HSU, M. *et al.* 2005. Neural systems responding to degrees of uncertainty in human decision-making. Science **310:** 1680–1683.
26. ROGERS, R.D. *et al.* 1999. Dissociable deficits in the decision-making cognition of chronic amphetamine abusers, opiate abusers, patients with focal damage to prefrontal cortex, and tryptophan-depleted normal volunteers: evidence for monoaminergic mechanisms. Neuropsychopharmacology **20:** 322–339.
27. SHIV, B. *et al.* 2005. Investment behavior and the negative side of emotion. Psychol. Sci. **16:** 435–439.
28. BAYLIS, L.L. & D. GAFFAN. 1991. Amygdalectomy and ventromedial prefrontal ablation produce similar deficits in food choice and in simple object discrimination learning for an unseen reward. Exp. Brain Res. **86:** 617–622.
29. FELLOWS, L.K. & M.J. FARAH. 2007. The role of ventromedial prefrontal cortex in decision making: judgment under uncertainty, or judgment per se? Cereb. Cortex **17:** 2669–2674.
30. FELLOWS, L.K. 2006. Deciding how to decide: ventromedial frontal lobe damage affects information acquisition in multi-attribute decision making. Brain **129:** 944–952.

Neuronal Activity Related to Anticipated Reward in Frontal Cortex

Does It Represent Value or Reflect Motivation?

MATTHEW R. ROESCH[a] AND CARL R. OLSON[b]

[a]Department of Anatomy and Neurobiology, University of Maryland School of Medicine, Baltimore, Maryland 21201, USA

[b]Department of Neuroscience and Center for the Neural Basis of Cognition, University of Pittsburgh and Carnegie Mellon University, Pittsburgh, Pennsylvania 15213, USA

ABSTRACT: It is thought that neuronal activity in orbitofrontal cortex (OFC) represents the value of anticipated reward; however activity in many other brain areas also seems to reflect expected reward value. For example, we have shown that in monkeys performing a memory-guided saccade task for a reward of variable size, activity in numerous areas of frontal cortex is stronger when the monkey anticipates a larger reward. The activity of these neurons might be related to the value of the expected reward or to the degree of motivation induced by expectation of the reward. Anticipation of a more valued reward leads to stronger motivation, as evidenced by measures of arousal, attention, and intensity of motor output. On the assumption that motivated behavior depends on influences arising in the limbic system and acting on the motor system, we hypothesized that neuronal signals representing reward value are unique to OFC, whereas signals arising from other frontal areas, those more closely tied the motor system, reflect the degree of motivation. To test this hypothesis, we recorded from single neurons in OFC and premotor cortex while two monkeys performed a task in which we dissociated value from motivation. Neuronal activity in premotor cortex reflected the monkey's degree of motivation, presumably related to the monkey's level of motor readiness and movement preparation, whereas neuronal activity in OFC represented the value of expected reward.

KEYWORDS: orbitofrontal; value; motivation; reward

INTRODUCTION

Orbitofrontal cortex (OFC) is thought to play a critical role in the evaluation of anticipated rewards. This view is based on the fact that lesions of

Address for correspondence: Matthew R. Roesch, Department of Anatomy and Neurobiology, University of Maryland School of Medicine, Baltimore, MD 21201. Voice: 410-706-8910; fax: 410-706-2512.

mroes001@umaryland.edu

Ann. N.Y. Acad. Sci. 1121: 431–446 (2007). © 2007 New York Academy of Sciences.
doi: 10.1196/annals.1401.004

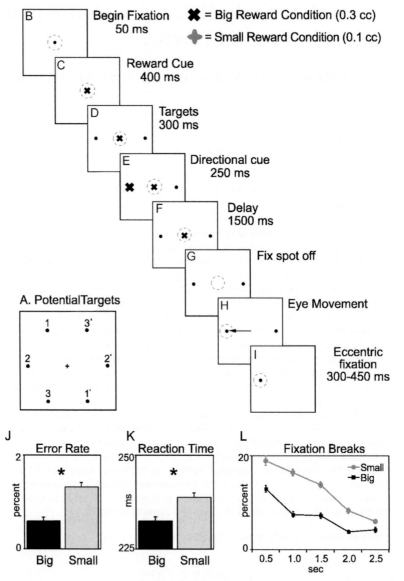

FIGURE 1. Variable-reward task. **(A)** All potential targets were at 10° eccentricity. One pair of diametrically opposed targets was used during each recording session (*1* and *1'*, *2* and *2'*, or *3* and *3'*). The pair was selected to include target at neuron's preferred location. *B–I*: screen in front of monkey during successive epochs of single representative trial. Center of *dashed circle* indicates monkey's direction of gaze during corresponding trial epoch; *arrow* indicates direction of eye movement and drops indicate reward. All other

OFC interfere with reward evaluation (see this issue)[5-15] and is supported by results of microelectrode recording studies demonstrating that neuronal activity is influenced by the value of an expected reward (see this issue).[2,3,16-26] Recently, reward-related activity has also been described in a number of other areas.[20,21,25,27-46] It is widely assumed that reward-related activity in these areas, as in OFC, corresponds to an internal representation of the incentive value. Here we suggest an alternative explanation, that reward-related activity may reflect the motivational modulation of control signals for motor preparation and motor output.

Motivation serves to "prime, facilitate, or potentiate a response mechanism that leads to the appetitive or consummatory behavior."[47] A commonly cited example is the tendency of rats to run faster down an alleyway in pursuit of a more valued reward.[48] In experiments of the sort alluded to above, there are a number of ways in which the value of an expected reward might exert motivational control over neuronal activity.

The fact that monkeys are faster and more accurate when working for a more valued reward suggests that neuronal activity representing the planned action or generalized readiness (e.g., arousal, attention, motor preparedness) may be enhanced when the anticipated reward is more valuable.[27,31,38,40,42,46] Neuronal activity that governs overt behaviors that accompany response planning, such as increased axial tonus, may be enhanced when the more valued reward is as stake. In accordance with this scenario, we have recently shown

←——

items represent images visible to monkey. **(B)** White fixation spot appeared at center of screen and monkey achieved foveal fixation. **(C)** After 50 ms, fixation spot was replaced by cue whose shape and color signified magnitude of upcoming reward. Pairing of cues with reward size was reversed after each block of 40 successful trials. **(D)** After 400 ms two targets appeared at diametrically opposed locations. **(E)** Flashed cue was then presented for 250 ms in superimposition on one target. **(F)** Delay period of 1500 ms ensued. **(G)** Fixation spot was extinguished. **(H)** Monkey was required to make saccade directly to previously cued target. **(I)** After maintaining fixation on target for 300–450 ms, monkey received reward of predicted magnitude. **J–L:** Impact of size of expected reward on behavior. **(J)** Error rate. Height of each bar indicates mean across all recording sessions in all monkeys (TABLE 1) of error rates on big-reward (black) and small-reward (gray) trials. Each value was obtained by first computing mean for each session and then taking average of session means. Error bars indicate SE for latter step. $*P < 0.0001$. **(K)** Mean behavioral reaction times on big-reward (black) and small-reward (gray) trials were computed similarly. $*P < 0.0001$. **(L)** Distribution of fixation breaks across 2500-ms period extending from initiation of fixation (in **B**) to offset of fixation spot (in **G**). For each 500-ms epoch in big-reward (*black square*) and small-reward (*gray circle*) trials, height of symbol indicates percentage of all fixation breaks that occurred during that epoch. The sum of 10 values is thus 100. Each value was obtained by first computing mean for each session and then taking average of session means. Error bars indicate SE for latter step. (Adapted from Roesch and Olson, *J. Neurophysiol.*, 2003.)

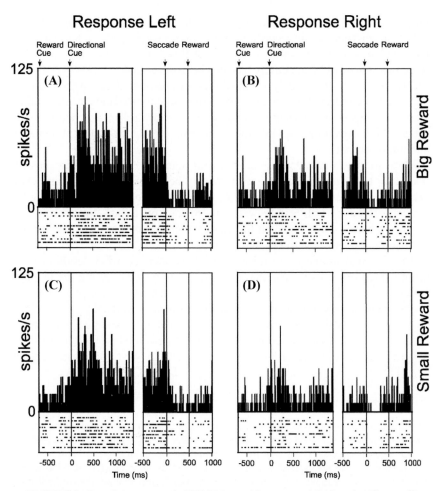

FIGURE 2. Data from neuron in FEF/PM transition zone exhibiting significant effects of reward-size. With response direction held constant, firing was significantly stronger on big-reward than on small-reward trials (**A** versus **C** and **B** versus **D**). With reward-size held constant, firing was significantly stronger on left-response than on right-response trials (**A** versus **B** and **C** versus **D**). Finally, there was a significant interaction between reward size and response direction such that directional signal (firing rate on left-response trials minus firing rate on right-response trials) was stronger under the big-reward than under the small-reward condition. (From Roesch and Olson, *J. Neurophysiol.*, 2003.)

that muscle tone in the neck is elevated in monkeys working for larger or more immediate reward.[1,4] Finally, the occurrence, in some contexts, of anticipatory licking[31,49] indicates that ingestive movements tend to be programmed prior to reward delivery. Reward-related activity may reflect any one of these processes.

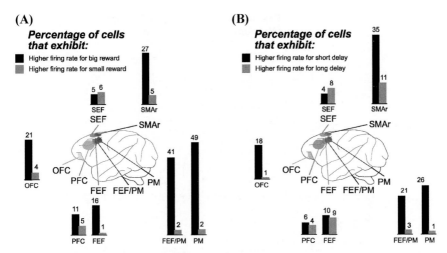

FIGURE 3. Frequency with which neuronal activity, as measured across entire trial, dependent on reward (**A**) or delay (**B**). (**A**) Black(or gray) bars indicate percentage of neurons by area in which firing rate was significantly higher (or lower) under the big-reward condition. (**B**) Black (or gray) bars indicate percentage of neurons by area in which firing rate was significantly higher (or lower) under the short-delay condition. (Adapted from Roesch and Olson, *J. Neurophysiol.*, 2003, 2005.)

The distinction between neuronal activity representing the value of an expected reward and neuronal activity reflecting motivational modulation of motor planning and performance has been acknowledged in principle by previous authors.[50] However, little consideration has been given to the question of how to distinguish between them in practice.

NEURONAL ACTIVITY IN WIDESPREAD AREAS REFLECTS ANTICIPATED VALUE

As a first step to resolving this issue, we extended our analysis of reward-related activity beyond OFC into adjacent frontal areas, including prefrontal cortex (PFC), frontal eye field (FEF), supplementary eye field (SEF), rostral supplementary motor area (SMAr), and premotor cortex (PM).[1,3] These areas differ from OFC in that they are not heavily interconnected with the limbic system, and inactivating them has no impact on reward evaluation. Instead, they are closely tied to the motor system and are directly involved in occulomotor and skeletomotor control. If reward-related activity reflects motivation-dependent variations in the monkey's level of motor readiness and motor output, then it should be prominent in these areas.

We first manipulated motivation by varying the magnitude of the reward expected after successful completion of a memory-guided saccade. The specifics of the task are illustrated in FIGURE 1.[1,3] Essentially, monkeys were required

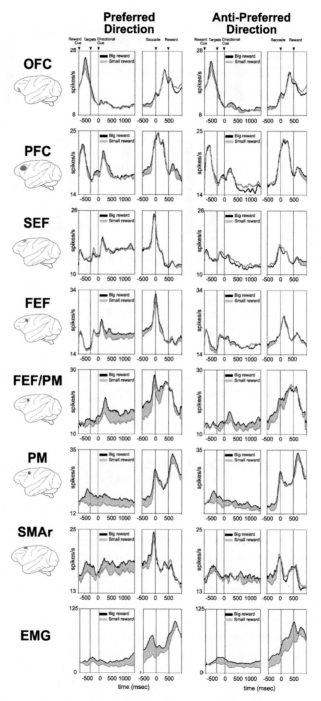

FIGURE 4.

to remember the spatial location of a flashed cue for 1.5 s while fixating at a central spot. When the fixation spot was extinguished, the monkey responded by making a saccade to the previously cued location. The size of the expected reward on a given trial was indicated by the color and shape of the fixation stimulus. As expected, cues that predicted the larger reward were more motivating, leading to faster reaction times and fewer errors (FIG. 1J–L).[1,3]

After training, we recorded from the frontal regions described above, each confirmed by microstimulation and structural MRI. The activity of neurons in most areas was modulated by anticipated reward size. Reward-related activity commonly took the form of a main effect with net firing rate higher on big-reward trials and less frequently took the form of an interaction effect with the strength of the directional signal stronger on large reward trials.[1,3] Both kinds of effect were present and significant in the neuron illustrated in FIGURE 2. Its net firing rate was clearly higher when a large reward was expected (top row versus bottom row). In addition, its directional signal, the difference in firing rate between trials requiring a leftward response (left column) and those requiring a rightward response (right column), was greater under the big-reward condition.

In line with our hypothesis, the impact of reward was most profound in posterior frontal areas affiliated with the motor system (FIG. 3).[1,3] To promote comparisons across areas, we constructed population histograms for each brain region (FIG. 4). In each plot, black and gray curves represent firing rate as a function of time during trials when the anticipated reward was large and small, respectively. Directional selectivity is evident in the difference between left and right columns, which represent saccades made into (preferred) or away from (antipreferred) each cell's response field. Effects of the predicted reward are manifest as differences in firing rate between trials in which the response direction was the same but reward level (indicated by gray level) was different. This difference (highlighted in gray) was most prominent in posterior areas (FEF/PM, PM, and SMAr) in accordance with the notion that anticipating a better reward leads to enhanced motor signals.

Although the activity of neurons in most frontal areas was influenced by the size of the expected reward, several interesting differences emerge. Most

---

FIGURE 4. Impact of magnitude of expected reward on neuronal activity in OFC, PFC, SEF, FEF, FEF/PM, and PM, and on muscle activation (EMG) in the neck (splenius capitus). Population curves representing mean population firing rate as function of time under four task conditions defined by two levels of reward (big = black, small = gray) and two directions (preferred = left column, antipreferred = right column). Data to *left* are aligned on onset of directional cue (FIG. 1E). Data to *right* are aligned on saccade initiation (FIG. 1H). Gray indicates enhanced activity in anticipation of large reward. (Adapted from Roesch and Olson, *J. Neurophysiol.*, 2003, 2005.)

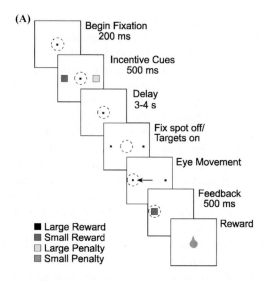

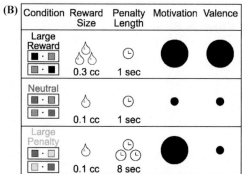

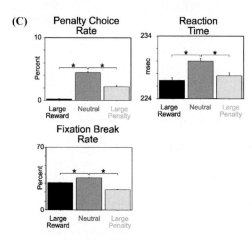

FIGURE 5.

notable is the timing of reward modulation. Activity in OFC was modulated during cue evaluation, whereas motor-related areas exhibited modulation throughout the period of increased motivation. These results, combined with the observation that that reward-related activity was most prominent in areas affiliated with the motor system, suggests that anticipation of reward can lead to the modulation of cognitive and/or motor signals in areas outside OFC when animals are motivated to perform better and faster. Importantly, these results were not specific to manipulations of motivation based on reward size. In a second experiment, instead of manipulating reward size, we varied how quickly the reward would come.[3,4] The task was identical in all respects except that the reward was of uniform size and the cue at the beginning of the trial indicated only whether there would be a long or short delay period. Monkeys were more motivated to work for rewards to be delivered after a short delay. This manipulation had a similar impact on neuronal activity as varying reward size (FIG. 3B). Moreover, the two effects were strongly correlated across neurons studied in both tasks.

DISTINGUISHING BETWEEN SIGNALS THAT REPRESENT VALUE AND REFLECT MOTIVATION

The results described above indicate that neuronal activity correlated with the value of an anticipated reward is widespread in frontal cortex. However, because the monkey's level of motivation was correlated with the value of the impending reward, the results do not allow any conclusion regarding whether neuronal activity in any given area represented anticipated value or merely reflected the monkey's level of motivation. To resolve this issue, we designed a novel task in which we manipulated motivation independently of promised reward value.[2] The monkeys performed a memory-guided saccade task, as in the previous experiments, but in this case, two cues presented at the beginning of the trial indicated both the size of the reward the monkey would receive in the event of success (one or three drops of juice) and the size of a penalty that

---

FIGURE 5. (A) Sequence of events in the reward-penalty task. Hatched circle indicates direction of gaze. (B) Trials fell into three categories defined by reward-penalty combination: large reward (large reward and small penalty), neutral (small reward and small penalty), and large penalty (small reward and large penalty). Incentive cues were distinguished by color. (C to E) Performance measures sensitive to reward and penalty size. Penalty choice rate: trials on which the monkeys chose penalty expressed as a fraction of all trials on which they chose reward or penalty. Fixation break rate: trials terminated by a fixation break expressed as a percentage of all trials. Reaction time: average interval between fixation spot offset and saccade initiation on all trials in which the monkey made a saccade in the rewarded direction. Asterisks (all planned comparisons): statistically significant differences at $P < 0.001$. (Adapted from Roesch and Olson, *Science*, 2004.)

would be incurred in the event of failure (a 1 s or 8 s time-out). The details of the task are given in FIGURE 5. Behavioral measures indicated that the monkeys (a) were motivated by the threat of a large penalty and (b) found it aversive (FIG. 5). The use of threatened penalties thus allowed dissociating motivation from value.

We expected that neurons sensitive to the degree of motivation would respond with similar changes in firing rate to increasing the size of either the promised reward or the threatened penalty. In contrast, we expected that neurons sensitive to anticipated value would be affected only by promised reward size (if they encoded the expected outcome of success) or would be affected in opposite ways by promised reward size and threatened penalty size (if they encoded a weighted average of the outcomes associated with success and failure). On the assumption that motivated behavior depends on influences arising in the limbic system and acting on the motor system, we predicted that neuronal signals representing reward value would predominate in OFC, whereas signals reflecting the degree of motivation would predominate in PM.

In OFC, the firing rate obviously depended on the size of the predicted reward and penalty.[2] For example, the neuron shown in FIGURE 6A responded to the cue display with stronger firing when a larger reward was promised (large-reward versus neutral condition) and weaker firing when a larger penalty was threatened (large-penalty versus neutral condition). Thus the strength of its response reflected the value conveyed by the combination of reward and penalty cues, not the motivational impact of the display. This was also true for the population as a whole (FIG. 6B). Recent data from Padoa-Schioppa and Assad. have also demonstrated that some neurons in OFC encode the composite value of what is offered, however they also show that other neurons encode the relative value of individual rewards within a specific offer (see this issue).[18] Their results provide further support for the idea that OFC neurons carry the representations of reward value on the basis of which decisions are made. On the assumption that OFC mediates emotional processes, this finding fits with idea that decisions are based on the anticipatory emotions that accompany picturing possible outcomes.[51]

Neurons in PM, unlike those in OFC, did not represent value (FIG. 6C, D).[2] Instead, their firing rate depended on the monkeys' degree of motivation. PM neurons fired continuously during the delay period between onset of the cues and execution of the saccade, maintaining a higher rate when either a large reward or a large penalty was at stake than under the neutral condition in which both reward and penalty were small, reflecting the motivational impact of the incentive-cue display, not the value conveyed by the display.

To quantify these effects, we computed, for each neuron, indices reflecting the dependence of its firing rate on reward and penalty size during the 500-ms period when the cues were visible. The reward index $(R - N)/(R + N)$, where R and N were the firing rates on large-reward and neutral trials, respectively, was positive in the case of any neuron firing more strongly when reward

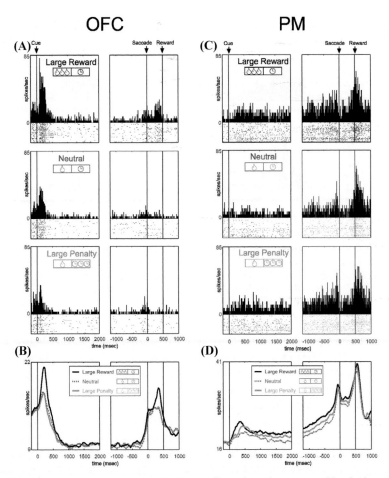

FIGURE 6. (A) Neuronal activity in OFC reflects the value conveyed by the incentive cues. Shown are data from a single neuron firing during the cue period at a rate that was especially high for large reward and especially low for large penalty. (B) Mean firing rate as a function of time under the three incentive conditions for all 176 OFC neurons. (C) Neuronal activity in PM reflects the motivational impact of the incentive cues. Shown are data from a single neuron firing throughout the trial at a rate that was high for large reward and large penalty. (D) Mean firing rate as a function of time under the three incentive conditions for all 135 PM neurons. (Adapted from Roesch and Olson, *Science*, 2004.)

size increased. The distribution of reward indices (FIG. 7A, B) was shifted significantly above zero for both OFC and PM (sign test; $P < 0.0001$). Thus both areas increased firing in anticipation of a large reward.

The penalty index, $(P - N)/(P + N)$, where P and N were the firing rates on large-penalty and neutral trials, respectively, was negative in the case of any neuron firing less strongly when penalty size increased. In OFC, the

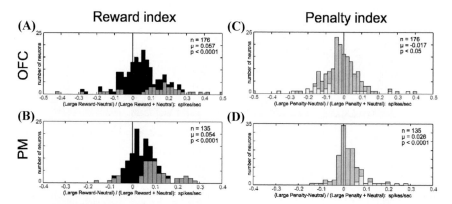

FIGURE 7. (A-B) Distribution of reward indices for all neurons in OFC **(A)** and PM **(B)**. The number of observations (n), mean of the distribution (μ), and level of significance at which it differed from zero (P) are shown. Pale bars represent neurons in which the dependence of firing rate on reward size achieved statistical significance (analysis of variance, $P < 0.05$). **(C-D)** Distribution of penalty indices for all neurons in OFC and PM. Conventions as in **(A–B)**. (Adapted from Roesch and Olson, *Science*, 2004.)

distribution of penalty indices (FIG. 7C) was shifted significantly below zero (sign test; $P < 0.05$) indicating that OFC neurons fired less strongly when the threatened penalty was larger. To the contrary, PM neurons fired more strongly when the threatened penalty was larger. In this case the distribution of penalty indices (FIG. 7D) was shifted away from zero in a positive direction, indicating that the majority of neurons fired more strongly when the penalty was larger (sign test; $P < 0.001$). We conclude that neuronal activity in OFC represents the value of the expected reward, whereas neuronal activity in PM reflects the degree of motivation that is induced by either a large reward or a large penalty.[2]

While it is clear that neuronal activity in PM does not represent "goods value"—the value of the goods to be delivered upon successful completion of the trial[18]—it might nevertheless be argued that it represents "action value"—the value that attaches to performing the required action.[52,53] According to this argument, the value of the action is high in the large-reward condition because it will lead to a substantial gain and high in the large-penalty condition because it will prevent a substantial loss. This interpretation, while logically consistent, seems dubious in light of the following three considerations. 1) Neurons representing action value must, by definition, be upstream from the value-based decision process. If they represent value in a meaningful sense, then the monkey must base on its activity the decision whether or how intensely to perform an action. Neurons exhibiting motivational modulation must, by definition, be downstream from the value-based decision process. They put into execution the monkey's decision. 2) There are cases in which activity correlated with action value certainly does not represent action value and instead is the product of motivational modulation. Electromyographic activity in the neck muscles is correlated with action value (FIG. 4).[1,4] No reasonable person would argue that the monkey decides to work harder because the neck muscles are more tense. Rather, the muscles are more tense because the monkey has decided to work harder. In other words, the neck muscles are downstream from the decision process and their reward-related activity is a product of motivational modulation. What is true of the neck muscles could equally well be true of neurons in PM. 3) There are strong reasons for supposing that animals choose a goal on the basis of its goods value and only then plan a course of action on the basis of its leading to the chosen goal. The major role of goods value in guiding decisions is evident in the fact that devaluing certain goods (for example producing satiation for certain foodstuffs) leads to cessation of behaviors required for obtaining them.[14,54] The minor role of action value in guiding decisions is evident in the fact that rats trained to run a maze through one set of alleys will, when the old alleys are inaccessible, run through a new set of alleys, executing a new set of turns, so as to get to the old goal.[55] These considerations weigh heavily against the notion that neuronal signals in PM represent action value in an economically meaningful sense. They favor instead the idea that neurons in PM carry motor preparation signals that are subject to modulation in accordance with the animal's motivational state. On one hand, PM neurons do carry a distant echo of goods-value signals in OFC. On the other hand, their signals, unlike those in OFC, do not inform value-based decisions. If this is true of PM, then it could well be true of other frontal and parietal areas in which neuronal activity varies with the strength of an anticipated reward.

CONCLUSION

Reward-related activity in OFC and PM appears to reflect the two extremes of a continuum. The first, manifest in OFC, involves representing the value of the reward. The second, manifest in PM, involves maintaining a degree of motivation commensurate with the value of the reward. These results are consistent with the idea that anticipated reward leads to motivated behavior through a series of steps originating in the limbic system and terminating in the motor system. However, it is not entirely clear by what stages the representation of reward value in the limbic system is transformed into motivational modulation of the motor system because the approach of independently manipulating reward size and motivation has not yet been applied to intervening areas where neurons exhibit reward-related activity. Although we have focused on single-unit studies in monkeys, the issue exists in connection with data obtained by other experimental procedures such as functional imaging. To understand fully the neural steps involved in goal-directed behavior will require distinguishing between signals related to attention, motivation or motor preparation, on one hand, and reward-value representation, on the other.

REFERENCES

1. ROESCH, M.R. & C.R. OLSON. 2003. Impact of expected reward on neuronal activity in prefrontal cortex, frontal and supplementary eye fields and premotor cortex. J. Neurophysiol. **90:** 1766–1789.
2. ROESCH, M.R. & C.R. OLSON. 2004. Neuronal activity related to reward value and motivation in primate frontal cortex. Science **304:** 307–310.
3. ROESCH, M.R. & C.R. OLSON. 2005. Neuronal activity in primate orbitofrontal cortex reflects the value of time. J. Neurophysiol. **94:** 2457–2471.
4. ROESCH, M.R. & C.R. OLSON. 2005. Neuronal activity dependent on anticipated and elapsed delay in macaque prefrontal cortex, frontal and supplementary eye fields, and premotor cortex. J. Neurophysiol. **94:** 1469–1497.
5. BAYLIS, L.L. & D. GAFFAN. 1991. Amygdalectomy and ventromedial prefrontal ablation produce similar deficits in food choice and in simple object discrimination learning for an unseen reward. Exp. Brain Res. **86:** 617–622.
6. BUTTER, C.M. & D.R. SNYDER. 1972. Alterations in aversive and aggressive behaviors following orbital frontal lesions in rhesus monkeys. Acta. Neurobiol. Exp. Wars **32:** 525–565.
7. BUTTER, C.M., J.A. MCDONALD & D.R. SNYDER. 1969. Orality, preference behavior, and reinforcement value of nonfood object in monkeys with orbital frontal lesions. Science **164:** 1306–1307.
8. GAFFAN, D. & E.A. MURRAY. 1990. Amygdalar interaction with the mediodorsal nucleus of the thalamus and the ventromedial prefrontal cortex in stimulus-reward associative learning in the monkey. J. Neurosci. **10:** 3479–3493.
9. DIAS, R., T.W. ROBBINS & A.C. ROBERTS. 1996. Dissociation in prefrontal cortex of affective and attentional shifts. Nature **380:** 69–72.
10. IVERSEN, S.D. & M. MISHKIN. 1970. Perseverative interference in monkeys following selective lesions of the inferior prefrontal convexity. Exp. Brain Res. **11:** 376–386.
11. IZQUIERDO, A., R.K. SUDA & E.A. MURRAY. 2004. Bilateral orbital prefrontal cortex lesions in rhesus monkeys disrupt choices guided by both reward value and reward contingency. J. Neurosci. **24:** 7540–7548.
12. JONES, B. & M. MISHKIN. 1972. Limbic lesions and the problem of stimulus–reinforcement associations. Exp. Neurol. **36:** 362–377.
13. MEUNIER, M., J. BACHEVALIER, & M. MISHKIN. 1997. Effects of orbital frontal and anterior cingulate lesions on object and spatial memory in rhesus monkeys. Neuropsychologia **35:** 999–1015.
14. PICKENS, C.L. et al. 2003. Different roles for orbitofrontal cortex and basolateral amygdala in a reinforcer devaluation task. J. Neurosci. **23:** 11078–11084.
15. SCHOENBAUM, G. et al. 2002. Orbitofrontal lesions in rats impair reversal but not acquisition of go, no-go odor discriminations. Neuroreport **13:** 885–890.
16. CRITCHLEY, H.D. & E.T. ROLLS. 1996. Hunger and satiety modify the responses of olfactory and visual neurons in the primate orbitofrontal cortex. J. Neurophysiol. **75:** 1673–1686.

17. HIKOSAKA, K. & M. WATANABE. 2000. Delay activity of orbital and lateral prefrontal neurons of the monkey varying with different rewards. Cereb. Cortex **10:** 263–271.
18. PADOA-SCHIOPPA, C. & J.A. ASSAD. 2006. Neurons in the orbitofrontal cortex encode economic value. Nature **441:** 223–226.
19. ROLLS, E.T. 1996. The orbitofrontal cortex. Philos. Trans. R. Soc. Lond. B. Biol. Sci. **351:** 1433–1443; discussion 1443–1444.
20. SCHOENBAUM, G., A.A. CHIBA & M. GALLAGHER. 1998. Orbitofrontal cortex and basolateral amygdala encode expected outcomes during learning. Nat. Neurosci. **1:** 155–159.
21. SCHOENBAUM, G., A.A. CHIBA & M. GALLAGHER. 1999. Neural encoding in orbitofrontal cortex and basolateral amygdala during olfactory discrimination learning. J. Neurosci. **19:** 1876–1884.
22. SCHOENBAUM, G. & M. ROESCH. 2005. Orbitofrontal cortex, associative learning, and expectancies. Neuron. **47:** 633–636.
23. TREMBLAY, L. & W. SCHULTZ. 1999. Relative reward preference in primate orbitofrontal cortex. Nature **398:** 704–708.
24. TREMBLAY, L. & W. SCHULTZ. 2000. Reward-related neuronal activity during go-nogo task performance in primate orbitofrontal cortex. J. Neurophysiol. **83:** 1864–1876.
25. WALLIS, J.D. & E.K. MILLER. 2003. Neuronal activity in primate dorsolateral and orbital prefrontal cortex during performance of a reward preference task. Eur. J. Neurosci. **18:** 2069–2081.
26. FEIERSTEIN, C.E. *et al.* 2006. Representation of spatial goals in rat orbitofrontal cortex. Neuron **51:** 495–507.
27. SCHULTZ, W. 2000. Multiple reward signals in the brain. Nat. Rev. Neurosci. **1:** 199–207.
28. HIKOSAKA, O., M. SAKAMOTO & S. USUI. 1989. Functional properties of monkey caudate neurons. III. Activities related to expectation of target and reward. J. Neurophysiol. **61:** 814–832.
29. APICELLA, P., E. SCARNATI & W. SCHULTZ. 1991. Tonically discharging neurons of monkey striatum respond to preparatory and rewarding stimuli. Exp. Brain Res. **84:** 672–675.
30. APICELLA, P., E. LEGALLET & E. TROUCHE. 1997. Responses of tonically discharging neurons in the monkey striatum to primary rewards delivered during different behavioral states. Exp. Brain Res. **116:** 456–466.
31. HASSANI, O.K., H.C. CROMWELL & W. SCHULTZ. 2001. Influence of expectation of different rewards on behavior-related neuronal activity in the striatum. J. Neurophysiol. **85:** 2477–2489.
32. SHIDARA, M. & B.J. RICHMOND. 2002. Anterior cingulate: single neuronal signals related to degree of reward expectancy. Science **296:** 1709–1711.
33. SHIDARA, M., T. MIZUHIKI & B.J. RICHMOND. 2005. Neuronal firing in anterior cingulate neurons changes modes across trials in single states of multitrial reward schedules. Exp. Brain Res. **163:** 242–245.
34. SETLOW, B., G. SCHOENBAUM & M. GALLAGHER. 2003. Neural encoding in ventral striatum during olfactory discrimination learning. Neuron **38:** 625–636.
35. NISHIJO, H., T. ONO & H. NISHINO. 1988. Single neuron responses in amygdala of alert monkey during complex sensory stimulation with affective significance. J. Neurosci. **8:** 3570–3583.

36. PLATT, M.L. & P.W. GLIMCHER. 1999. Neural correlates of decision variables in parietal cortex. Nature **400:** 233–238.
37. MCCOY, A.N. *et al.* 2003. Saccade reward signals in posterior cingulate cortex. Neuron **40:** 1031–1040.
38. WATANABE, T. & H. NIKI. 1985. Hippocampal unit activity and delayed response in the monkey. Brain Res. **325:** 241–254.
39. AMADOR, N., M. SCHLAG-REY & J. SCHLAG. 2000. Reward-predicting and reward-detecting neuronal activity in the primate supplementary eye field. J. Neurophysiol. **84:** 2166–2170.
40. HOLLERMAN, J.R., L. TREMBLAY & W. SCHULTZ. 1998. Influence of reward expectation on behavior-related neuronal activity in primate striatum. J. Neurophysiol. **80:** 947–963.
41. KAWAGOE, R., Y. TAKIKAWA & O. HIKOSAKA. 1998. Expectation of reward modulates cognitive signals in the basal ganglia. Nat. Neurosci. **1:** 411–416.
42. LAUWEREYNS, J. *et al.* 2002. A neural correlate of response bias in monkey caudate nucleus. Nature **418:** 413–417.
43. LAUWEREYNS, J. *et al.* 2002. Feature-based anticipation of cues that predict reward in monkey caudate nucleus. Neuron **33:** 463–473.
44. TAKIKAWA, Y. *et al.* 1998. Presaccadic omnidirectional burst activity in the basal interstitial nucleus in the monkey cerebellum. Exp. Brain Res. **121:** 442–450.
45. KOBAYASHI, S. *et al.* 2002. Influence of reward expectation on visuospatial processing in macaque lateral prefrontal cortex. J. Neurophysiol. **87:** 1488–1498.
46. TAKIKAWA, Y., R. KAWAGOE & O. HIKOSAKA. 2002. Reward-dependent spatial selectivity of anticipatory activity in monkey caudate neurons. J. Neurophysiol. **87:** 508–515.
47. STELLAR, J.R. & E. STELLAR. 1985. The Neurobiology of Motivation and Reward. Springer-Verlag. New York.
48. STELLAR, E. 1982. The Physiological Mechanisms of Motivation and Reward: 377–407. Springer-Verlag. New York.
49. WATANABE, M. *et al.* 2001. Behavioral reactions reflecting differential reward expectations in monkeys. Exp. Brain Res. **140:** 511–518.
50. MAUNSELL, J.H. 2004. Neuronal representations of cognitive state: reward or attention? Trends Cogn. Sci. **8:** 261–265.
51. MELLERS, B.A. & A.P. MCGRAW. 2001. Anticipated emotions as guides to choice. Curr. Dir. Psychol. Sci. **10:** 210–214.
52. DORRIS, L. *et al.* 2004. Mind-reading difficulties in the siblings of people with Asperger's syndrome: evidence for a genetic influence in the abnormal development of a specific cognitive domain. J. Child. Psychol. Psychiatry **45:** 412–418.
53. SUGRUE, L.P., G.S. CORRADO & W.T. NEWSOME. 2004. Matching behavior and the representation of value in the parietal cortex. Science **304:** 1782–1787.
54. DICKINSON, A. & B. BALLEINE. 1994. Motivational control of goal-directed action. Anim. Learn. and Behav. **22:** 1–14.
55. TOLMAN, E.C. 1948. Cognitive maps in rats and men. Psychol. Rev. **55:** 189–208.

Neuronal Mechanisms in Prefrontal Cortex Underlying Adaptive Choice Behavior

JONATHAN D. WALLIS

*University of California at Berkeley, Helen Wills Neuroscience Institute,
Berkeley, California 94720, USA*

ABSTRACT: This chapter aims to address two questions relating to the
role of the prefrontal cortex (PFC) in reward-guided choice behavior.
First, do PFC neurons encode rewards per se, or are they encoding
behavioral sequelae of reward? To address this, we recorded simultaneously from multiple PFC subregions, with the rationale that neuronal
selectivity that directly encoded the reward outcome should occur before
selectivity that reflected reward-related sequelae. Our results indicate
that neurons in the orbitofrontal cortex (OFC) encode reward information before neurons in the dorsolateral PFC (DLPFC). Furthermore,
whereas DLPFC neurons encoded both the upcoming response as well
as the expected reward, OFC neurons encoded the reward alone. Our
interpretation of these results is that the OFC encodes the reward and
passes this information to the DLPFC, which uses it to determine the
behavioral response. The second question is whether the encoding is specific to the reward outcome or reflective of a more abstract value signal
that could facilitate decision making. We examined this by determining
whether the PFC encodes other types of information relevant to decision
making, such as probability of success and effort. We found that many
PFC neurons encoded at least one of these variables, but neurons in the
OFC and the medial PFC (MPFC) encoded combinations of the variables
indicative of encoding an abstract value signal. This signal could provide decision making with flexibility and a capacity to deal with novelty,
which are two of the hallmark features of prefrontal function. Future
research will focus on delineating the differential contributions of the
OFC and the MPFC to decision making.

KEYWORDS: monkey; neurophysiology; prefrontal; orbitofrontal; dorsolateral; reward; probability; decision making; choice

Address for correspondence: Jonathan D. Wallis, University of California at Berkeley, Helen Wills
Neuroscience Institute, 132 Barker Hall, Berkeley, CA, 94720.
wallis@berkeley.edu

Ann. N.Y. Acad. Sci. 1121: 447–460 (2007). © 2007 New York Academy of Sciences.
doi: 10.1196/annals.1401.009

INTRODUCTION

Making a bad choice can be serious. For example, the beta monkey that attacks the alpha male has to weigh the risk of injury or death against the biological need to procreate. How does the brain make such decisions? How does it ensure that it consistently selects the action most likely to realize the needs of the organism and to enhance the organism's survival prospects? The orbitofrontal cortex (OFC) is a key region in this regard, since damage to this area produces a relatively specific deficit in choice behavior. For example, consider the case of Elliott, a happily married young man in his 30s.[1,2] Elliott excelled in college and rose rapidly through the ranks of a home-building firm to become its chief accountant at the age of 32. Then, when Elliott was 35, doctors diagnosed him with a brain tumor. The operation to remove the tumor was successful, but the surgery left Elliot with bilateral damage to his OFC and the ventral portion of his medial prefrontal cortex (MPFC). However, neuropsychological tests of intelligence, memory, and language detected no evidence of brain damage. Even tests designed specifically to tax frontal lobe processes, such as working memory and rule switching, failed to reveal any deficits. Despite this, Elliot's life quickly spiraled out of control as he made a series of disastrous life decisions. He quit his job, lost a large sum of money to a scam artist, divorced his wife, lost contact with family and friends, and remarried a prostitute he had known for a month. His second marriage ended in divorce 6 months later, and he moved in with his parents. Thus, there is a paradox with the OFC: damage to this area leaves many of our cognitive abilities intact, yet it devastates our ability to make everyday decisions. In this chapter, we will focus on the underlying neuronal mechanisms that might help explain this paradox.

OFC NEURONS ENCODE EXPECTED REWARDS

The first neurophysiological studies of the OFC noted the frequency of neurons that showed responses to the delivery of juice rewards.[3,4] Subsequent studies showed that the neurons showed differential activity to two visual stimuli. One stimulus predicted the delivery of fruit juice, and the other predicted the delivery of saline.[4] Such neurons were not simply encoding the visual properties of the stimulus; when the reward contingencies were reversed, the neuronal selectivity also would reverse. Thus, the neurons appeared to be encoding the reward predicted by the stimulus and expected by the monkey. It was clear that these neuronal properties might be useful for decision making: encoding what reward to expect from a given action would allow the motor system to choose consistently the action that would lead to the largest reward.

However, the results of later studies countered the notion that these properties were unique to the OFC. For example, a series of studies demonstrated that neurons showing differential activity dependent on the expected reward were also in the dorsolateral prefrontal cortex (DLPFC).[5-11] Particularly challenging was a study by Roesch and Olson, which examined the influence of expected reward magnitude on neurons throughout the frontal lobe.[12] Neurons showing a difference in firing rate depending on whether the subject expected a large or small reward were more prevalent in motor areas, such as the premotor cortex, than they were in the PFC. Similar neurons were also present in the posterior cortex, including the perirhinal cortex,[13] the parietal cortex,[14-16] and even the primary visual cortex.[17] We must be careful in interpreting these results, however. A neuron is not necessarily encoding a reward just because its firing rate correlates with some parameters of that reward. This is because many behavioral and cognitive measures also correlate with expected reward. For example, an animal's muscles often tense when it expects a large reward, and its behavior is quicker and more accurate.[12] An animal also pays more attention to cues that predict reward[18] and enters a state of higher autonomic arousal. Any of these processes may be driving neuronal firing rates.

How, then, do we determine whether OFC neurons are encoding the expected reward value or one of the correlates of reward? Our approach has been to compare the latency at which neurons encode expected rewards across various brain regions. Our rationale is that we must first determine that an animal expects a large reward before it can activate other cognitive processes, such as increased attention, arousal, and motor readiness. Thus, neurons that encode the expected reward will show differential activity dependent on the reward before neurons that encode cognitive processes that correlate with expected reward. In our first experiment, we recorded simultaneously from the DLPFC and the OFC to examine whether we could use this rationale to specify more precisely the contribution that both areas make to reward processing.

EXPERIMENT 1: COMPARISON OF REWARD ENCODING IN THE DLPFC AND THE OFC

In our first experiment we trained two monkeys to choose between different pictures associated with delivery of different amounts of fruit juice.[19] The subject would fixate on a central point on the screen, and two pictures would sequentially appear (one on the left and one on the right) separated by a delay (FIG. 1). The subject would then select one of the pictures by making a saccade to the location where that picture had appeared. Each picture was associated with the delivery of a specific amount of juice (0, 2, 4, or 8 drops). We used new pictures each day, and subjects learned by trial and error to maximize their reward by selecting pictures associated with larger juice amounts. Once subjects were consistently selecting the pictures associated with the largest reward (that is, they selected the largest reward on 27 out of the last 30 trials), we reversed the picture–reward contingencies. Thus, the picture that previously was associated with 8 drops of juice now was associated with 0 drops of juice,

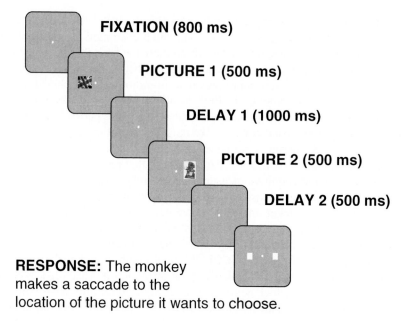

FIGURE 1. Illustration of the behavioral task that we used in Experiment 1.

the picture that previously was associated with 4 drops of juice now was associated with 2 drops of juice, and so on. This ensured that when a picture appeared on the screen, we could determine whether a neuron was encoding the reward that the picture predicted or was encoding the visual properties of the picture. For our present discussion, the most important neuronal activity was the one that occurred once the second picture appeared. At this point, the subject could predict what reward he would receive, as well as what motor response he would need to make in order to receive that reward.

We recorded neuronal activity simultaneously from multiple electrodes implanted in the DLPFC and the OFC. Recording simultaneously (as opposed to sequentially) from the two areas has the advantage that we are measuring the areas' neuronal activity during the exact same behavior, thereby controlling for subtle changes in behavior such as practice effects across recording sessions. We recorded the activity of 167 DLPFC neurons and 134 OFC neurons. FIGURE 2 illustrates two examples of OFC neurons that encoded the expected reward. FIGURE 2A and B show an example of an OFC neuron that encoded whether the subject expected to receive 4 drops of juice. The graphs show a higher firing rate on these trials compared to those in which the subject expected to receive either 2 or 8 drops. Its firing rate, however, was the same irrespective of whether the monkey made a left (FIG. 2A) or a right saccade (FIG. 2B). FIGURE 2C and D show an example an OFC neuron that encoded the expected reward in a parametric fashion. It showed a depression in its firing

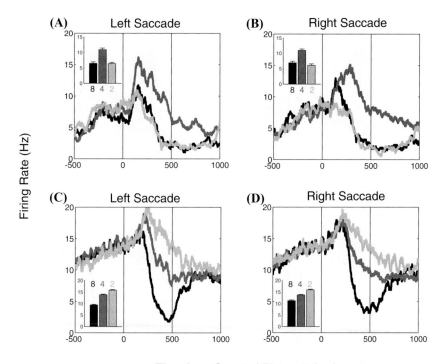

FIGURE 2. Spike density histograms from two OFC neurons indicating how the neuronal firing rate changed according to the expected payoff and the monkey's response (a left or right saccade). Inset bar graphs indicate the mean firing rate ($\pm$ standard error) during the presentation of the reward-predictive cue (the first 500 ms). Black indicates that the cue predicted the delivery of 8 drops of juice, dark gray 4 drops, and light gray 2 drops. **(A, B)** OFC neuron showing a higher firing rate on trials in which the monkey expects to receive 4 drops of juice. **(C, D)** OFC neuron encoding the predicted reward in a parametric fashion. It showed a depression in its firing rate that was greatest for 8 drops of juice, less for 4 drops, and least for 2 drops. The upcoming saccade did not affect the firing rate of either neuron.

rate that was greatest for 8 drops of juice, less for 4 drops, and least for 2 drops. Again, the pattern of activity was independent of the direction of the saccade.

In contrast, DLPFC neurons tended to show complex responses that related to both the expected reward and the direction of the upcoming saccade. FIGURE 3 illustrates two representative DLPFC neurons. During the picture epoch, the neuron in FIGURE 3A and B discriminated between the different expected reward amounts when the monkey made a rightward saccade; it showed a high firing rate when 8 drops of juice was expected. (In contrast, during the subsequent delay period, the same neuron was reward-selective only when the

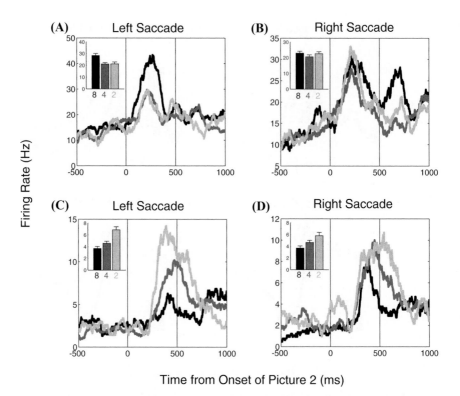

Time from Onset of Picture 2 (ms)

FIGURE 3. Spike density histograms from two DLPFC neurons, illustrated in the same manner as FIGURE 2. **(A, B)** During the time period that the picture was on the screen, the neuron discriminated between the different expected reward amounts, but only when the monkey made a rightward saccade. **(C, D)** The neuron encoded the reward in a parametric fashion, increasing its firing rate as the amount of expected reward increased. However, this effect was much greater when the subject was about to make a leftward saccade as opposed to a rightward saccade.

monkey made a leftward saccade.) The activity of the neuron in FIGURE 3C and D also was affected by both the upcoming saccade and the amount of juice that the subject expected. In this case, the neuron encoded the reward in a parametric fashion, increasing its firing rate as the amount of expected reward increased. However, this effect was much greater when the subject was about to make a leftward saccade as opposed to a rightward saccade.

These single neurons were representative of the properties of OFC and DLPFC neurons. To determine the proportion of these different types of neurons across the population, we performed a two-way ANOVA on the neuron's mean firing rate during the presentation of the second picture, using the factors of Reward (2, 4, or 8 drops of juice) and Saccade (leftward or rightward) (FIG. 4). In the OFC, 28% of the neurons showed a significant main

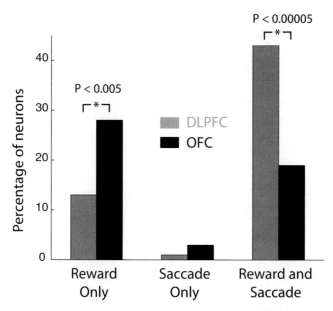

FIGURE 4. Bar chart illustrating the prevalence of neurons that encoded the expected payoff alone, the upcoming saccade alone, or an interaction between the payoff and the saccade. For every neuron that we recorded, we determined what it was encoding by performing a two-way ANOVA on the neuron's mean firing rate during the period that the picture was on the screen assessed at $P < 0.05$ (we saw similar results for the subsequent delay epoch). OFC neurons tended to encode the reward alone, while neurons in DLPFC encoded a combination of the reward and the upcoming saccade. Very few neurons in either area encoded the saccade alone.

effect of Reward (assessed at $P < 0.05$) with no main effect or interaction with Saccade, in comparison to 13% of DLPFC neurons ($\chi^2 = 9.8$, $P < 0.005$). In contrast, 43% of DLPFC neurons showed a significant Reward–Saccade interaction, compared to 19% of OFC neurons ($\chi^2 = 19$, $P < 0.00005$). Neurons in both areas encoded reward in a variety of ways. Some showed a parametric increase in firing rate as the expected reward size increased (27%). Others showed a parametric decrease (15%). Yet others encoded a specific reward (59%). These proportions were similar for both the OFC and the DLPFC.

A sliding receiver operating characteristic (ROC) analysis of the time-course of the selectivity revealed further differences in the encoding of reward between the two areas. Starting from 500 ms prior to the presentation of the second picture, we calculated an ROC value for a 200-ms time window. We then stepped this window forward in 10-ms increments until we had analyzed the rest of the trial. Briefly, the ROC analysis measured the degree of overlap between two response distributions. For each neuron, we defined the expected reward amount that yielded the highest firing rate as the preferred reward amount, and the expected reward amount that elicited the lowest mean firing rate as the non-preferred reward amount. For trials in which the subject expected either the preferred or the non-preferred reward amount, we determined the total number of spikes that occurred in the 200-ms time window. This yielded two distributions of neuronal activity for trials in which the monkey expected either the preferred (P) or the non-preferred (N) reward. We then generated an ROC curve by taking each observed neuronal firing rate and plotting the proportion of P that exceeded the value of that observation against the proportion of N that exceeded the value of that observation. The area under this curve was then calculated. A value of 0.5 would indicate that the two distributions completely overlapped (since for each value of the neuron's firing rate the proportions of P and N exceeding that value are equal), and as such the neuron would not be selective. A value of 1.0, on the other hand, would indicate that the two distributions are completely separate (that is, every value drawn from N is exceeded by the entire distribution of P). In somewhat simpler terms, it is the probability that if I told you the firing rate of the neuron, you could predict which volume of juice the monkey expected to receive.

We used this analysis to compute the latency at which selectivity appeared. We defined this latency as the point at which the ROC curve exceeded 0.6. We chose the criterion as one that yielded a close approximation to the time at which we judged selectivity to appear from the spike density histograms. This measure did not differ between the two areas: 36% (60/167) of the DLPFC neurons reached criterion in a mean time of 467 ms, while 39% (52/134) of the OFC neurons reached criterion in a mean time of 426 ms (t-test $= 1.0$, $d.f. = 110$, $P > 0.1$). However, while selectivity for the reward tended to appear at about the same time in both areas, it then rose more rapidly and peaked earlier in the OFC than in the DLPFC (FIG. 5A). Therefore, for neurons that reached criterion, we calculated the value and time of the peak ROC value between the onset of the second picture and the start of the behavioral response. There was no difference between the two areas in the mean peak ROC value (DLPFC $= 0.654$, OFC $= 0.646$, t-test $= 0.89$, $d.f. = 110$, $P > 0.1$), but the peak was reached significantly earlier in the OFC than in the DLPFC. FIG-URE 5B shows a distribution of the times at which each neuron reached its peak ROC value for the upcoming reward. On average, this occurred about 80 ms earlier in the OFC (510 ms after the onset of picture 2) than in the DLPFC (592 ms after the onset of picture 2; t-test $= 2.1$, $d.f. = 110$, $P < 0.05$).

In conclusion, we found neurons sensitive to the expected reward in both the DLPFC and the OFC. However, there was evidence for functional specialization. OFC neurons only encoded the expected reward, whereas DLPFC neurons encoded the upcoming saccade in addition to the expected reward. Further, OFC neurons encoded reward information 80 ms earlier than neurons in the DLPFC. The OFC is heavily and reciprocally connected with gustatory and olfactory cortices,[20,21] as well as the basolateral amygdala that might provide the OFC with information as to the value of the reward.[22,23] Thus, the OFC is conceivably the first prefrontal region that would receive information

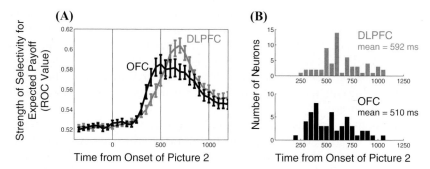

FIGURE 5. **(A)** Time-course of selectivity for the expected payoff (amount of reward) across the DLPFC (gray) and OFC (black) population of neurons. The thick line indicates the mean selectivity of the neurons, while the error bars indicate the standard error of the mean. Both populations began to encode the expected payoff at about the same time, but selectivity reached its peak value in the OFC before the DLPFC. The measure of selectivity is derived from the ROC of each neuron's firing rate. The ROC is the probability that an independent observer could correctly identify the payoff given the firing rate of the neuron. No selectivity equates to an ROC value of 0.5. (In practice it is slightly higher than this because we rectify the ROC value during its calculation. Small fluctuations due to noise push the value to about 0.52). Maximal selectivity equates to a value of 1.0. **(B)** Distribution of peak selectivity across the population of DLPFC and OFC neurons. The OFC population reached its peak selectivity approximately 80 ms before the DLPFC population (Wilcoxon's rank-sum test, $P < 0.05$).

about the value of the forthcoming juice reward. Our observation that reward value information peaks sooner in the OFC than in the DLPFC is consistent with that notion. In contrast, the timing of reward information in the DLPFC, along with these neurons' tendency to encode the upcoming response, suggest that this area may be where information about reward value converges with information about the subject's actions, thus allowing the subject to choose between the two different reward amounts. Thus, our hypothesis is that information about expected rewards enters the PFC through the OFC and then is relayed to the DLPFC. If this hypothesis is true, inactivation of the DLPFC should not affect reward information in the OFC, whereas inactivation of the OFC should attenuate reward information in the DLPFC. Future experiments will test this hypothesis.

EXPERIMENT 2: ENCODING OF OTHER IMPORTANT DECISION PARAMETERS

Thus far, we have seen that OFC neurons show differential activity depending upon the reward that the subject expects for a given choice. We have also seen that the timing of this activity is more consistent with the OFC neuronal response reflecting the encoding of the reward, rather than reflecting a cognitive process that merely correlates with the reward. We have suggested that this neuronal response would make an important contribution to decision making by indicating to the motor system the action that would lead to the larger reward. However, decision making is more complex than simply always choosing the maximal reward. For example, a large reward may be obtainable, but if it is difficult to obtain it may be better to aim for a smaller, more readily obtainable reward.

Evolutionary biologists and economists have constructed detailed models of how we integrate different parameters to make effective decisions. These models emphasize the consideration of three basic parameters: the expected reward or payoff, the cost in terms of time and energy, and the probability of success.[24–26] Determining the value of a choice involves calculating the difference between the payoff and the cost and multiplying this by the probability of success. An obvious question, therefore, is to what extent OFC neurons also encode these other decision parameters. Do OFC neurons perform the calculations that are necessary for making an ideal choice, and is this their critical contribution to decision making? Recent results from neuroimaging studies suggest that this might be the case. The OFC (and sometimes the MPFC) is activated by manipulations of various decision variables—including probability,[27–29] payoff,[30–32] or the combination of these two variables—to create a set of integrated expected values.[33–37] These observations have led to the hypothesis that the OFC might integrate all variables relevant to making a decision to derive an abstract value signal, the so-called neuronal currency.[38]

A recent study in our own laboratory directly tested whether neurons in any of the major PFC regions were capable of responding to multiple parameters that underlie decisions. We trained monkeys to choose between pictures while we simultaneously recorded from the OFC, the MPFC, and the lateral PFC (LPFC).[39] Each picture was associated with a specific outcome. Some pictures were associated with a fixed amount of juice, but only on a certain proportion of trials (probability manipulation). Other pictures were associated with varying amounts of juice (payoff manipulation). Finally, some pictures were associated with a fixed amount of juice, but the subject had to earn the juice by pressing a lever a number of times (effort manipulation). About one-third of the PFC neurons responded parametrically to manipulations of just one of the decision parameters. These neurons occurred with equal prevalence in the three PFC areas from which we recorded. Furthermore, some neurons responded to a combination of two or more parameters. There was a progressive increase in the proportion of these neurons from the LPFC (16%) to the OFC (27%) to the MPFC (48%). Given these results, it is not surprising that the most severe decision-making deficits in humans occur after combined damage to the OFC and the MPFC.

We speculate that an important function of the OFC and the MPFC is to combine the multiple variables necessary to make a decision in order to derive an abstract value signal. This simplifies the task of the motor system, which at any given instant should select the action with the highest value. This encoding scheme offers distinct computational advantages. When faced with two choices, A and B, one might imagine it would be simpler to compare them directly rather than going through an additional step of assigning them an abstract value. The problem with this is that as the number of available choices increases, the number of direct comparisons increases exponentially. Thus, choosing among A, B, and C would require three comparisons (AB, AC, and BC), while choosing among A, B, C, and D requires six comparisons (AB, AC, AD, BC, BD, and CD). The solution quickly suffers from combinatorial explosion as the number of choices increases. In contrast, valuing each choice along a common reference scale provides a linear solution to the problem.

An abstract representation provides important additional behavioral advantages, such as flexibility and a capacity to deal with novelty, both of which are hallmarks of prefrontal function. For example, suppose an animal encounters a new food type. In order to determine whether it is worth choosing relative to other potential food sources, the animal must determine the value of that food. If the animal relies on making direct comparisons, it can only determine the new food's relative worth by iteratively comparing it with all previously encountered foods. On the other hand, if the animal calculates an abstract value, it has to perform only a single calculation. By assigning the new food a value on the common reference scale, the animal knows the value of this foodstuff relative to all other foods. Second, it is often unclear how to compare directly very different outcomes. How does a monkey decide between grooming a conspecific and eating a banana? Valuing the alternatives along a common reference scale can help. For example, although I have never needed to value my car in terms of bananas, I can readily do so because I can assign the bananas and the car an abstract, monetary value.

Recent neuropsychological studies of decision making in patients with OFC and MPFC damage are consistent with this interpretation of our findings. Patients show unusual patterns of decision making when faced with complex choices that require the consideration and integration of multiple attributes.[40] For example, in choosing among different apartments, the patient might need to consider each apartment's size, neighborhood, and noise level. Some of these considerations might involve a trade-off between disparate variables, such as a large apartment in a so-so neighborhood or a small apartment in a good neighborhood, and thus would benefit from valuation along an abstract scale. Behavioral data suggested that controls attempted to make the choice that maximized as many of the attributes as possible, whereas patients followed a somewhat simpler strategy of assessing each apartment against some standard of acceptability, a strategy termed *satisficing*.

It is not just complex decisions that are impaired, however. Patients with OFC and MPFC damage also show erratic performance on a task that requires preference judgments between stimuli presented two at a time, such as pictures of food, famous people, or even just colored swatches. Unlike controls, the patients showed erratic choices. For example, if they preferred A over B and B over C, they did not necessarily prefer A over C.[41] Thus, simple preference judgments also seem to benefit from the signals provided by the OFC and the MPFC.

CONCLUSION

Damage to the OFC produces a unique deficit. It impairs everyday decision making while leaving other cognitive capabilities intact. An extensive literature implicates the OFC in processing reward information, but in interpreting the area's neuronal responses, we must be careful to differentiate between responses that directly relate to the encoding of the reward's value and responses that only indirectly relate to the reward, via their encoding of cognitive and behavioral processes that covary with reward. Our findings from the first experiment suggest that the OFC is indeed encoding the reward's value, given the short latency of the neuronal reward-related responses. In contrast, the DLPFC appears to encode reward information as it relates to the guidance of behavioral responses. In addition, PFC neurons appear to encode other factors relevant to a decision, such as the effort required to obtain the reward and the probability of the reward's occurrence. Furthermore, we suggest that PFC neurons, particularly those in the OFC and the MPFC, are responsible for integrating the different decision variables to derive an abstract value signal. In turn, this signal would facilitate our capacity to make flexible and effective decisions in novel situations. Future research will aim to determine the precise contributions that the OFC and the MPFC make to decision making.

ACKNOWLEDGMENTS

Grants from NIDA R01-DA019028 and the Hellman Family Faculty Fund support our work. I would like to thank Earl Miller, in whose laboratory much of the work for the first experiment was completed. I would also like to thank Steven Kennerley for valuable conversations that went into the development of many of the ideas in this manuscript.

REFERENCES

1. ESLINGER, P.J. & A.R. DAMASIO. 1985. Severe disturbance of higher cognition after bilateral frontal lobe ablation: patient EVR. Neurology 35: 1731–1741.
2. DAMASIO, A.R. 1994. Descartes' Error: Emotion, Reason, and the Human Brain. Putman. New York.

3. ROSENKILDE, C.E., R.H. BAUER & J.M. FUSTER. 1981. Single cell activity in ventral prefrontal cortex of behaving monkeys. Brain Res. **209:** 375–394.

4. THORPE, S.J., E.T. ROLLS & S. MADDISON. 1983. The orbitofrontal cortex: neuronal activity in the behaving monkey. Exp. Brain Res. **49:** 93–115.

5. HIKOSAKA, K. & M. WATANABE. 2000. Delay activity of orbital and lateral prefrontal neurons of the monkey varying with different rewards. Cereb. Cortex **10:** 263–271.

6. AMEMORI, K. & T. SAWAGUCHI. 2006. Contrasting effects of reward expectation on sensory and motor memories in primate prefrontal neurons. Cereb. Cortex **16:** 1002–1015.

7. KOBAYASHI, S. *et al.* 2002. Influence of reward expectation on visuospatial processing in macaque lateral prefrontal cortex. J. Neurophysiol. **87:** 1488–1498.

8. LEON, M.I. & M.N. SHADLEN. 1999. Effect of expected reward magnitude on the response of neurons in the dorsolateral prefrontal cortex of the macaque. Neuron **24:** 415–425.

9. WATANABE, M. 1990. Prefrontal unit activity during associative learning in the monkey. Exp. Brain Res. **80:** 296–309.

10. WATANABE, M. 1992. Frontal units of the monkey coding the associative significance of visual and auditory stimuli. Exp. Brain Res. **89:** 233–247.

11. WATANABE, M. 1996. Reward expectancy in primate prefrontal neurons. Nature **382:** 629–632.

12. ROESCH, M.R. & C.R. OLSON. 2003. Impact of expected reward on neuronal activity in prefrontal cortex, frontal and supplementary eye fields and premotor cortex. J. Neurophysiol. **90:** 1766–1789.

13. LIU, Z. & B.J. RICHMOND. 2000. Response differences in monkey TE and perirhinal cortex: stimulus association related to reward schedules. J. Neurophysiol. **83:** 1677–1692.

14. PLATT, M.L. & P.W. GLIMCHER. 1999. Neural correlates of decision variables in parietal cortex. Nature **400:** 233–238.

15. MUSALLAM, S. *et al.* 2004. Cognitive control signals for neural prosthetics. Science **305:** 258–262.

16. SUGRUE, L.P., G.S. CORRADO & W.T. NEWSOME. 2004. Matching behavior and the representation of value in the parietal cortex. Science. **304:** 1782–1787.

17. SHULER, M.G. & M.F. BEAR. 2006. Reward timing in the primary visual cortex. Science **311:** 1606–1609.

18. MAUNSELL, J.H. 2004. Neuronal representations of cognitive state: reward or attention? Trends Cogn. Sci. **8:** 261–265.

19. WALLIS, J.D. & E.K. MILLER. 2003. Neuronal activity in primate dorsolateral and orbital prefrontal cortex during performance of a reward preference task. Eur. J. Neurosci. **18:** 2069–2081.

20. MORECRAFT, R.J., C. GEULA & M.M. MESULAM. 1992. Cytoarchitecture and neural afferents of orbitofrontal cortex in the brain of the monkey. J. Comp. Neurol. **323:** 341–358.

21. CARMICHAEL, S.T. & J.L. PRICE. 1995. Sensory and premotor connections of the orbital and medial prefrontal cortex of macaque monkeys. J. Comp. Neurol. **363:** 642–664.

22. BAXTER, M.G. & E.A. MURRAY. 2002. The amygdala and reward. Nat. Rev. Neurosci. **3:** 563–573.

23. CARDINAL, R.N. *et al.* 2002. Emotion and motivation: the role of the amygdala, ventral striatum, and prefrontal cortex. Neurosci. Biobehav. Rev. **26:** 321–352.

24. KAHNEMAN, D. & A. TVERSKY. 2000. Choices, Values and Frames. Cambridge University Press. New York.
25. LOEWENSTEIN, G. & J. ELSTER. 1992. Choice Over Time. Russel Sage Foundation. New York.
26. STEPHENS, D.W. & J.R. KREBS. 1986. Foraging Theory. Princeton University Press. Princeton.
27. ABLER, B. et al. 2006. Prediction error as a linear function of reward probability is coded in human nucleus accumbens. Neuroimage **31**: 790–795.
28. CRITCHLEY, H.D., C.J. MATHIAS & R.J. DOLAN. 2001. Neural activity in the human brain relating to uncertainty and arousal during anticipation. Neuron **29**: 537–545.
29. HUETTEL, S.A. et al. 2006. Neural signatures of economic preferences for risk and ambiguity. Neuron. **49**: 765–775.
30. BREITER, H.C. et al. 2001. Functional imaging of neural responses to expectancy and experience of monetary gains and losses. Neuron **30**: 619–639.
31. ELLIOTT, R. et al. 2003. Differential response patterns in the striatum and orbitofrontal cortex to financial reward in humans: a parametric functional magnetic resonance imaging study. J. Neurosci. **23**: 303–307.
32. KNUTSON, B. et al. 2001. Anticipation of increasing monetary reward selectively recruits nucleus accumbens. J. Neurosci. **21**: RC159.
33. YACUBIAN, J. et al. 2006. Dissociable systems for gain- and loss-related value predictions and errors of prediction in the human brain. J. Neurosci. **26**: 9530–9537.
34. TOBLER, P. N. et al. 2007. Reward value coding distinct from risk attitude-related uncertainty coding in human reward systems. J. Neurophysiol. **97**: 1621–1632.
35. O'DOHERTY, J. et al. 2001. Abstract reward and punishment representations in the human orbitofrontal cortex. Nat Neurosci. **4**: 95–102.
36. KNUTSON, B. et al. 2005. Distributed neural representation of expected value. J Neurosci. **25**: 4806–4812.
37. DREHER, J.C., P. KOHN & K.F. BERMAN. 2006. Neural coding of distinct statistical properties of reward information in humans. Cereb. Cortex. **16**: 561–573.
38. MONTAGUE, P.R. & G.S. BERNS. 2002. Neural economics and the biological substrates of valuation. Neuron **36**: 265–284.
39. KENNERLEY, S.W., A.H. LARA & J.D. WALLIS. 2005. Prefrontal neurons encode an abstract representation of value. Society For Neuroscience. 194.16.
40. FELLOWS, L.K. 2006. Deciding how to decide: ventromedial frontal lobe damage affects information acquisition in multi-attribute decision making. Brain. **129**: 944–952.
41. FELLOWS, L.K. & M.J. FARAH. 2007. The role of ventromedial prefrontal cortex in decision making: judgment under uncertainty or judgment per se? Cereb. Cortex. **17**: 2669–2674.

Dysfunctions of Medial and Lateral Orbitofrontal Cortex in Psychopathy

R. J. R. BLAIR

Mood and Anxiety Program, National Institute of Mental Health, National Institutes of Health, Department of Health and Human Services, Bethesda, Maryland, USA

ABSTRACT: Psychopathy is a developmental disorder marked by emotional hypo-responsiveness and an increased risk for instrumental and reactive aggression. In this paper, it will be argued that the developmental origins of psychopathy do not lie in orbitofrontal cortex (OFC) dysfunction. This is because the key functional impairments seen in psychopathy are associated with amygdala damage, not with OFC damage. However, it will be argued that the role played by the integrated functioning of the amygdala and medial OFC in stimulus–reinforcement learning and decision making is disrupted in psychopathy. Impaired learning of stimulus–reinforcement associations and representation of reinforcement expectations are thought to underlie the impairments in socialization and appropriate decision making seen in psychopathy. It is suggested that the impairment in the role of medial OFC in prediction error signaling and the detection of contingency change may underlie the impairments in flexible behavioral change seen in psychopathy.

KEYWORDS: psychopathy; orbitofrontal cortex; amygdala

INTRODUCTION

The goal of this paper is to consider whether there is dysfunction within orbitofrontal cortex (OFC) in individuals with psychopathy. First, the disorder will be briefly described. Then, three questions will be addressed: (1) Whether psychopathy is a developmental form of "acquired sociopathy"/pseudo-psychopathy; (2) Whether there is medial OFC dysfunction in psychopathy;

Address for correspondence: James Blair, Mood and Anxiety Program, National Institute of Mental Health, Room 206, 15K North Drive, MSC 2670, Bethesda, MD 20892. Voice: (301) 496 5198; fax: 301-594-9959.

blairj@intra.nimh.nih.gov

Ann. N.Y. Acad. Sci. 1121: 461–479 (2007). © 2007 New York Academy of Sciences.
doi: 10.1196/annals.1401.017

and (3) Whether there is lateral OFC or ventrolateral prefrontal cortex dysfunction in psychopathy.

THE DISORDER OF PSYCHOPATHY

Psychopathy is a developmental disorder involving two core components: emotional dysfunction and antisocial behavior.[1–3] The emotional dysfunction involves reduced guilt and empathy as well as reduced attachment to significant others. The antisocial behavior component involves a predisposition to antisocial behavior from an early age. It is identified in children with the antisocial process screening device[4] and in adults with the revised psychopathy checklist.[3,5] Recent work has confirmed the stability of psychopathy from childhood into adulthood; childhood psychopathy is significantly associated with adulthood psychopathy.[6] Importantly, this disorder is not equivalent to the psychiatric diagnoses of conduct disorder (CD) or antisocial personality disorder (ASPD) (DSM-IV) or CD and dissocial personality disorder (ICD 10). These psychiatric diagnoses are relatively poorly specified and concentrate almost entirely on the antisocial behavior shown by the individual rather than any potential cause for this behavior, such as the emotion dysfunction seen in psychopathy.[7]

A distinctive feature of psychopathy is that it confers an increased risk for both instrumental and reactive aggression.[8–10] Instrumental aggression (also referred to as proactive aggression) is purposeful and goal directed. The aggression is used instrumentally to achieve a specific desired goal.[11] Reactive aggression (also referred to as affective or impulsive aggression) is triggered by a frustrating or threatening event which frequently also induces anger. Importantly, the aggression is not goal directed. Many emotional disorders conditions (e.g., childhood bipolar disorder and Post Traumatic Stress Disorder) confer an increased risk for reactive aggression.[7] However, psychopathy is the only psychiatric condition to also confer an increased risk for instrumental aggression. This paper will concentrate on the implications of OFC dysfunction in psychopathy for the increased risk for instrumental and reactive aggression seen in this disorder.

One of the major strengths of the Psychopathy Checklist-Revised (PCL-R) in the classification of psychopathy has been its utility in risk assessment. This is in rather striking contrast to the diagnoses of CD and ASPD. Considerable work has shown the predictive power of scores on the PCL-R with respect to recidivism.[12–14] Moreover, this work has shown that the correlation between recidivism and psychopathy is significantly higher than that of the DSM diagnoses of CD and ASPD.[15] In recent work with children, the importance of the classification is beginning to be recognized with respect to treatment also. Hawes and Dadds found that amongst boys referred for conduct problems to a 10-week behavioral parent-training intervention, callous and unemotional

(CU) traits uniquely predicted clinical outcomes when analyzed in relation to conduct-problem severity, other predictors of antisocial behavior, and parents' implementation of treatment. Specifically, they found that boys with high CU traits were less responsive to treatment than boys with conduct problems but low CU traits.[16]

THE BASIS OF THE DISORDER

There have been suggestions that psychopathy might be due to early physical/sexual abuse or early neglect.[17] This now appears unlikely. Animal and human work has examined the impact of extreme stressors on the development of the brain. For example, animal work has precisely shown that neglect and other stressors increase emotional responsiveness to threatening stimuli.[18,19] Similarly, in humans, early physical/sexual abuse is a significant risk factor for the emergence of Post Traumatic Stress Disorder. This anxiety disorder is also associated with increased emotional responsiveness.[20] However, psychopathy is a disorder marked by reduced rather than increased emotional responsiveness.

Several recent studies have suggested a genetic contribution to the disorder.[21,22] In one of the largest of these, involving around 3500 twin pairs, CU traits were shown to be strongly heritable (67% heritability) at 7 years.[21] However, an understanding of psychopathy at the molecular genetic level remains in its infancy. Importantly though, our increased understanding of the pathophysiology of psychopathy, in particular the dysfunction within the amygdala and medial OFC (see below), allows for some suggestive possibilities. Recent work has shown that several different genetic polymorphisms impact the functioning of these structures.[23-25] For example, several studies have reported that individuals who are long/long homozygotes for the serotonin transporter (5-HTTLPR) gene show significantly reduced amygdala responding to emotional expressions relative to those who have the short form polymorphism of the gene.[23] In addition, such individuals show weaker performance on some emotional learning tasks reliant on the interaction of the amygdala and medial frontal cortex.[26] It is possible that there is an array of genes whose polymorphisms affect the functional integrity of the amygdala and medial frontal cortex. The basic genetic risk for psychopathy may emerge if an individual possesses a sufficient number of polymorphisms predisposing the individual to reduced emotional and amygdala responsiveness.

While it is clear that psychopathy is under considerable genetic influence, this does not imply that social factors do not influence its development. They clearly do. For example, socioeconomic status is associated with the emergence of the full syndrome; it is significantly less likely to appear in individuals of higher social status.[27] This is unsurprising. As noted above, one of the distinct features of psychopathy is the increased risk for goal-directed instrumental aggression. An individual is less likely to be motivated to commit many types of antisocial behavior (e.g., mugging) if they already have the material resources to achieve their goals through other means.

IS PSYCHOPATHY DEVELOPMENTAL PSEUDO-PSYCHOPATHY?

In the early 1990s, Damasio and colleagues described a series of neurological patients who had suffered lesions to regions of ventromedial prefrontal cortex that include OFC.[28] In particular, they noted that, following the lesion, these patients were under increased risk for inappropriate and sometimes antisocial behavior. They also noted that these patients presented with decision-making impairments, particularly on the Iowa gambling task.[29,30] On the basis of these data, they suggested that the "acquired sociopathy" following such lesions might be considered to model the impairment seen in individuals with psychopathy.[28,31] They argued that psychopathy might be a developmental consequence of early OFC damage.[28]

This view remains popular. However, it faces two serious problems. First, while OFC damage increases an individual's risk for frustration-based reactive aggression, it does not increase an individual's risk for goal-directed instrumental aggression even if the damage occurs early in life.[32,33] OFC is involved in the regulation of the neural architecture that mediates the basic response to threat, i.e., the amygdala, hypothalamus, and periaqueductal gray.[7,34,35] Lesions of OFC presumably disrupt the downregulation of this architecture such that the individual is more likely to express the extreme reaction to a threat (reactive aggression) rather than a more appropriate reaction, such as freezing.[7] However, lesions of OFC do not increase the risk for instrumental aggression, which is the core behavioral feature seen in psychopathy. Of course, the impact of this criticism is tempered by the knowledge that there is no neurological condition that gives rise to patients who present with a condition similar to psychopathy.[36] This should not be considered surprising. Psychopathy is a developmental condition related to disturbances in the integrated functioning of specific neural regions, not a consequence of ablation to any specific area.

The second problem for the view that psychopathy might be a developmental consequence of early OFC damage is far more serious. Psychopathy is associated with a series of core functional impairments. However, these impairments are not seen following lesions of OFC. In contrast, they are seen in patients with amygdala lesions. For example, patients with psychopathy and neurological patients with lesions of the amygdala or OFC have been tested on similar aversive-conditioning paradigms. While patients with psychopathy[37] and patients with amygdala lesions[30] show impairment in aversive conditioning, patients with OFC lesions do not.[30] Similarly, all three patient groups have been tested on very similar expression-recognition paradigms.

All three groups show impairment, but while for patients with psychopathy[38] and patients with amygdala lesions[39] the impairment is particularly marked for fearful expressions, it is notably generalized for all negative emotional expressions in patients with OFC lesions.[40]

Moreover, the idea that there is amygdala pathology in psychopathy is supported by the imaging literature. In studies with adult forensic populations, individuals with psychopathy have been found to show reduced amygdala responding to emotional words in the context of emotional-memory paradigms[41] and during aversive conditioning.[37] Work with sub-clinical populations has found that individuals with psychopathic traits show reduced amygdala responses to emotional expressions[42] and less amygdala differentiation in responding when making cooperation choices relative to defection choices in a prisoner's dilemma paradigm.[43] In short, it is unlikely that OFC dysfunction can be considered the *cause* of psychopathy (the primary deficits seen in the disorder are not consequences of OFC dysfunction). However, it is important to note that this does not imply that OFC is not dysfunctional in psychopathy (see below).

THE AMYGDALA, STIMULUS–REINFORCEMENT LEARNING, AND THE DEVELOPMENT OF PSYCHOPATHY

A considerable literature implicates the role of the amygdala in the formation and processing of stimulus–reinforcement associations.[44,45] The core deficits seen in psychopathy all relate to this functional role of the amygdala.[46] Impairment in the formation of aversive stimulus–reinforcement associations would give rise to the observed deficits in individuals with psychopathy in aversive conditioning, the augmentation of the startle reflex following the presentation of visual threat primes and passive avoidance learning.[47–49]

One important class of aversive stimuli for socialization is the distress of other individuals, the expressions of fear and sadness.[50] The amygdala is crucially involved in the response to these stimuli.[39,50,51] In line with suggestions of a specific form of empathy deficit, individuals with psychopathy show reduced autonomic responses to the distress cues of other individuals and impaired fearful facial and vocal expression recognition.[50]

The argument has been made that the expressions of fear and sadness serve as social reinforcers.[50] As such, they allow caregivers to teach the societal valence of objects and actions to the developing individual[50]; stimuli associated with the sadness/fear of others, in healthy developing children, are to be avoided. As such, they represent a particular form of outcome with respect to stimulus-outcome processing. A considerable body of work attests to the power of facial expressions to transmit valence information in both humans and other primates.[50,52,53]

With respect to psychopathy, it is argued that because of their impairment in the response to other individuals' displays of sadness and fear and in the formation of stimulus–reinforcement associations, individuals with psychopathy are less able to take advantage of this "moral" social referencing. They are less likely to learn to avoid actions that might harm others. In line with this, several studies have demonstrated that individuals with psychopathy are more difficult to socialize through standard parenting techniques.[54,55]

It is interesting to note here that while the role of the amygdala in the formation and processing of stimulus–reinforcement associations is disrupted in psychopathy, it is not clear that all functions of the amygdala are similarly disturbed. Neuropsychological and neuroimaging work in humans has suggested a role for the amygdala in some aspects of social cognition.[56] While the functional details of this role remain underspecified, it appears that the amygdala plays a role in affect-related judgments based on facial stimuli.[56,57] Thus, the amygdala has been implicated in the ability to make trustworthiness judgments on the basis of neuropsychological[58] and neuroimaging data.[59] The amygdala has also been implicated in the ability to judge complex social emotions based only on information from the eye region[60] by both neuropsychological[61,62] and neuroimaging work.[63] Individuals with psychopathy show no significant impairment in making trustworthiness judgments[64] or during performance on the eyes task.[65] These data suggest that the amygdala's role in performing these tasks remains intact in individuals with psychopathy.

It should also be noted that these data complete a double dissociation with data from individuals with autism. Amygdala-centric models of the development of autism have also been proposed.[57] Individuals with autism appear to show deficits in making trustworthiness judgments,[66] though this is debated.[67] They certainly show deficits on the eyes task.[60] In contrast, their capacity to form stimulus–reinforcement associations appears intact though there may be some inappropriate generalization[68] and they also show appropriate augmentation of the startle reflex.[69]

MEDIAL OFC

Studies have indicated a role for medial OFC (including, in some studies, more superior regions of BA 10) in encoding the value of Pavlovian conditioned stimuli[70,71] (see also Refs. 72–74). Similar regions of medial OFC have also been implicated in goal-directed instrumental action selection whether the task requires the learning of stimulus–outcome[75–78] or response–outcome associations[79] or if the outcome information is explicitly supplied to the participant in the form of a decision-making task.[80–82]

In line with animal work,[83–85] the amygdala appears involved if the value to be represented is determined through prior stimulus–reinforcement learning, whether in the context of a Pavlovian conditioning[70,71] or instrumental learning task.[75,77,86] In line with suggestions that the amygdala is not necessary for stimulus–response learning,[44] the amygdala may *not* be involved if the value to be represented is determined through prior stimulus–response association learning.[79] The basic suggestion is that the amygdala feeds forward reinforcement information associated with stimuli to medial OFC, which then represents this outcome information. This idea is a core component of the Integrated Emotion Systems (IES) model of psychopathy,[46] and this component of the IES model was derived principally from the work of Schoenbaum and colleagues.[83–85]

The function of this representation of reinforcement information within OFC is becoming clearer. There have been suggestions that OFC normalizes the value of competing outcomes so that the value of differing rewards, such as apples and oranges can be compared[87] (see also Ref. 88). In line with these suggestions, recent recording work demonstrated the existence of cells in OFC that encode the value of offered and chosen goods. They show greater activity to smaller amounts of a more desirable object relative to greater amounts of a less desirable object.[89]

Considerable progress is being made regarding the functional roles of OFC for decision making in relation to other important structures, such as dorsomedial frontal cortex.[90] An issue of particular relevance to psychopathy is the degree to which OFC's role in the representation of outcome information allows the *comparison* of values.[46,88,91] This suggestion was driven by the finding of a significant correlation of OFC activity and subjective reports of choice difficulty.[91] But if OFC is involved in the comparison of values, it should show differential responsiveness to parameters that increase choice difficulty on the basis of value information. Two parameters that increase choice difficulty are: (1) the degree of difference in reinforcement associated with the chosen and non-chosen object (the greater the differential in value, the easier the decision making); and (2) the number of objects to choose among (the fewer objects with different values to choose between, the easier the decision making). However, neither the degree of difference in reinforcement associated with the chosen and non-chosen object[76] nor the number of objects to choose among[75] had a significant impact on OFC activity. In both these studies, medial OFC activity was seen to vary as a function of the reinforcement associated with the chosen stimulus.[75,76] Indeed, there was evidence that OFC was involved in the representation of the reinforcement associated with the non-chosen stimulus also.[76] But OFC as such does not appear to be involved in the *comparison* of values.

Dorsal regions of anterior cingulate cortex did show significant activity in response both to the degree of difference in reinforcement associated with the chosen and non-chosen object and to the number of objects among which to choose.[75,76] This is consistent with suggestions that dorsal anterior cingulate cortex is involved in the monitoring and resolution of response conflict.[92–95] It is plausible that the representation of outcome information by medial OFC allows reinforcement expectancies to be translated as approach or avoidance tendencies. Response options that are close in reinforcement value should be associated with approach or avoidance tendencies of similar strength and greater response conflict than in cases where options are more dissimilar.[76] Similarly, the greater the number of response options, the greater should be the response conflict.[75] Individuals with psychopathy show general impairment on tasks involving deciding between objects on the basis of stimulus–reinforcement information,[96] consistent with the suggestion that the role of medial OFC in the representation of outcome information is impaired (see below). However, their level of impairment is not significantly affected by reinforcement distance. This is consistent with the suggestion that the role of dorsal anterior cingulate in the monitoring and resolution of response conflict is intact in psychopathy.

In short, the suggestion here, following Schoenbaum and Roesch,[88] is that medial OFC codes reinforcement expectancies, potentially normalizing the value of competing outcomes (see also Ref. 87). This region itself does not directly select between responses but rather allows the representation of value information crucial for stimulus selection. Dorsal anterior cingulate cortex operates on the translation of this information into response tendencies.

MEDIAL OFC AND PSYCHOPATHY

As noted above, the amygdala feeds forward reinforcement information associated with stimuli to medial OFC, which then represents this outcome information.[83–85] Given the suggestion made above that the amygdala's role in stimulus–reinforcement learning is disrupted in psychopathy, it might be expected that individuals with psychopathy will show anomalous medial OFC activity in the context of tasks which activate the amygdala. This is exactly what is seen. In Kiehl and colleagues' study of emotional memory, individuals with psychopathy not only showed reduced amygdala responses to the emotional words but also reduced rostral anterior cingulate cortex/medial OFC activation.[41] There was also reduced medial OFC activity in the individuals with psychopathy during aversive conditioning,[37] as well as less medial OFC differentiation in responding when making cooperation choices relative to defection choices in the prisoner's dilemma paradigm.[43]

Of course, it is impossible to determine on the basis of these imaging results whether the reduced medial OFC activity reflects dysfunction in this region or simply reduced input to this region from the amygdala. As noted above, considerable animal work has stressed the importance of the interaction of the amygdala and OFC.[88,97] Damage to the amygdala has a detrimental impact on OFC functioning.[88] However, it is important to note that animal work also suggests that early amygdala dysfunction disrupts the appropriate development of OFC.[98] It thus appears likely that psychopathy is associated with both amygdala and medial OFC dysfunction. However, to demonstrate this conclusively it will be necessary to demonstrate anomalous activity in medial frontal cortex in a task which does not implicate the amygdala.

Medial OFC and, to a lesser extent, the amygdala have been consistently identified in neuroimaging studies of moral reasoning.[99–101] For example, Greene and colleagues reported increased medial OFC activity to personal as opposed to impersonal moral choices[100]; the difference between these two situations effectively relates to the salience of the victim. Similarly, Luo and colleagues demonstrated increased amygdala and medial OFC activity to more severe relative to less severe moral transgressions.[99]

Much of the moral reasoning has been relatively vague regarding the functional roles of the neural regions implicated. For example, Greene and colleagues related the areas they identified to "emotional processing."[100] Moll and colleagues have argued that medial OFC is implicated in representing social and emotional structured-event complexes.[102] These social and emotional structured-event complexes are considered to be long-term memories of event sequences that guide the perception and execution of goal-oriented activities, such as going to a concert or giving a dinner party.[102] However, the functional specifics of these structured-event complexes remain underspecified, particularly with respect as to how they interact with emotional processing and limbic system activity.

However, by referring to the animal literature it is possible to understand the functional role of the interaction of the amygdala and medial OFC in moral reasoning in more detail.[88] This literature allows greater specification of the roles of these structures with respect to moral reasoning and, when dysfunctional, the development of psychopathy. It is argued here that the amygdala plays a role in morality by allowing the association of representations of transgressions that harm others (e.g., interpersonal violence, property damage/theft) with the emotional response to the victim's fear/sadness.[7,103] The individual's "automatic moral attitude" to a moral transgression involves the activation of the amygdala by the conditioned stimulus that is the individual's representation of the moral transgression. The amygdala then provides expected reinforcement information (both positively and negatively valenced), which is represented as a valenced outcome within medial OFC. This information is crucial for determining the individual's "attitude" towards the action, their tendency to approach or avoid it.

This suggests that damage to medial OFC should disrupt moral reasoning. In some interesting recent work, Hauser and colleagues examined the performance of patients with lesions of medial OFC on variants of the trolley problem used in Greene and colleagues' neuroimaging study.[104] In the trolley problem, the participant has to decide whether to save one or five people. If the salience of the one and the five are relatively similar, participants, unsurprisingly, are significantly more likely to save the five. However, if the salience of the one is increased (e.g., because it is necessary to actively push the one in front of the train to save the five), healthy participants are significantly more likely to choose to save the one rather than the five. In contrast, however, patients with medial OFC lesions are more likely to save the five no matter the emotional salience of the one's predicament.[104]

In psychopathy, disruption of the functioning of the amygdala and medial OFC means that the guidance of behavior provided by the integrated functioning of the amygdala and medial OFC is dysfunctional. The individual is more likely to harm others because they less well represent the aversive outcome of the victim's distress and so are less likely to avoid performing the moral transgression. The individual with psychopathy shows impaired moral reasoning[103] and is also impaired in decision making more generally; there is reduced avoidance of actions associated with expected punishment.[48,96,105]

LATERAL ORBITAL/VENTROLATERAL FRONTAL CORTEX AND PSYCHOPATHY

Individuals with psychopathy have been found to show impairment in reversal-learning paradigms.[105–108] In reversal-learning paradigms, the individual initially learns to make a response to gain a reward. The reinforcement contingency then changes so that the correct response no longer results in reward, and a new response must be learned to achieve the reward.

The impairment in reversal learning seen in psychopathy is not thought to relate to the development of psychopathy *per se.*[46] Reversal-learning impairments have been seen in other clinical populations; e.g., children with bipolar disorder.[109] Instead, the reversal-learning impairment is thought to relate to an increased risk for reactive aggression.[46] An increased risk for reactive aggression is seen in both childhood bipolar disorder and psychopathy.[110,111] As noted above, reactive aggression is associated with frustration as well as perceived threat. An individual who cannot change their behavior to accommodate to changing real-life contingencies, an individual who cannot perform reversal learning, is at increased risk for frustration. As such, they are at increased risk for reactive aggression.[7]

Early neuroimaging work consistently suggested the importance of lateral regions of OFC/ventrolateral frontal cortex in reversal learning.[112–114] Given this early neuroimaging literature and the consistent findings of reversal-learning impairment in psychopathy, it was suggested that psychopathy was associated with dysfunction within lateral regions of OFC/ventrolateral frontal cortex.[46,107] However, it now appears that these early suggestions regarding lateral OFC/ventrolateral frontal cortex dysfunction may have been wrong.

In contrast to the neuroimaging work, the human and, to a greater extent, the animal neuropsychological work considering reversal learning has demonstrated that lesions in more *medial* regions, orbital and medial prefrontal cortex, are associated with impairments in reversal learning.[115–118] Indeed, minimal animal work has investigated the impact of ventrolateral prefrontal cortex for reversal learning.

Part of the problem with the human neuroimaging literature may have been the frequent use of serial reversal paradigms; i.e., the advantageous response becomes the disadvantageous response and then becomes the advantageous response and so on throughout the study.[112,119–121] Such serial reversal paradigms may emphasize the motor control aspects of reversal learning (the selection of the appropriate motor response to achieve the goal) at the expense of those aspects of reversal learning relating to the computation of reinforcement expectancies.

A recent fMRI study of reversal learning used a number of different pairs of stimuli.[122] For those pairs of stimuli where the response contingencies changed, they only changed once. Moreover, the response contingencies did not change for all stimuli. This study replicated previous findings that a punished reversal error was associated with significantly increased activity in ventrolateral and dorsomedial prefrontal cortex.[112,119,123] Importantly though, the activation in ventrolateral prefrontal cortex could not be related to the inhibition of a previously prepotent response[112] or the representation of punishment information.[121,123,124] One of the reasons for this was that both ventrolateral and dorsomedial prefrontal cortex showed strong activation to rewarded *incorrect* responses during *acquisition*. In other words, these regions could show significant activity *before a prepotent response had been established* to a response that engendered *reward*. The argument developed by Budhani and colleagues[122] was that response conflict occurred following punishment information to a reversal error or an accidental mistake during acquisition and that this led to dorsomedial frontal cortex activation[92–94] (see also Ref. 95). This response conflict was resolved via the recruitment of ventrolateral prefrontal cortex.

Budhani et al.[122] also observed that punished reversal errors had a significant impact on medial OFC activity; specifically, they were associated with significantly reduced activity in these regions. The function ascribed to OFC in reversal learning within the animal literature has not been clearly specified. There have been suggestions that it might mediate behavioral inhibition, however recent data indicate that this is not the case.[125] The Budhani et al.[122] data suggested that the function of medial OFC in reversal learning might relate directly to its role in outcome representation. Previous work has implicated medial OFC in prediction error signaling; i.e., it has demonstrated a decrease in neuronal firing and blood-oxygen-level dependent response following an unexpected punishment or the absence of an expected reward.[74,126,127] It is possible that this prediction error signaling in medial OFC may be important for the rapid detection of contingency change and consequent reversal learning.

The Budhani et al.[122] study thus suggested that the reversal-learning impairment seen in individuals with psychopathy might relate to dysfunction either in systems putatively signaling unexpected reinforcement (medial OFC) or in those implicated in processing response conflict and implementing response changes (dorsomedial and ventrolateral frontal cortex). A recent study investigating this issue using a paradigm very similar to that of Budhani et al.[122] indicated that the impairment might relate to medial OFC dysfunction (Finger et al., submitted). Children with Disruptive Behavior Disorders and elevated CU traits (the emotional component of psychopathy) failed to show reduced activity in medial OFC to punished reversal errors. This was in marked contrast to healthy children and children with Attention Deficit and Hyperactivity Disorder (Finger et al., submitted).

CONCLUSIONS

Psychopathy is a developmental disorder marked by a significantly increased risk for goal-directed instrumental aggression and frustration-based reactive aggression that occurs the context of a specific form of emotional hypo-responsiveness. It does not appear to be a developmental form of the pseudo-psychopathy that can be seen following lesions of medial OFC. This is because the core functional impairments seen in individuals with psychopathy do not rely on the integrity of OFC. Instead, the core functional impairments rely on the integrity of the amygdala. Importantly, though, this does not suggest that psychopathy can simply be considered to reflect amygdala dysfunction. Certain functions of the amygdala, particularly those reflecting social cognition, appear intact in individuals with psychopathy.

Considerable animal and human neuroimaging work attests to the important integrated role played by the amygdala and medial OFC with respect to stimulus–reinforcement learning and decision making. It is this integrated function that appears disrupted in individuals with psychopathy. This disrupts their capacity for socialization and makes them significantly more likely to engage in instrumental actions that may give rise to others' harm.

There have been suggestions that lateral regions of OFC/ventrolateral prefrontal cortex might be disrupted in individuals with psychopathy. This was based on repeated human neuroimaging findings that indicated an important role for these regions but not for more medial regions of OFC in reversal learning. Reversal learning is impaired in psychopathy. It is thought that this deficit in being able to flexibly alter behavior following changes in reinforcement contingencies is causally related to the increased risk for frustration-based reactive aggression seen in this disorder. However, more recent imaging work has indicated that medial OFC does play an important role in reversal learning, consistent with previous animal work. These imaging data have suggested that the role of this region in the representation of reinforcement information and consequent signaling of prediction errors if this reinforcement does not occur is crucial for reversal learning. Current neuroimaging work with children with the emotional deficit seen in psychopathy indicates that dysfunction in medial OFC may underpin their impairment in reversal learning.

REFERENCES

1. FRICK, P.J. 1995. Callous-unemotional traits and conduct problems: a two-factor model of psychopathy in children. Issues in Criminological and Legal Psychology **24**: 47–51.
2. HARPUR, T.J., A.R. HAKSTIAN & R.D. HARE. 1988. The factor structure of the Psychopathy Checklist. Journal of consulting and clinical psychology **56**: 741–747.
3. HARE, R.D. 1991. The Hare Psychopathy Checklist-Revised. Multi-Health Systems. Toronto, Ontario.
4. FRICK, P.J. & R.D. HARE. 2001. The Antisocial Process Screening Device. Multi-Health Systems. Toronto.
5. HARE, R.D. 2003. Hare Psychopathy Checklist-Revised (PCL-R; 2nd Ed). Multi Health Systems. Toronto.
6. LYNAM, D.R. et al. 2007. Longitudinal evidence that psychopathy scores in early adolescence predict adult psychopathy. J. Abnorm. Psychol. **116**: 155–165.
7. BLAIR, R.J.R., D.G.V. MITCHELL & K.S. BLAIR. 2005. The Psychopath: emotion and the Brain. Blackwell. Oxford.
8. FRICK, P.J. et al. 2005. Callous-unemotional traits in predicting the severity and stability of conduct problems and delinquency. Journal of Abnormal Child Psychology **33**: 471–487.
9. CORNELL, D.G. et al. 1996. Psychopathy in instrumental and reactive violent offenders. Journal of Consulting and Clinical Psychology **64**: 783–790.
10. WILLIAMSON, S., R.D. HARE & S. WONG. 1987. Violence: criminal psychopaths and their victims. Canadian Journal of Behavioral Science **19**: 454–462.
11. BERKOWITZ, L. 1993. Aggression: its Causes, Consequences, and Control. Temple University Press. Philadelphia.
12. HART, S., P.R. KROPP & R.D. HARE. 1988. Performance of male psychopaths following conditional release from prison. Journal of Consulting and Clinical Psychology **56**: 227–232.
13. KAWASAKI, H. et al. 2001. Single-neuron responses to emotional visual stimuli recorded in human ventral prefrontal cortex. Nat. Neurosci. **4**: 15–16.
14. HARE, R.D. et al. 2000. Psychopathy and the predictive validity of the PCL-R: an international perspective. Behavioral Sciences and the Law **18**: 623–645.
15. HEMPHILL, J.F., R.D. HARE & S. WONG. 1998. Psychopathy and recidivism: a review. Legal and Criminological Psychology **3**: 139–170.
16. HAWES, D.J. & M.R. DADDS. 2005. The treatment of conduct problems in children with callous-unemotional traits. J. Consult. Clin. Psychol. **73**: 737–741.
17. RUTTER, M. 2005. Commentary: what is the meaning and utility of the psychopathy concept? J. Abnorm. Child. Psychol. **33**: 499–503.
18. RILLING, J.K. et al. 2001. Neural correlates of maternal separation in rhesus monkeys. Biol. Psychiatry **49**: 146–157.
19. BREMNER, J.D. & E. VERMETTEN. 2001. Stress and development: behavioral and biological consequences. Development and Psychopathology **13**: 473–489.

20. RAUCH, S.L., L.M. SHIN & E.A. PHELPS. 2006. Neurocircuitry models of post-traumatic stress disorder and extinction: human neuroimaging research–past, present, and future. Biological Psychiatry **60**: 376–382.
21. VIDING, E. *et al.* 2005. Evidence for substantial genetic risk for psychopathy in 7-year-olds. Journal of Child Psychology and Psychiatry **46**: 592–597.
22. BLONIGEN, D.M. *et al.* 2005. Psychopathic personality traits: heritability and genetic overlap with internalizing and externalizing psychopathology. Psychological Medicine **35**: 637–648.
23. HARIRI, A.R. *et al.* 2002. Serotonin transporter genetic variation and the response of the human amygdala. Science **297**: 400–403.
24. MEYER-LINDENBERG, A. *et al.* 2006. Neural mechanisms of genetic risk for impulsivity and violence in humans. Proc. Natl. Acad. Sci. USA **103**: 6269–6274.
25. PEZAWAS, L. *et al.* 2005. 5-HTTLPR polymorphism impacts human cingulate-amygdala interactions: a genetic susceptibility mechanism for depression. Nat. Neurosci. **8**: 828–834.
26. FINGER, E.C. *et al.* 2007. The impact of tryptophan depletion and 5-HTTLPR genotype on passive avoidance and response reversal instrumental learning tasks. Neuropsychopharmacology **32**: 206–215.
27. SILVERTHORN, P. & P.J. FRICK. 1999. Developmental pathways to antisocial behavior: the delayed-onset pathway in girls. Dev. Psychopathol. **11**: 101–126.
28. DAMASIO, A.R. 1994. Descartes' Error: emotion, Rationality and the Human Brain. Putnam (Grosset Books). New York.
29. BECHARA, A. *et al.* 2001. Decision-making deficits, linked to a dysfunctional ventromedial prefrontal cortex, revealed in alcohol and stimulant abusers. Neuropsychologia **39**: 376–389.
30. BECHARA, A. *et al.* 1999. Different contributions of the human amygdala and ventromedial prefrontal cortex to decision-making. Journal of Neuroscience **19**: 5473–5481.
31. DAMASIO, A. 1998. The somatic marker hypothesis and the possible functions of the Prefrontal Cortex. *In* The Prefrontal Cortex. A.C. Roberts, T.W. Robbins & L. Weiskrantz, Eds.: 36–50. Oxford University Press. New York.
32. GRAFMAN, J. *et al.* 1996. Frontal lobe injuries, violence, and aggression: a report of the Vietnam head injury study. Neurology **46**: 1231–1238.
33. ANDERSON, S.W. *et al.* 1999. Impairment of social and moral behaviour related to early damage in human prefrontal cortex. Nature Neuroscience **2**: 1032–1037.
34. PANKSEPP, J. 1998. Affective Neuroscience: the Foundations of Human and Animal Emotions. Oxford University Press. New York.
35. GREGG, T.R. & A. SIEGEL. 2001. Brain structures and neurotransmitters regulating aggression in cats: implications for human aggression. Prog. Neuropsychopharmacol Biol. Psychiatry **25**: 91–140.
36. BLAIR, R.J.R. 2006. The emergence of psychopathy: implications for the neuropsychological approach to developmental disorders. Cognition **101**: 414–442.
37. BIRBAUMER, N. *et al.* 2005. Deficient fear conditioning in psychopathy: a functional magnetic resonance imaging study. Arch. Gen. Psychiatry **62**: 799–805.
38. BLAIR, R.J.R. *et al.* 2004. Reduced sensitivity to other's fearful expressions in psychopathic individuals. Personality & Individual Differences **37**: 1111–1121.
39. ADOLPHS, R. 2002. Neural systems for recognizing emotion. Curr. Opin. Neurobiol. **12**: 169–177.

40. HORNAK, J. *et al.* 2003. Changes in emotion after circumscribed surgical lesions of the orbitofrontal and cingulate cortices. Brain **126:** 1691–1712.
41. KIEHL, K.A. *et al.* 2001. Limbic abnormalities in affective processing by criminal psychopaths as revealed by functional magnetic resonance imaging. Biological Psychiatry **50:** 677–684.
42. GORDON, H.L., A.A. BAIRD & A. END. 2004. Functional differences among those high and low on a trait measure of psychopathy. Biological Psychiatry **56:** 516–521.
43. RILLING, J.K. *et al.* 2007. Neural correlates of social cooperation and non-cooperation as a function of psychopathy. Biol Psychiatry **61:** 1260–1271.
44. BAXTER, M.G. & E.A. MURRAY. 2002. The amygdala and reward. Nat. Rev. Neurosci. **3:** 563–573.
45. EVERITT, B.J. *et al.* 2003. Appetitive behavior: impact of amygdala-dependent mechanisms of emotional learning. Annals New York Academy of Sciences **985:** 233–250.
46. BLAIR, R.J.R. 2004. The roles of orbital frontal cortex in the modulation of antisocial behavior. Brain and Cognition **55:** 198–208.
47. FLOR, H. *et al.* 2002. Aversive Pavlovian conditioning in psychopaths: peripheral and central correlates. Psychophysiology **39:** 505–518.
48. NEWMAN, J.P. & D.S. KOSSON. 1986. Passive avoidance learning in psychopathic and nonpsychopathic offenders. Journal of Abnormal Psychology **95:** 252–256.
49. LEVENSTON, G.K. *et al.* 2000. The psychopath as observer: emotion and attention in picture processing. Journal of Abnormal Psychology **109:** 373–386.
50. BLAIR, R.J.R. 2003. Facial expressions, their communicatory functions and neuro-cognitive substrates. Philos. Trans. R. Soc. Lond. B. Biol. Sci. **358:** 561–572.
51. HOFFMAN, K.L. *et al.* 2007. Facial-expression and gaze-selective responses in the monkey amygdala. Curr. Biol. **17:** 766–772.
52. MINEKA, S. & M. COOK. 1993. Mechanisms involved in the observational conditioning of fear. Journal of Experimental Psychology: General **122:** 23–38.
53. KLINNERT, M.D. *et al.* 1987. Social referencing: the infant's use of emotional signals from a friendly adult with mother present. Annual Progress in Child Psychiatry and Child Development **22:** 427–432.
54. WOOTTON, J.M. *et al.* 1997. Ineffective parenting and childhood conduct problems: the moderating role of callous-unemotional traits. Journal of Consulting and Clinical Psychology **65:** 292–300.
55. OXFORD, M., T.A. CAVELL & J.N. HUGHES. 2003. Callous-unemotional traits moderate the relation between ineffective parenting and child externalizing problems: a partial replication and extension. Journal of Clinical Child and Adolescent Psychology **32:** 577–585.
56. ADOLPHS, R. 2003. Is the human amygdala specialized for processing social information? Ann. N. Y. Acad. Sci. **985:** 326–340.
57. BARON-COHEN, S. *et al.* 2000. The amygdala theory of autism. Neuroscience Biobehavior Review **24:** 355–364.
58. ADOLPHS, R., D. TRANEL & A.R. DAMASIO. 1998. The human amygdala in social judgment. Nature **393:** 470–474.
59. WINSTON, J.S. *et al.* 2002. Automatic and intentional brain responses during evaluation of trustworthiness of faces. Nat. Neurosci. **5:** 277–283.
60. BARON-COHEN, S., S. WHEELWRIGHT & T. JOLIFFE. 1997. Is there a "language of the eyes"? Evidence from normal adults, and adults with autism or Asperger syndrome. Visual Cognition **4:** 311–331.

61. ADOLPHS, R., S. BARON-COHEN & D. TRANEL. 2002. Impaired recognition of social emotions following amygdala damage. J. Cogn. Neurosci. **14:** 1264–1274.

62. STONE, V.E. *et al.* 2003. Acquired theory of mind impairments in individuals with bilateral amygdala lesions. Neuropsychologia **41:** 209–220.

63. BARON-COHEN, S. *et al.* 1999. Social intelligence in the normal and autistic brain: an fMRI study. European Journal of Neuroscience **11:** 1891–1898.

64. RICHELL, R.A. *et al.* 2005. Trust and distrust: the perception of trustworthiness of faces in psychopathic and non-psychopathic offenders. Personality and Individual Differences **38:** 1735–1744.

65. RICHELL, R.A. *et al.* 2003. Theory of mind and psychopathy: can psychopathic individuals read the 'language of the eyes'? Neuropsychologia **41:** 523–526.

66. ADOLPHS, R., L. SEARS & J. PIVEN. 2001. Abnormal processing of social information from faces in autism. Journal of Cognitive Neuroscience **13:** 232–240.

67. WHITE, S. *et al.* 2006. An islet of social ability in Asperger syndrome: judging social attributes from faces. Brain Cogn. **61:** 69–77.

68. GAIGG, S.B. & D.M. BOWLER. 2007. Differential fear conditioning in Asperger's syndrome: implications for an amygdala theory of autism. Neuropsychologia **45:** 2125–2134.

69. BERNIER, R. *et al.* 2005. Individuals with autism spectrum disorder show normal responses to a fear potential startle paradigm. J. Autism. Dev. Disord. **35:** 575–583.

70. GOTTFRIED, J.A. & R.J. DOLAN. 2004. Human orbitofrontal cortex mediates extinction learning while accessing conditioned representations of value. Nature Neuroscience **7:** 1144–1152.

71. GOTTFRIED, J.A., J. O'DOHERTY & R.J. DOLAN. 2003. Encoding predictive reward value in human amygdala and orbitofrontal cortex. Science **301:** 1104–1107.

72. KNUTSON, B. & J.C. COOPER. 2005. Functional magnetic resonance imaging of reward prediction. Curr. Opin. Neurol. **18:** 411–417.

73. KNUTSON, B. *et al.* 2005. Distributed neural representation of expected value. J. Neurosci. **25:** 4806–4812.

74. KNUTSON, B. *et al.* 2001. Dissociation of reward anticipation and outcome with event-related fMRI. Neuroreport **12:** 3683–3687.

75. MARSH, A.A. *et al.* 2007. Response options and expectations of reward in decision-making: the differential roles of dorsal and rostral anterior cingulate cortex. Neuroimage **35:** 979–988.

76. BLAIR, K.S. *et al.* 2006. Choosing the lesser of two evils, the better of two goods: specifying the roles of ventromedial prefrontal cortex and dorsal anterior cingulate cortex in object choice. Journal of Neuroscience **26:** 11379–11386.

77. KOSSON, D.S. *et al.* 2006. The role of the amygdala and rostral anterior cingulate in encoding expected outcomes during learning. Neuroimage **29:** 1161–1172.

78. KIM, H., S. SHIMOJO & J.P. O'DOHERTY. 2006. Is avoiding an aversive outcome rewarding? Neural substrates of avoidance learning in the human brain. PLoS Biol. **4:** e233.

79. VALENTIN, V.V., A. DICKINSON & J.P. O'DOHERTY. 2007. Determining the neural substrates of goal-directed learning in the human brain. J. Neurosci. **27:** 4019–4026.

80. ERNST, M. *et al.* 2004. Choice selection and reward anticipation: an fMRI study. Neuropsychologia **42:** 1585–1597.

81. PAULUS, M.P. *et al.* 2002. Error rate and outcome predictability affect neural activation in prefrontal cortex and anterior cingulate during decision-making. Neuroimage **15**: 836–846.
82. ROGERS, R.D. *et al.* 2004. Distinct portions of anterior cingulate cortex and medial prefrontal cortex are activated by reward processing in separable phases of decision-making cognition. Biological Psychiatry **55**: 594–602.
83. SCHOENBAUM, G. *et al.* 2003. Encoding predicted outcome and acquired value in orbitofrontal cortex during cue sampling depends upon input from basolateral amygdala. Neuron **39**: 855–867.
84. SCHOENBAUM, G. *et al.* 2002. Orbitofrontal lesions in rats impair reversal but not acquisition of go, no-go odor discriminations. Neuroreport **13**: 885–890.
85. GALLAGHER, M., R.W. MCMAHAN & G. SCHOENBAUM. 1999. Orbitofrontal cortex and representation of incentive value in associative learning. Journal of Neuroscience **19**: 6610–6614.
86. IZQUIERDO, A. & E.A. MURRAY. 2007. Selective bilateral amygdala lesions in rhesus monkeys fail to disrupt object reversal learning. J. Neurosci. **27**: 1054–1062.
87. MONTAGUE, P.R. & G.S. BERNS. 2002. Neural economics and the biological substrates of valuation. Neuron **36**: 265–284.
88. SCHOENBAUM, G. & M. ROESCH. 2005. Orbitofrontal cortex, associative learning, and expectancies. Neuron **47**: 633–636.
89. PADOA-SCHIOPPA, C. & J.A. ASSAD. 2006. Neurons in the orbitofrontal cortex encode economic value. Nature **441**: 223–226.
90. RUSHWORTH, M.F. *et al.* 2007. Contrasting roles for cingulate and orbitofrontal cortex in decisions and social behaviour. Trends Cogn. Sci. **11**: 168–176.
91. ARANA, F.S. *et al.* 2003. Dissociable contributions of the human amygdala and orbitofrontal cortex to incentive motivation and goal selection. J. Neurosci. **23**: 9632–9638.
92. CARTER, C.S. *et al.* 2000. Parsing executive processes: strategic vs. evaluative functions of the anterior cingulate cortex. Proc. Natl. Acad. Sci. USA **97**: 1944–1948.
93. COHEN, J.D., M. BOTVINICK & C.S. CARTER. 2000. Anterior cingulate and prefrontal cortex: who's in control? Nat. Neurosci. **3**: 421–423.
94. KERNS, J.G. *et al.* 2004. Anterior cingulate conflict monitoring and adjustments in control. Science **303**: 1023–1026.
95. BOTVINICK, M.M., J.D. COHEN & C.S. CARTER. 2004. Conflict monitoring and anterior cingulate cortex: an update. Trends in Cognitive Science **8**: 539–546.
96. BLAIR, K.S. *et al.* 2006. Impaired decision making on the basis of both reward and punishment information in individuals with psychopathy. Personality and Individual Differences **41**: 155–165.
97. MURRAY, E.A. & A. IZQUIERDO. In press. Orbitofrontal cortex and amygdala contributions to affect and action in primates. Ann. N. Y. Acad. Sci.
98. DIERGAARDE, L. *et al.* 2005. Early amygdala damage disrupts performance on medial prefrontal cortex-related tasks but spares spatial learning and memory in the rat. Neuroscience **130**: 581–590.
99. LUO, Q. *et al.* 2006. The neural basis of implicit moral attitude–an IAT study using event-related fMRI. Neuroimage **30**: 1449–1157.
100. GREENE, J.D. *et al.* 2001. An fMRI investigation of emotional engagement in moral judgment. Science **293**: 1971–1972.

101. MOLL, J. *et al.* 2002. Functional networks in emotional moral and nonmoral social judgments. Neuroimage **16:** 696–703.
102. MOLL, J. *et al.* 2005. Opinion: the neural basis of human moral cognition. Nat. Rev. Neurosci. **6:** 799–809.
103. BLAIR, R.J.R. 1995. A cognitive developmental approach to morality: investigating the psychopath. Cognition **57:** 1–29.
104. KOENIGS, M. *et al.* 2007. Damage to the prefrontal cortex increases utilitarian moral judgements. Nature **446:** 908–911.
105. MITCHELL, D.G.V. *et al.* 2002. Risks decisions and response reversal: is there evidence of orbitofrontal cortex dysfunction in psychopathic individuals? Neuropsychologia **40:** 2013–2022.
106. BLAIR, R.J., E. COLLEDGE & D.G. MITCHELL. 2001. Somatic markers and response reversal: is there orbitofrontal cortex dysfunction in boys with psychopathic tendencies? J. Abnorm. Child. Psychol. **29:** 499–511.
107. BUDHANI, S. & R.J. BLAIR. 2005. Response reversal and children with psychopathic tendencies: success is a function of salience of contingency change. J. Child. Psychol. Psychiatry **46:** 972–981.
108. BUDHANI, S., R.A. RICHELL & R.J. BLAIR. 2006. Impaired reversal but intact acquisition: probabilistic response reversal deficits in adult individuals with psychopathy. J. Abnorm. Psychol. **115:** 552–558.
109. GORRINDO, T. *et al.* 2005. Deficits on a probabilistic response-reversal task in patients with pediatric bipolar disorder. Am. J. Psychiatry **162:** 1975–1977.
110. LEIBENLUFT, E. *et al.* 2003. Irritability in pediatric mania and other childhood psychopathology. Annals New York Academy of Sciences **1008:** 201–218.
111. FRICK, P.J. *et al.* 2003. Callous-unemotional traits and conduct problems in the prediction of conduct problem severity, aggression, and self-report delinquency. Journal of Abnormal Child Psychology **31:** 457–470.
112. COOLS, R. *et al.* 2002. Defining the neural mechanisms of probabilistic reversal learning using event-related functional magnetic resonance imaging. J. Neurosci. **22:** 4563–4567.
113. ROGERS, R.D. *et al.* 2000. Contrasting cortical and subcortical activations produced by attentional-set shifting and reversal learning in humans. J. Cogn. Neurosci. **12:** 142–162.
114. KRINGELBACH, M.L. & E.T. ROLLS. 2003. Neural correlates of rapid reversal learning in a simple model of human social interaction. NeuroImage **20:** 1371–1383.
115. IVERSEN, S.D. & M. MISHKIN. 1970. Perseverative interference in monkeys following selective lesions of the inferior prefrontal convexity. Exp. Brain Res. **11:** 376–386.
116. DIAS, R., T.W. ROBBINS & A.C. ROBERTS. 1996. Dissociation in prefrontal cortex of affective and attentional shifts. Nature **380:** 69–72.
117. IZQUIERDO, A., R.K. SUDA & E.A. MURRAY. 2004. Bilateral orbital prefrontal cortex lesions in rhesus monkeys disrupt choices guided by both reward value and reward contingency. J. Neurosci. **24:** 7540–7548.
118. FELLOWS, L.K. & M.J. FARAH. 2003. Ventromedial frontal cortex mediates affective shifting in humans: evidence from a reversal learning paradigm. Brain **126:** 1830–1837.
119. REMIJNSE, P.L. *et al.* 2005. Neural correlates of a reversal learning task with an affectively neutral baseline: an event-related fMRI study. Neuroimage **26:** 609–618.

120. O'DOHERTY, J. *et al.* 2003. Dissociating valence of outcome from behavioral control in human orbital and ventral prefrontal cortices. Journal of Neuroscience **23:** 7931–7939.
121. O'DOHERTY, J. *et al.* 2001. Abstract reward and punishment representations in the human orbitofrontal cortex. Nat. Neurosci. **4:** 95–102.
122. BUDHANI, S. *et al.* 2007. Neural correlates of response reversal: considering acquisition. Neuroimage **34:** 1754–1765.
123. KRINGELBACH, M.L. 2005. The human orbitofrontal cortex: linking reward to hedonic experience. Nat. Rev. Neurosci. **6:** 691–702.
124. KRINGELBACH, M.L. & E.T. ROLLS. 2004. The functional neuroanatomy of the human orbitofrontal cortex: evidence from neuroimaging and neuropsychology. Progressive Neurobiology **72:** 341–372.
125. CHUDASAMA, Y., J.D. KRALIK & E.A. MURRAY. 2007. Rhesus monkeys with orbital prefrontal cortex lesions can learn to inhibit prepotent responses in the reversed reward contingency task. Cereb. Cortex **17:** 1154–1159.
126. YACUBIAN, J. *et al.* 2006. Dissociable systems for gain- and loss-related value predictions and errors of prediction in the human brain. J. Neurosci. **26:** 9530–9537.
127. O'DOHERTY, J.P. *et al.* 2003. Temporal difference models and reward-related learning in the human brain. Neuron **38:** 329–337.

The Orbitofrontal Cortex, Real-World Decision Making, and Normal Aging

NATALIE L. DENBURG,[a] CATHERINE A. COLE,[b] MICHAEL HERNANDEZ,[a] TORRICIA H. YAMADA,[a] DANIEL TRANEL,[a] ANTOINE BECHARA,[c] AND ROBERT B. WALLACE[d]

[a]Department of Neurology, Division of Cognitive Neuroscience, University of Iowa Roy J. and Lucille A. Carver College of Medicine, Iowa City, Iowa, USA

[b]Department of Marketing, University of Iowa, Iowa City, Iowa, USA

[c]Department of Psychology, University of Southern California, Los Angeles, California, USA

[d]Department of Epidemiology, University of Iowa College of Public Health, Iowa City, Iowa, USA

ABSTRACT: The present series of three studies aims at investigating the hypothesis that some seemingly normal older persons have deficits in reasoning and decision making due to dysfunction in a neural system which includes the ventromedial prefrontal cortices. This hypothesis is relevant to the comprehensive study of aging, and also addresses the question of why so many older adults fall prey to fraud. To our knowledge, this work represents the first of its kind to begin to identify, from an individual-differences perspective, the behavioral, psychophysiological, and consumer correlates of defective decision making among healthy older adults. Our findings, in a cross-sectional sample of community-dwelling participants, demonstrate that a sizeable subset of older adults (approximately 35–40%) perform disadvantageously on a laboratory measure of decision making that closely mimics everyday life, by the manner in which it factors in reward, punishment, risk, and ambiguity. These same poor decision makers display defective autonomic responses (or somatic markers), reminiscent of that previously established in patients with acquired prefrontal lesions. Finally, we present data demonstrating that poor decision makers are more likely to fall prey to deceptive advertising, suggesting compromise of real-world judgment and decision-making abilities.

KEYWORDS: aging; frontal lobe; decision making

Address for correspondence: Natalie L. Denburg, Ph.D., Assistant Professor, #2007 RCP, Department of Neurology, University of Iowa Hospitals and Clinics, 200 Hawkins Drive, Iowa City, IA 52242-1053. Voice: 319-356-7619; fax: 319-384-7199.
natalie-denburg@uiowa.edu

Ann. N.Y. Acad. Sci. 1121: 480–498 (2007). © 2007 New York Academy of Sciences.
doi: 10.1196/annals.1401.031

INTRODUCTION

This article presents a series of three studies that begin to identify, from an individual-differences perspective, the behavioral,[1] psychophysiological,[2] and consumer (Denburg *et al.*, manuscript submitted for publication) correlates of defective decision making among seemingly healthy older adults. The basic hypothesis for these studies involves the idea that some normal older persons, who are free of obvious neurologic or psychiatric disease, have deficits in reasoning and decision making on account of dysfunction in a neural system which includes the ventromedial prefrontal cortices (VMPC).

It is important to be clear right from the outset about our anatomic terminology, because some confusion tends to surround the use of the terms orbitofrontal and ventromedial regions of the prefrontal cortex. The orbitofrontal region includes the rectus gyrus and orbital gyri, which constitute the inferior surface of the frontal lobes lying immediately above the orbital plates. In humans, lesions that involve this region are not usually restricted to the orbitofrontal cortex, but they extend into neighboring cortex and involve different sectors of the medial and ventral regions of the prefrontal cortex, as well as the subgenual part of the anterior cingulate (i.e., Brodmann's areas 25, lower 24, 32, medial aspect of 11, 12, and 10, and the white matter adjacent to all of these areas). Therefore, in most of our studies of patients with lesions in this region, we refer to the damage as involving the VMPC regions, and not strictly the orbitofrontal region.

Our hypothesis is relevant to the comprehensive study of aging, and it is also relevant to the pressing practical issue of why so many older adults fall prey to fraud. The theoretical framework that guides this work is built around the "frontal lobe hypothesis" of cognitive aging,[3,4] which in broad terms implies that some older adults have disproportionate age-related change of prefrontal brain structures, and, concomitantly, of associated cognitive functions. The frontal lobe hypothesis is supported by multiple sources of evidence that are steadily mounting, involving neuropsychological,[5–14] neuroanatomic,[15–21] and functional neuroimaging[22,23] studies. The hypothesis has not been without its critics,[24,25] but it provides a plausible and testable account of at least some age-related neurocognitive phenomena.[4]

SIGNIFICANCE

Older adulthood has been characterized as a period of critical and complex decision making, and for many of the decisions that older adults make, there is a lot at stake. For example, the elderly deal with such issues as investment of savings and retirement income, purchase of insurance and living trusts, estate planning, anticipating and planning possible nursing home placement, purchase of a burial site, funeral costs, out-of-pocket medical costs, and sudden changes in financial roles following the death of a spouse. For most, these decisions are made while the person is on a fixed income. Such decisions would be a challenge even for intelligent young adults; however, when one considers possible executive dysfunction, in conjunction with fraudulent and vicious marketing extant in the social system, the degree of decision-making difficulty is greatly augmented in older adults.

Beginning in 1996 and continuing to the present, the U.S. Senate and House of Representatives have held numerous hearings focused on the fact that a sizable proportion of the elderly are falling prey to both misleading and fraudulent advertising.[26] Despite recent legislative emphasis on this issue, research efforts examining older consumers' vulnerability to fraud are sorely lacking. In the studies that follow, we argue that cognitive vulnerability generally, and impairments in decision-making ability specifically, even in the context of relatively intact memory and intellect, can explain why older adults are frequently the victims of unscrupulous business activities.

STUDY 1: BEHAVIORAL CORRELATES OF DEFECTIVE DECISION MAKING

Researchers at the University of Iowa, Division of Behavioral Neurology and Cognitive Neuroscience, have been long interested in a critical set of functions associated with prefrontal brain structures, especially the processes of reasoning, decision making, and how these interface with emotional processing. It has been shown that younger patients with acquired VMPC damage manifest notable real-world decision-making impairments[28] and, moreover, have impaired self-awareness of such deficits. Thus, guided by rationale derived from our work with lesion patients, we examined the possibility that a sizable number of elderly suffer from a decline in cognitive functions critical for decision making, in spite of relatively intact memory and general intellect. In turn, the first manifestation of this cognitive decline may be exercising poor judgment and decision making in many important real-life matters.

In the initial study in this series, neurologically and psychiatrically healthy older and younger adults were administered a well-validated decision-making paradigm, called the Iowa Gambling Task (IGT). The IGT provides a close analogue to real-world decision making in the manner in which it factors reward, punishment, and unpredictability,[29] and taxes decision-making functions mediated by the VMPC region.[30-33] Here, we hypothesized that a subset of older adults would manifest decision-making deficits on the IGT.

An age- and sex-stratified community-dwelling sample of 80 adults was dichotomized on age, using a conventional demarcation point,[33] to form a Younger Group (aged 26–55 years [$M = 41.0$ years]; 50% female) and an Older Group (aged 56–85 years [$M = 70.4$ years]; 53% female). Each participant was tested individually in a 3-hour session that included the IGT and a battery of standard neuropsychological tests. A structured interview (as in Tranel et al.[34]) was used to determine that all participants enrolled in the study were deemed exceptionally healthy. Exclusionary criteria included major surgeries with complications; neurological events, such as cerebrovascular insults, seizures, or head injury with loss of consciousness exceeding 5 min; medications, especially those that might produce untoward effects on cognition; and a history of significant psychiatric disease necessitating inpatient treatment and/or interfering with daily functioning.

The computerized IGT was administered in the standard fashion,[30] involving 100 card selections from four decks. Some card selections are followed by a reward only (monetary gain); others are followed by a reward and a punishment (monetary loss). The task is manipulated such that decks with lower immediate reward have lower long-term punishment, and thus yield an overall net gain (decks C and D, referred to as "Good" decks); decks with higher immediate reward have higher long-term punishment, and thus yield an overall net loss (decks A and B, referred to as "Bad" decks). Participants are not informed about the number of trials or the reward/punishment schedules, and the schedules cannot be deduced mathematically. To quantify performance on the IGT, the 100 choices are divided into five discrete blocks of 20 cards each, and for each Trial Block, we calculate a performance score by subtracting the number of disadvantageous deck choices (A and B) from the number of advantageous deck choices (C and D), $[(C + D)-(A + B)]$. Scores below zero thus indicate "disadvantageous" performance (an overall loss of money), and scores greater than zero indicate "advantageous" performance (an overall gain of money).

The normal pattern of performance in healthy, non-elderly individuals is to begin the first Trial Block by selecting more from the Bad decks than from the Good decks, because the Bad decks have the appeal of more immediate reward. As the game progresses, however, steep penalties are encountered in the Bad decks, and participants gradually shift their selections toward the Good decks. By the final couple of Trial Blocks, participants select predominantly from the Good decks. FIGURE 1 depicts such a positively sloped performance, graphed as a function of Trial Block, which begins a bit below the zero mark and gradually rises into the positive range as participants begin selecting cards in a more and more advantageous manner. By contrast, in patients with neurologic damage to the VMPC, the ability to shift decision making in a favorable direction is impaired, and the patients continue to choose preferentially from the Bad decks for the duration of the game (FIG. 1).[30]

IGT performances of the Younger and Older Groups were analyzed with a 2×5 ANOVA using Age Group (Younger versus Older) as the between-subjects factor, and Trial Block (1–5) as the within-subjects factor. It was our expectation that this analysis would yield an interaction: the Younger Group was expected to show the typical positively sloped line, whereas the Older Group, which we believed would contain a subset of participants who performed disadvantageously, was expected to show a flatter slope across Trial Blocks. We also looked at individual performance profiles in each of the Groups. We collapsed across Trial Blocks and calculated for each participant

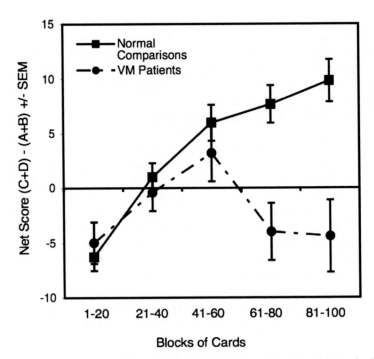

FIGURE 1.   Decision-making performance on the IGT in patients with acquired damage to VMPC and demographically matched normal comparisons participants, graphed as a function of Trial Block (±SEM, standard error of the mean).

a single index of performance, specifically, the sum of Good deck choices minus the sum of Bad deck choices [(C+D)–(A+B)]. Under the assumption that random behavior on the IGT would yield a score of zero in this formula, we categorized each participant as "unimpaired" or "impaired," based on whether the overall performance index differed significantly from zero (using the binomial test), and in which direction. Participants who had indices that were significantly different from zero in the positive direction were categorized as "unimpaired," and participants who had indices that were significantly different from zero in the negative direction were categorized as "impaired."

The Group results accorded with our predictions (FIG. 2): the Younger Group started below zero, and then gradually shifted toward the Good decks as the game progressed. The Older Group did not demonstrate this shift: after the first Trial Block, their performance hovered around the zero-line for the entire task. The statistical analysis of these data yielded the predicted two-way interaction between Age Group and Trial Block ($F(4,312) = 3.65$, $P < 0.05$). The Age Group ($F(1,78) = 11.89$, $P < 0.01$) and Trial Block ($F(4,312) = 14.00$, $P < 0.0001$) main effects were also significant.

Regarding performances of individual participants, in the Younger Group, 37 of 40 participants were "unimpaired," achieving overall indices significantly

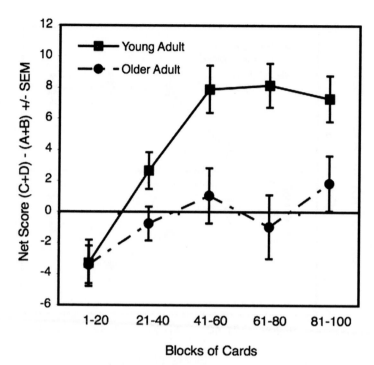

FIGURE 2. Decision-making performance on the IGT in Younger and Older participants, graphed as a function of Trial Block (±SEM).

above zero (3 were "impaired," obtaining indices significantly below zero). This outcome is consistent with our previous studies, which have indicated that nearly all younger normal participants perform in an advantageous manner on the IGT (cf.[30]). In the Older Group, we found that 15 participants were "unimpaired," obtaining overall indices significantly above zero (Mage = 70.3 years; 40% female), whereas 14 were "impaired," obtaining overall indices significantly below zero (Mage = 71.1 years; 50% female). (Another 11 participants were considered "borderline," because their indices did not differ significantly from zero in either the positive or negative direction. Because this outcome is inconclusive, we will not consider this subgroup any further.) Thus, consistent with our expectation, a subset of the Older participants performed abnormally on the IGT, failing to shift their selections toward advantageous outcomes. In regard to the proportion of participants in each Age Group who were unimpaired versus impaired, there was a significant difference between the Younger and Older Groups ($\chi^2 = 18.80$, $P < 0.0001$), reflecting the much higher rate of impaired performance in the Older participants.

We conducted a follow-up analysis, focused specifically on the Older-Unimpaired and Older-Impaired Groups. The performance profiles of these two Groups diverged markedly (FIG. 3). The Older-Unimpaired Group began

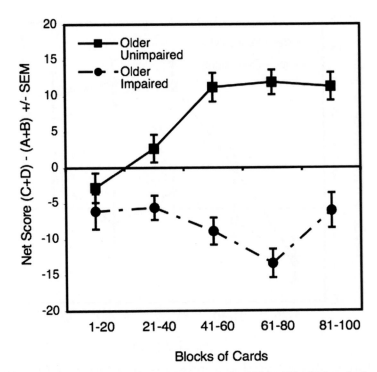

FIGURE 3. Decision-making performance on the IGT in Older-Unimpaired participants and Older-Impaired participants, graphed as a function of Trial Block ($\pm$SEM).

by selecting more cards from the Bad decks, but then demonstrated a strong and sustained shift toward the Good decks as the task progressed. The Older-Impaired Group did not show this shift, as they chose predominantly from the Bad decks all the way through the task (in a manner reminiscent of patients with ventromedial prefrontal lesions). A 2×5 ANOVA using Group (Older-Unimpaired versus Older-Impaired) as a between-subjects factor and Trial Block (Blocks 1–5) as a within-subjects factor yielded a significant two-way interaction $[F(4,108) = 10.53, P < 0.0001]$, substantiating the trends evident in FIGURE 3.[a] (The Group $(F(1,27) = 104.83, P < 0.0001)$ and Trial Block $[F(4, 108) = 3.91, P < 0.05]$ main effects were also significant.)

In summary, the findings from this study support the notion that a subset of older individuals has significant difficulty with reasoning and decision making, as indexed by the IGT. This impairment occurred in the absence of any frank neurologic or psychiatric disease, and there was no evidence that it could be explained by pre-morbid factors (e.g., educational level),

---

[a] Because the two Groups differed slightly in Trial Block 1, we used the Block 1 score as a covariate in a 2×4 ANCOVA using the same factors as in the primary ANOVA. The Group x Trial Block interaction remained significant $(F(3,78) = 8.16, P < 0.0001)$.

overall health status, or weaknesses in other cognitive realms such as attention, memory, or language (confirmed by detailed neuropsychological testing of the participants). Moreover, within the age range subsumed by our Older participant sample (56–85), there was no indication that age per se accounted for the decision-making impairment. The rate of impairment in our sample was not trivial: 14 of 40 older participants were deficient, compared to only 3 of 40 younger participants.

STUDY 2: PSYCHOPHYSIOLOGICAL CORRELATES OF DEFECTIVE DECISION MAKING

Defective decision making in patients with acquired VMPC damage has been discussed in the framework of the *somatic marker hypothesis*, which posits that decision making is often assisted by emotional processes and somatic "markers," originating not only from the body itself, but also from several large-scale cortical and subcortical brain networks, including the VMPC, amygdala, insular cortices/somatosensory cortices, and possibly the basal ganglia, as well as signals from the peripheral nervous system.[30,36,37] In previous studies, electrodermal activity, specifically the skin conductance response (SCR), has been used in our laboratory as a dependent measure of somatic state activation and somatic "signaling" activity.[38]

In previous work, we have shown that healthy, non-elderly individuals generate anticipatory SCRs prior to a Bad deck selection, while age-matched VMPC patients (mean age $\cong$ 44 years) fail to generate such SCRs.[31] In other words, young participants generate discriminatory anticipatory SCRs during the IGT, with the largest SCRs observed just prior to a Bad deck selection, and smaller SCRs just prior to a Good deck selection. By contrast, VMPC patients generate small and relatively equivalent SCRs to both types of selections, and thus do not display such discrimination.[39] These findings have been taken as evidence that the somatic "signaling" that normally facilitates decision making under conditions of uncertainty and risk is disrupted in VMPC patients.

In another study in the current series, our objective was to add an investigation of the psychophysiological correlates of decision making in older adults, to determine whether the integrity of anticipatory SCRs might be compromised in the subset of older individuals that demonstrates impaired IGT performance. We hypothesized that the "somatic signaling" process would be attenuated in the impaired decision makers, but not in the unimpaired ones. Specifically, we predicted that (1) Older-Impaired participants would not generate discriminatory anticipatory SCRs during the IGT; and (2) Older-Unimpaired participants would generate discriminatory anticipatory SCRs during the IGT.

Using the same rationale and procedures as in the previous study (Study 1: Behavioral Correlates of Defective Decision Making), 40 new older adult participants were recruited. Thus, the overall sample comprised 80 healthy, community-dwelling older adults, aged 56–85 (40 previous participants, 40 new participants). The two samples did not differ with respect to demographic variables, such as age, education, and gender distribution ($Ps > 0.05$).

The IGT was administered according to the standard protocol of our laboratory, involving computer administration and psychophysiological (i.e., SCR) measurement. As before, we carried out the following analysis of the IGT behavioral data. Under the assumption that random behavior on the IGT would yield a score of zero for the formula, $[(C + D)–(A + B)]$, we categorized each older adult participant as "Unimpaired" or "Impaired," based on whether their IGT performance score collapsed across the five Trial Blocks differed significantly from zero, and in which direction, using the binomial test. Participants who had overall performance scores that were significantly different from zero in the positive direction were categorized as "Unimpaired" on the IGT, and participants who had performance scores that were significantly different from zero in the negative direction were categorized as "Impaired" on the IGT. (As in the previous study, this left a middle group of participants whose scores did not significantly differ from zero in either direction, and we refer to this group as "Borderline.")

While playing the IGT, participants were connected to a polygraph. SCRs were recorded from two Ag/AgCl electrodes attached to the thenar and hypothenar eminences of each hand. Every turn of a card from any deck coincided with a mark on the SCR polygram. The inter-trial interval was set to 6 s, although, given time for deliberation, the average time between card choices was approximately 10 s.[39] For the present study, we were interested in anticipatory SCRs generated during the IGT, and this corresponds to the time window between the *end* of the 5-s period following the choice of a card and *before* the next click of a card (i.e., the time period during which participants are pondering their choice).

The SCR data were acquired through an MP100 WS system (BIOPAC Systems, Inc., Santa Barbara, CA) at the rate of 100 samples per second. The IGT SCR data were analyzed using AcqKnowledge III software (BIOPAC Systems, Inc.) for the MP100 WS system. Quantification of the SCR wave involved elimination of the downward drift using a mathematical transformation function named "Difference," followed by visual inspection of the wave for experimental artifacts. The primary dependent SCR variable was "area under the curve" in microSiemens per second ($\mu S/s$), during the "anticipation phase"; again, this was the time window between the end of the 5-s period following choice of a card and before the next click of a card.

Initial descriptive statistics on the SCR data revealed that, within participant group, the means and standard deviations were similar in magnitude (as is common for electrodermal data of this type).[40] We also noted that, between participant groups, the variances were unequal (i.e., heterogeneity of variance). For these reasons, the SCR data were analyzed with non-parametric techniques. Specifically, we utilized the Wilcoxon matched-pairs signed-ranks test and the

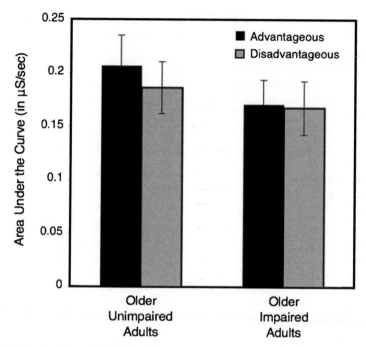

FIGURE 4. Mean (±SEM) anticipatory SCRs in microSiemens (μS) as measured during the IGT. Data are presented by Group (Older-Unimpaired versus Older-Impaired) and by Deck Type (Good versus Bad).

Mann–Whitney U test as non-parametric alternatives to the t test and F test, respectively, to analyze the SCR data.

The results of the binomial test revealed 24 Older-Impaired participants and 36 Older-Unimpaired participants. The data from six participants were excluded, in three cases secondary to a lack of measurable SCRs (2 men, 1 woman), and in three cases secondary to experimenter error (3 men). One of those excluded was "Impaired" and five were "Unimpaired," which left 23 Older-Impaired decision makers and 31 Older-Unimpaired decision makers in the final sample of psychophysiological data.

The first prediction was confirmed. Using Wilcoxon paired samples signed-ranks test, we found that the Older-Impaired participants failed to generate discriminatory anticipatory SCRs ($P = 0.93$); in fact, their anticipatory SCRs were nearly identical for the advantageous and disadvantageous decks. The second prediction was also confirmed. The Older-Unimpaired participants demonstrated discriminatory anticipatory SCRs ($P < 0.05$). Specifically, this Group generated larger amplitude (i.e., greater area under the curve) SCRs to the advantageous decks compared to the disadvantageous decks, as shown in FIGURE 4.

It is important to explore whether these findings can be explained by a basic between-Group difference in overall SCR responsivity. A Mann–Whitney U

test failed to demonstrate any reliable between-Group differences ($Ps > 0.05$), as the magnitude of SCRs was generally comparable between the Impaired and Unimpaired participants.

This study provides an extension of our previous work exploring the nature of decision making in healthy older adults.[1] Specifically, we demonstrated that the decision-making defect has a psychophysiological correlate; namely, Older-Impaired participants lacked discriminatory SCRs to advantageous versus disadvantageous choices, whereas Older-Unimpaired participants demonstrated reliable anticipatory psychophysiological discrimination of good and bad choices.

The psychophysiological findings supported our basic hypothesis regarding the absence of somatic "signaling" in the impaired participants. Specifically, the Older-Impaired participants failed to generate discriminatory anticipatory SCRs. It was interesting, though, that the pattern of results was different from that observed previously in patients with bilateral VMPC damage.[39] Those patients failed to acquire anticipatory SCRs to either the advantageous or disadvantageous choices. By contrast, the Older-Impaired participants *did* acquire anticipatory SCRs, although those responses did not discriminate good from bad choices.

Interestingly, the Older-Unimpaired participants generated discriminatory anticipatory SCRs, consistent with our second prediction. However, the direction of the anticipatory SCR discrimination was reversed in the Older-Unimpaired participants compared to that found in previous studies involving healthy, non-elderly (young) participants. That is, the Older-Unimpaired participants produced higher-amplitude SCRs to the advantageous decks, while young participants produce higher-amplitude SCRs to the disadvantageous decks. Taken at face value, the pattern of anticipatory discrimination during successful IGT performance differs in important ways for young and older adults.

In conclusion, older adults with strong decision-making abilities, as measured by the IGT, show discriminatory anticipatory SCRs, and it appears that positive (rather than negative) somatic markers play a significant role in shaping their advantageous decisions. By contrast, older adults with poor decision-making abilities do not appear to be differentially influenced by either positive or negative somatic markers, although they may be influenced by both types of markers in a manner unlike patients with acquired VMPC lesions.

STUDY 3: CONSUMER CORRELATES OF DEFECTIVE DECISION MAKING

A growing body of literature in marketing examines age differences in consumer reactions to printed marketing materials, primarily from an information-processing perspective.[41–46] Such studies have suggested that under certain environmental conditions, older consumers are more likely than younger consumers to miscomprehend and incorrectly use printed marketing information. For example, not only are older adults less likely to decipher implied claims, but older adults are more vulnerable to the "truth effect" (the tendency to believe repeated information more than new information) because older adults have relatively poor context or source memory, but relatively intact familiarity of repeated claims.[43,44] Furthermore, there is preliminary evidence linking the integrity of the prefrontal cortex to frequently studied consumer behaviors, such as comprehension, information search, and decision making.[46-48]

In the last study in the current series, we questioned how age differences in reactions to deceptive advertising are related to decision making ability (and potentially the integrity of VMPC structures) (Denburg *et al.*, manuscript submitted for publication). We proposed that IGT performance would predict susceptibility to the influence of deceptive advertising. Specifically, it was predicted that Older-Impaired decision makers would be more vulnerable to deceptive advertising than either Older-Unimpaired or Younger comparison participants. By adopting this neuroscientific perspective, we hoped to understand age differences in consumer behavior at a more fundamental (neural) level, and to refine existing theories.[49]

Using the same rationale, procedures, and participants as in the previous study (Study 1: Behavioral Correlates of Defective Decision Making), 20 Unimpaired Younger adults participated. Additionally, from the earlier study, the 15 Older Adult participants that were labeled as "Unimpaired" and the 14 Older Adults that were "Impaired" also participated. In all, then, there were three Groups: (1) Younger; (2) Older-Unimpaired (good IGT decision makers); and (3) Older-Impaired (bad IGT decision makers). The samples did not differ with respect to demographic variables, such as age, education, and gender distribution ($P > 0.05$). There were two dependent measures, IGT behavioral performance and vulnerability to deceptive advertising.

In a preliminary session, participants individually came to the laboratory to perform the IGT and a battery of neuropsychological tests. At a second testing session on a separate day, we invited each participant to participate in an "advertising study." In this study, prior to looking through an advertising booklet, they learned that they could take as long as they liked to review the booklet and that we would ask about their opinions of the advertisements later in a written questionnaire.

Participants were exposed to actual advertisements with deceptive and non-deceptive claims. The deceptive claims have been drawn from those cases deemed problematic by the Federal Trade Commission (FTC) as published in *FTC Decisions*, and hence, the advertisements we used had documented external validity. For each FTC advertisement, non-deceptive counterparts were created. Deceptive and non-deceptive advertisements were admixed to create two advertising booklets. A deceptive advertisement is one in which a discrepancy arises between the factual performance of the product and consumers' beliefs about the product.[42,50]

Each advertising booklet contained five advertisements, plus two "control" ads (one at the beginning and the other at the end, in an effort to minimize primary and recency effects). After incidental reading of the advertisement booklet, a questionnaire was administered which examined participants' (a) purchase intentions and (b) comprehension of claims.[52] All the advertisements were in color and were professionally designed; none specifically mentioned price. A short paragraph description separated the advertisements. For example, "Please read the following advertisement. It will appear in magazines such as *Women's Day* and *Sports Illustrated* during the Fall." To better illustrate how the advertisements differed based on manipulation, we offer the Luggage advertisement as an example and present the Group results.

The manipulation for the Luggage advertisement involved disclosure that the luggage is made in Mexico versus no such disclosure. Both the deceptive and non-deceptive Luggage advertisements contained color pictures and a verbal description of the three-piece luggage set. Both versions started with the headline "Legacy brings you the finest American Quality Luggage." The FTC wrote that an advertisement that bears the headline "American Quality" is "likely to convey to consumers a claim that the product is of US origin," and thus would not be compliant with the "Made in the USA standard" if it were of foreign origin, unless the advertisement disclosed where the product was manufactured. So, the non-misleading advertisement contained the statement "After manufacture in Mexico, each piece is carefully inspected in Tennessee at our corporate headquarters before it is shipped to you." The misleading version made the same claim but omitted the words "in Mexico."

The comprehension-of-claims variable for the Legacy Luggage was analyzed with a 2×3 ANOVA using advertisement version (Limited Disclosure versus Full Disclosure) as the within-subjects factor and Group (Younger versus Older-Impaired versus Older-Unimpaired) as the between-subjects factor (FIG. 5). We found a significant effect for version [$F(1,43) = 37.27, P < 0.01$] as well as a significant version by Group interaction [$F(2,43) = 3.68, P < 0.03$]. We conducted follow-up t tests and found that the Groups who viewed the Legacy Luggage ad that made a full disclosure about where the luggage was made did not differ in their comprehension of claims for the luggage set. However, among the Groups who viewed the deceptive Legacy Luggage ad, which did not disclose where the luggage was made, the Older-Impaired Group was significantly more likely than the Older-Unimpaired Group ($t = 3.44$, $P < 0.01$) or the Younger Group ($t = 3.56, P < 0.01$) to believe that the Legacy Luggage set was made in the United States.

Similarly, the purchase intentions variable for the Legacy Luggage was analyzed with a 2×3 ANOVA using advertisement version (Limited Disclosure versus Full Disclosure) as the within-subjects factor and Group (Younger versus Older-Impaired versus Older-Unimpaired) as the between-subjects factor (FIG. 6). We found a significant effect for version [$F(1,43) = 5.64, P < 0.03$] as well as a significant version by Group interaction [$F(2,43) = 4.31, P < 0.02$].

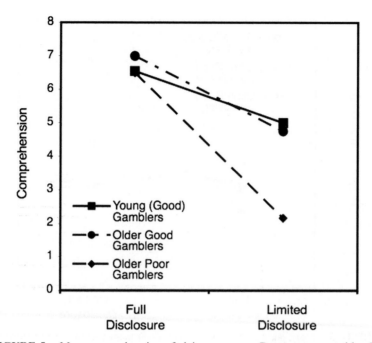

FIGURE 5. Mean comprehension of claims response. Data are presented by Group (Older-Unimpaired versus Older-Impaired versus Younger) and by Advertisement Version (Full Disclosure versus Limited Disclosure).

We conducted follow-up t tests and found that the Groups who viewed the Legacy Luggage ad that made a full disclosure about where the luggage was made did not differ in their purchase intentions for the luggage set. However, among the Groups who viewed the deceptive Legacy Luggage ad that did not disclose where the luggage was made, the Older-Impaired Group was significantly more likely than the Older-Unimpaired Group ($t = 2.7$, $P < 0.02$) or the Younger Group ($t = 1.99$, $P < 0.06$) to indicate higher purchase intentions for deceptively advertised luggage. Therefore, we conclude that the Older-Unimpaired participants and the Younger participants responded more similarly to deceptive advertising than the Older-Impaired participants.

This research begins to identify a neuroscientific explanation for age differences in responses to deceptive advertising. Future research is needed to pin down more closely the relationship between decision making performance and age-associated changes in vulnerable brain regions. An important area for future neurobiological and consumer research is to identify the extent to which bad decision makers can recruit or be trained to use compensatory processing to improve accuracy of beliefs and judgments.[42,45,52]

From a marketing context, these studies suggest that there is considerable heterogeneity in the older consumer market. Prior research has suggested the need for segmenting markets according to lifestyle and other demographic

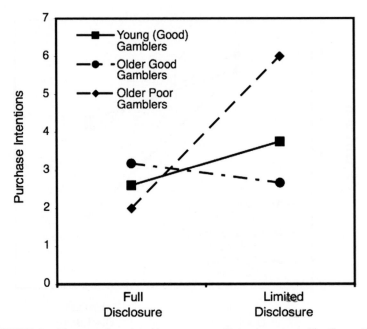

FIGURE 6. Mean purchase intentions response. Data are presented by Group (Older-Unimpaired versus Older-Impaired versus Younger) and by advertisement version (Full Disclosure versus Limited Disclosure).

variables using something called "gerontographics."[54] Our research suggests that the integrity of prefrontal cortex functioning may be one important segmenting variable. Indexing the integrity of prefrontal cortex functioning is not simple, but as neuroscience develops, it may be possible to identify otherwise healthy older adults who have dysfunction in prefrontal cortex. These individuals could be made aware that they may be particularly susceptible to misleading advertising.

CONCLUDING COMMENT

Given the well-documented association between decision making on the IGT and integrity of ventromedial prefrontal structures, we take the current findings as suggestive of the possibility that some ostensibly normal older adults have disproportionate aging of VMPC. To the extent that this turns out to be correct, it has some very important implications. Perhaps the most alarming example is older adults' heightened vulnerability to advertising fraud. In fact, the Federal Bureau of Investigation (FBI) has estimated that there are 14,000 fraudulent telemarketing firms operating in the United States, with 80% of these aiming their activities at older individuals.[54] Our own work in this area has already provided preliminary suggestion of a link between ventromedial prefrontal dysfunction, faulty decision making, and vulnerability to misleading advertising.

The issue of whether a sizable number of older individuals have decision-making deficits has provocative societal implications. These include not only the aforementioned problem of older persons being targeted by fraudulent advertising, but also the fact that, at a time of heightened vulnerability, these older persons face a host of critical life decisions ranging from driving and housing decisions to choice of medical care and allocation of personal wealth. In fact, it is hard to overemphasize the ramifications of impaired decision making for older adults. From a public policy perspective, our research has immediate implications for the voluntary and regulatory control of advertising.

The series of studies summarized here provides strong support for the notion that some neurologically and psychiatrically healthy older adults can have decision making impairments in the absence of other neuropsychological defects. Whether this finding turns out to have a structural or functional neurologic correlate remains to be seen, but the finding is at least broadly consistent with the frontal lobe hypothesis of aging, articulated by West[4] and others, and further supported by several recent lines of evidence.[56,57]

It will be important to tackle these open questions with other neuroscience approaches, including functional imaging (e.g., fMRI), and it will also be important to identify the neuropathologic process or processes that are giving rise to VMPC dysfunction in some older persons. For instance, is this dysfunction a harbinger of a progressive degenerative disease, such as Alzheimer's disease or Pick's disease? Longitudinal work and postmortem neuropathology studies will be needed to help answer such questions. Another intriguing and open question concerns sex differences. Recent work has provided preliminary evidence of sex-related functional asymmetry of the VMPC, whereby in men the right-sided VMPC sector is more important than the left for functions, such as complex decision making, emotional regulation, and social conduct, whereas in women the left-sided VMPC sector appears to be more important than the right for such functions.[58] Future work in older adults should take into account possible sex differences, and we would predict that such differences may turn out to be a lot more than trivial, at both behavioral and neural levels.

ACKNOWLEDGMENTS

Preparation of this article was supported by a National Institute on Aging Career Development Award (K01 AG022033) and by fellowship funding from the Iowa Scottish Rite Masonic Foundation to N.L.D., and by NIDA Grant R01 DA022549 to D.T.

REFERENCES

1. DENBURG, N.L., D. TRANEL & A. BECHARA. 2005. The ability to decide advantageously declines prematurely in some normal older persons. Neuropsychologia **43:** 1099–1106.
2. DENBURG, N.L., E.C. RECKNOR, A. BECHARA & D. TRANEL. 2006. Psychophysiological anticipation of positive outcomes promotes advantageous decision making in normal older persons. Int. J. Psychophysiol. **61:** 19–25.
3. WEST, R.L. 1996. An application of prefrontal cortex function theory to cognitive aging. Psychol. Bull. **120:** 272–292.
4. WEST, R.L. 2000. In defense of the frontal lobe hypothesis of cognitive aging. J. Int. Neuropsychol. Soc. **6:** 727–729.
5. DAIGNEAULT, S., C.M.J. BRAUN & H.A. WHITAKER. 1992. Early effects of normal aging on perseverative and non-perseverative prefrontal measures. Dev. Neuropsychol. **8:** 99–114.
6. DEMPSTER, F.N. 1992. The rise and fall of the inhibitory mechanism: toward a unified theory of cognitive development and aging. Dev. Rev. **12:** 45–75.
7. HARTLEY, A.A. 1993. Evidence for the selective preservation of spatial selective attention in old age. Psychol. Aging **8:** 371–379.
8. HAALAND, K.Y., L. PRICE & LARUE, A. 2003. What does the WMS-III tell us about memory changes with normal aging. J. Int. Neuropsychol. Soc. **9:** 89–96.
9. MITTENBERG, W., M. SEIDENBERG, D.S. O'LEARY & D.V. DIGIULIO. 1989. Changes in cerebral functioning associated with normal aging. J. Clin. Exp. Neuropsychol. **11:** 918–932.
10. MOSCOVITCH, M. & G. WINOCUR. 1992. The neuropsychology of memory and aging. *In* The Handbook of Aging and Cognition. F.I.M. Craik & T.A. Salthouse, Eds.: 315–372. Lawrence Erlbaum. Hillsdale, NJ.
11. ROBBINS, T.W., M. JAMES, A.M. OWEN, *et al.* 1998. A study of performance on tests from the CANTAB battery sensitive to frontal lobe dysfunction in a large sample of normal volunteers: implications for theories of executive functioning and cognitive aging. J. Int. Neuropsychol. Soc. **4:** 474–490.
12. SHIMAMURA, A.P. & P.J. JURICA. 1994. Memory interference effects and aging: findings from a test of frontal lobe function. Neuropsychology **8:** 408–412.
13. WEST, R.L., K.J. MURPHY, M.L. ARMILIO, *et al.* 2002. Lapses in attention and performance variability reveal age-related increases in fluctuations in executive control. Brain Cogn. **49:** 402–419.
14. WHELIHAN, W.M. & E.L. LESHER. 1985. Neuropsychological changes in frontal functions with age. Dev. Neuropsychol. **1:** 371–380.
15. COFFEY, C.E., W.E. WILKINSON, I.A. PARASHOS, *et al.* 1992. Quantitative cerebral anatomy of the aging human brain: a cross-sectional study using magnetic resonance imaging. Neurology **42:** 527–536.
16. COWELL, P.E., B.I. TURETSKY, R.C. GUR, *et al.* 1994. Sex differences in aging of the human frontal and temporal lobes. J. Neurosci. **14:** 4748–4755.
17. JERNIGAN, T.L., S.L. ARCHIBALD, C. FENNEMA-NOTESTINE, *et al.* 2001. Effects of age on tissues and regions of the cerebrum and cerebellum. Neurobiol. Aging **22:** 581–594.
18. RAZ, N., F.M. GUNNING, D. HEAD, *et al.* 1997. Selective aging of the human cerebral cortex observed in vivo: differential vulnerability of the prefrontal gray matter. Cereb. Cortex **7:** 268–282.

19. RAZ, N., F.M. GUNNING-DIXON & J.D. ACKER. 1998. Neuroanatomical correlates of cognitive aging: evidence from structural magnetic resonance imaging. Neuropsychology **12:** 95–114.
20. RESNICK, S.M., D.L. PHAM, M.A. KRAUT, *et al.* 2003. Longitudinal magnetic resonance imaging studies of older adults: a shrinking brain. J. Neurosci. **23:** 3295–3301.
21. SALAT, D.H., J.A. KAYE & J.S. JANOWSKY. 2001. Selective preservation and degeneration within the prefrontal cortex in aging and Alzheimer's disease. Arch. Neurol. **58:** 1403–1408.
22. GUR, R.C., R.E. GUR, W.D. ORBIST, *et al.* 1987. Age and regional cerebral blood flow at rest and during cognitive activity. Arch. Gen. Psychiat. **44:** 617–621.
23. MELAMED, E., S. LAVY, B. SHLOMO, *et al.* 1980. Reduction in regional cerebral blood flow during normal aging in man. Stroke **11:** 31–34.
24. BAND, G.P.H., K.R. RIDDERINKOF & S. SEGALOWITZ. 2002. Explaining neurocognitive aging: Is one factor enough? Brain Cogn. **49:** 259–267.
25. GREENWOOD, P.M. 2000. The frontal aging hypothesis evaluated. J. Int. Neuropsychol. Soc. **6:** 705–726.
26. Protecting Seniors from Fraud, Hearing before the Special Committee on Aging, United States Senate, 106th Congress, 2nd Sess. 2000. U.S. Government Printing Office. Washington, DC.
27. ESLINGER, P.J. & A.R. DAMASIO. 1985. Severe disturbance of higher cognition after bilateral frontal lobe ablation: Patient EVR. Neurology **35:** 1731–1741.
28. BECHARA, A., A.R. DAMASIO, H. DAMASIO & S.W. ANDERSON. 1994. Insensitivity to future consequences following damage to human prefrontal cortex. Cognition **50:** 7–15.
29. BECHARA, A., H. DAMASIO & A.R. DAMASIO. 2000. Emotion, decision making, and the orbitofrontal cortex. Cereb. Cortex **10:** 295–307.
30. BECHARA, A., D. TRANEL & H. DAMASIO. 2000. Characterization of the decision making deficit of patients with ventromedial prefrontal cortex lesions. Brain **123:** 2189–2202.
31. ERNST, M., K. BOLLA, M. MOURATIDIS, *et al.* 2002. decision making in a risk-taking task: A PET study. Neuropsychopharmacology **26:** 682–691.
32. SCHMITT, W.A., C.A. BRINKLEY & J.P. NEWMAN. 1999. Testing Damasio's somatic marker hypothesis with psychopathic individuals: risk takers or risk averse? J. Abnorm. Psychol. **108:** 538–543.
33. SCHAIE, K.W. 1996. Intellectual development in adulthood. *In* Handbook of Psychology and Aging. J.E. Birren & K.W. Schaie, Eds.: 266–286. Academic Press. San Diego, CA.
34. TRANEL, D., A. BENTON & K. OLSON. 1997. A 10-year longitudinal study of cognitive changes in elderly persons. Dev. Neuropsychol. **13:** 87–96.
35. DAMASIO, A.R. 1994. Descartes' Error: emotion, Reason, and the Human Brain. Grosset/Putnam. New York.
36. DAMASIO, A.R. 1996. The somatic marker hypothesis and the possible functions of the prefrontal cortex. Phil. Trans. Roy. Soc. London Biol. **351:** 1413–1420.
37. TRANEL, D. 2000. Electrodermal activity in cognitive neuroscience: neuroanatomical and neuropsychological correlates. *In* Cognitive Neuroscience of Emotion. R.D. Lane & L. Nadel, Eds.: 192–224. Oxford University Press. New York.
38. BECHARA, A., D. TRANEL, H. DAMASIO & A.R. DAMASIO. 1996. Failure to respond autonomically to anticipated future outcomes following damage to prefrontal cortex. Cereb. Cortex **6:** 215–225.

39. VENABLES, P.H. & M.J. CHRISTIE. 1973. Mechanisms and techniques. *In* Electrodermal Activity in Psychological Research. W.F. Prokasy & D.C. Raskin, Eds.: 1–123. Academic Press. New York.

40. COLE, C. & G. GAETH. 1990. Cognitive and age-related differences in the ability to use nutritional information in a complex environment. J. Market. Res. **27:** 175–184.

41. COLE, C. & M. HOUSTON. 1987. Encoding and medial effects on consumer learning deficiencies in the elderly. J. Market. Res. **24:** 55–63.

42. GAETH, G. & T.B. HEATH. 1987. The cognitive processing of misleading advertising in young and old adults: assessment and training. J. Consum. Res. **14:** 43–54.

43. LAW, S., S.A. HAWKINS & F.I.M. CRAIK. 1998. Repetition-induced belief in the elderly: rehabilitating age-related memory deficits. J. Consum. Res. **25:** 91–107.

44. SKURNIK, I., C. YOON, D.C. PARK, N. SCHWARZ. 2005. How warnings about false claims become recommendations. J. Consum. Res. **31:** 713–724.

45. YOON, C. 1997. Age differences in consumers' processing strategies: an investigation of moderating influences. J. Consum. Res. **24:** 329–342.

46. MARTIN-LOECHES, M., P. CASADO, J.A. HINOJOSA, *et al.* 2005. Higher-order activity beyond the word level: cortical dynamics of simple transitive sentence. Brain Lang. **92:** 332–348.

47. FELLOWS, L.K. 2006. Deciding how to decide: ventromedial frontal lobe damage affects information acquisition in multi-attribute decision making. Brain **129:** 944–952.

48. JOHNSON, M.K., K.J. MITCHELL, C.L. RAYE & E.J. GREENE. 2004. An gge-related deficit in prefrontal cortical function associated with refreshing information. Psychol. Sci. **15:** 127–132.

56. SHIV, B., G. LOEWENSTEIN, A. BECHARA, *et al.* 2005. Investment behavior and the dark side of emotion. Psychol. Sci. **16:** 435–439.

50. ADITYA, R.N. 2001. The psychology of deception in marketing: a conceptual framework for research and practice. Psychol. Market. **18:** 735–761.

51. OLSON, J.C. & P.A. DOVER. 1978. Cognitive effects of deceptive advertising. J. Market. Res. **15:** 29–38.

52. WILLIAMS, P. & A. DROLET. 2005. Age-related differences in responses to emotional advertisements. J. Consum. Res. **32:** 343–354.

53. MOSCHIS, G.P. 1996. Gerontographics: Life-Stage Segmentation for Marketing Strategy Development. Greenwood Publishing. Westport, CT.

54. AMERICAN ASSOCIATION OF RETIRED PERSONS. 1996. Telemarketing Fraud and Older Americans: An AARP Survey. AARP. Washington, DC.

55. HEAD, D., A.Z. SNYDER, L.E. GIRTON, *et al.* 2005. Frontal-hippocampal double dissociation between normal aging and Alzheimer's disease. Cereb. Cortex **15:** 732–739.

56. LAMAR, M., & S.M. RESNICK. 2004. Aging and prefrontal functions: dissociating orbitofrontal and dorsolateral abilities. Neurobiol. Aging **25:** 553–558.

57. TRANEL, D., H. DAMASIO, N.L. DENBURG & A. BECHARA. 2005. Does gender play a role in functional asymmetry of ventromedial prefrontal cortex? Brain **128:** 2872–2881.

Orbitofrontal Cortex Function and Structure in Depression

WAYNE C. DREVETS

Section on Neuroimaging in Mood and Anxiety Disorders, National Institute of Mental Health, National Institutes of Health, Bethesda, Maryland, USA

ABSTRACT: The orbitofrontal cortex (OFC) has been implicated in the pathophysiology of major depression by evidence obtained using neuroimaging, neuropathologic, and lesion analysis techniques. The abnormalities revealed by these techniques show a regional specificity, and suggest that some OFC regions which appear cytoarchitectonically distinct also are functionally distinct with respect to mood regulation. For example, the severity of depression correlates inversely with physiological activity in parts of the posterior lateral and medial OFC, consistent with evidence that dysfunction of the OFC associated with cerebrovascular lesions increases the vulnerability for developing the major depressive syndrome. The posterior lateral and medial OFC function may also be impaired in individuals who develop primary mood disorders, as these patients show grey-matter volumetric reductions, histopathologic abnormalities, and altered hemodynamic responses to emotionally valenced stimuli, probabilistic reversal learning, and reward processing. In contrast, physiological activity in the anteromedial OFC situated in the ventromedial frontal polar cortex increases during the depressed versus the remitted phases of major depressive disorder to an extent that is positively correlated with the severity of depression. Effective antidepressant treatment is associated with a reduction in activity in this region. Taken together these data are compatible with evidence from studies in experimental animals indicating that some orbitofrontal and medial prefrontal cortex regions function to inhibit, while others function to enhance, emotional expression. Alterations in the functional balance between these regions and the circuits they form with anatomically related areas of the temporal lobe, striatum, thalamus, and brain stem thus may underlie the pathophysiology of mood disorders, such as major depression.

KEYWORDS: major depressive disorder; bipolar disorder; anterior cingulate cortex; PET; MRI

Address for correspondence: Wayne C. Drevets, M.D., Mood and Anxiety Disorders Program, NIH NIMH/MIB, 15K North Dr., MSC 2670, Bethesda, MD 20892-2670. Voice: 301-594-1367; fax: 301-402-6100.

drevetsw@intra.nimh.nih.gov

Ann. N.Y. Acad. Sci. 1121: 499–527 (2007). © 2007 New York Academy of Sciences.
doi: 10.1196/annals.1401.029

INTRODUCTION

Major depressive disorder (MDD) is ranked by the World Health Organization as the leading cause of years-of-life lived with disability.[1] Despite many psychological and biological theories regarding the pathogenesis of MDD, its etiology remains unknown. The intrusive, spontaneous, and perseverative nature of this condition's symptoms and the responsiveness of these symptoms to antidepressant drugs suggest that abnormal brain processes underlie and maintain the major depressive syndrome. Consistent with this expectation a variety of neurophysiological, neuropathologic, and neurochemical abnormalities have been found within neural systems that modulate emotional behavior in both MDD and the other major primary mood disorder, bipolar disorder (BD, which is associated with manic as well as depressive episodes). These abnormalities implicate the extended neural networks formed by the orbitofrontal cortex (OFC) and medial prefrontal cortex (mPFC) and their anatomic connections with the temporal lobe, striatum, thalamus, and brain stem.[2,3]

Consistent with the implication of these networks in MDD and BD, the clinical and neuropsychological phenomena of mood disorders can be characterized by disturbances in functional domains linked to the OFC and mPFC. The syndrome common to both MDD and BD, the major depressive episode (MDE), is best known as a pathologic mood state characterized by persistently sad or depressed mood. However, MDEs also are generally accompanied by: (1) altered incentive and reward processing, evidenced by amotivation, apathy, and anhedonia; (2) impaired modulation of anxiety and worry, manifested by generalized, social and panic anxiety, and oversensitivity to negative feedback; (3) inflexibility of thought and behavior in association with changing reinforcement contingencies, apparent as ruminative thoughts of self-reproach, pessimism, and guilt, and inertia toward initiating goal-directed behavior; (4) altered integration of sensory and social information, as evidenced by mood-congruent processing biases; (5) impaired attention and memory, shown as performance deficits on tests of attention set-shifting and maintenance, and autobiographical and short-term memory; and 6) visceral disturbances, including altered weight, appetite, sleep, and endocrine and autonomic function.[4,5] As reviewed by the other articles in this volume, most of these symptom complexes involve functional domains mediated in part by the OFC, suggesting that dysfunction within neural circuits involving the OFC play major roles in the pathophysiology of mood disorders.

This hypothesis receives support from studies of MDE arising secondarily to neurologic disorders, with respect to their effects on OFC function. Individuals who develop an MDE within the context of cerebrovascular disease differ from control cases with a similar extent of cerebrovascular disease by having lesions in the OFC.[6,7] In addition, depressed patients with Parkinson's disease (PD) differ from non-depressed patients with PD by showing abnormally reduced metabolism or CBF in the OFC.[8,9] Nevertheless, each of these neurologic conditions affects other brain systems as well, limiting the specificity of these findings for implicating the OFC in mood disorders.

NEUROIMAGING CORRELATES
OF PRIMARY MOOD DISORDERS

In primary idiopathic MDD and BD (i.e., arising spontaneously in the absence of other medical or psychiatric antecedents) neuroimaging and neuropathologic studies also have identified abnormalities of structure and function in the OFC, as well as in mPFC structures which share extensive anatomic connections with the OFC, and which function together with the OFC as part of a "visceromotor network" which is thought to modulate endocrine, autonomic, behavioral, and experiential aspects of emotional behavior.[2] While whole-brain and entire frontal lobe volumes generally do not differ between depressed and healthy control samples,[10] reductions of grey-matter volume and cortex thickness have been demonstrated more specifically in the posterolateral OFC (BA 47, caudal BA 11),[11–14] as well as in mPFC regions, such as the subgenual anterior cingulate cortex (sgACC; BA 24, 25)[15–19] and ventrolateral PFC (BA 45)[20] (FIG. 1). The best characterized of these structural imaging abnormalities involves the sgACC, where the reduction in grey-matter volume has been shown to persist across episodes of illness,[15, 17] to correlate with a more severe course of illness course, to be evident early in the course of illness, and to arise at least partly prior to onset of illness in subjects at high familial risk for MDD.[21] Although the relationship between course of illness and volumetric changes in the OFC has not been established, one study reported that this relationship may be complex, with volume being larger at illness onset, and then declining with multiple episodes.[22]

Neurophysiological imaging studies of MDD and BD have identified abnormalities of regional cerebral blood flow (CBF) and glucose metabolism in the regions where structural and histopathologic abnormalities exist in mood disorders (FIG. 2). In most cases, these functional abnormalities appear mood-state-dependent, with respect to showing increased metabolism in the depressed phase relative to the remitted phase of illness,[2, 15, 23–27] as shown, for example, by longitudinal studies of patients imaged both before and after treatment,[26] and challenge studies of patients imaged both in remission and during depressive relapse[24] (TABLE 2). Since local glucose metabolism and CBF reflect summations of the energy utilization associated with terminal field synaptic transmission,[28] the increasing physiological activity in these regions during depression presumably reflects areas where neuronal activity increases to mediate or respond to the emotional and cognitive manifestations of the depressive syndrome.

In contrast, abnormalities that persist independently of the mood state instead may reflect neuropathologic sequelae of recurrent illness or

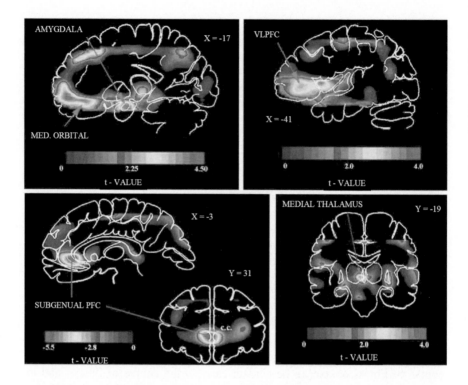

FIGURE 1. Areas of abnormally increased physiological activity in familial MDD shown as images of unpaired t-values, which were computed using a statistical parametric mapping approach to compare activity between depressives and controls.[25, 145] The abnormal activity in these regions was replicated using glucose metabolism imaging in independent subject samples.[26,37,38] *Upper left:* The positive t-values in this sagittal section at 17 mm left of midline (X = −17) show areas were CBF is increased in the depressives in the amygdala and medial (MED) orbital cortex. Anterior is to the left. (From Price *et al.*[146] Reproduced by permission.). *Upper right:* Positive t-values in a sagittal section 41 mm left of midline (X = −41) show areas where CBF is increased in the depressives in the left ventrolateral PFC (VLPFC), lateral orbitofrontal C, and anterior insula. (From Drevets *et al.*[10] Reproduced by permission.). *Lower right:* Positive t-values in a coronal section 19 mm posterior to the anterior commissure (Y = −19) show an area of increased CBF in the depressives in the left medial thalamus. (From Drevets and Todd.[4] Reproduced by permission). *Lower left:* Coronal (31 mm anterior to the anterior commissure; Y = 31) and sagittal (3 mm left of midline; X = −3) sections showing negative voxel *t*-values where glucose metabolism is decreased in depressives versus controls. The reduction in activity in this prefrontal cortex (PFC) region located in the anterior cingulate gyrus ventral to the genu of the corpus callosum (i.e., subgenual) appeared to be accounted for by a corresponding reduction in cortical volume (TABLE 2). Anterior (or left) is to *left.* (From Drevets *et al.*[145] Reproduced by permission.) The PET images from which the t-image was generated have been stereotaxically transformed to the coordinate system of Talairach and Tournoux,[147] from whose atlas the corresponding outline is shown.

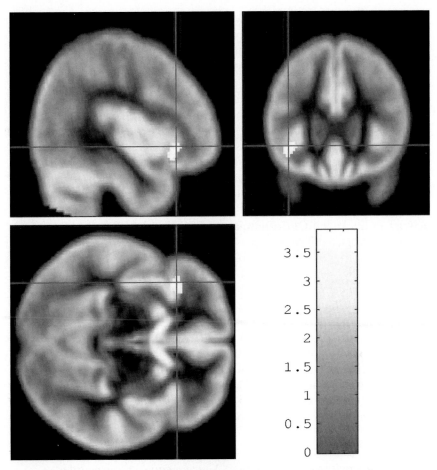

FIGURE 2. Lateral orbitofrontal cortical area (approximately BA 47*l*)[3] where peak effect size of grey-matter reduction was located in bipolar disorder. The image sections shown are from a voxel-based morphometric analysis which compared MRI measures of grey-matter volume between depressed subjects with bipolar disorder versus healthy controls. (From Nugent *et al.*[11] Reproduced by permission.)

neurodevelopmental abnormalities that confer vulnerability to MDD (e.g., in cases where they are evident in otherwise healthy individuals at high familial risk for developing mood disorders). Such abnormalities in CBF and metabolism may reflect pathologic changes in synaptic transmission associated with altered neurotransmitter receptor function, cerebrovascular disease, changes in neuronal arborization or synapse formation, or abnormalities in cellular viability or proliferation. For example, in the sgACC the CBF and metabolism increased during the depressed relative to the remitted phases of illness, yet in both phases flow and metabolism were *decreased* relative to controls.[15,24] This abnormality was subsequently associated with tissue reductions and histopathologic changes in MRI-based morphometric and postmortem neuropathologic studies of MDD and BD.[15,19] The dorsomedial/dorsal anterolateral PFC (DM/DALPFC) also shows persistently decreased metabolism in depressed patients relative to healthy controls (TABLE 2),[29] and this region also contains histopathologic changes that include reductions in neuronal size and in neuronal and glial cell counts.[12,30]

Finally, functional imaging studies comparing depressives and controls while performing neuropsychological tasks demonstrate altered activation of the OFC. For example, during exposure to emotionally valenced stimuli and performance of reward-processing tasks, neurophysiological activity is altered in the OFC (e.g., see FIG. 3). Moreover, while performing a probabilistic reversal-learning task, unipolar depressives demonstrated attenuated hemodynamic activity in the lateral OFC/ventrolateral PFC, and DMPFC relative to both healthy controls and bipolar depressives on trials in which misleading negative feedback triggered a behavioral response reversal, compared to trials in which misleading negative feedback did not precipitate reversal (Taylor Tavares et al., article under review). This physiological difference was associated with an increased likelihood for the unipolar depressives to switch their behavioral responses as a result of the misleading negative feedback. Nevertheless, the MDD, BD, and control groups did not differ significantly on errors per rule reversal, number of correct responses, reaction time on correct responses, or spontaneous errors, suggesting that basic object reversal learning is intact in depression. Another study showed an increased hemodynamic response in the posterior orbital cortex in depressed versus non-depressed BD subjects imaged while performing a color-word Stroop task.[31]

Sensitivity and Specificity of Neuroimaging Abnormalities

The neuroimaging abnormalities discovered to date lack the sensitivity and specificity needed to provide diagnostic utility. Their effect sizes have been relatively small, and although their specificity to mood disorders has not been entirely established, in some cases similar abnormalities exist in the anxiety disorders which occur co-morbidly with mood disorders (e.g., see Refs. 32 and 33). Moreover, the psychiatric imaging literature remains in disagreement regarding the specific location and direction of some abnormalities.

Some discrepancies in the results across studies likely reflect technical issues of image acquisition and/or analysis (reviewed in Refs. 10 and 34). For example, the spatial resolution of imaging technology generally is low relative to the size of brain structures of interest, but varies widely across scanning and data analysis techniques. With respect to morphometric assessments of grey-matter volume, the volumetric resolution of state-of-the-art image data is in the

(A)

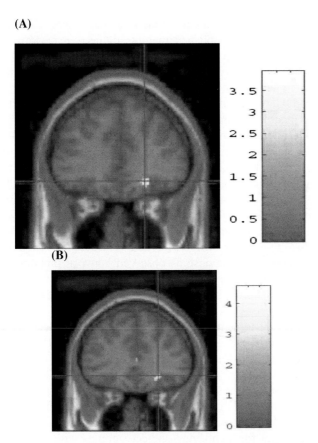

(B)

FIGURE 3. Area of the orbitofrontal cortex where hemodynamic activity in depressives exceeds that in controls during (**A**) anticipated loss and (**B**) anticipated reward trials of the Monetary Incentive Delay task of Knutson *et al.*,[148] as described in Wang *et al.*[147] The coronal image sections shown are from a statistical parametric mapping image comparing the fMRI blood oxygen level dependency (BOLD) signal between the anticipation of a cue to which the subject must respond quickly to either avoid a loss (**A**) or gain a reward (**B**), relative to anticipation of a cue which has no monetary significance. Twelve depressed patients (10 with MDD plus 2 with BD) are compared against 11 healthy controls. In the same contrast, the BOLD response was increased in depressives versus controls in the anterior insula, amygdala and hippocampal subiculum, but was decreased in the depressives in the anteroventral striatum. The *color bar* indicates voxel values for the unpaired t-statistic. The stereotaxic coordinates for the peak voxel t-values in **A** are x = 24, y = 34, z = −12, and in **B** are x = 26, y = 33, z = −10, with positive x indicating mm to the right of the midline, positive y indicating mm anterior to the anterior commissure, and negative z indicating mm ventral to a plane containing both the anterior and posterior commissures. These peak differences are separated by a distance smaller than the spatial resolution of the fMRI images analyzed, implying that the same orbitofrontal cortex area shows exaggerated neural activity in response to both anticipated gain and anticipated loss in depression. (In color in *Annals* online.)

range of 0.5–1 mm^3, which compares with the average cortex thickness of only 3 mm. Nevertheless, many published imaging studies were performed at spatial resolutions even lower than this, and such studies generally proved insensitive for detecting the neuromorphometric abnormalities reported by other studies performed at higher resolution.

Another problem related to the limited spatial resolution is that reductions in grey-matter volume in mood disorders may be sufficiently prominent to produce partial volume effects in functional brain images, yielding complex relationships between physiological measures and depression severity. For example, relative to controls, depressed MDD and BD subjects show metabolic activity that appears *reduced* in the sgACC.[15] However, when the reduction in grey-matter volume in MDD and BD is taken into account by correcting the PET measures for partial volume-averaging effects, metabolism during depression instead appears *increased* in the sgACC.[2] The volumetric reductions in the OFC and ventrolateral PFC also may account for the complex relationships observed between metabolism and illness severity, as metabolism appears elevated in samples of depressives with mild-to-moderate severity, but reduced in more severe, treatment-refractory cases.[10, 35]

In other cases disagreements in the literature may reflect differences in subject-selection criteria, as the diagnostic criteria for MDD encompass a group of conditions which is heterogeneous with respect to pathophysiology and etiology.[4] Neuroimaging abnormalities generally appear specific to subsets of unmedicated MDD subjects.[34] For example, the requirements that, in addition to meeting MDD criteria, subjects have been recently unmedicated and show familial aggregation of illness and an early age at onset of illness improves sensitivity for identifying subject samples with reproducible neuroimaging abnormalities.[36-38] Clinical differences related to the capacity for developing mania or psychosis or to the age at illness onset also have been shown to influence neuroimaging data. For example, elderly MDD subjects with a late age at onset of depression have an elevated prevalence of MRI signal hyperintensities (evident in T_2-weighted MRI scans as putative correlates of cerebrovascular disease within this clinical context) in the deep and periventricular white matter, which is not the case for elderly depressives with an early age at onset of depression.[10] Similarly, both elderly MDD cases with a late-life onset and delusional MDD cases have been shown to have lateral ventriclular enlargement, a finding which has not been present in MDD cases who are elderly but have an early age at onset of MDD or in midlife depressives who are not delusional.[10]

The neurophysiological imaging data further suggest that MDE can be associated with an assortment of distinct patterns of abnormal CBF and metabolism within the limbic-cortical-striatal-pallido-thalamic circuitry. For example, the lesions involving the PFC (i.e., tumors or infarctions) and the diseases of the basal ganglia which increase the risk for developing depression to a greater extent than other similarly debilitating conditions result in dysfunction at distinct points within these circuits and affect synaptic transmission in diverse ways (reviewed in Ref. 39). Imaging studies of depressive syndromes arising secondary to these conditions generally show results that differ from those reported for primary mood disorders. For example, in contrast to the findings of increased CBF or metabolism in parts of the OFC in primary depressives (TABLE 2), the OFC flow is decreased or not significantly different in subjects with depressive syndromes arising secondary to PD, Huntington's disease, or basal ganglia infarction relative to non-depressed subjects with the same illnesses.[8,9,39,40] Primary and secondary depressive syndromes may thus involve the same neural network, although the direction of the physiological abnormalities within individual structures may differ across conditions. A common substrate in these cases may be dysfunction of the prefrontal cortical–striatal modulation of limbic and visceral functions, as the neuropathologic changes evident in the OFC, mPFC, and ventral striatum in primary mood disorders (see above), and those associated with lesions of the OFC and striatum or with some neurodegenerative conditions of the basal ganglia, appear capable of inducing depressive syndromes.

Clinical Correlations with Neuroimaging Abnormalities

In the lateral OFC, ventrolateral PFC, and anterior insula, the resting CBF and metabolism have been abnormally increased in *unmedicated* subjects with primary, early-onset, recurrent MDD (reviewed in Ref. 10; see TABLE 2 and FIG. 2). The elevated activity in these areas in MDD appears mood-state-dependent[25] and, during treatment with somatic antidepressant therapies, flow and metabolism decreases in these regions (reviewed in Ref. 10; see TABLE 2). The relationship between severity of depression and physiological activity in the lateral OFC/ventrolateral PFC is complex, however. While CBF and metabolism increase in these areas in the depressed relative to the remitted phases of MDD, the magnitude of these measures is inversely correlated with ratings of depressive ideation and severity.[25,38] Moreover, while metabolic activity is abnormally increased in these areas in treatment-responsive unipolar and bipolar depressives, more severely ill or treatment-refractory patients show CBF and metabolic values lower than or not different from those of controls.[35,41,42] This inverse relationship between OFC/ventrolateral PFC activity and ratings of depression severity extends to some other emotional states as well. Posterolateral OFC flow also increases in subjects with obsessive–compulsive disorder or simple animal phobias during exposure to phobic stimuli and in healthy subjects during induced sadness, and the change in posterolateral orbital CBF in these conditions correlates inversely with changes in obsessive thinking, anxiety, and sadness, respectively.[32,43,44]

These data appear consistent with electrophysiological and lesion analysis data showing that parts of the OFC participate in modulating behavioral and visceral responses associated with defensive, emotional, and reward-directed behavior as reinforcement contingencies change[45–48] (as detailed below). For example, the OFC modulates the effects of the amygdala in organizing emotional expression via direct projections to the amygdala and to the hypothalamic and brain stem structures to which the central nucleus of the amygdala projects.[45,46,48] Activation of these OFC areas during depression may thus reflect compensatory attempts to attenuate emotional expression or experience or to interrupt unreinforced aversive thought and emotion.

This hypothesis is consistent with the evidence reviewed above that lesions of the OFC increase the risk for developing depression,[6] and that OFC activity is decreased to a greater extent in depressed versus non-depressed subjects with PD.[8,9] Moreover, experimental challenges that reduce central serotonin and catecholamine neurotransmission (achieved via tryptophan depletion and alpha-methyl-*para*-tyrosine [AMPT] administration, respectively) induce a reduction in metabolism in the OFC which is associated with depressive relapse in remitted subjects with MDD.[24,49,50] Both serotonergic and catecholaminergic transmission appear necessary for optimal PFC function, so depleting these neurotransmitters may impair OFC function.[51,52]

These observations also suggest that while CBF and metabolism decrease in the lateral OFC and ventrolateral PFC during antidepressant drug treatment (TABLE 2), these effects may not be a primary mechanism through which such agents ameliorate depressive symptoms. Instead, direct inhibition of pathologic limbic activity in areas, such as the amygdala and sgACC may instead be critical for attenuating expression of depressive symptoms.[23,26,53] The OFC neurons may thus return to basal levels of activity, as reflected by the return of metabolism to normal levels, as antidepressant drug therapy attenuates the pathologic limbic activity to which OFC neurons respond.[54]

In contrast to these data pertaining to the posterior lateral and medial areas of the OFC, an anteromedial OFC region in the ventromedial frontal polar cortex (classified by Ongur *et al.* as BA 10o)[3] shows positive correlations between metabolism and depression severity, along with the amygdala and the sgACC[2,25,38,55,56] (Hasler *et al.* in review). Metabolism and flow also decrease in this anteromedial OFC region during *effective* treatment with antidepressant drugs or deep brain stimulation of the sgACC.[23,26] Under experimental conditions involving serotonin or catecholamine depletion, recovered MDD cases who experience depressive relapse show *increased* metabolism in this region and the sgACC, with the extent of change in the anteromedial OFC correlating positively with depression severity[24,49,50] (Hasler *et al.* in review).

Activity in this anteromedial OFC region may additionally or alternatively relate to symptoms of MDD other than depressed mood. For example, during anxiety provocation in patients with obsessive–compulsive disorder, the CBF in the right anteromedial OFC increased in direct correlation with the change in obsession ratings.[32] These data were compatible with evidence in experimental animals that parts of the ventromedial PFC play critical roles in mediating the expression of emotions, such as learned fear, putatively by integrating information from sensory and contextual inputs and regulating expression of fear memories via projections to the basal nucleus of the amygdala.[57,58] Another study implicated the left anteromedial OFC in anger, showing that during anger induction the blood flow increased in this region in healthy humans, and that the extent of this change was significantly greater in healthy control subjects compared to depressed subjects who manifested anger attacks (possibly because this region was already physiologically activated at baseline in the MDD group).[25,59]

NEUROPATHOLOGIC CORRELATES OF STRUCTURAL IMAGING ABNORMALITIES

Postmortem studies have characterized the histopathologic correlates of the grey-matter volumetric abnormalities found in primary mood disorders. These studies demonstrated abnormal reductions in *glial* cell counts, density and markers, and in glial cell-to-neuron ratios in MDD and BD in the OFC, sgACC, pregenual ACC, frontal polar cortex (BA 10), and DM/DALPFC (BA 9).[12,19,30,60–69] In the sgACC the reduction in volume also was associated with an increased neuronal density.[19] In contrast, the density of *nonpyramidal* neurons was decreased in the ACC and hippocampus in BD[61] and in the DALPFC (BA 9) in MDD.[30] Reductions in synapses and synaptic proteins also were evident in BD subjects in the ACC and in the hippocampal subiculum/ventral CA1 region.[70–72] Finally, the mean *size of neurons* was abnormally reduced in the DALPFC (BA 9) in MDD[12] and in the lateral amygdala in BD.[73]

The glial cell type that differed between MDD and control samples in most studies which subtyped glia was the oligodendrocyte.[62,65,66,74] Myelinating oligodendroglia were implicated by findings that myelin basic protein concentration was decreased in the frontal polar cortex (BA 10) in MDD.[64] Compatible with this finding, several reports of deficits in glia in the cerebral cortex depended upon laminar analysis, with the greatest effects localizing to layers III, V, and VI.[12,62,63,68] The intracortical plexuses of myelinated fibers known as "bands of Baillarger" generally are concentrated in layers III and V. The size of these plexuses varies across cortical areas, so if the oligodendroglia related to these plexuses were affected, different areas would be expected to show greater or lesser deficits. Layer VI in particular contains a large component of myelinated fibers running between the grey and white matter.

Satellite oligodendrocytes also have been implicated in BD by an electron microscopic study which revealed decreased nuclear size, clumping of chromatin, and indications of both apoptotic and necrotic degeneration.[65,75] Satellite oligodendroglia appear to participate in maintaining the extracellular environment for surrounding neurons that resembles the functions mediated by astroglia. These oligodendrocytes are immunohistochemically reactive for glutamine synthetase, suggesting they function like astrocytes to take up synaptically released glutamate for conversion to glutamine and cycling back into neurons.[75]

Factors that conceivably may contribute to a loss of oligodendroglia in mood disorders include the abnormal elevation of glucocorticoid secretion and glutamatergic transmission during depression. Glucocorticoids affect glia as well as neurons,[76] and elevated glucocorticoid levels decrease the proliferation of oligodendrocyte precursors.[77] Moreover, oligodendrocytes express AMPA and kainite-type glutamate receptors, and are sensitive to excitotoxic damage from excess glutamate as well as to oxidative stress (reviewed in Ref. 74). The targeted nature of the reductions in grey-matter volume and glial cells to specific areas of the limbic–cortical circuits that show increased glucose metabolism during depressive episodes is noteworthy given the evidence that the glucose metabolic signal is dominated by glutamatergic transmission.[28, 78, 79]

Correlations with Rodent Models of Repeated Stress

In regions that appear homologous to the areas where grey-matter reductions are evident in depressed humans (i.e., mPFC and hippocampus), repeated stress results in dendritic atrophy and reductions in synapses and glial cell counts or proliferation in rodents.[80,81] These dendritic reshaping processes depend on interactions between the increased N-methyl-D-aspartate (NMDA) receptor stimulation and glucocorticoid secretion associated with repeated stress,[81] and notably both of these neurochemical processes are abnormally elevated in depression (see below). Dendritic atrophy would decrease the volume of the neuropil, which occupies most of the grey-matter volume. The histopathogic changes that accompany stress-induced dendritic atrophy in rats may thus appear similar to those found in humans suffering from depression. In rats the stress-induced dendritic atrophy in the mPFC was associated with impaired extinction learning of behavioral responses to fear-conditioned stimuli,[82] potentially analogous to the findings that volumetric reductions are associated with pathologic emotional states in depressed humans.

NEUROCHEMICAL SYSTEMS IMPLICATED IN THE OFC IN DEPRESSION

Of the numerous neurotransmitter systems which modulate neurotransmission within the OFC, mood disorders have been associated with abnormalities in serotonergic, dopaminergic, noradrenergic, cholinergic, glutamatergic, GABAergic, glucocorticoid, and peptidergic (e.g., corticotrophin-releasing factor [CRF]) function. The monoamine neurotransmitter systems have particularly received attention because most antidepressant drugs exert their primary receptor pharmacologic effects through these systems, although the delayed onset of antidepressant effects during treatment with such agents suggests that changes in gene expression likely underlie the therapeutic mechanisms of these drugs. Mechanisms hypothesized to serve as final common pathways for antidepressant responses include: (1) increases in the gene expression of brain-derived neurotrophic factor (BDNF) and other neurotrophic/neuroprotective factors[83,84]; (2) enhancement of postsynaptic serotonin type 1A receptor (5-HT$_{1A}$R) function[85]; and (3) reductions in the sensitivity or transmission of NMDA-glutamatergic receptors.[86,87]

Serotonergic System

The central serotonin (5-HT) system received particular interest in depression research because selective serotonin reuptake inhibitors (SSRIs) exerted antidepressant effects, and most other antidepressant drugs also increased 5-HT transmission. This effect was thought to compensate for deficient serotonergic function in MDD, since postmortem neuroimaging and pharmacologic challenge studies of depression showed abnormalities in the density and sensitivity of some 5-HT receptor types.[88] Compatible with this hypothesis, about one-half of remitted MDD subjects who are unmedicated or are being treated with SSRI agents experience depressive relapse under acute tryptophan depletion, which putatively decreases central serotonergic function.[24]

The most promising evidence for a serotonin system deficiency that is compensated by antidepressant pharmacotherapy involves the post-synaptic 5-HT$_{1A}$R. Chronic administration of antidepressant drugs with diverse primary pharmacologic actions enhances postsynaptic 5-HT$_{1A}$R function.[85] The postsynaptic 5-HT$_{1A}$R binding in the OFC, anterior insula, ACC, posterior cingulate cortex and parieto-occipital cortex are abnormally decreased in most studies of MDD and BD.[20,89–91] This abnormality appears to affect function, as depressed subjects show blunted thermic and endocrine responses to 5-HT$_{1A}$R agonist challenge (reviewed in Ref. 89). The magnitude of 5-HT$_{1A}$R binding in the OFC predicted treatment outcome during SSRI treatment, with treatment non-responders showing higher baseline binding than responders.[92] These data suggested that patients who have reduced 5-HT$_{1A}$R binding in the OFC are more likely to benefit from treatments that enhance postsynaptic 5-HT$_{1A}$R function. Compatible with this hypothesis, the reduction in central 5-HT transmission achieved experimentally via tryptophan depletion resulted in impaired function and reduced metabolism in the OFC.[24,49,50,52]

Another link between depression, OFC function, and the serotonergic system is provided by studies of the functional effects of the 5-HT transporter promoter region length polymorphism (5-HTT LPR). The short ("s") allelic form of this single nucleotide polymorphism increases the risk for depression within the context of stressful events, an effect which is particularly prominent for s homozygotes.[93] Notably, monkeys which are homozygous for the orthologous structural variant of the 5-HTT LPR s allele show reduced cognitive flexibility while performing object discrimination reversal-learning and instrumental extinction tasks.[94] The behaviors indexed by these tasks depend upon OFC and/or ventromedial PFC function, suggesting the hypothesis that the risk this polymorphism confers for developing depression in the context of stress is mediated by reduced prefrontal cortical flexibility in the face of changing reinforcement contingencies under duress.

Catecholaminergic Systems

The central dopaminergic and noradrenergic systems also have been implicated in the pathophysiology of depression and the mechanisms of antidepressant drugs.[95] Selective norepinephrine reuptake inhibitors (e.g., reboxetine), dopamine (DA) reuptake inhibitors (e.g., nomifensine), and DA receptor agonists (e.g., pramipexole) exert antidepressant effects in placebo-controlled studies.[96] In MDD the cerebrospinal fluid (CSF) and jugular vein plasma levels of the DA metabolite, homovanillic acid, are abnormally decreased, suggesting decreased DA turnover.[96,97] In contrast, the levels of norepinephrine metabolite concentrations were decreased in some,[97] but increased in other[98] studies. Neuroimaging studies of MDD showed reduced striatal DA transporter binding and [^{11}C]l-DOPA uptake across the blood–brain barrier, consistent with reduced DA neurotransmission.[95]

Consistent with these observations, the reduction in catecholaminergic function induced by administration of reserpine or AMPT is associated with depressive relapse in recovered MDD subjects, and the degeneration of DA neurons in PD is associated with increased vulnerability for developing MDE.[49,99] Each of these conditions was associated with effects on OFC function. In both healthy and recovered MDD subjects, glucose metabolism in the OFC decreased under catecholamine depletion achieved via AMPT administration,[24,49,50] and activity in the OFC was decreased to a greater extent in depressed versus non-depressed subjects with PD.[8,9]

The mesolimbic DA projections from the ventral tegmental area (VTA) to the nucleus accumbens shell and the OMPFC play major roles in learning associations between operant behaviors or sensory stimuli and reward, and in mediating the reinforcing properties of drugs of abuse and natural rewards, such as food and sex.[100] Thus the evidence suggesting that DA release is reduced in depression gave rise to hypotheses that deficient mesolimbic DA function underlies the anhedonia, amotivation, and psychomotor slowing associated with MDE.[100,101] During performance of reward-related tasks, which have been shown to be sensitive to catecholamine depletion, neurophysiological responses were abnormal in the OFC, accumbens, anterior insula, amygdala, and hippocampal subiculum (FIG. 3).

Glutamatergic and GABAergic Systems

The function of the major excitatory and inhibitory neurotransmitters, glutamate and gamma-amino-butyric acid (GABA), respectively, also appears altered in mood disorders. Early studies reported that GABA concentrations were abnormally decreased in the plasma and CSF in MDD subjects (reviewed in Ref. 102). In contrast, postmortem studies of the NMDA receptor complex in depressed suicide victims found evidence of increased glutamatergic transmission in the PFC, and implicated disturbances in glutamate metabolism and in the glutamatergic NMDA and mGluR1,5 receptors in depression and suicide.[86,87] Moreover, antidepressant and mood-stabilizing drugs, which have diverse primary pharmacological actions, generally reduce NMDA receptor sensitivity and/or transmission, and many of these agents also increase GABA levels or transmission.[86,87]

The neurophysiological activation of visceromotor circuits in depression is putatively mediated by elevated glutamatergic transmission within limbic-thalamo-cortical circuits. For example, the abnormally increased CBF and metabolism in the OFC and ventrolateral PFC, ventral ACC, amygdala, ventral striatum, and medial thalamus evident in depression (FIG. 2) implicate a limbic-thalamo-cortical circuit involving the amygdala, mediodorsal nucleus of the thalamus and OMPFC, and a limbic-cortical-striatal-pallidal-thalamic circuit involving related parts of the striatum and the ventral pallidum along with the components of the other circuit.[25] The first of these circuits can be conceptualized as an excitatory triangular circuit whereby the basolateral nucleus of the amygdala and the OMPFC are interconnected by excitatory projections with each other and with the mediodorsal nucleus.[103–106] The elevated metabolism evident in limbic-thalamo-cortical circuits in depression would be expected to reflect increased excitatory transmission in these circuits, as cerebral glucose metabolism predominately reflects the energetic requirements associated with glutamatergic transmission.[28,78] During effective antidepressant drug or electroconvulsive therapy, metabolic activity decreases in these regions (TABLE 1),[10,26] compatible with evidence that these treatments result in desensitization of NMDA receptors in the PFC.[87]

The limbic-cortical-striatal-pallidal-thalamic circuit constitutes a disinhibitory side loop between the amygdala or PFC and the mediodorsal nucleus. The amygdala and the PFC send excitatory projections to overlapping parts of the ventromedial striatum.[107] This part of the striatum sends an inhibitory projection to the ventral pallidum, which in turn sends GABAergic, inhibitory fibers to the mediodorsal nucleus.[104,108]

Magnetic resonance spectroscopic (MRS) studies of MDD demonstrate abnormalities of glutamate (measured together with glutamine as the combined

TABLE 1.   Neuroimaging and postmortem evidence implicating the orbitofrontal cortex in the pathophysiology of major depression

- Glucose metabolism/CBF
  - Increased in medial, lateral OFC in depressed versus remitted phase
  - Decreased in medial OFC in remitted phase
- Grey-matter volume reduced in lateral OFC
- Glial cell counts reduced in lateral OFC
- Glutamate + glutamine ("Glx") MRS spectra reduced
- 5-HT1 A receptor binding to WAY100635 reduced
- Lesions increase vulnerability to depression
- Hemodynamic responses altered during:
  - Reward/loss processing
  - Spurious negative feedback during probabalistic reversal learning

"Glx" peak in the MRS spectra) and GABA concentrations in depressed subjects in the anteromedial OFC, mPFC, and DALPFC.[102] These MRS spectra reflect the combined intracellular and extracellular pools of glutamate, glutamine, and GABA, but are dominated overwhelmingly by the intracellular pools. These data would thus be compatible with findings of reduced glia in these regions because of the prominent role played by glia in glutamate–glutamine cycling. Depressed MDD subjects show abnormally reduced GABA levels in the DM/DALPFC and occipital cortex in depressed MDD subjects.[102, 109] The GABA pool predominantly exists within GABAergic neurons, so the reduction in GABA in the DALPFC would be compatible with the report of reduced GABAergic neurons in this region (BA 9) in MDD.[30]

Glucocorticoid System

Severe depression is associated with hypersecretion of cortisol, pituitary and adrenal gland enlargement, and CSF levels of CRF that are increased to an extent that is inappropriate to the plasma cortisol levels (i.e., implying that negative feedback systems are impaired and/or that the central drive on the release of CRF or other ACTH secretagogues is increased).[10, 110, 111] Depressed subjects also show blunted ACTH responses to CRF *in vivo*, and a reduction in the CRF receptor density in the PFC and increased corticotrophic cell size and mRNA levels in the pituitary gland post mortem, indicating the HPA axis has been chronically activated.[110–112] Some moderately depressed subjects also show reduced sensitivity to dexamethasone negative feedback,[113] and moderately and abnormally increased cortisol secretion under stress.[37, 89] The elevation of cortisol secretion in depression is thought to contribute to elevated body temperature, mitochondrial dysfunction, premature osteoporosis and aging, other medical morbidities, and the neuropathologic changes described above.[81, 114]

IMPLICATIONS FOR CIRCUIT-BASED MODELS
OF DEPRESSION

The neuromorphometric, neuropathologic, and neurophysiological abnormalities found in the OFC and mPFC also extend to regions that share extensive, reciprocal, monosynaptic anatomic connections with these PFC areas, and which are considered part of a "visceromotor network" (TABLE 2).[3,46,115] These structures include the amygdala, ventromedial striatum, mediodorsal and midline thalamic nuclei, mid- and posterior cingulate cortex, hippocampus, parahippocampal gyrus, superior temporal gyrus, temporopolar cortex, and medial cerebellum. In most of these regions metabolic activity also was reported to be abnormally elevated in the depressed phase of MDD and BD, to decrease during antidepressant pharmacotherapy, and to increase in recovered MDD patients during experimentally induced depressive relapse (reviewed in Refs. 2, 10, and 26; TABLE 2). Neurophysiological responses to emotionally valenced stimuli and reward-processing tasks also are altered in MDD and BD in the amygdala, ventral stiatum, mid- and posterior cingulate cortex, superior temporal gyrus, and hippocampus.[116–121] Finally, anatomic MRI and/or postmortem studies of MDD or BD demonstrated reductions of grey-matter volume, cell counts, or cellular processes in the amygdala, ventral striatum, posterior cingulate cortex, hippocampus, parahippocampal cortex, superior temporal gyrus, temporopolar cortex, and cerebellum.[2,11,20,70,74,122–126]

This extended "visceromotor" network functions to regulate endocrine, autonomic, neurotransmitter, and behavioral responses to aversive and rewarding stimuli and contexts, by directly modulating neuronal activity within the limbic and brain stem structures that mediate and organize emotional expression.[3] For example, the basolateral amygdala sends anatomic projections to the central nucleus of the amygdala (ACe) and the bed nucleus of the stria terminalis (BNST), and projections from these structures to the hypothalamus, periaqueductal grey (PAG), nucleus basalis, locus ceruleus, raphe, and other diencencephalic and brain stem nuclei play major roles in organizing the neuroendocrine, neurotransmitter, autonomic, and behavioral responses to stressors and emotional stimuli (FIG. 4).[127,128] The OFC and mPFC send overlapping projections to each of these structures and to the amygdala, which function to modulate each component of emotional expression.[3] The neuropathologic changes evident in the OFC and mPFC in mood disorders thus may impair their modulatory role over emotional expression, disinhibiting or dysregulating limbic responses to stressors and emotional stimuli, and giving rise to the clinical signs and symptoms of depression. Compatible with this hypothesis, pharmacologic, neurosurgical, and electrical stimulation treatments for mood disorders appear to inhibit pathologic activity within visceromotor network structures which may specifically play roles in mediating emotional expression, such as the amygdala and sgACC (e.g., Ref. 2, 23, 26).

Reciprocal functional relationships between structures that mediate emotional expression (e.g., amygdala) and PFC regions which modulate emotional expression have been evidenced by electrophysiological and lesion analysis studies in experimental animals. In rats stimulation of projections from the amygdala to the mPFC inhibits neuronal ensemble activity in the mPFC, and stimulation of projections from the mPFC to the amygdala excites GABAergic projections which *inhibit* neuronal activity in the ACe.[129,130] Moreover, rats exposed to fear-conditioned stimuli show reduced mPFC neuronal firing activity, and the magnitude of this decrement correlates inversely with the corresponding increase in amygdala neuron activity and fear behavior.[131] Conversely, lesions of the right or bilateral mPFC enhance behavioral, sympathetic, and endocrine responses to stressors or fear-conditioned stimuli.[132,133]

In depressed humans and nonhuman primates reciprocal relationships also are evident between PFC and amygdala function with respect to emotional expression. As reviewed above, in MDD severity of depression correlates positively with amygdala activity, but negatively with activity in the left ventrolateral PFC/posterolateral OFC.[10,25,38] Lesions of the left OFC increase the risk for developing depression,[6] whereas electrical stimulation of the amygdala can produce fear, anxiety, dysphoria, sympathetic autonomic arousal, social withdrawal, and cortisol release in humans and/or nonhuman primates (reviewed in Ref. 36). In monkeys, lesions of the OFC also induce divergent effects from lesions of the amygdala on the emotional response to other monkeys or human intruders, with OFC lesions specifically enhancing emotional expression in social interactions with other monkeys or toward novel humans,[134,135] compatible with the hypothesis that the OFC exerts a modulatory or inhibitory role over emotional expression.

In human mood disorders impaired OFC function, which disinhibits amygdala function, also may contribute to the endocrine, autonomic, neurochemical, and cognitive abnormalities associated with MDE (FIG. 4). For example, the amygdala mediates the *stressed component* of glucocorticoid hormone secretion by disinhibiting CRF release from the hypothalamic paraventricular nucleus.[136] Conversely the glucocorticoid responses to stress are inhibited by stimulation of glucocorticoid receptors in the ventral ACC, and lesioning this cortex in rats increases ACTH and CORT secretion during stress.[137] Excessive amygdala activity combined with reduced OMPFC function may thus contribute to the excessive cortisol response to stress seen in depressed humans.

Dysfunction of the OFC and mPFC coupled with amygdala hyperactivity also may contribute to the anhedonia, amotivation, and inattention manifest in depression. The mPFC receives extensive dopaminergic innervation from the VTA, and sends projections to the VTA which regulate phasic DA release. In rats, stimulation of mPFC areas elicits burst firing patterns in the VTA–DA neurons, while inactivation of the mPFC converts burst firing patterns to pacemaker-like firing activity (reviewed in Ref. 60). The burst firing patterns increase DA release in the accumbens, which appears to encode information regarding reward prediction.[139] If the neuropathologic changes extant within the PFC in mood disorders interfere with its drive on VTA–DA neuronal burst firing activity they may impair reward *perception*,

TABLE 2. Neuroimaging and neuropathologic abnormalities within the extended visceromotor network in unmedicated samples with primary, early-onset, major depressive disorder and bipolar disorder

Brain region	Grey-matter volume Depressive vs. Control	Cell counts, cell markers Depressive vs. Control	Glucose metabolism, CBF Depressive vs. Control	Glucose metabolism, CBF Depressive vs. Remitted
Dorsal medial/anterolateral PFC (BA9)	↓	↓	↓	↑
Frontal polar C (BA 10)			↓	↑
Subgenual anterior cingulate C	↓	↓	↓/↑[a]	↑
Pregenual anterior cingulate C	↓	↓	↑	↑
Orbital C/ventrolateral PFC	↓	↓	↑	↑
Posterior cingulate	↓		↑	↑
Parahippocampal C			↑	↑
Amygdala	↓/↑[b]	↓ BD	↑	↑
Ventromedial striatum	↓	↓ MDD	↑	↑
Hippocampus	↓		n.s.	n.s.
Superior temporal G/temporopolar C	↓	↓ BD		↑
Medial thalamus			↑	↑

NOTE: The structures that compose this network generally show increased metabolic activity in the depressed phase relative to the remitted phase of illness, together with histopathologic and/or volumetric deficits relative to healthy controls.

Arrows indicate the presence and direction of replicated abnormalities in mood disorders relative to controls in the first three columns, and the direction of change between the depressed relative to the remitted condition in the fourth column (see text for explanation and references). Empty cells indicate where insufficient data exist.

[a] In the subgenual anterior cingulate cortex the apparent reduction in CBF and metabolism in PET images of depressed subjects is thought to be accounted for by the reduction in tissue volume in the corresponding cortex, as after partial volume correction for the reduction in grey matter, the metabolism appears increased compared to controls.

[b] The literature has disagreed regarding amygdala volume in mood disorders, and the reduction in volume may be limited to chronically or intermittently ill subjects with MDD and pediatric cases of BD.

ABBREVIATIONS: BA = Brodmann area; BD = bipolar disorder; C = cortex; Dep vs Con: Unmedicated depressives versus healthy controls; Dep vs Rem: Unmedicated depressives versus themselves in either the medicated or unmedicated remitted phases; G = gyrus; MDD = major depressive disorder; n.s.: differences generally not significant; PFC = prefrontal cortex.

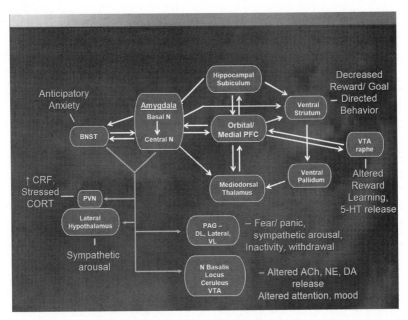

FIGURE 4. Anatomic circuits involving the orbitomedial PFC (OMPFC) and amygdala reviewed within the context of a model in which OMPFC dysfunction results in disinhibition of limbic activity through the amygdala, yielding the emotional, endocrine, autonomic, neurochemical, and cognitive manifestations of depression. See text for references. The basolateral amygdala sends efferent projections to the central nucleus of the amygdala (ACe) and the bed nucleus of the stria terminalis (BNST). The efferent projections from these structures to the hypothalamus, periaqueductal grey (PAG), nucleus basalis, locus ceruleus, raphe and other diencencephalic and brain stem nuclei then organize the neuroendocrine, neurotransmitter, autonomic, and behavioral responses to stressors and emotional stimuli.[127,128] The OMPFC shares reciprocal projections with these limbic, hypothalamic and brain stem structures (although only the connections with the amygdala are shown), which function to modulate each component of emotional expression.[3] Impaired OMPFC function thus may disinhibit or dysregulate the efferent transmission through the ACe and BNST. *Solid white lines* indicate some of the major anatomic connections between structures, with closed *arrowheads* indicating the direction of projecting axons. *Solid yellow lines* show efferent pathways of the ACe and BNST, which generally are monosynaptic, but in some cases are bisynaptic connections.[136] 5-HT, serotonin; Ach, acetylcholine; DA, dopamine; DL, dorsolateral column of PAG; N, nucleus; NE, norepinephrine; NTS, nucleus tractus solitarius; PVN, paraventricular N of the hypothalamus; VL, ventrolateral column of PAG; VTA, ventral tegmental area. (From Drevets and Furey.[5] Reproduced by permission.) (In color in *Annals* online.)

conceivably experienced as a loss of the pleasure and behavioral reinforcement derived from normally rewarding activities. Dysfunction involving the OFC also may interfere with assessments of the relative value of potentially rewarding stimuli and the integration of this information into behavioral incentive in depression.[140–142]

Furthermore, the cognitive and behavioral response patterns supporting goal- or reward-directed behavior involve PFC inputs to the ventral striatum, which are maintained or "gated" by projections from the hippocampal subiculum to the accumbens.[143] Stimulation of amygdalar projections to the ventral striatum interrupts the maintenance of cortically driven response patterns, providing an adaptive, limbic override that interrupts goal-directed thought or behavior in response to threatening or novel stimuli. Nevertheless, in MDE the excessive amygdala activity conceivably may interfere with cognitive performance and goal-directed behavior to an extent that becomes maladaptive.

Nevertheless, in some other cases the relationships between the amygdala and OFC/mPFC regions with respect to their effects on emotional behavior appear facilitatory or synergistic, rather than reciprocal. For example, monkeys with lesions which include the medial OFC also show blunted innate fear responses to rubber snakes.[134] In addition, lesions of the anterior cingulate gyrus in monkeys result in decreases in social interactions, time spent in proximity with other individuals, and vocalizations.[141, 144] Finally, in rats physiological activity within the prelimbic cortex is necessary for mediating the expression of learned fears.[57] These data thus appear potentially consistent with the evidence reviewed above that in depressed humans physiological activity correlates positively with depression severity in some areas of the medial OFC/ventromedial PFC.

SUMMARY

Normal emotional and social behavior depends upon integrated interactions between several brain areas, including the OFC, mPFC, and amygdala. Within the OFC and mPFC some regions appear to play roles in inhibiting or modulating emotional expression, while others appear to promote or facilitate emotional expression. Both types of areas may participate in the pathophysiology of depression, as neuroimaging, lesion analysis, and postmortem data converge to support models in which the signs and symptoms of MDE result from dysfunction within a neural network involving the OFC, mPFC, amygdala, and anatomically related areas of the temporal lobe, striatum, thalamus and brain stem, which interferes with this system's adaptive modulation of emotional behavior. Antidepressant and mood-stabilizing therapies may compensate for this dysfunction by attenuating the pathologic limbic activity which mediates expression of depressive symptoms,[26] and by increasing expression of neurotrophic/neuroprotective factors which restore or preserve modulatory PFC function.[83] Cognitive-behavioral strategies for managing depressive symptoms may instead rely upon enhancing the function of modulatory PFC systems via top-down mechanisms, thereby restoring the adaptive role of cortico-limbic circuits in organizing emotional processing and experience.

REFERENCES

1. WHO. 2001. The World Health Report. www.who.int. Chapters 2 and 4.
2. DREVETS, W.C. & PRICE, J.L. 2005. Neuroimaging and neuropathological studies of mood disorders. *In* Biology of Depression: from Novel Insights to Therapeutic Strategies, Vol. 1. J.W.M. Licinio, Ed.: 427–466. Wiley–VCH Verlag GmbH. Weinheim, Germany.
3. ONGUR, D., A.T. FERRY & J.L. PRICE. 2003. Architectonic subdivision of the human orbital and medial prefrontal cortex. J. Comp. Neurol. **460:** 425–49.
4. DREVETS, W.C. & R.D. TODD. 2005. Depression, mania and related disorders. *In* Adult Psychiatry, 2nd ed. E. Rubin & C. Zorumski, Ed.: 91–129. Blackwell Publishing, Ltd. Oxford.
5. DREVETS, W.C. & M.L. FUREY. 2007. Emotional disorders: depression and the Brain. *In* New Encyclopedia of Neuroscience. L.R. Squire, Ed. Elsevier Publishing, Inc. Oxford, UK. In press.
6. MACFALL, J.R. *et al.* 2001. Medial orbital frontal lesions in late-onset depression. Biol. Psychiatry **49:** 803–806.
7. RAJKOWSKA, G. *et al.* 2005. Prominent reduction in pyramidal neurons density in the orbitofrontal cortex of elderly depressed patients. Biol. Psychiatry **58:** 297–306.
8. RING, H.A. *et al.* 1994. Depression in Parkinson's disease: a positron emission study. Br. J. Psychiatry **165:** 333–339.
9. MAYBERG, H.S. *et al.* 1990. Selective hypometabolism in the inferior frontal lobe in depressed patients with Parkinson's disease. Ann. Neurol. **28:** 57–64.
10. DREVETS, W.C., K. GADDE & K.R.R. KRISHNAN. 2004. Neuroimaging studies of depression. *In* The Neurobiological Foundation of Mental Illness, 2nd ed. D.S. Charney, E. Nestler, B.J. Bunney, Ed.: 461–490. Oxford University Press. New York.
11. NUGENT, A.C. *et al.* 2005. Cortical abnormalities in bipolar disorder investigated with MRI and voxel-based morphometry. Neuroimage **30:** 485–497.
12. RAJKOWSKA, G. *et al.* 1999. Morphometric evidence for neuronal and glial prefrontal cell pathology in major depression. Biol. Psychiatry **45:** 1085–1098.
13. LYOO, I.K. *et al.* 2004. Frontal lobe gray matter density decreases in bipolar I disorder. Biol. Psychiatry **55:** 648–651.
14. TAYLOR, W.D. *et al.* 2007. Orbitofrontal cortex volume in late life depression: influence of hyperintense lesions and genetic polymorphisms. Psychol. Med. 1–11 [Epub ahead of print].
15. DREVETS, W.C. *et al.* 1997. Subgenual prefrontal cortex abnormalities in mood disorders. Nature **386:** 824–827.
16. HIRAYASU, Y. *et al.* 1999. Subgenual cingulate cortex volume in first-episode psychosis. Am. J. Psychiatry **156:** 1091–1093.
17. CORYELL, W. *et al.* 2005. Subgenual prefrontal cortex volumes in major depressive disorder and schizophrenia: diagnostic specificity and prognostic implications. Am. J. Psychiatry **162:** 1706–1712.
18. BOTTERON, K.N. *et al.* 2002. Volumetric reduction in left subgenual prefrontal cortex in early onset depression. Biol. Psychiatry **51:** 342–344.
19. ONGUR, D., W.C. DREVETS & J.L. PRICE. 1998. Glial reduction in the subgenual prefrontal cortex in mood disorders. Proc. Natl. Acad. Sci. USA **95:** 13290–13295.

20. BOWEN, D.M. *et al.* 1989. Circumscribed changes of the cerebral cortex in neuropsychiatric disorders of later life. Proc. Natl. Acad. Sci. USA **86:** 9504–9508.

21. DREVETS, W.C. *et al.* 2004. Subgenual prefrontal cortex volume decreased in healthy humans at high familial risk for mood disorders. Soc. Neurosci. Abstr. 799.19.

22. ADLER, C.M. *et al.* 2005. Changes in gray matter volume in patients with bipolar disorder. Biol. Psychiatry **58:** 151–157.

23. MAYBERG, H.S. *et al.* 2005. Deep brain stimulation for treatment-resistant depression. Neuron **45:** 651–660.

24. NEUMEISTER, A. *et al.* 2004. Neural and behavioral responses to tryptophan depletion in unmedicated patients with remitted major depressive disorder and controls. Arch. Gen. Psychiatry **61:** 765–773.

25. DREVETS, W.C. *et al.* 1992. A functional anatomical study of unipolar depression. J. Neurosci. **12:** 3628–3641.

26. DREVETS, W.C., W. BOGERS & M.E. RAICHLE. 2002. Functional anatomical correlates of antidepressant drug treatment assessed using PET measures of regional glucose metabolism. Eur. Neuropsychopharmacol. **12:** 527–544.

27. MAYBERG, H.S. *et al.* 1999. Reciprocal limbic-cortical function and negative mood: converging PET findings in depression and normal sadness. Am. J. Psychiatry **156:** 675–682.

28. MAGISTRETTI, P.L. 1999. Cellular mechanisms of brain imaging metabolism and their relevance to functional brain imaging. Phil. Trans. R. Soc. London Ser. B, Biol. Sci. **354:** 1155–1163.

29. BAXTER, L.R. *et al.* 1989. Reduction of prefrontal cortex glucose metabolism common to three types of depression. Arch. Gen. Psychiatry **46:** 243–250.

30. RAJKOWSKA, G. *et al.* 2007. GABAergic neurons immunoreactive for calcium binding proteins are reduced in the prefrontal cortex in major depression. Neuropsychopharmacology **32:** 471–482.

31. BLUMBERG, H.P. *et al.* 2003. A functional magnetic resonance imaging study of bipolar disorder: state- and trait-related dysfunction in ventral prefrontal cortices. Arch. Gen. Psychiatry **60:** 601–609.

32. RAUCH, S.L. *et al.* 1994. Regional cerebral blood flow measured during symptom provocation in obsessive-compulsive disorder using oxygen 15-labeled carbon dioxide and positron emission tomography. Arch. Gen. Psychiatry **51:** 62–70.

33. KESSLER, R.C. *et al.* 2005. Prevalence, severity, and comorbidity of 12-month DSM-IV disorders in the National Comorbidity Survey Replication. Arch. Gen. Psychiatry **62:** 617–627.

34. DREVETS, W. 2000. Neuroimaging studies of mood disorders. Biol. Psychiatry **48:** 813–829.

35. KETTER, T.A. & W.C. DREVETS. 2002. Neuroimaging studies of bipolar depression: functional neuropathology, treatment effects, and predictors of clinical response. Clin. Neurosci. Res. **2:** 182–192.

36. DREVETS, W.C. 2001. Neuroimaging and neuropathological studies of depression: implications for the cognitive-emotional features of mood disorders. Curr. Opin. Neurobiol. **11:** 240–249.

37. DREVETS, W.C. *et al.* 2002. Glucose metabolism in the amygdala in depression: relationship to diagnostic subtype and plasma cortisol levels. Pharmacol. Biochem. Behav. **71:** 431–447.

38. DREVETS, W., E. SPITZNAGEL & M. RAICHLE. 1995. Functional anatomical differences between major depressive subtypes. J. Cereb. Blood Flow Metab. **15:** S93.
39. DREVETS, W.C. & R. TODD. 2005. Depression, mania and related disorders. *In* Adult Psychiatry, 2nd ed. E. Rubin & C. Zorumski, Eds.: 91–129. Blackwell Publishing, Ltd. Oxford, UK.
40. MAYBERG, H.S., *et al.* 1992. Paralimbic frontal lobe hypometabolism in depression associated with Huntington's disease. Neurology **42:** 1791–1797.
41. MAYBERG, H.S. *et al.* 1997. Cingulate function in depression: a potential predictor of treatment response. Neuroreport **8:** 1057–1061.
42. MAYBERG, H.S. *et al.* 1994. Paralimbic hypoperfusion in unipolar depression. J. Nucl. Med. **35:** 929–934.
43. SCHNEIDER, F. *et al.* 1995. Mood effects on limbic blood flow correlate with emotional self-rating: a PET study with oxygen-15 labeled water. Psychiatry Res. **61:** 265–283.
44. DREVETS, W.C., J.R. SIMPSON & M.E. RAICHLE. 1995. Regional blood flow changes in response to phobic anxiety and habituation. J. Cereb. Blood Flow Metab. **15:** S856.
45. MOGENSON, G.J. *et al.* 1993. From motivation to action: a review of dopaminergic regulation of limbic → nucelus accumbens → ventral pallidum → pedunculopontine nucleus circuitries involved in limbic motor integration. *In* Limbic Motor Circuits and Neuropsychiatry. P.W. Kalivas & C.D. Barnes, Eds. CRC Press. London.
46. ONGUR, D. & J.L. PRICE. 2000. The organization of networks within the orbital and medial prefrontal cortex of rats, monkeys and humans. Cereb. Cortex **10:** 206–219.
47. ROLLS, E.T. 1995. A theory of emotion and consciousness, and its application to understanding the neural basis of emotion. *In* The Cognitive Neurosciences. M.S. Gazzaniga, Ed.: 1091–1106. MIT Press. Cambridge, MA.
48. TIMMS, R.J. 1977. Cortical inhibition and facilitation of the defence reaction [proceedings]. J. Physiol. **266:** 98P–99P.
49. BREMNER, J.D. *et al.* 2003. Regional brain metabolic correlates of alpha-methylparatyrosine-induced depressive symptoms: implications for the neural circuitry of depression. JAMA **289:** 3125–3134.
50. BREMNER, J.D., *et al.* 1997. Positron emission tomography measurement of cerebral metabolic correlates of tryptophan depletion-induced depressive relapse. Arch. Gen. Psychiatry **54:** 364–374.
51. BROZOSKI, T.J. *et al.* 1979. Cognitive deficit caused by regional depletion of dopamine in prefrontal cortex of rhesus monkey. Science **205:** 929–932.
52. ROGERS, R.D. *et al.* 1999. Dissociable deficits in the decision-making cognition of chronic amphetamine abusers, opiate abusers, patients with focal damage to prefrontal cortex, and tryptophan-depleted normal volunteers: evidence for monoaminergic mechanisms. Neuropsychopharmacology **20:** 322–339.
53. MAYBERG, H.S. *et al.* 1999. Reciprocal limbic-cortical function and negative mood: converging PET findings in depression and normal sadness. Am. J. Psychiatry **156:** 675–682.
54. GARCIA, R. *et al.* 1999. The amygdala modulates prefrontal cortex activity relative to conditioned fear. Nature **402:** 294–296.
55. ABERCROMBIE, H.C. *et al.* 1998. Metabolic rate in the right amygdala predicts negative affect in depressed patients. Neuroreport **9:** 3301–3307.

56. Osuch, E. 1999. Regional cerebral metabolism unique to anxiety symptoms in affective disorder patients. Biol. Psychiatry **45:**417.
57. Corcoran, K.A. & G.J. Quirk. 2007. Activity in prelimbic cortex is necessary for the expression of learned, but not innate, fears. J. Neurosci. **27:** 840–844.
58. Sierra-Mercado, D., Jr. et al. 2006. Inactivation of the ventromedial prefrontal cortex reduces expression of conditioned fear and impairs subsequent recall of extinction. Eur. J. Neurosci. **24:** 1751–1758.
59. Dougherty, D.D. et al. 2004. Ventromedial prefrontal cortex and amygdala dysfunction during an anger induction positron emission tomography study in patients with major depressive disorder with anger attacks. Arch. Gen. Psychiatry **61:** 795–804.
60. Drevets, W.C., D. Ongur & J.L. Price. 1998. Neuroimaging abnormalities in the subgenual prefrontal cortex: implications for the pathophysiology of familial mood disorders. Mol. Psychiatry **3:** 220–226, 190–191.
61. Benes, F.M., S.L. Vincent & M. Todtenkopf. 2001. The density of pyramidal and nonpyramidal neurons in anterior cingulate cortex of schizophrenic and bipolar subjects. Biol. Psychiatry **50:** 395–406.
62. Cotter, D. et al. 2002. Reduced neuronal size and glial cell density in area 9 of the dorsolateral prefrontal cortex in subjects with major depressive disorder. Cereb. Cortex **12:** 386–394.
63. Cotter, D. et al. 2001. Reduced glial cell density and neuronal size in the anterior cingulate cortex in major depressive disorder. Arch. Gen. Psychiatry **58:** 545–553.
64. Honer, W.G. et al. 1999. Synaptic and plasticity-associated proteins in anterior frontal cortex in severe mental illness. Neuroscience **91:** 1247–1255.
65. Uranova, N. et al. 2001. Electron microscopy of oligodendroglia in severe mental illness. Brain Res. Bull. **55:** 597–610.
66. Uranova, N.A. et al. 2004. Oligodendroglial density in the prefrontal cortex in schizophrenia and mood disorders: a study from the Stanley Neuropathology Consortium. Schizophr. Res. **67:** 269–275.
67. Rajkowska, G., A. Halaris & L.D. Selemon. 2001. Reductions in neuronal and glial density characterize the dorsolateral prefrontal cortex in bipolar disorder. Biol. Psychiatry **49:** 741–752.
68. Johnston-Wilson, N.L. et al. 2000. Disease-specific alterations in frontal cortex brain proteins in schizophrenia, bipolar disorder, and major depressive disorder. Stanley Neuropathology Consortium. Mol. Psychiatry **5:** 142–149.
69. Eastwood, S.L. & P.J. Harrison. 2000. Hippocampal synaptic pathology in schizophrenia, bipolar disorder and major depression: a study of complexin mRNAs. Mol. Psychiatry **5:** 425–432.
70. Rosoklija, G. et al. 2000. Structural abnormalities of subicular dendrites in subjects with schizophrenia and mood disorders: preliminary findings. Arch. Gen. Psychiatry **57:** 349–356.
71. Eastwood, S.L. & P.J. Harrison. 2001. Synaptic pathology in the anterior cingulate cortex in schizophrenia and mood disorders: a review and a Western blot study of synaptophysin, GAP-43 and the complexins. Brain Res. Bull. **55:** 569–578.
72. Bezchlibnyk, Y.B. et al. 2007. Neuron somal size is decreased in the lateral amygdalar nucleus of subjects with bipolar disorder. J. Psychiatry Neurosci. **32:** 203–210.

73. HAMIDI, M., W.C. DREVETS & J.L. PRICE. 2004. Glial reduction in amygdala in major depressive disorder is due to oligodendrocytes. Biol. Psychiatry **55:** 563–569.
74. D'AMELIO, F., L.F. ENG & M.A. GIBBS. 1990. Glutamine synthetase immunoreactivity is present in oligodendroglia of various regions of the central nervous system. Glia **3:** 335–341.
75. CHENG, J.D. & J. DE VELLIS. 2000. Oligodendrocytes as glucocorticoids target cells: functional analysis of the glycerol phosphate dehydrogenase gene. J. Neurosci. Res. **59:** 436–445.
76. ALONSO, G. 2000. Prolonged corticosterone treatment of adult rats inhibits the proliferation of oligodendrocyte progenitors present throughout white and gray matter regions of the brain. Glia **31:** 219–231.
77. SHULMAN, R.G. et al. 2004. Energetic basis of brain activity: implications for neuroimaging. Trends Neurosci. **27:** 489–495.
78. NOWAK, G., G.A. ORDWAY & I.A. PAUL. 1995. Alterations in the N-methyl-D-aspartate (NMDA) receptor complex in the frontal cortex of suicide victims. Brain Res. **675:** 157–164.
79. CZEH, B. et al. 2006. Astroglial plasticity in the hippocampus is affected by chronic psychosocial stress and concomitant fluoxetine treatment. Neuropsychopharmacology **31:** 1616–1626.
80. MCEWEN, B.S. & A.M. MAGARINOS. 2001. Stress and hippocampal plasticity: implications for the pathophysiology of affective disorders. Hum. Psychopharmacol. **16:** S7–S19.
81. IZQUIERDO, A., C.L. WELLMAN & A. HOLMES. 2006. Brief uncontrollable stress causes dendritic retraction in infralimbic cortex and resistance to fear extinction in mice. J. Neurosci. **26:** 5733–5738.
82. MANJI, H.K., W.C. DREVETS & D.S. CHARNEY. 2001. The cellular neurobiology of depression. Nat. Med. **7:** 541–547.
83. SANTARELLI, L. et al. 2003. Requirement of hippocampal neurogenesis for the behavioral effects of antidepressants. Science **301:** 805–809.
84. HADDJERI, N., P. BLIER & C. DE MONTIGNY. 1998. Long-term antidepressant treatments result in a tonic activation of forebrain 5-HT1 A receptors. J. Neurosci. **18:** 10150–10156.
85. KRYSTAL, J.H. et al. 2002. Glutamate and GABA systems as targets for novel antidepressant and mood-stabilizing treatments. Mol. Psychiatry 7(Suppl. 1): S71–S80.
86. PAUL, I.A. & P. SKOLNICK. 2003. Glutamate and depression: clinical and preclinical studies. Ann. N.Y. Acad. Sci. **1003:** 250–272.
87. STOCKMEIER, C.A. 2003. Involvement of serotonin in depression: evidence from postmortem and imaging studies of serotonin receptors and the serotonin transporter. J. Psychiatr. Res. **37:** 357–373.
88. DREVETS, W.C. et al. 1999. PET imaging of serotonin 1A receptor binding in depression. Biol. Psychiatry **46:** 1375–1387.
89. SARGENT, P.A. et al. 2000. Brain serotonin1 A receptor binding measured by positron emission tomography with [11C]WAY-100635: effects of depression and antidepressant treatment. Arch. Gen. Psychiatry **57:** 174–180.
90. LOPEZ, J.F. et al. 1998. A.E. Bennett Research Award. Regulation of serotonin1 A, glucocorticoid, and mineralocorticoid receptor in rat and human hippocampus: implications for the neurobiology of depression. Biol. Psychiatry **43:** 547–573.

91. MOSES-KOLKO, E.L., *et al.* 2007. Measurement of 5-HT(1A) receptor binding in depressed adults before and after antidepressant drug treatment using positron emission tomography and [(11)C]WAY-100635. Synapse **61:** 523–530.

92. CASPI, A. *et al.* 2003. Influence of life stress on depression: moderation by a polymorphism in the 5-HTT gene. Science **301:** 386–389.

93. IZQUIERDO, A. *et al.* 2007. Genetic modulation of cognitive flexibility and socioemotional behavior in rhesus monkeys. Proc. Natl. Acad. Sci. USA **104:** 14128–14133.

94. NUTT, D.J. 2006. The role of dopamine and norepinephrine in depression and antidepressant treatment. J. Clin. Psychiatry **67**(Suppl 6): 3–8.

95. WILLNER, P. 1995. Dopaminergic mechanisms in depression and mania. *In* Psychopharmacology: the Fourth Generation of Progress. F.E. Bloom & D.J. Kupfer, Eds.: 921–932. Raven Press. New York.

96. LAMBERT, G. *et al.* 2000. Reduced brain norepinephrine and dopamine release in treatment-refractory depressive illness: evidence in support of the catecholamine hypothesis of mood disorders. Arch. Gen. Psychiatry **57:** 787–793.

97. VEITH, R.C. *et al.* 1994. Sympathetic nervous system activity in major depression: basal and desipramine-induced alterations in plasma norepinephrine kinetics. Arch. Gen. Psychiatry **51:** 411–422.

98. SANTAMARIA, J., E. TOLOSA & A. VALLES. 1986. Parkinson's disease with depression: a possible subgroup of idiopathic parkinsonism. Neurology **36:** 1130–1133.

99. NESTLER, E.J. & W.A. CARLEZON, JR. 2006. The mesolimbic dopamine reward circuit in depression. Biol. Psychiatry **59:** 1151–1159.

100. SWERDLOW, N.R. & G.F. KOOB. 1987. Dopamine, schizophrenia, mania, and depression: toward a unified hypothesis of cortico-striato-thalamic function. Behav. Brain Sci. **10:** 197–245.

101. HASLER, G. *et al.* 2007. Reduced prefrontal glutamate/glutamine and gamma-aminobutyric acid levels in major depression determined using proton magnetic resonance spectroscopy. Arch. Gen. Psychiatry **64:** 193–200.

102. AMARAL, D.G. & R. INSAUSTI. 1992. Retrograde transport of D-[3H]-aspartate injected into the monkey amygdaloid complex. Exp. Brain Res. **88:** 375–88.

103. KURODA, M. & J.L. PRICE. 1991. Synaptic organization of projections from basal forebrain structures to the mediodorsal thalamic nucleus of the rat. J. Comp. Neurol. **303:** 513–533.

104. BACON, S.J. *et al.* 1996. Amygdala input to medial prefrontal cortex (mPFC) in the rat: a light and electron microscope study. Brain Res. **720:** 211–219.

105. AMARAL, D.G. & J.L. PRICE. 1984. Amygdalo-cortical projections in the monkey (*Macaca fascicularis*). J. Comp. Neurol. **230:** 465–496.

106. RUSSCHEN, F.T. *et al.* 1985. The amygdalostriatal projections in the monkey: an anterograde tracing study. Brain Res. **329:** 241–257.

107. GRAYBIEL, A.M. 1990. Neurotransmitters and neuromodulators in the basal ganglia. Trends Neurosci. **13:** 244–254.

108. SANACORA, G. *et al.* 1999. Reduced cortical gamma-aminobutyric acid levels in depressed patients determined by proton magnetic resonance spectroscopy. Arch. Gen. Psychiatry **56:** 1043–1047.

109. GOLD, P.W. & G.P. CHROUSOS. 2002. Organization of the stress system and its dysregulation in melancholic and atypical depression: high vs low CRH/NE states. Mol. Psychiatry **7:** 254–275.

110. SWAAB, D.F., A.M. BAO & P.J. LUCASSEN. 2005. The stress system in the human brain in depression and neurodegeneration. Ageing Res. Rev. **4:** 141–194.
111. LOPEZ, J.F. *et al.* 1992. Localization and quantification of pro-opiomelanocortin mRNA and glucocorticoid receptor mRNA in pituitaries of suicide victims. Neuroendocrinology **56:** 491–501.
112. YOUNG, E.A. *et al.* 1993. Dissociation between pituitary and adrenal suppression to dexamethasone in depression. Arch. Gen. Psychiatry **50:** 395–403.
113. GOLD, P.W., W.C. DREVETS & D.S. CHARNEY. 2002. New insights into the role of cortisol and the glucocorticoid receptor in severe depression. Biol. Psychiatry **52:** 381–385.
114. ÖNGÜR, D. & J.L. PRICE. 2000. Intrinsic and extrinsic connections of networks within the orbital and medial prefrontal cortex. Cerebral Cortex.
115. SHELINE, Y.I. *et al.* 2001. Increased amygdala response to masked emotional faces in depressed subjects resolves with antidepressant treatment: an fMRI study. Biol Psychiatry **50:** 651–658.
116. FU, C.H. *et al.* 2004. Attenuation of the neural response to sad faces in major depression by antidepressant treatment: a prospective, event-related functional magnetic resonance imaging study. Arch. Gen. Psychiatry **61:** 877–889.
117. ELLIOTT, R. *et al.* 2002. The neural basis of mood-congruent processing biases in depression. Arch. Gen. Psychiatry **59:** 597–604.
118. NEUMEISTER, A. *et al.* 2006. Effects of a alpha(2C)-adrenoreceptor gene polymorphism on neural responses to facial expressions in depression. Neuropsychopharmacology **31:** 1750–1756.
119. SIEGLE, G.J. *et al.* 2002. Can't shake that feeling: event-related fMRI assessment of sustained amygdala activity in response to emotional information in depressed individuals. Biol. Psychiatry **51:** 693–707.
120. THOMAS, K.M. *et al.* 2001. Amygdala response to fearful faces in anxious and depressed children. Arch. Gen. Psychiatry **58:** 1057–1063.
121. ALTSHULER, L.L. *et al.* 1991. Reduction of temporal lobe volume in bipolar disorder: a preliminary report of magnetic resonance imaging. Arch. Gen. Psychiatry **48:** 482–483.
122. BAUMANN, B., *et al.* 1999. Reduced volume of limbic system-affiliated basal ganglia in mood disorders: preliminary data from a post mortem study. J. Neuropsych. Clin. Neurosci. **11:** 71–78.
123. ONGUR, D. & J.L. PRICE. 1997. Distribution of glucocorticoid receptors in the Macaque central nervous system. Soc. Neurosci. Abstr. **1494.**
124. BOWLEY, M.P. *et al.* 2002. Low glial numbers in the amygdala in major depressive disorder. Biol. Psychiatry **52:** 404–412.
125. EASTWOOD, S.L. & P.J. HARRISON. 2000. Hippocampal synaptic pathology in schizophrenia, bipolar disorder and major depression: a study of complexin mRNAs. Mol. Psychiatry **5:** 425–432.
126. DAVIS, M. & C. SHI. 1999. The extended amygdala: are the central nucleus of the amygdala and the bed nucleus of the stria terminalis differentially involved in fear versus anxiety? Ann. N. Y. Acad. Sci. **877:** 281–291.
127. LEDOUX, J. 2003. The emotional brain, fear, and the amygdala. Cell Mol. Neurobiol. **23:** 727–738.
128. LIKHTIK, E. *et al.* 2005. Prefrontal control of the amygdala. J. Neurosci. **25:** 7429–7437.

129. PEREZ-JARANAY, J.M. & F. VIVES. 1991. Electrophysiological study of the response of medial prefrontal cortex neurons to stimulation of the basolateral nucleus of the amygdala in the rat. Brain Res. **564:** 97–101.

130. GARCIA, R. *et al*. 1999. The amygdala modulates prefrontal cortex activity relative to conditioned fear. Nature **402:** 294–296.

131. MORGAN, M.A. & J.E. LEDOUX. 1995. Differential contribution of dorsal and ventral medial prefrontal cortex to the acquisition and extinction of conditioned fear in rats. Behav. Neurosci. **109:** 681–688.

132. SULLIVAN, R.M. & A. GRATTON. 1999. Lateralized effects of medial prefrontal cortex lesions on neuroendocrine and autonomic stress responses in rats. J. Neurosci. **19:** 2834–2840.

133. IZQUIERDO, A., R.K. SUDA & E.A. MURRAY. 2005. Comparison of the effects of bilateral orbital prefrontal cortex lesions and amygdala lesions on emotional responses in rhesus monkeys. J. Neurosci. **25:** 8534–8542.

134. MACHADO, C.J. & J. BACHEVALIER. 2006. The impact of selective amygdala, orbital frontal cortex, or hippocampal formation lesions on established social relationships in rhesus monkeys (*Macaca mulatta*). Behav. Neurosci. **120:** 761–786.

135. HERMAN, J.P. & W.E. CULLINAN. 1997. Neurocircuitry of stress: central control of the hypothalamo-pituitary-adrenocortical axis. Trends Neurosci. **20:** 78–84.

136. DIORIO, D., V. VIAU & M.J. MEANEY. 1993. The role of the medial prefrontal cortex (cingulate gyrus) in the regulation of hypothalamic-pituitary-adrenal responses to stress. J. Neurosci. **13:** 3839–3847.

137. SCHULTZ, W., P. DAYAN & P.R. MONTAGUE. 1997. A neural substrate of prediction and reward. Science **275:** 1593–1599.

138. SCHULTZ, W. 1997. Dopamine neurons and their role in reward mechanisms. Curr. Opin. Neurobiol. **7:** 191–197.

139. RUDEBECK, P.H. *et al*. 2006. A role for the macaque anterior cingulate gyrus in social valuation. Science **313:** 1310–1312.

140. IZQUIERDO, A., R.K. SUDA & E.A. MURRAY. 2004. Bilateral orbital prefrontal cortex lesions in rhesus monkeys disrupt choices guided by both reward value and reward contingency. J. Neurosci. **24:** 7540–7548.

141. GOTO, Y. & A.A. GRACE. 2005. Dopaminergic modulation of limbic and cortical drive of nucleus accumbens in goal-directed behavior. Nat. Neurosci. **8:** 805–812.

142. HADLAND, K.A. *et al*. 2003. The effect of cingulate lesions on social behaviour and emotion. Neuropsychologia **41:** 919–931.

143. DREVETS, W.C. *et al*. 1997. Subgenual prefrontal cortex abnormalities in mood disorders. Nature **386:** 824–827.

144. PRICE, J.L., S.T. CARMICHAEL & W.C. DREVETS. 1996. Networks related to the orbital and medial prefrontal cortex; a substrate for emotional behavior? Prog. Brain Res. **107:** 523–536.

145. TALAIRACH, J. & P. TOURNOUX. 1988. Co-Planar Stereotaxic Axis of the Human Brain. Thieme. Stuttgart, Germany.

146. KNUTSON, B. *et al*. 2001. Anticipation of increasing monetary reward selectively recruits nucleus accumbens. J. Neurosci. **21,** RC **159:** 1–5.

147. WANG, H. *et al*. Differential BOLD response to a monetary incentive delay task in healthy versus depressed subjects. Presented at the Annual Meeting of the Organization of Human Brain Mapping, Chicago, June 10–14, 2007.

Symptoms of Frontotemporal Dementia Provide Insights into Orbitofrontal Cortex Function and Social Behavior

INDRE V. VISKONTAS, KATHERINE L. POSSIN, AND BRUCE L. MILLER

Memory and Aging Center, Department of Neurology, University of California, San Francisco, California, USA

ABSTRACT: Recent investigations into the brain substrates of behavioral changes in frontotemporal dementia (FTD) demonstrate that the orbitofrontal cortex (OFC) plays a crucial role in normal social and emotional behavior. The initial symptoms of FTD reflect the early involvement of OFC as well as the disruption of an associated network involving the insula, striatum, and medial frontal lobes. As predicted by patients with other types of OFC lesions, FTD patients show impairments involving stimulus-reward reversal learning, response inhibition, and ability to judge the appropriateness of their behavior in the social context. While the natural reward system remains intact in these patients, that is, patients will seek out directly rewarding stimuli, such as food and sex, with progressive OFC dysfunction they lose the ability to process complex stimulus-reward contingencies. These abnormalities are apparent in their social interactions, which break down early in the disease. Also, deficits in emotion recognition and empathy have been directly linked to OFC atrophy in these patients. In contrast, some patients with early FTD show intact cognitive skills, including memory and executive functioning. Here, we review the behavioral and neuropsychological changes that accompany OFC atrophy in FTD and argue that phylogenetically new neurons found in this region, called von Economo neurons, are selectively vulnerable in FTD.

KEYWORDS: orbitofrontal cortex; frontotemporal dementia; social behavior

Frontal-variant frontotemporal dementia (FTD) is a devastating neurodegenerative disease in which the first brain region to show atrophy is the orbitofrontal cortex (OFC)[1] (see FIG. 1). In keeping with this anatomy, the first symptoms of FTD typically involve behavioral alterations, changes in personality, and impairments in social interactions. This disorder progresses slowly and is associated with gradual atrophy and dysfunction of the frontal and/or anterior temporal lobes with a relative sparing of the posterior brain. Once considered

Address for correspondence: Bruce Miller, M.D., Memory and Aging Center, University of California, San Francisco, 350 Parnassus Avenue, Suite 706, San Francisco, CA 94143-1207. Voice: 415-476-6880; fax: 415-476-4800.
bmiller@memory.ucsf.edu

Ann. N.Y. Acad. Sci. 1121: 528–545 (2007). © 2007 New York Academy of Sciences.
doi: 10.1196/annals.1401.025

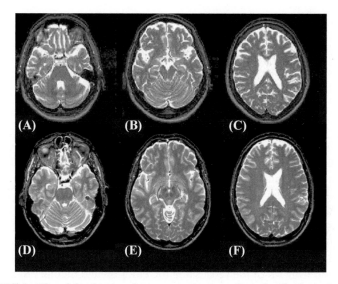

FIGURE 1. T2-weighted magnetic resonance images of a patient in the early stages of FTD (**A-C**) showing relatively selective OFC atrophy and a healthy age-matched control subject (**D-F**) for comparison.

rare, it is now accepted that FTD is at least as common as Alzheimer's disease (AD) in patients under 65 years of age[2-4] On post-mortem examination, FTD shows selective atrophy, gliosis, and neuronal loss in the frontal and anterior temporal regions. Histologically, FTD has two main subtypes, one associated with tau inclusions (Pick's disease) and the other with ubiquitin-TDP-43 positive/tau-negative inclusions.[5]

In this paper, we review the behavioral and neuropsychological changes that accompany OFC atrophy in FTD and argue that phylogenetically new neurons found in this region, called von Economo neurons, are selectively vulnerable in FTD.

CHARACTERISTICS OF FTD

The Neary Criteria[6] for FTD define this syndrome as a behavioral disorder characterized by early decline in social and personal conduct, emotional blunting, and loss of insight. Neuroimaging studies suggest that early in the illness, FTD patients show predominantly right frontal, anterior insular, and anterior cingulate involvement with pronounced OFC atrophy.[2,7,8] FTD has a strong male predominance (about 64%), often begins before the age of 60 years, and shows a fast but variable progression to death, with mean estimates ranging from 2.3 to 8.7 years from first symptoms.[2,9,10] These patients are frequently misdiagnosed with psychiatric disorders or other neurological diseases.[11] Rankin *et al.*,[12] however, demonstrated that examiner ratings of patient behavior after only 1 hour of testing were useful for discriminating FTD patients from other types of dementia. FTD patients exhibited excessive calmness or ease during the evaluation, a subset exhibited disinhibited behavior, and many lost respect for personal boundaries.

ANATOMY OF THE OFC

The OFC occupies the ventral portion of the prefrontal cortex (PFC) and is made up of five cytoarchitectonic sub-regions: frontopolar area 10, area 11 in the anterior boundary, area 13 at the posterior boundary, area 14 medially, and area 47/12 at the lateral boundary.[13] The OFC is also among the few brain regions, and the only frontal region, that receives projections from all the sensory modalities.[14] It is extensively connected to the limbic system, receiving direct projections from the amygdala, cingulate gyrus, parahippocampal cortex, and hippocampus.[15] Therefore, its anatomical placement gives the OFC information from all of the senses and the emotion and memory systems.

The OFC is selectively vulnerable in FTD: in a study of 12 FTD patients, the three mildest patients showed no detectable frontal atrophy, while six patients with moderate atrophy showed significant atrophy in the OFC and right insula[1] (see FIG. 2). The patients with the most severe atrophy showed diffuse involvement of the entire frontal region, including white matter. These results support the hypothesis that the OFC and insula are the most vulnerable regions in FTD. In addition, the behavioral symptoms that are seen early in FTD include functions that are known to rely on intact OFC, such as complex decision making and perseveration, as discussed below.

OFC AND REWARD PROCESSING

Patients with OFC damage or dysfunction show two characteristic behaviors: perseverative responses to previously rewarding stimuli and deficits in complex decision making. Perseveration is one of the first deficits to be described in monkeys with OFC lesions, such that lesioned monkeys are unable to inhibit responding to an object that was previously associated with a reward when the reward contingencies are reversed and a previously unrewarded stimulus is now the key to the reward.[16] This deficit in stimulus-reward reversal learning is found in patients with OFC damage,[17] but not in patients with damage limited to the dorsolateral PFC.[18] Perseveration also disrupts performance on the Iowa gambling task by patients with OFC lesions.[19] In this task, participants are asked to choose cards from one of four decks, with some cards winning and some losing hypothetical money. Two of the decks consistently yield small gains and smaller losses, while the other two yield large gains but even greater losses. Healthy controls quickly learn that the best strategy is to stick to the

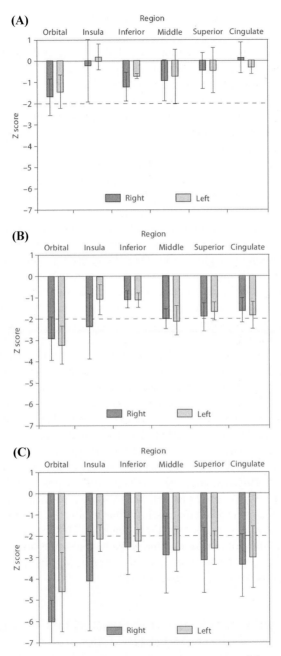

FIGURE 2. Mean regional volumes by patient subgroup: **(A)** mild atrophy (n = 3), **(B)** moderate atrophy (n = 6), and **(C)** severe atrophy (n = 3). Values are expressed in z scores derived from control mean and standard deviation values. Error bars indicate plus or minus two standard errors of the mean. Reprinted with permission from Perry *et al.* (2006).[1]

more conservative decks, but patients with OFC damage continue to choose cards from the risky decks until they lose all their "money." Recently, this task was administered to 20 patients with FTD who also showed impairments similar to those seen in OFC patients relative to age-matched controls.[20] Furthermore, in a study of autonomic responses during the Iowa gambling task, control participants showed an increase in skin conductance just before they chose a card from one of the high-risk decks, while OFC patients failed to show any anticipatory response.[21] Once the choice was rewarded or punished, however, patients showed skin conductance responses that were equivalent to those seen in controls. Bechara et al.[22] further demonstrated that autonomic responses can still be affected by learning in OFC patients, suggesting that the deficit seen in the patients stems from an inability to associate patterns of environmental stimuli with autonomic responses.

Accounting for these findings, the OFC is thought to bind situations with consequences, or, more specifically, to learn how stimuli will affect the organism emotionally and physically. Thus it can predict and create a resultant autonomic state in the presence of particular circumstances. This theory, which proposes that the OFC contributes to decision making by integrating and evaluating bodily signals is known as the somatic marker hypothesis.[23] In the presence of OFC impairment, patients are unable to choose between alternatives because the emotional consequences are not differentiable: the patient can no longer use "gut feelings" when weighing options, and all decisions, regardless of their importance or triviality, become arbitrary. This deficit in the ability to predict emotional consequences of behavior may explain why patients with FTD can often describe the consequences of their actions with complete emotional neutrality. For example, in our FTD population, one patient was able to describe in perfect detail the distressed emotional reaction that his spouse displayed when he said something injurious to her, without remorse or any indication that he realized he could avoid hurting her in the future by monitoring his language. FTD patients are also unable to judge the relative seriousness of consequences. For example, another patient used company funds to purchase illicit materials online because he did not want his wife to find out about his penchant for lewd material. This example demonstrates that the patient did not realize that the consequences of embezzling money at work were far more serious than his wife's anger, highlighting the deficit in weighing options seen in patients with FTD.

DIRECT MEASURES OF CHANGING STIMULUS-REWARD CONTINGENCIES

As predicted by patients with OFC lesions, early FTD patients show impairments in shifting strategies based on changing stimulus-reward associations. For example, in a recent study of FTD patients who were unimpaired on classic frontal-executive tests, the patients demonstrated a select impairment on the "flanker" test of attentional control.[24] On this test, participants indicated the direction of a centrally presented arrow as quickly and as accurately as possible. The central arrow was flanked on both sides by arrows either pointing in the same direction (congruent condition) or opposite direction (incongruent condition). FTD patients showed reduced accuracy and speed on incongruent trials. In another study of early FTD patients with intact performance on frontal-executive tests, the patients showed difficulty in reversing previously learned visual discriminations when reinforcement contingencies changed.[25] These same patients also showed slowed deliberation times and increased risk taking on a decision-making task. The deficits demonstrated by the early FTD patients in these two studies may arise from impairment in adjusting strategies based on trial-by-trial changes in stimuli and their associated reinforcement value, with reinforcement value defined as the emotional response associated with correct and incorrect responding. This process was attributed to OFC activity based on the results of a recent functional magnetic resonance imaging (fMRI) study of brain activity during various conditions of the flanker test.[26]

INABILITY TO ADAPT TO CHANGING REINFORCEMENT MAY LEAD TO DISINHIBITION

Based on their reviews of OFC functional and lesion studies, Kringelbach and Rolls[27] propose that the OFC flexibly processes reward and punishment values of stimuli in the environment and adapts behaviors contingent on the changing nature of these reinforcers. Based on their model, patients with OFC damage, such as early FTD patients, may produce socially inappropriate actions or comments because they are unable to adapt their behavior when there is a conflict between immediate personal and delayed gratification values, particularly when social reward cues must be inferred from minimal or complex input.[28] Socially inappropriate behavior is common in FTD and can include sexually charged comments or otherwise offensive speech, theft, and public urination or masturbation.[29] Additional evidence for a direct role of OFC in disinhibition comes from studies of patients with OFC lesions[30] and from a study by Peters and colleagues[31] that reported a specific association between disinhibition and posterior orbitofrontal hypometabolism in FTD.

NATURAL REWARD SYSTEM

The natural reward system modulates the drive to seek out directly rewarding stimuli, such as food, sex, and water, by monitoring internal cues (satiety) and external cues in the surrounding environment. OFC lesions have been shown to leave the natural reward system intact: animals with complete re-moval of OFC will still work for natural rewards[32] and will learn that a neutral stimulus predicts reward.[33] Without the ability to code and react to chang-ing values of reinforcement, however, OFC atrophy may lead to behaviors, such as overeating. In fact, alterations in eating behavior have frequently been observed in patients with FTD, including an increased preference for sweet foods,[34] and recent research by Woolley and colleagues[35] suggests that a right orbitofrontal-insula-striatal circuit may be necessary for normal regulation of feeding and satiety. Patients with FTD, semantic dementia (SD), progressive non-fluent aphasia, progressive supranuclear palsy, AD, and normal controls were presented with a constant volume of sandwiches for 1 hour at lunchtime. Six of the patients with FTD, but none of the other participants, overate. Five of these six patients spontaneously reported to the experimenter that they were full during the lunch but nevertheless continued to eat, and all six showed nor-mal primary taste processing. These overeating patients showed the greatest preference for the sweet jelly sandwich from among the other five sandwich choices. The overeating patients did not differ from the other patients on any cognitive variables, including tests of language and executive functioning, but they did show greater behavioral disturbances, as rated by their caregivers, in-volving euphoria, apathy, disinhibition, aberrant motor behavior, and aberrant sleep behavior. Using voxel-based morphometry (VBM) to compare cortical atrophy in the overeating patients to the non-overeating patients and the con-trols, the authors identified greater atrophy in right rostral OFC, right ventral insula, and right striatum in the overeating patients.

These findings are supported by a study conducted by Whitwell and col-leagues,[34] in which the neural correlates of altered eating behavior in 13 pa-tients with FTD and three with SD, as rated by their caregivers, were measured. Increased preference for sweet foods was associated with marked gray-matter reductions in OFC bilaterally and right anterior insula, and increased food consumption was associated with OFC bilaterally. Based on single-neuron recording studies in the macaque and functional neuroimaging studies in hu-mans, Rolls has proposed that the OFC represents the reward value of taste, and further, that the reward value declines when the individual has eaten to satiety.[36,37] The abnormal eating behaviors frequently observed in FTD, such as a change in food preference toward sweet foods and continued eating after satiety is experienced, are likely manifestations of the early OFC involvement associated with this disease.

EMOTION RECOGNITION AND EMPATHY: DISRUPTIONS IN REWARD PROCESSING IMPAIR SOCIAL COGNITION IN FTD

Arguably the most complex web of reinforcement schedules is found in social interactions. Our ability to recognize emotions in others and to infer their mental states provides us with social cues for appropriate behavior and allows us to receive social rewards and avoid punishment. Patients with FTD are particularly insensitive to social cues and their rewarding or punishing values. FTD patients are impaired in the recognition of both facial and vocal expressions of emotions,[38] and this impairment is more severe than in patients with AD.[39] Tests tapping the cognitive processes important for recognizing these cues show some promise for the early diagnosis of FTD.[40]

Empathy is a complex cognitive and emotional process involving the ability to recognize and feel the emotional response of another individual. Empathy promotes social engagement, provides cues important for appropriate social conduct, and has been shown to be lacking in FTD patients.[41] Using VBM-determined cortical atrophy, Rankin and colleagues[42] provided evidence that the OFC may be required for normal empathy. They demonstrated that right medial OFC volume was strongly related to loss of cognitive and emotional empathy in a sample of 123 patients with neurodegenerative disease, including 30 with FTD. If patients are unable to evoke or process the autonomic responses inherent during emotional experiences in themselves, their capacity to feel or recognize emotions in others would necessarily be impoverished. This disconnection between "gut feelings" and reward processing in FTD may explain how empathy is lost with OFC atrophy.

Empathy is a complex process, however, and there are multiple dissociable systems involved in the experience of empathy and related social processes.[43] For example, empathy may be disrupted after amygdala damage because of an impairment in both the recognition and experience of emotion,[44] and dorsomedial PFC may be particularly important for the mental attribution of intentions.[45]

Gregory and colleagues[46] showed that the related concept of theory of mind (i.e., the ability to infer other people's mental states, thoughts, and feelings) was impaired in FTD and that the degree of impairment showed a strong concordance with OFC damage. The FTD patients studied by Gregory and colleagues were impaired on several tests of theory of mind, with about half of patients impaired on tests that tap the ability to make cognitive inferences about what story characters were thinking (e.g., "what does character x think character y knows?") and 74% impaired on a more complex "faux pas" detection test that requires integrating the mental and emotional states of two individuals in order to process embarrassment (e.g., recognizing that character x should not have unintentionally done something because it may be hurtful to character y). Patients with bilateral OFC lesions and intact medial PFC tested using a similar battery showed a select impairment in the more complex "faux pas" detection test.[47] These results suggest that the OFC may play a role in inferring the mental state of another person from external cues and likely plays a critical role in comparing the emotional value of an inferred mental state with the value of other internal or external stimuli. The disruption of these cognitive mechanisms in FTD may explain why patients with this disease commonly seem unconcerned about the feelings of their loved ones.

OFC ATROPHY IN THE CONTEXT
OF A LARGER NETWORK

Increasing the complexity of this story, the initial symptoms of FTD may reflect the early involvement of an associated network involving the insula, striatum, and medial frontal lobes, in addition to the OFC. Recently, direct correlations between OFC atrophy and the behavioral changes in FTD have been reported. In a study of 62 patients with FTD and SD, Rosen and colleagues[48] examined the neural correlates of caregiver ratings of behavior with regional differences in cortical atrophy using VBM. Specific behaviors in FTD, including apathy, disinhibition, repetitive compulsive behaviors, and overeating, correlated with atrophy in the right frontal, insular, striatal, and anterior temporal regions. The average of these four behavioral disturbances also correlated with tissue loss in right inferior and medial frontal cortex, including OFC, as well as with tissue loss in the right caudate head and the right anterior insula. Additional unique effects were observed for apathy with the ventromedial superior frontal gyrus, disinhibition with the subgenual cingulate gyrus, and aberrant motor behavior with the right dorsal anterior cingulate cortex (ACC). The brain-behavior correlations observed in this study suggest that the right OFC regulates behavior in concert with predominantly right-sided network involving the insula and striatum.

Apathy, defined as a lack of interest, lethargy, social and emotional withdrawal, and reduced speech output, is almost universally prevalent in FTD patients to some degree[49] and seems to rely mainly on medial PFC function. While apathy is almost universally present, other behavioral disturbances vary considerably among patients, reflecting the heterogeneity of the pathology and its anatomical distribution. In an effort to characterize different manifestations of the disease, two distinct behavioral syndromes have been described, including an apathetic subtype, characterized by a generalized loss of interest in activities and volition, loss of social emotions, and decreased pain response; and a disinhibited subtype, characterized by an increased preference for sweet foods, hyperorality, exaggerated sensory responses, repetitive motor behavior, and increased apathy.[50] Other behaviors include stereotyped or ritualized behaviors, such as repetitive organization of objects into groups, hoarding, or repetition of a story or catch phrase. Caregivers report personality changes, such as increased submissiveness or rigidity, or shifts in their attitudes or values, such as a change in religious beliefs.[51–53] As the disease progresses and atrophy encompasses more and more frontal and temporal regions, the number and severity of behavioral impairments increase, and impairments in executive functioning emerge.[49,54,55] With relatively spared medial temporal and parietal lobes, FTD patients retain their visuospatial skills and the ability to learn new information, in contrast to the classic presentation of AD.[56,57]

INTACT COGNITIVE SKILLS EARLY IN THE DISEASE

Like patients with OFC lesions, early in the disease, many FTD patients show few measurable cognitive deficits. Widely used bedside cognitive screening instruments, such as the Mini-Mental State Examination (MMSE), are insensitive to the early stage impairments of FTD.[58] Certain newer batteries have shown minimal success in differentiating early FTD patients, as a group, from early AD patients.[59-61] These batteries have been less successful in differentiating frontal variant patients and AD patients than batteries that include caregiver-rating scales of behavior.[62,63]

Like patients with OFC lesions, early FTD patients can perform in the normal range on traditional "frontal executive" tests, such as tests of concept formation, working memory, verbal fluency, planning, or complex sequencing. As the disease progresses, however, impairments on frontal-executive tests typically emerge and can be useful for differential diagnosis.[54,57,64] The approach patients take and the errors they make may be more useful for diagnosis than the overall achievement scores.[65] Normal performance on these executive tests relies heavily on the functioning of lateral PFC.[66] When performance on these tests is preserved in FTD, the disease process may be predominantly affecting orbitofrontal or dorsomedial areas.[55]

SELECTIVELY VULNERABLE CELLS: VON ECONOMO NEURONS AND FTD

Compelling evidence regarding the exact locus of early degeneration has recently been reported by Seeley *et al.*[67] (see FIGS. 3 and 4). Von Economo neurons (VENs), formerly called "spindle cells," are a group of recently evolved neurons primarily in the ACC and the frontoinsular (FI) cortex in humans, great apes, and whales, all creatures with complex social behaviors. These cells are large bipolar cells, found in cortical layer Vb, with only a single large basal dendrite, and thus are easily distinguished from pyramidal cells. Extensively described and mapped by von Economo and Koskinas,[68] these neurons have arisen only within the last 15 million years in hominids. As a result, they may be particularly vulnerable to disease and dysfunction. They are largest and most numerous in humans, declining in density in hominids with approximately the phylogenetic distance from humans; that is, the larger the distance between the hominid and humans, the fewer VENs are found in that species.[69]

The right FI cortex has about 30% more VENs than the left FI,[70] leading to the hypothesis that VENs are involved in processes that are more reliant on right than left hemisphere activity. These functions include emotional and social processes. In fact, this right-sided bias in VEN numbers may account for the MRI-based findings that cortical gray matter is greater in the right

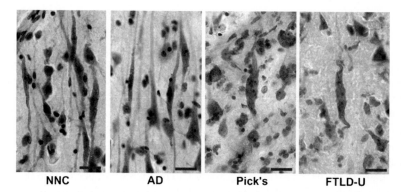

FIGURE 3. VEN swelling and dysmorphism in FTD. VENs in non-neurological control subjects (NNC) and AD patients showed prominent clustering, smooth contours, and slender, tapering somata. In FTD, VENs were often solitary, swollen (especially in Pick's disease), or showed twisting and kinking of proximal dendrites (both Pick's and frontotemporal lobar degeneration with ubiquitin inclusions (FTLD-U)). Cresyl violet stain. Scale bars = 20 μm. Photomicrographs are oriented with the pial surface at the top. Reprinted with permission from Seeley et al. (2007).[8]

than the left frontal cortex.[71,72] VENs also appear later in development—only about 15% of them are present at birth—and they continue to migrate and differentiate until age four.[73] At birth, the right hemisphere shows only 6% more VENs than the left, reinforcing the notion that VENs play a special role in social and emotional behavior.

In humans, VENs have a large, elongated, symmetrical cell body with an apical dendrite extending toward the pial surface of the cortex and a single basal dendrite extending toward the underlying white matter.[69] In the ACC, VENs are about four times larger than their neighboring pyramidal cells.[74] This large size suggests that the cells are involved in the rapid relay of information to and from the frontal cortex. VENs cluster close to small arterioles, suggesting that they have high metabolic requirements and may be more prone to injury from oxidation over time.[67]

As mentioned above, the FI is one of the key areas in which VENs have been found. Further evidence underscoring the role of the FI in social behavior can be found in fMRI studies: Bartels and Zeki[75] found that when participants viewed images of loved ones, there was more neural activity in the FI than when they viewed images of mere acquaintances, while Lamm, Batson, and Decety[76] found that greater activity in the insular cortex correlated with greater empathy. In addition, the medial part of Brodmann's Area 10 has been shown to be preferentially active when participants are required to choose a course of action affecting the lives of others.[77]

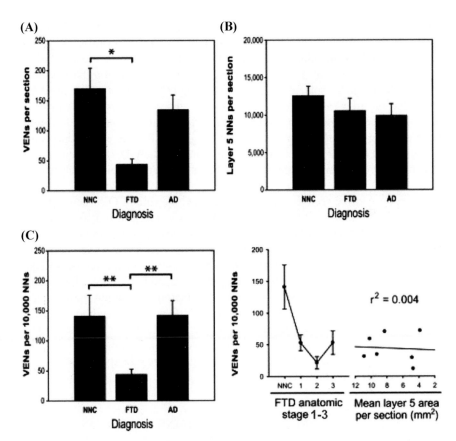

FIGURE 4. Severe, selective, disease-specific, and early loss of VENs in FTD. **(A)** VENs per section were reduced by 74% in FTD compared with non-neurological subjects (NNC) (*$P < 0.005$, Tukey's test after F-test for three-group analysis of variance [ANOVA]). **(B)** Layer 5 neighboring neurons (NNs), in contrast, showed a mild, statistically nonsignificant reduction in FTD, similar to that seen in AD. **(C)** VEN per 10,000 NN estimates indicated selective VEN depletion in FTD compared with NNC subjects and patients with AD (**$P < 0.05$, Tukey's tests after F-test for three-group ANOVA). **(D)** Even mild stages of FTD-related atrophy were accompanied by marked VEN dropout. Mean Layer 5 area per ACC section, used here as a local marker for disease severity, had no bearing on the VEN/10,000 NN ratio, further suggesting that VEN selectivity occurred across FTD stages. Error bars reflect the standard error of the mean. Reprinted with permission from Seeley *et al.* (2007).[8]

NEUROTRANSMITTERS: VASOPRESSIN, DOPAMINE, AND SEROTONIN

Receptors expressed on VENs include the vasopressin 1a receptor, the dopamine D3 receptor, and the serotonin 2b receptor. Vasopressin is a neurotransmitter that has been strongly linked to the formation of social bonds.[78] The dopamine D3 receptor has been implicated in reward-seeking behavior, including drug addiction.[79] Though not playing a direct role in creating the rewarding effects of psychostimulants, D3 receptors seem to be involved in the motivation to self-administer drugs where significant effort must be expended in order to receive the drug, that is, where the cost of the drug is high. D3 receptors seem to modulate the effect that environmental stimuli have on drug-seeking behavior, while having no influence on natural reinforcers, such as food or sex.[79] Finally, serotonin in the OFC has been shown to contribute to cognitive flexibility.[80] When serotonin is depleted selectively from the PFC, perseverative responses to previously rewarding stimuli are observed.[81] A more recent study has confirmed the role of OFC serotonin in inhibition of prepotent reponses.[82] The serotonin 2b receptor is also numerous in the human stomach and intestines, where it contributes to peristalsis.[83] The activation of these receptors in the gut, then, may contribute to the signaling of danger or threat, and this information may be rapidly integrated by VENs.

Recent work has demonstrated severe, selective, and early loss of VENs in patients with FTD[67] (see FIGS. 3 and 4). Compared to healthy age-matched controls, patients showed a 74% reduction in VENs, while neighboring layer V pyramidal cells were not significantly depleted. While a previous study has shown that VENs are lost in AD as well, Seeley et al.[67] showed that early in AD, this VEN loss is not detectable, suggesting that the selective loss of VENs in FTD is a defining feature of the disease.

FUTURE DIRECTIONS

Patients with early FTD show marked behavioral changes and functional declines, and as such, it follows that there are impaired underlying processes that could theoretically be tapped by objective measures. There is a clear clinical need to develop neuropsychological tests that are sensitive to the impaired cognitive processes of early FTD, both to improve methods for early and accurate diagnosis and to better evaluate the efficacy of new treatments. Some initial progress toward this goal has involved adapting tests with demonstrated sensitivity to OFC dysfunction, specifically tests of emotion recognition, theory of mind, attention, and decision making. These tests measure various aspects of processing emotional or social cues, their reinforcement value, and the flexible use of those cues to guide behavior.

In addition, finding a direct link between VEN activity and social behavior will allow scientists to develop computational models of OFC function. FTD offers a unique window into the mechanisms by which these cells facilitate social interactions and complex behavior. Understanding how OFC damage affects decision-making processes will not only inform neuroscientists about the OFC itself, but will also be of interest to economists, anthropologists, psychologists, and individuals who hope to understand how humans are able to function in a world of seemingly infinite choices.

ACKNOWLEDGEMENTS

We would like to thank all of the patients and their caregivers who have participated in studies at the Memory & Aging Center. We would also like to acknowledge grants to Bruce L. Miller from the National Institute of Aging, including a Program Project Grant (PO1AG19724) and an Alzheimer's Disease Research Center (P50-AG023501), and a Network grant from the Hillblom Foundation. Indre Viskontas is supported by Fellowship from the McBean Foundation. Finally, we would like to thank Kate Rankin and Joel Kramer for their comments on earlier drafts of this paper.

REFERENCES

1. PERRY, R.J. *et al.* 2006. Patterns of frontal lobe atrophy in frontotemporal dementia: a volumetric MRI study. Dement. Geriatr. Cogn. Disord. **22:** 278–287.
2. HODGES, J.R. *et al.* 2003. Survival in frontotemporal dementia. Neurology **61:** 349–354.
3. RATNAVALLI, E. *et al.* 2002. The prevalence of frontotemporal dementia. Neurology **58:** 1615–1621.
4. KNOPMAN, D.S. *et al.* 2004. The incidence of frontotemporal lobar degeneration in Rochester, Minnesota, 1990 through 1994. Neurology **62:** 506–508.
5. JOHNSON, J.K. *et al.* 2005. Frontotemporal lobar degeneration: demographic characteristics of 353 patients. Arch. Neurol. **62:** 925–930.
6. NEARY, D. *et al.* 1998. Frontotemporal lobar degeneration: a consensus on clinical diagnostic criteria. Neurology **51:** 1546–1554.
7. ROSEN, H.J. *et al.* 2002. Patterns of brain atrophy in frontotemporal dementia and semantic dementia. Neurology **58:** 198–208.
8. SEELEY, W.W. *et al.* 2007. Frontal paralimbic network atrophy in very mild behavioral variant frontotemporal dementia. Arch. Neurol. In press.
9. ROBERSON, E.D. *et al.* 2005. Frontotemporal dementia progresses to death faster than Alzheimer disease. Neurology **65:** 719–725.
10. JOSEPHS, K.A. *et al.* 2005. Survival in two variants of tau-negative frontotemporal lobar degeneration: FTLD-U vs FTLD-MND. Neurology **65:** 645–647.
11. PASSANT, U. *et al.* 2005. Psychiatric symptoms and their psychosocial consequences in frontotemporal dementia. Alzheimer Dis. Assoc. Disord. **19**(Suppl 1): S15–S18.
12. RANKIN, K.P. *et al.* 2007. Spontaneous social behaviors discriminate behavioral dementias from psychiatric disorders or other dementias. J. Clin. Psychiatry In press.
13. WALLIS, J.D. 2007. Orbitofrontal Cortex and Its Contribution to Decision-Making. Annu. Rev. Neurosci. **30:** 31–56.
14. CARMICHAEL, S.T. & J.L. PRICE. 1995. Sensory and premotor connections of the orbital and medial prefrontal cortex of macaque monkeys. J. Comp. Neurol. **363:** 642–664.

15. CARMICHAEL, S.T. & J.L. PRICE. 1995. Limbic connections of the orbital and medial prefrontal cortex in macaque monkeys. J. Comp. Neurol. **363:** 615–641.
16. MISHKIN, M. 1964. Perseveration of central sets after frontal lesions in monkeys. *In* The Frontal Granular Cortex and Behavior. J.M. Warren & K. Akert, Eds.: 219–241. McGraw-Hill. New York.
17. ROLLS, E.T. *et al.* 1994. Emotion-related learning in patients with social and emotional changes associated with frontal lobe damage. J. Neurol. Neurosurg. Psychiatry **57:** 1518–1524.
18. FELLOWS, L.K. & M.J. FARAH. 2003. Ventromedial frontal cortex mediates affective shifting in humans: evidence from a reversal learning paradigm. Brain **126**(Pt 8): 1830–1837.
19. BECHARA, A. *et al.* 1994. Insensitivity to future consequences following damage to human prefrontal cortex. Cognition **50:** 7–15.
20. TORRALVA, T. *et al.* 2007. The relationship between affective decision-making and theory of mind in the frontal variant of fronto-temporal dementia. Neuropsychologia **45:** 342–349.
21. BECHARA, A. *et al.* 1997. Deciding advantageously before knowing the advantageous strategy [see comments]. Science **275:** 1293–1295.
22. BECHARA, A. *et al.* 1999. Different contributions of the human amygdala and ventromedial prefrontal cortex to decision-making. J. Neurosci. **19:** 5473–5481.
23. DAMASIO, A.R. 1996. The somatic marker hypothesis and the possible functions of the prefrontal cortex. Philos. Trans. R. Soc. Lond. B. Biol. Sci. **351:** 1413–1420.
24. KRAMER, J., *et al.* 2007. Inhibition Deficits in Very Early Frontotemporal Dementia. American Academy of Neurology. Boston, MA.
25. RAHMAN, S. *et al.* 1999. Specific cognitive deficits in mild frontal variant frontotemporal dementia. Brain **122**(Pt 8): 1469–1493.
26. LUKS, T.L. *et al.* 2007. Preparatory allocation of attention and adjustments in conflict processing. Neuroimage **35:** 949–958.
27. KRINGELBACH, M.L. & E.T. ROLLS. 2004. The functional neuroanatomy of the human orbitofrontal cortex: evidence from neuroimaging and neuropsychology. Prog. Neurobiol. **72:** 341–372.
28. RANKIN, K. 2007. Social cognition in frontal injury. *In* The Human Frontal Lobes. B.L. Miller & J.L. Cummings, Eds.: 345–360. Guilford Press. New York.
29. MILLER, B.L. *et al.* 1997. Aggressive, socially disruptive and antisocial behaviour associated with fronto-temporal dementia. Br. J. Psychiatry **170:** 150–154.
30. STARKSTEIN, S.E. & R.G. ROBINSON. 1997. Mechanism of disinhibition after brain lesions. J. Nerv. Ment. Dis. **185:** 108–114.
31. PETERS, F. *et al.* 2006. Orbitofrontal dysfunction related to both apathy and disinhibition in frontotemporal dementia. Dement. Geriatr. Cogn. Disord. **21:** 373–379.
32. IZQUIERDO, A., R.K. SUDA & E.A. MURRAY. 2004. Bilateral orbital prefrontal cortex lesions in rhesus monkeys disrupt choices guided by both reward value and reward contingency. J. Neurosci. **24:** 7540–7548.
33. PICKENS, C.L. *et al.* 2003. Different roles for orbitofrontal cortex and basolateral amygdala in a reinforcer devaluation task. J. Neurosci. **23:** 11078–11084.
34. WHITWELL, J.L. *et al.* 2007. VBM signatures of abnormal eating behaviours in frontotemporal lobar degeneration. Neuroimage **35:** 207–213.
35. WOOLLEY, J.D. *et al.* 2007. Binge eating is associated with right orbitofrontal-insular-striatal atrophy in frontotemporal dementia. Neurology **69:** 1424–1433.

36. ROLLS, E.T. 2004. The functions of the orbitofrontal cortex. Brain Cogn. **55:** 11–29.
37. ROLLS, E.T., Z.J. SIENKIEWICZ & S. YAXLEY. 1989. Hunger modulates the responses to gustatory stimuli of single neurons in the caudolateral orbitofrontal cortex of the macaque monkey. Eur. J. Neurosci. **1:** 53–60.
38. KEANE, J. *et al.* 2002. Face and emotion processing in frontal variant frontotemporal dementia. Neuropsychologia **40:** 655–665.
39. LAVENU, I. *et al.* 1999. Perception of emotion in frontotemporal dementia and Alzheimer disease. Alzheimer Dis. Assoc. Disord. **13:** 96–101.
40. NARVID, J.R.K., M.L. GORNO-TEMPINI, Y.H. CHA, *et al.* Frontal lobes, Theories of Mind and Exostoses. Neurocase, in press.
41. RANKIN, K.P., J.H. KRAMER & B.L. MILLER. 2005. Patterns of cognitive and emotional empathy in frontotemporal lobar degeneration. Cogn. Behav. Neurol. **18:** 28–36.
42. RANKIN, K.P. *et al.* 2006. Structural anatomy of empathy in neurodegenerative disease. Brain **129**(Pt 11): 2945–2956.
43. DECETY, J. & P.L. JACKSON. 2004. The functional architecture of human empathy. Behav. Cogn. Neurosci. Rev. **3:** 71–100.
44. ADOLPHS, R. *et al.* 1995. Fear and the human amygdala. J. Neurosci. **15:** 5879–5891.
45. GALLAGHER, H.L. & C.D. FRITH. 2003. Functional imaging of 'theory of mind'. Trends Cogn. Sci. **7:** 77–83.
46. GREGORY, C. *et al.* 2002. Theory of mind in patients with frontal variant frontotemporal dementia and Alzheimer's disease: theoretical and practical implications. Brain **125**(Pt 4): 752–764.
47. STONE, V.E., S. BARON-COHEN & R.T. KNIGHT. 1998. Frontal lobe contributions to theory of mind. J. Cogn. Neurosci. **10:** 640–656.
48. ROSEN, H.J. *et al.* 2005. Neuroanatomical correlates of behavioural disorders in dementia. Brain **128:** 2612–2625.
49. DIEHL-SCHMID, J. *et al.* 2006. Behavioral disturbances in the course of frontotemporal dementia. Dement. Geriatr. Cogn. Disord. **22:** 352–357.
50. SNOWDEN, J.S. *et al.* 2001. Distinct behavioural profiles in frontotemporal dementia and semantic dementia. J. Neurol. Neurosurg. Psychiatry **70:** 323–332.
51. MILLER, B.L. *et al.* 2001. Neuroanatomy of the self: Evidence from patients with frontotemporal dementia. Neurology **57:** 817–821.
52. RANKIN, K.P. *et al.* 2003. Double dissociation of social functioning in frontotemporal dementia. Neurology **60:** 266–271.
53. RANKIN, K.P. *et al.* 2004. Right and left medial orbitofrontal volumes show an opposite relationship to agreeableness in FTD. Dement Geriatr. Cogn. Disord. **17:** 328–332.
54. KRAMER, J.H. *et al.* 2003. Distinctive neuropsychological patterns in frontotemporal dementia, semantic dementia, and Alzheimer disease. Cogn. Behav. Neurol. **16:** 211–218.
55. HODGES, J.R. *et al.* 1999. The differentiation of semantic dementia and frontal lobe dementia (temporal and frontal variants of frontotemporal dementia) from early Alzheimer's disease: a comparative neuropsychological study. Neuropsychology **13:** 31–40.
56. HARCIAREK, M. & K. JODZIO. 2005. Neuropsychological differences between frontotemporal dementia and Alzheimer's disease: a review. Neuropsychol. Rev. **15:** 131–145.

57. PERRY, R.J. & J.R. HODGES. 2000. Differentiating frontal and temporal variant frontotemporal dementia from Alzheimer's disease. Neurology **54:** 2277–2284.
58. GREGORY, C.A., J. SERRA-MESTRES & J.R. HODGES. 1999. Early diagnosis of the frontal variant of frontotemporal dementia: how sensitive are standard neuroimaging and neuropsychologic tests? Neuropsychiatry Neuropsychol. Behav. Neurol. **12:** 128–135.
59. GREGORY, C.A. *et al.* 1997. Can frontotemporal dementia and Alzheimer's disease be differentiated using a brief battery of tests? Int. J. Geriatr. Psychiatry **12:** 375–383.
60. LISCIC, R.M. *et al.* 2007. Clinical and psychometric distinction of frontotemporal and Alzheimer dementias. Arch. Neurol. **64:** 535–540.
61. MATHURANATH, P.S. *et al.* 2000. A brief cognitive test battery to differentiate Alzheimer's disease and frontotemporal dementia. Neurology **55:** 1613–1620.
62. ROSEN, H.J. *et al.* 2002. Utility of clinical criteria in differentiating frontotemporal lobar degeneration (FTLD) from AD. Neurology **58:** 1608–1615.
63. PERRI, R. *et al.* 2005. Alzheimer's disease and frontal variant of frontotemporal dementia– a very brief battery for cognitive and behavioural distinction. J. Neurol. **252:** 1238–1244.
64. RASCOVSKY, K. *et al.* 2002. Cognitive profiles differ in autopsy-confirmed frontotemporal dementia and AD. Neurology **58:** 1801–1808.
65. THOMPSON, J.C. *et al.* 2005. Qualitative neuropsychological performance characteristics in frontotemporal dementia and Alzheimer's disease. J. Neurol. Neurosurg. Psychiatry **76:** 920–927.
66. KNIGHT, R.T. & D.T. STUSS. 2002. Prefrontal cortex: the present and the future. *In* Principles of Frontal Lobe Function. D.T. Stuss & R.T. Knight, Eds.: 573–597. Oxford University Press. Oxford.
67. SEELEY, W.W. *et al.* 2006. Early frontotemporal dementia targets neurons unique to apes and humans. Ann. Neurol. **60:** 660–667.
68. VON ECONOMO, C. & G. KOSKINAS. 1925. Die Cytoarchitectonik der Hirnrinde des erwaschsenen Menschen. Springer. Berlin.
69. ALLMAN, J., A. HAKEEM & K. WATSON. 2002. Two phylogenetic specializations in the human brain. Neuroscientist **8:** 335–346.
70. BENOWITZ, L.I. *et al.* 1983. Hemispheric specialization in nonverbal communication. Cortex **19:** 5–11.
71. WATKINS, K.E. *et al.* 2001. Structural asymmetries in the human brain: a voxel-based statistical analysis of 142 MRI scans. Cereb. Cortex **11:** 868–877.
72. ALLMAN, J.M. *et al.* 2005. Intuition and autism: a possible role for Von Economo neurons. Trends Cogn. Sci. **9:** 367–373.
73. WEICKERT, C.S. *et al.* 2000. Localization of epidermal growth factor receptors and putative neuroblasts in human subependymal zone. J. Comp. Neurol. **423:** 359–372.
74. NIMCHINSKY, E.A. *et al.* 1999. A neuronal morphologic type unique to humans and great apes. Proc. Natl. Acad. Sci. U.S.A. **96:** 5268–5273.
75. BARTELS, A. & S. ZEKI. 2004. The neural correlates of maternal and romantic love. Neuroimage **21:** 1155–1166.
76. LAMM, C., C.D. BATSON & J. DECETY. 2007. The neural substrate of human empathy: effects of perspective-taking and cognitive appraisal. J. Cogn. Neurosci. **19:** 42–58.
77. GREENE, J.D. *et al.* 2001. An fMRI investigation of emotional engagement in moral judgment. Science **293:** 2105–2108.

78. INSEL, T.R. & L.J. YOUNG. 2001. The neurobiology of attachment. Nat. Rev. Neurosci. **2:** 129–136.
79. LE FOLL, B., S.R. GOLDBERG & P. SOKOLOFF. 2005. The dopamine D3 receptor and drug dependence: effects on reward or beyond? Neuropharmacology **49:** 525–541.
80. CLARKE, H.F. *et al.* 2004. Cognitive inflexibility after prefrontal serotonin depletion. Science **304:** 878–880.
81. DIAS, R., T.W. ROBBINS & A.C. ROBERTS. 1996. Dissociation in prefrontal cortex of affective and attentional shifts. Nature **380:** 69–72.
82. CLARKE, H.F. *et al.* 2007. Cognitive inflexibility after prefrontal serotonin depletion is behaviorally and neurochemically specific. Cereb. Cortex **17:** 18–27.
83. BORMAN, R.A. *et al.* 2002. 5-HT(2B) receptors play a key role in mediating the excitatory effects of 5-HT in human colon in vitro. Br. J. Pharmacol. **135:** 1144–1151.

The Role of the Orbitofrontal Cortex in Anxiety Disorders

MOHAMMED R. MILAD[a] AND SCOTT L. RAUCH[a,b]

[a]Department of Psychiatry, Massachusetts General Hospital and Harvard Medical School, Charlestown, Massachusetts 02129, USA

[b]McLean Hospital, Belmont, Massachusetts 02478, USA

ABSTRACT: Advances in neuroimaging techniques over the past two decades have allowed scientists to investigate the neurocircuitry of anxiety disorders. Such research has implicated the orbitofrontal cortex (OFC). Characterizing the role of OFC in anxiety disorders, however, is principally complicated by two factors–differences in underlying pathophysiology across the anxiety disorders and heterogeneity in function across different OFC sub-territories. Contemporary neurocircuitry models of anxiety disorders have primarily focused on amygdalo-cortical interactions. The amygdala is implicated in generating fear responses, whereas cortical regions, specifically the medial OFC (mOFC) and the ventromedial prefrontal cortex (vmPFC), are implicated in fear extinction. In contrast to mOFC, anterolateral OFC (lOFC) has been associated with negative affects and obsessions and thus dysfunctional lOFC may underlie different aspects of certain anxiety disorders. Herein, we aim to review the above-mentioned theories and provide a heuristic model for conceptualizing the respective roles of mOFC and lOFC in the pathophysiology and treatment of anxiety disorders. We will also review the role of the OFC in fear extinction and the implications of this role to the pathophysiology of anxiety disorders.

KEYWORDS: amygdala; fear extinction; conditioning; ventromedial prefrontal cortex; neuroimaging

INTRODUCTION

The orbitofrontal cortex (OFC) is implicated in a variety of functions, particularly higher-order executive functions. These executive functions include control and inhibition of inappropriate behavioral and emotional responses, decision making, maintaining behavioral flexibility to switch between different problem solving strategies, and evaluation of contingencies between

Address for correspondence: Mohammed R. Milad, Ph.D., Department of Psychiatry, Massachusetts General Hospital, Bldg 149, 13th Street, 2nd Floor, Charlestown, MA 02129. Voice: 617-724-8533; fax: 617-726-4078.

milad@nmr.mgh.harvard.edu

Ann. N.Y. Acad. Sci. 1121: 546–561 (2007). © 2007 New York Academy of Sciences.
doi: 10.1196/annals.1401.006

different stimuli to guide future behaviors to maximize reward and minimize punishment (for example, see Refs. 1–4). Inappropriate function of the OFC, therefore, could lead to an array of behavioral deficits and psychopathology, ranging from making a wrong financial decision to disabling anxiety. Here, we focus on the role of OFC in anxiety disorders. Specifically, we will address: 1) the pertinent neuroanatomical connections of the OFC, 2) the contribution of different sub-regions of the OFC to specific pertinent functions, and 3) the implications of OFC anatomy and function to anxiety disorders. In this review, we will outline findings from studies relevant to these three points with specific emphasis on the human OFC and its contribution to anxiety disorders.

ANATOMICAL CONNECTIONS OF THE OFC

The detailed inputs and outputs of the OFC have been well characterized in rats, non-human primates, and to some degree in humans.[5–9] Though this material will be covered in greater detail elsewhere in this volume, we will summarize the connections that we believe are most pertinent to anxiety disorders. The OFC is part of the prefrontal cortex and receives projections from the magnocellular division of the mediodorsal nucleus of the thalamus.[10] Based on connections and architectonics of the OFC and parts of the medial prefrontal cortex (mPFC), Price and colleagues[5,6] proposed two functional networks: orbital and medial networks of the orbitomedial prefrontal cortex (OMPFC).

According to this classification, the orbital network is composed of mostly lateral orbitofrontal structures that receive input from all sensory modalities and is proposed to be critical for sensory integration and food intake. Lateral OFC projects to more central and dorsal regions of the striatum[11] that may influence behaviors in response to punishment, as well as automated or ritualized behaviors evolved to escape or otherwise mitigate danger. The medial network of the OMPFC includes parts of the ventral medial prefrontal cortex (vmPFC) and anterior cingulate (including BA 25, and parts of BA 32 and 24), as well as parts of the medial division of the OFC. This medial network has projections to visceromotor structures critical to modulate behavior. For example, medial OFC (mOFC, which is part of the medial network) projects massively to the ventral striatum,[12] and these projections are thought to subserve the modulation of reward-related behaviors. Furthermore, mOFC projects to the amygdala[6,13] as well as to the lateral hypothalamus,[14] the periaqueductal gray,[14] and the hippocampus.[9] These projections are thought to influence emotional expression.[13,15] Thus, the anatomical connections to and from the OFC clearly support its overall function in the integration of different sensory modalities and in using this information along with previous experiences to guide future behavioral outcome with maximum benefit to the organism.

OFC FUNCTIONS RELEVANT TO ANXIETY DISORDERS

Lateral versus Medial OFC Function in Reward and Punishment

The function of the OFC in reward and goal-directed behavior has been extensively studied in rodents and in non-human primates (for reviews, see Refs. 2, 16–18). Herein, we will primarily focus on human neuroimaging studies. Several recent neuroimaging studies have shown that the mOFC increases its activity during the anticipation of reward,[19–22] when evaluating attractive faces,[23–25] and during the consumption of chocolate.[26] On the other hand, anterolateral OFC (lOFC) appears to increase its activity in response to cues signaling the absence of reward,[19,27] unpleasant smell and touch,[28,29] anticipation of viewing aversive pictures,[30] and aversion to eating excessive chocolate.[26] Recall of positive affect preferentially activates the mOFC, whereas negative affects preferentially activate the lOFC.[27] Thus, a theme has emerged emphasizing the role of the mOFC in evaluating and mediating responses to positive affective states, whereas the lOFC appears to play a role in evaluating and mediating responses to negative affective states.[31,32] Several other studies have provided additional support for this dichotomous role of the mOFC and lOFC in valence-specific responses.[33,34] Finally, Kringelbach and Rolls[1] have conducted an extensive meta-analysis in which they reviewed 87 published articles that have examined the role of the OFC in rewards and punishments; the results provided support to this heuristic theme dichotomizing the OFC into medial versus lateral subdivisions, associated with positive versus negative valence, respectively. This is pertinent to models of anxiety disorders, given that such conditions are characterized by imbalance toward negatively valenced cognitions, such as anticipation of adverse of outcomes. Thus one might hypothesize that subjects with anxiety disorders would exhibit excessive lOFC and/or deficient mOFC function.

Medial OFC and Fear Extinction

In addition to the above-mentioned functions of the OFC, several animal studies along with recent human neuroimaging studies also implicate the mOFC and the vmPFC in the extinction of conditioned fear responding.[35–40] Several studies have shown that the rat vmPFC is implicated in the extinction of cued fear conditioning.[41–50] Lesions or inactivation of the vmPFC do not prevent short-term extinction learning, but they do impair recall of extinction after a delay.[45,47,49,51] Furthermore, interfering with NMDA receptors, protein kinases, or protein synthesis in vmPFC impairs consolidation of extinction learning.[52,53] Consistent with extinction-related plasticity in vmPFC, neurons in the infralimbic sub-region of vmPFC increase their activity when rats are recalling extinction, as evidenced by single-unit recording,[54] evoked potential recording,[55,56] and metabolic mapping.[42]

Recent neuroimaging studies have specifically linked the human vmPFC to extinction recall after fear conditioning and extinction training. Specifically, using functional MRI, two recent studies showed that vmPFC activity increased during extinction recall.[57,58] Using structural MRI, we recently demonstrated that thickness of the vmPFC in healthy humans was positively correlated with the magnitude of extinction recall expressed in the first two extinction trials during test.[59] Moreover, consistent with the previous neuroimaging studies, we observed increased vmPFC activity to an extinguished conditioned stimulus during extinction recall that was positively correlated with extinction success (measured by skin conductance response).[60] Thus, these recent human neuroimaging data strongly support the role of the mOFC and adjacent vmPFC in expressing extinction memory and therefore reducing conditioned fear to a previously conditioned stimulus.

Challenges to a Parsimonious Account of OFC in Anxiety Disorders

The data are vast regarding functions of OFC across animals and man. We have chosen two popular heuristics that we believe help to organize data pertinent to the role of OFC in anxiety disorders. Nonetheless, we wish to acknowledge and underscore that substantial data exist that do not fit neatly into these conceptualizations and some even contradict these models. In many instances, lack of clarity regarding the precise regions involved highlights the importance of such details, given these heuristics that posit opposite effects based on fine anatomy within OFC. For example, surgically severing cortical (including OFC)-subcortical connections results in the reduction of anxiety symptoms.[61] In a pediatric population examined after traumatic brain injury, the number of lesions within the OFC inversely correlated with anxiety symptoms and post-traumatic stress disorder (PTSD).[62] In rats, whereas inactivation of the infralimbic region reduced anxiety-like defensive responding, inactivation of the ventromedial orbital region had the opposite effect,[63] suggesting that different sub-regions within the vmPFC may have antagonistic effects on anxiety-like behaviors.

CLINICAL CHARACTERISTICS OF ANXIETY DISORDERS

Anxiety disorders are characterized by exaggerated anxiety and inappropriate fear responses to relatively harmless stimuli. Anxiety disorders include PTSD, panic disorder (PD), phobias including social anxiety disorder (SAD) and specific phobia (SP), and obsessive-compulsive disorder (OCD). The pathogenesis of these anxiety disorders remains unknown, though the etiology of PTSD is nominally defined. In the aftermath of a severe traumatic event, PTSD patients develop a constellation of symptoms including re-experiencing phenomena, avoidance, and hyperarousal. PD is characterized by recurrent panic episodes that typically occur spontaneously. Panic attacks entail a rapid escalation to extreme anxiety that is accompanied by physical symptoms including rapid breathing, palpitations, sweating, and dizziness. Emotional and cognitive symptoms, such as the feeling that something catastrophic is about to happen, also accompany panic attacks. Individuals with PD often develop anticipatory anxiety, repeated panic episodes, and avoidance of places or situations where they believe panic attacks are more likely to occur.

Phobias are characterized by exaggerated anxiety responses to innocuous stimuli, such as small animals, or social situations, such as public speaking. The critical phenomenological features across the phobias are that: A) the cause of fear reactions are generally circumscribed and specific, and B) the objects of phobias tend to be stimuli that do in fact pose some degree of threat or risk in a particular setting. OCD is characterized by intrusive, unwanted thoughts (i.e., obsessions) and ritualized, repetitive behaviors (i.e., compulsions). The obsessions are commonly accompanied by anxiety that drives the compulsions. The compulsions, therefore, are performed to neutralize and attenuate the obsessions and anxiety.

CURRENT HYPOTHESES AND FINDINGS REGARDING PATHOPHYSIOLOGY OF ANXIETY DISORDERS: SUPPORT FROM NEUROIMAGING STUDIES

In the following section of this review, we will summarize neuroimaging studies pertaining to the pathophysiology of anxiety disorders. Given the massive literature published in this arena, we will focus on findings related to the medial and lateral regions of the OFC.

Post-traumatic Stress Disorder

One of the hypotheses regarding the development of PTSD is that hyper-conditionability (forming abnormally strong associations between the trauma-induced emotions and stimuli present during trauma exposure),[64,65] along with failure to extinguish these fear responses, may underlie the emotional perseveration commonly observed in PTSD.[38,66-69] This led investigators to hypothesize that the exaggerated fear and anxiety in PTSD may result from hyper-responsivity within the amygdala to threat-related stimuli, with inadequate top-down governance over the amygdala by the vmPFC and mOFC (for example, see Ref. 35).

Indeed, this hypothesis is supported by a substantial body of neuroimaging data. For example, the majority of studies comparing PTSD to non-PTSD control groups have consistently shown diminished mPFC activation (see FIG. 1). Symptom provocation studies indicate that when exposed to reminders of

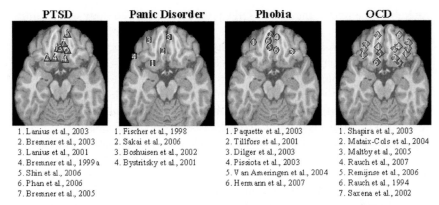

PTSD	Panic Disorder	Phobia	OCD
1. Lanius et al., 2003	1. Fischer et al., 1998	1. Paquette et al., 2003	1. Shapira et al., 2003
2. Bremner et al., 2003	2. Sakai et al., 2006	2. Tillfors et al., 2001	2. Mataix-Cols et al., 2004
3. Lanius et al., 2001	3. Boshuisen et al., 2002	3. Dilger et al., 2003	3. Maltby et al., 2005
4. Bremner et al., 1999a	4. Bystritsky et al., 2001	4. Pissiota et al., 2003	4. Rauch et al., 2007
5. Shin et al., 2006		5. Van Ameringen et al., 2004	5. Remijnse et al., 2006
6. Phan et al., 2006		6. Herrmann et al., 2007	6. Rauch et al., 1994
7. Bremner et al., 2005			7. Saxena et al., 2002

FIGURE 1. Summary of neuroimaging studies across all anxiety disorders showing increases in activity in comparison with controls or associated with anxiety symptoms (illustrated in red across all the anxiety disorders) and decreases in activity in comparison with controls or associated with anxiety symptoms (illustrated in blue across all anxiety disorders).

traumatic events, PTSD patients exhibit attenuated responses within mPFC areas.[70-75] Shin and colleagues[71] observed decreases in mPFC activity that were inversely correlated with increases in amygdala activity in PTSD. Additional support for the involvement of prefrontal areas in PTSD comes from morphometric MRI studies, where PTSD patients showed smaller mPFC volumes in comparison with non-PTSD controls; in some instances, these diminished prefrontal volumes have included mOFC structures. While many of the frontal structural and functional abnormalities in PTSD extend beyond the OFC, several studies have reported such findings that are referable to the mOFC regions as well as adjacent areas. For example, PTSD patients exhibit attenuated mOFC and subcallosal cortical activation during retrieval of emotionally valenced words[76] and during exposure to reminders of traumatic events.[77,78]

Panic Disorder

One hypothesis indicates that panic attacks evolve in the context of what should be minor anxiety episodes because of failures in the systems responsible for limiting such normal responses, similar to the model of PTSD.[38] Alternatively, panic episodes could reflect anxiety responses mediated by structures, such as the amygdala, at the subconscious level. Activation of the amygdala without the awareness of the threat-related stimulus has in fact been documented.[79,80] Thus, this model might characterize PD by fundamental amygdala hyper-responsivity to subtle environmental cues, thereby initiating full-scale threat-related responses in the absence of conscious awareness of the initial triggers. We have previously proposed that the basis for the development of PD resembles the pathogenesis of PTSD, regardless of the etiology of the initial panic attacks.[81]

Data from neuroimaging studies have indicated dysfunctional mOFC and amygdala activity in PD (for example, see Refs. 82, 83, FIG. 1). Some of these studies used symptom-provocation techniques in which the panic episode was pharmacologically induced. For example, Woods and colleagues[84] employed single photon emission computed tomography and yohimbine infusions and found that PD subjects experienced increased anxiety and exhibited decreased regional cerebral blood flow (rCBF) in bilateral frontal cortex. Fischer and colleagues[85] captured a spontaneous panic attack during positron emission tomography (PET) acquisition in a single case and reported data showing decreased rCBF in right mOFC and anterior cingulate cortex during the acute event. Neutral state studies have found increased OFC activity at rest in PD, whereas, successful treatment with imipramine was accompanied by an attenuation of this OFC hyperactivity.[86] Interestingly, an inverse correlation was observed between OFC resting activity in the treated PD patients and their anxiety levels, suggesting again that OFC may be recruited to dampen anxiety in a compensatory fashion. A recent PET study comparing glucose consumption before and after cognitive behavioral therapy showed that successful treatment was accompanied by increased glucose consumption in medial prefrontal areas.[87]

Phobias

Note that, although specific (animal) phobias and SAD represent discrete disorders, we have summarized them beneath the same heading here. This was done pragmatically, due to the limited body of OFC findings for each condition, as well as the convergence of results and phenomenological similarities between these disorders. In phobias, the offending stimuli are generally more circumscribed and of a stereotypic nature. Thus, it has been previously proposed that the clinical features of phobias may reflect hypersensitivity in the pathways that mediate innate fear, responses to stimuli that evolution has made source for this type of fear, such as snakes and spiders.[88] This would most likely involve exaggerated activity of the amygdala along with dysfunction within the OFC.[89] Further, such dysfunction might only be evident during exposure to specific phobic stimuli. Neuroimaging data have in fact supported this view (see FIG. 1). Specifically, OFC dysfunction has been implicated in SAD as well as SP, and these aberrant responses are observed to occur only in the setting of exposure to the phobic object.[90,91] For example, one PET symptom-provocation study contrasting public versus private speaking conditions found decreases in mOFC in the SAD relative to the non-phobic group.[92] Another PET symptom-provocation study reported deactivation of mOFC in SAD during exposure to phobia-inducing events.[93] A recent fMRI study also reported decreased activity of the mOFC in phobic patients upon exposure to phobia-inducing pictures.[94]

Analogous studies have conversely found increased activation in lOFC regions when spider-phobic subjects viewed phobia-related pictures.[95]

Obsessive-Compulsive Disorder

OCD appears to be distinct from the other anxiety disorders in several respects. In general, pathophysiological models of this disorder have focused on cortico-striato-thalamo-cortical circuitry.[96–101] One hypothesis suggests that the primary pathology is within the striatum, which leads to inefficient gating at the level of the thalamus. This leads to hyperactivity within OFC (corresponding to the intrusive thoughts) and hyperactivity within anterior cingulate cortex (corresponding to anxiety, in a non-specific manner).[89,96,102–104] It is important to note that OCD is a highly heterogeneous condition, such that its subtypes may be characterized by somewhat different pathophysiological profiles.

With respect to neuroimaging data and OCD, hyperactivity in the OFC has been the most consistent finding across many studies using different experimental paradigms (for example, see Refs. 96, 105–107, see FIG. 1). Pre/post-treatment studies have likewise indicated attenuation of abnormal regional brain activity within OFC, anterior cingulate cortex, and caudate nucleus associated with successful treatment.[97,108–110] Moreover, similar changes have been observed for both pharmacological and behavioral therapies.[97,111] Treatment studies have also consistently indicated that the magnitude of OFC activity prior to pharmacotherapy predicts subsequent response to serotonin reuptake inhibitors,[97,111,112] such that lesser magnitude of OFC hyperactivity predicts better response to treatment. Symptom provocation studies using PET[113,114] and fMRI[115,116] have also shown increased OFC activation along with increased activation in other brain regions including the anterior cingulate cortex and caudate nucleus; such increases in activity were associated with the OCD symptomatic state. A recent fMRI study has shown that improvement of OCD symptoms either due to pharmacological or behavioral therapy interventions, reduced symptom-provocation increases in the OFC.[117]

Interestingly, increased activation in the lOFC and caudate appear to be specific to OCD. On the other hand, dysfunctional mOFC activity is generally observed across all anxiety disorders.[67] Note that in a symptom-provocation study, Rauch and colleagues[113] showed that whereas OCD symptom severity was directly correlated with lOFC activation, severity of anxiety in OCD was inversely correlated with posteromedial OFC activity (see FIG. 1). It has also been shown that activity within OFC correlated directly with subsequent response to cognitive behavior therapy,[111] consistent with the concept that magnitude of mOFC function may be associated with the capacity for patients to benefit from an extinction-based therapy.

THE ROLE OF THE OFC IN EXTINCTION: IMPLICATIONS FOR ANXIETY DISORDERS

Cognitive behavioral therapy is considered to be effective for essentially all anxiety disorders. As with fear extinction in rats, during behavioral therapy patients with anxiety disorders are exposed to the anxiety-inducing stimuli in the absence of any negative reinforcement.[118] After several sessions of exposure therapy, the majority of patients learn to inhibit their fear responses.[119] However, some patients with anxiety disorders fail to respond to exposure therapy,[120,121] consistent with the hypothesis that extinction learning may be especially deficient in these treatment-resistant patients.

Despite the direct link between OFC dysfunction in anxiety disorders, the role of OFC in fear extinction, and the fact that extinction forms the basis for exposure therapy used to treat anxiety disorders, the integrity of the OFC in anxiety disorders in the context of fear extinction, and specifically extinction recall, has not been thoroughly examined. Although the neuroimaging studies reviewed above have undoubtedly provided critical information regarding the neurocircuitry of anxiety disorders, most of those studies have employed experimental tools that did not directly assess the functional integrity of the OFC during fear extinction. Understanding the neural mechanisms of fear extinction may be fundamental to elucidating the pathophysiology of anxiety disorders. Such a line of inquiry could also enhance our understanding of the mechanism of action by which extinction-based treatments confer their therapeutic effects (e.g. see Refs. 35, 81).

SUMMARY AND CONCLUSIONS

We have presented a brief review, adopting popular schemes for subdividing OFC into mOFC and lOFC zones. This conceptualization provides a useful heuristic for considering the neurocircuitry pertinent to the pathophysiology and treatment of anxiety disorders. Specifically, we propose that the two extremes of OFC dysfunction are manifested in the anxiety disorders. On the one hand, across the anxiety disorders, hypoactive mOFC is detected where there is a failure to inhibit inappropriate fear and anxiety responses. On the other hand, hyperactive lOFC is most commonly detected when there are prominent anxiety-laden cognitions, such as in OCD. This simplistic model reconciles a large volume of initial neuroimaging findings, which otherwise appear superficially inconsistent, with a broad array of OFC increases and decreases. Further, this theoretical framework leads to straightforward testable hypotheses about regional brain function, severity of symptoms, and predictors of treatment response. Perhaps most importantly, this model suggests new targets for neuromodulatory treatments that might seek to enhance mOFC function in the service of fortifying extinction capacity, or to attenuate excessive lOFC activity to mitigate obsessions and worries.

ACKNOWLEDGMENTS

The authors of this review were supported in part by NIMH grants R21MH072156 and RO1MH60219.

REFERENCES

1. KRINGELBACH, M.L. & E.T. ROLLS. 2004. The functional neuroanatomy of the human orbitofrontal cortex: Evidence from neuroimaging and neuropsychology. Prog. Neurobiol. **72:** 341–372.
2. SCHOENBAUM, G. & M. ROESCH. 2005. Orbitofrontal cortex, associative learning, and expectancies. Neuron **47:** 633–636.
3. O'DOHERTY, J. 2003. Can't learn without you: predictive value coding in orbitofrontal cortex requires the basolateral amygdala. Neuron **39:** 731–733.
4. IZQUIERDO, A., R.K. SUDA & E.A. MURRAY. 2004. Bilateral orbital prefrontal cortex lesions in rhesus monkeys disrupt choices guided by both reward value and reward contingency. J. Neurosci. **24:** 7540–7548.
5. ONGUR, D., A.T. FERRY & J.L. PRICE. 2003. Architectonic subdivision of the human orbital and medial prefrontal cortex. J. Comp Neurol. **460:** 425–449.
6. ONGUR, D. & J.L. PRICE. 2000. The organization of networks within the orbital and medial prefrontal cortex of rats, monkeys and humans. Cereb. Cortex **10:** 206–219.
7. CARMICHAEL, S.T. & J.L. PRICE. 1994. Architectonic subdivision of the orbital and medial prefrontal cortex in the macaque monkey. J. Comp Neurol. **346:** 366–402.
8. BARBAS, H. 2000. Connections underlying the synthesis of cognition, memory, and emotion in primate prefrontal cortices. Brain Res Bull. **52:** 319–330.
9. CAVADA, C. *et al.* 2000. The anatomical connections of the macaque monkey orbitofrontal cortex. A review. Cereb. Cortex **10:** 220–242.
10. FUSTER, J.M. 2001. The prefrontal cortex–an update: Time is of the essence. Neuron **30:** 319–333.
11. FERRY, A.T., X.C. LU & J.L. PRICE. 2000. Effects of excitotoxic lesions in the ventral striatopallidal–thalamocortical pathway on odor reversal learning: Inability to extinguish an incorrect response. Exp. Brain Res. **131:** 320–335.
12. FERRY, A.T. *et al.* 2000. Prefrontal cortical projections to the striatum in macaque monkeys: Evidence for an organization related to prefrontal networks. J. Comp Neurol. **425:** 447–470.
13. BARBAS, H. *et al.* 2003. Serial pathways from primate prefrontal cortex to autonomic areas may influence emotional expression. BMC Neurosci. **4:** 25.
14. FLOYD, N.S. *et al.* 2000. Orbitomedial prefrontal cortical projections to distinct longitudinal columns of the periaqueductal gray in the rat. J. Comp Neurol. **422:** 556–578.
15. GUSNARD, D.A. *et al.* 2003. Persistence and brain circuitry. Proc. Natl. Acad. Sci. USA **100:** 3479–3484.
16. SCHULTZ, W. 2006. Behavioral theories and the neurophysiology of reward. Annu. Rev. Psychol. **57:** 87–115.
17. ROLLS, E.T. 2004. The functions of the orbitofrontal cortex. Brain Cogn. **55:** 11–29.

18. HOLLAND, P.C. & M. GALLAGHER. 2004. Amygdala-frontal interactions and reward expectancy. Curr. Opin. Neurobiol. **14:** 148–155.
19. URSU, S. & C.S. CARTER. 2005. Outcome representations, counterfactual comparisons and the human orbitofrontal cortex: implications for neuroimaging studies of decision-making. Brain Res. Cogn. Brain Res. **23:** 51–60.
20. COX, S.M., A. ANDRADE & I.S. JOHNSRUDE. 2005. Learning to like: a role for human orbitofrontal cortex in conditioned reward. J. Neurosci. **25:** 2733–2740.
21. GALVAN, A. *et al.* 2005. The role of ventral frontostriatal circuitry in reward-based learning in humans. J. Neurosci. **25:** 8650–8656.
22. KIM, H., S. SHIMOJO & J.P. O'DOHERTY. 2006. Is avoiding an aversive outcome rewarding? Neural substrates of avoidance learning in the human brain. PLoS Biol. **4:** e233.
23. O'DOHERTY, J. *et al.* 2003. Beauty in a smile: The role of medial orbitofrontal cortex in facial attractiveness. Neuropsychologia **41:** 147–155.
24. WINSTON, J.S. *et al.* 2007. Brain systems for assessing facial attractiveness. Neuropsychologia **45:** 195–206.
25. ISHAI, A. 2007. Sex, beauty and the orbitofrontal cortex. Int. J. Psychophysiol. **63:** 181–185.
26. SMALL, D.M. *et al.* 2003. Dissociation of neural representation of intensity and affective valuation in human gustation. Neuron **39:** 701–711.
27. MARKOWITSCH, H.J. *et al.* 2003. Engagement of lateral and medial prefrontal areas in the ecphory of sad and happy autobiographical memories. Cortex **39:** 643–665.
28. ROLLS, E.T., M.L. KRINGELBACH & I.E. DE ARAUJO. 2003. Different representations of pleasant and unpleasant odours in the human brain. Eur. J. Neurosci. **18:** 695–703.
29. ROLLS, E.T., J.V. VERHAGEN & M. KADOHISA. 2003. Representations of the texture of food in the primate orbitofrontal cortex: neurons responding to viscosity, grittiness, and capsaicin. J. Neurophysiol. **90:** 3711–3724.
30. NITSCHKE, J.B., I. SARINOPOULOS, K.L. MACKIEWICZ, *et al.* 2006. Functional neuroanatomy of aversion and its anticipation. Neuroimage **29:** 106–116.
31. ELLIOTT, R. *et al.* 2000. Selective attention to emotional stimuli in a verbal go/no-go task: an fMRI study. Neuroreport **11:** 1739–1744.
32. O'DOHERTY, J. *et al.* 2001. Abstract reward and punishment representations in the human orbitofrontal cortex. Nat. Neurosci. **4:** 95–102.
33. BLAIR, R.J. *et al.* 1999. Dissociable neural responses to facial expressions of sadness and anger. Brain **122**(Pt 5): 883–893.
34. ZALD, D.H. & J.V. PARDO. 2000. Functional neuroimaging of the olfactory system in humans. Int. J. Psychophysiol. **36:** 165–181.
35. MILAD, M.R. *et al.* 2006. Fear extinction in rats: implications for human brain imaging and anxiety disorders. Biol. Psychol. **73:** 61–71.
36. BARAD, M. 2005. Fear extinction in rodents: basic insight to clinical promise. Curr. Opin. Neurobiol. **15:** 710–715.
37. SOTRES-BAYON, F., C.K. CAIN & J.E. LEDOUX. 2006. Brain mechanisms of fear extinction: historical perspectives on the contribution of prefrontal cortex. Biol. Psychiatry **60:** 329–336.
38. RAUCH, S.L., L.M. SHIN & E.A. PHELPS. 2006. Neurocircuitry models of post-traumatic stress disorder and extinction: Human neuroimaging research–past, present, and future. Biol. Psychiatry **60:** 376–382.

39. QUIRK, G.J., R. GARCIA & F. GONZALEZ-LIMA. 2006. Prefrontal mechanisms in extinction of conditioned fear. Biol. Psychiatry **60:** 337–343.
40. DAVIS, M. *et al.* 2006. Pharmacological treatments that facilitate extinction of fear: relevance to psychotherapy. NeuroRx. **3:** 82–96.
41. BERRETTA, S. *et al.* 2005. Infralimbic cortex activation increases c-Fos expression in intercalated neurons of the amygdala. Neuroscience **132:** 943–953.
42. BARRETT, D. *et al.* 2003. Metabolic mapping of mouse brain activity after extinction of a conditioned emotional response. J. Neurosci. **23:** 5740–5749.
43. HERRY, C. & N. MONS. 2004. Resistance to extinction is associated with impaired immediate early gene induction in medial prefrontal cortex and amygdala. Eur. J. Neurosci. **20:** 781–790.
44. SIERRA-MERCADO, D. *et al.* 2006. Inactivation of ventromedial prefrontal cortex reduces expression of conditioned fear and impairs subsequent recall of extinction. Eur. J. Neurosci. **24:** 1751–1758.
45. CORCORAN, K.A. & G.J. QUIRK. 2007. Activity in prelimbic cortex is necessary for the expression of learned, but not innate, fears. J. Neurosci. **27:** 840–844.
46. QUIRK, G.J. *et al.* 2000. The role of ventromedial prefrontal cortex in the recovery of extinguished fear. J. Neurosci. **20:** 6225–6231.
47. LEBRON, K., M.R. MILAD & G.J. QUIRK. 2004. Delayed recall of fear extinction in rats with lesions of ventral medial prefrontal cortex. Learn. Mem. **11:** 544–548.
48. SANTINI, E. *et al.* 2004. Consolidation of fear extinction requires protein synthesis in the medial prefrontal cortex. J. Neurosci. **24:** 5704–5710.
49. MORGAN, M.A., L.M. ROMANSKI & J.E. LEDOUX. 1993. Extinction of emotional learning: contribution of medial prefrontal cortex. Neurosci. Lett. **163:** 109–113.
50. MILAD, M.R., I. VIDAL-GONZALEZ & G.J. QUIRK. 2004. Electrical stimulation of medial prefrontal cortex reduces conditioned fear in a temporally specific manner. Behav. Neurosci. **118:** 389–394.
51. SIERRA-MERCADO, D., JR. *et al.* 2006. Inactivation of the ventromedial prefrontal cortex reduces expression of conditioned fear and impairs subsequent recall of extinction. Eur. J. Neurosci. **24:** 1751–1758.
52. HUGUES, S., O. DESCHAUX & R. GARCIA. 2004. Postextinction infusion of a mitogen-activated protein kinase inhibitor into the medial prefrontal cortex impairs memory of the extinction of conditioned fear. Learn. Mem. **11:** 540–543.
53. BURGOS-ROBLES, A. *et al.* 2007. Consolidation of fear extinction requires NMDA receptor-dependent bursting in the ventromedial prefrontal cortex. Neuron **53:** 871–880.
54. MILAD, M.R. & G.J. QUIRK. 2002. Neurons in medial prefrontal cortex signal memory for fear extinction. Nature **420:** 70–74.
55. HERRY, C. & R. GARCIA. 2002. Prefrontal cortex long-term potentiation, but not long-term depression, is associated with the maintenance of extinction of learned fear in mice. J. Neurosci. **22:** 577–583.
56. FARINELLI, M. *et al.* 2006. Hippocampal train stimulation modulates recall of fear extinction independently of prefrontal cortex synaptic plasticity and lesions. Learn. Mem. **13:** 329–334.
57. KALISCH, R. *et al.* 2006. Context-dependent human extinction memory is mediated by a ventromedial prefrontal and hippocampal network. J. Neurosci. **26:** 9503–9511.

58. PHELPS, E.A. *et al.* 2004. Extinction learning in humans: role of the amygdala and vmPFC. Neuron **43:** 897–905.
59. MILAD, M.R. *et al.* 2005. Thickness of ventromedial prefrontal cortex in humans is correlated with extinction memory. Proc. Natl. Acad. Sci. USA **102:** 10706–10711.
60. MILAD, M.R. *et al.* 2007. Recall of fear extinction in humans activates the ventromedial prefrontal cortex and hippocampus in concert. Biol. Psychiatry **62:** 446–454.
61. WEINGARTEN, S. 1999. The Human Frontal Lobes: functions and Disorders. B. Miller & J. Cummings, Eds. Guilford Press. New York.
62. VASA, R.A. *et al.* 2004. Neuroimaging correlates of anxiety after pediatric traumatic brain injury. Biol. Psychiatry **55:** 208–216.
63. WALL, P.M. *et al.* 2004. Differential effects of infralimbic vs. ventromedial orbital PFC lidocaine infusions in CD-1 mice on defensive responding in the mouse defense test battery and rat exposure test. Brain Res **1020:** 73–85.
64. ORR, S.P. *et al.* 2000. De novo conditioning in trauma-exposed individuals with and without posttraumatic stress disorder. J. Abnorm. Psychol. **109:** 290–298.
65. ORR, S.P., L.J. METZGER & R.K. PITMAN. 2002. Psychophysiology of posttraumatic stress disorder. Psychiatr. Clin. North Am. **25:** 271–293.
66. LIBERZON, I. & B. MARTIS. 2006. Neuroimaging studies of emotional responses in PTSD. Ann. N. Y. Acad. Sci **1071:** 87–109.
67. RAUCH, S.L. *et al.* 1998. Neuroimaging and the neuroanatomy of PTSD. CNS Spectr. **3:** 30–41.
68. DAVIS, M. *et al.* 2006. Effects of d-cycloserine on extinction: translation from preclinical to clinical work. Biol. Psychiatry **60:** 369–375.
69. PITMAN, R.K., L.M. SHIN & S.L. RAUCH. 2001. Investigating the pathogenesis of posttraumatic stress disorder with neuroimaging. J. Clin. Psychiatry **62**(Suppl 17): 47–54.
70. PHAN, K.L. *et al.* 2006. Corticolimbic blood flow during nontraumatic emotional processing in posttraumatic stress disorder. Arch. Gen. Psychiatry **63:** 184–192.
71. SHIN, L.M. *et al.* 2004. Regional cerebral blood flow in the amygdala and medial prefrontal cortex during traumatic imagery in male and female Vietnam veterans with PTSD. Arch. Gen. Psychiatry **61:** 168–176.
72. SHIN, L.M. *et al.* 2001. An fMRI study of anterior cingulate function in posttraumatic stress disorder. Biol. Psychiatry **50:** 932–942.
73. SHIN, L.M. *et al.* 1999. Regional cerebral blood flow during script-driven imagery in childhood sexual abuse-related PTSD: a PET investigation. Am. J. Psychiatry **156:** 575–584.
74. LANIUS, R.A. *et al.* 2002. Brain activation during script-driven imagery induced dissociative responses in PTSD: a functional magnetic resonance imaging investigation. Biol. Psychiatry **52:** 305–311.
75. LIBERZON, I., J.C. BRITTON & K.L. PHAN. 2003. Neural correlates of traumatic recall in posttraumatic stress disorder. Stress **6:** 151–156.
76. BREMNER, J.D. *et al.* 2003. Neural correlates of declarative memory for emotionally valenced words in women with posttraumatic stress disorder related to early childhood sexual abuse. Biol. Psychiatry **53:** 879–889.
77. BREMNER, J.D. *et al.* 1999. Neural correlates of exposure to traumatic pictures and sound in Vietnam combat veterans with and without posttraumatic stress

disorder: a positron emission tomography study. Biol. Psychiatry **45:** 806–816.

78. BREMNER, J.D. 1999. Alterations in brain structure and function associated with post-traumatic stress disorder. Semin. Clin. Neuropsychiatry **4:** 249–255.

79. MORRIS, J.S., A. OHMAN & R.J. DOLAN. 1998. Conscious and unconscious emotional learning in the human amygdala. Nature **393:** 467–470.

80. WHALEN, P.J. *et al.* 1998. Masked presentations of emotional facial expressions modulate amygdala activity without explicit knowledge. J. Neurosci. **18:** 411–418.

81. RAUCH, S.L., L.M. SHIN & C.I. WRIGHT. 2003. Neuroimaging studies of amygdala function in anxiety disorders. Ann. N. Y. Acad. Sci. **985:** 389–410.

82. BYSTRITSKY, A. *et al.* 2001. Functional MRI changes during panic anticipation and imagery exposure. Neuroreport **12:** 3953–3957.

83. SAKAI, Y. *et al.* 2005. Cerebral glucose metabolism associated with a fear network in panic disorder. Neuroreport **16:** 927–931.

84. WOODS, S.W. *et al.* 1988. Carbon dioxide-induced anxiety. Behavioral, physiologic, and biochemical effects of carbon dioxide in patients with panic disorders and healthy subjects. Arch. Gen. Psychiatry **45:** 43–52.

85. FISCHER, H. *et al.* 1998. Brain correlates of an unexpected panic attack: a human positron emission tomographic study. Neurosci. Lett. **251:** 137–140.

86. NORDAHL, T.E. *et al.* 1998. Regional cerebral metabolic asymmetries replicated in an independent group of patients with panic disorders. Biol. Psychiatry **44:** 998–1006.

87. SAKAI, Y. *et al.* 2006. Changes in cerebral glucose utilization in patients with panic disorder treated with cognitive-behavioral therapy. Neuroimage **33:** 218–226.

88. OHMAN, A. & S. MINEKA. 2001. Fears, phobias, and preparedness: toward an evolved module of fear and fear learning. Psychol. Rev. **108:** 483–522.

89. AOUIZERATE, B. *et al.* 2004. Pathophysiology of obsessive-compulsive disorder: a necessary link between phenomenology, neuropsychology, imagery and physiology. Prog. Neurobiol. **72:** 195–221.

90. PISSIOTA, A. *et al.* 2003. Amygdala and anterior cingulate cortex activation during affective startle modulation: a PET study of fear. Eur. J. Neurosci. **18:** 1325–1331.

91. PAQUETTE, V. *et al.* 2003. "Change the mind and you change the brain": effects of cognitive-behavioral therapy on the neural correlates of spider phobia. Neuroimage **18:** 401–409.

92. TILLFORS, M. *et al.* 2001. Cerebral blood flow in subjects with social phobia during stressful speaking tasks: a PET study. Am. J. Psychiatry **158:** 1220–1226.

93. VAN AMERINGEN, M. *et al.* 2004. A PET provocation study of generalized social phobia. Psychiatry Res **132:** 13–18.

94. HERMANN, A. *et al.* 2007. Diminished medial prefrontal cortex activity in blood-injection-injury phobia. Biol. Psychol. **75:** 124–130.

95. DILGER, S. *et al.* 2003. Brain activation to phobia-related pictures in spider phobic humans: an event-related functional magnetic resonance imaging study. Neurosci. Lett. **348:** 29–32.

96. CANNISTRARO, P.A. & S.L. RAUCH. 2003. Neural circuitry of anxiety: evidence from structural and functional neuroimaging studies. Psychopharmacol. Bull. **37:** 8–25.

97. BAXTER, L.R., JR. 1992. Neuroimaging studies of obsessive compulsive disorder. Psychiatr. Clin. North Am. **15:** 871–884.
98. SAXENA, S. & S.L. RAUCH. 2000. Functional neuroimaging and the neuroanatomy of obsessive-compulsive disorder. Psychiatr. Clin. North Am. **23:** 563–586.
99. VAN DEN HEUVEL, O.A. *et al.* 2005. Disorder-specific neuroanatomical correlates of attentional bias in obsessive-compulsive disorder, panic disorder, and hypochondriasis. Arch. Gen. Psychiatry **62:** 922–933.
100. REMIJNSE, P.L. *et al.* 2006. Reduced orbitofrontal-striatal activity on a reversal learning task in obsessive-compulsive disorder. Arch. Gen. Psychiatry **63:** 1225–1236.
101. MALTBY, N. *et al.* 2005. Dysfunctional action monitoring hyperactivates frontal-striatal circuits in obsessive-compulsive disorder: an event-related fMRI study. Neuroimage **24:** 495–503.
102. GRAYBIEL, A.M. & S.L. RAUCH. 2000. Toward a neurobiology of obsessive-compulsive disorder. Neuron **28:** 343–347.
103. ZALD, D.H. & S.W. KIM. 1996. Anatomy and function of the orbital frontal cortex, I: anatomy, neurocircuitry; and obsessive-compulsive disorder. J. Neuropsychiatry Clin. Neurosci. **8:** 125–138.
104. ZALD, D.H. & S.W. KIM. 1996. Anatomy and function of the orbital frontal cortex, II: Function and relevance to obsessive-compulsive disorder. J. Neuropsychiatry Clin. Neurosci. **8:** 249–261.
105. SHAPIRA, N.A. *et al.* 2003. Brain activation by disgust-inducing pictures in obsessive-compulsive disorder. Biol. Psychiatry **54:** 751–756.
106. MATAIX-COLS, D. *et al.* 2004. Distinct neural correlates of washing, checking, and hoarding symptom dimensions in obsessive-compulsive disorder. Arch. Gen. Psychiatry **61:** 564–576.
107. RAUCH, S.L. *et al.* 2007. Functional magnetic resonance imaging study of regional brain activation during implicit sequence learning in obsessive-compulsive disorder. Biol. Psychiatry **61:** 330–336.
108. HURLEY, R.A. *et al.* 2002. Predicting treatment response in obsessive-compulsive disorder. J. Neuropsychiatry Clin. Neurosci. **14:** 249–253.
109. PERANI, D. *et al.* 1995. [18F]FDG PET study in obsessive-compulsive disorder. A clinical/metabolic correlation study after treatment. Br. J. Psychiatry **166:** 244–250.
110. SWEDO, S.E., H.L. LEONARD & J.L. RAPOPORT. 1992. Childhood-onset obsessive compulsive disorder. Psychiatr. Clin. North Am. **15:** 767–775.
111. BRODY, A.L. *et al.* 1998. FDG-PET predictors of response to behavioral therapy and pharmacotherapy in obsessive compulsive disorder. Psychiatry Res. **84:** 1–6.
112. RAUCH, S.L. *et al.* 2002. Predictors of fluvoxamine response in contamination-related obsessive compulsive disorder: A PET symptom provocation study. Neuropsychopharmacology **27:** 782–791.
113. RAUCH, S.L. *et al.* 1994. Regional cerebral blood flow measured during symptom provocation in obsessive-compulsive disorder using oxygen 15-labeled carbon dioxide and positron emission tomography. Arch. Gen. Psychiatry **51:** 62–70.
114. McGUIRE, P.K. *et al.* 1994. Functional anatomy of obsessive-compulsive phenomena. Br. J. Psychiatry **164:** 459–468.
115. ADLER, C.M. *et al.* 2000. fMRI of neuronal activation with symptom provocation in unmedicated patients with obsessive compulsive disorder. J. Psychiatr. Res. **34:** 317–324.

116. BREITER, H.C. *et al.* 1996. Functional magnetic resonance imaging of symptom provocation in obsessive-compulsive disorder. Arch. Gen. Psychiatry **53:** 595–606.
117. NAKAO, T. *et al.* 2005. [Duration effect on neuropsychological function and treatment response of OCD]. Seishin Shinkeigaku Zasshi **107:** 1286–1298.
118. WALD, J. & S. TAYLOR. 2003. Preliminary research on the efficacy of virtual reality exposure therapy to treat driving phobia. Cyberpsychol. Behav. **6:** 459–465.
119. DAVIDSON, J.R. & E.B. FOA. 1991. Refining criteria for posttraumatic stress disorder. Hosp. Community Psychiatry **42:** 259–261.
120. FOA, E.B. 2000. Psychosocial treatment of posttraumatic stress disorder. J. Clin. Psychiatry **61**(Suppl 5): 43–48.
121. VAN MINNEN, A. & M. HAGENAARS. 2002. Fear activation and habituation patterns as early process predictors of response to prolonged exposure treatment in PTSD. J. Trauma Stress **15:** 359–367.

Vulnerability of the Orbitofrontal Cortex to Age-Associated Structural and Functional Brain Changes

SUSAN M. RESNICK,[a] MELISSA LAMAR,[b] AND IRA DRISCOLL[a]

[a]Intramural Research Program, National Institute on Aging, Gerontology Research Center, Baltimore, Maryland 21224, USA

[b]Institute of Psychiatry, King's College London, De Crespigny Park, London, England SE5 8AH, United Kingdom

ABSTRACT: Cross-sectional and longitudinal findings from the Baltimore Longitudinal Study of Aging (BLSA) neuroimaging study indicate that the orbitofrontal cortex (OFC) is among those regions vulnerable to age-associated tissue loss in older adults without dementia. Neuropathologic and recent *in vivo* amyloid imaging studies indicate that the OFC is also among the earliest neocortical regions to show deposition of amyloid plaques in aging and Alzheimer's disease. We performed behavioral and imaging studies to investigate age effects on specific aspects of OFC function. We compared performance in young (age 20–40) and old (age 60 and older) adults on cognitive tasks selected for differential sensitivity to OFC versus dorsolateral prefrontal cortex (DLPFC). Overall, greater age differences were seen in the OFC tasks compared to DLPFC tasks, with Delayed Match and Non-Match to Sample tasks showing the greatest effect size among OFC tasks and Self-Ordered Pointing Task showing the greatest effect size among DLPFC tasks. A functional magnetic resonance imaging study was conducted in parallel to probe the neural underpinnings of age differences in OFC function using the Delayed Match and Non-Match to Sample paradigm. Young but not old adults showed the expected OFC activation. Older compared with young adults showed greater activation in association with successful performance for several posterior regions, perhaps indicating compensation in the face of OFC deficits. Together, these findings indicate a vulnerability of the OFC to age-related decline in brain structure and function. Future studies using new *in vivo* imaging probes will help determine whether neuropathologic changes underlie the structural and functional changes.

KEYWORDS: orbitofrontal cortex; aging; cognition; MRI; longitudinal studies

Address for correspondence: Susan M. Resnick, LPC/NIA/NIH, Box 3, 5600 Nathan Shock Drive, Baltimore, MD 21224–6825. Voice: 410-558-8618; fax: 410-558-8674.
susan.resnick@nih.gov

Ann. N.Y. Acad. Sci. 1121: 562–575 (2007). © 2007 New York Academy of Sciences.
doi: 10.1196/annals.1401.027

INTRODUCTION

Longitudinal studies from the Baltimore Longitudinal Study of Aging (BLSA)[1] and other samples[2] have shown that some aspects of memory and other cognitive functions show age-related changes in older adults without dementia. Numerous studies attest to the fact that normal age-related decline is not unique to humans and is commonly observed in normally aging non-human animals as well.[3–5] However, only specific aspects of cognition may show age-related declines, and the rates of decline may vary among cognitive domains. In humans, crystallized abilities or overlearned skills, such as vocabulary and other language skills, show little change with normal aging, but fluid or more novel and complex cognitive skills, including executive functions (complex organization, planning, and judgment), spatial abilities, and memory show marked age-related changes in average performance.

Similarly, both global and regional changes with age in brain structure and function are well documented.[6–10] Using magnetic resonance imaging (MRI) to measure brain structure in older individuals without dementia, many investigations have shown age-related decreases in brain volume and increases in cerebrospinal fluid (CSF), an indirect measure of brain atrophy. Functional MRI (fMRI) studies using a variety of different paradigms also indicate the effects of age on regional brain activation patterns, with many studies showing different patterns of activation in older compared with younger persons even in the face of comparable behavioral task performance.[11,12] These shifts in the neural networks underlying successful performance have been interpreted as functional compensation in older individuals.

To understand how age may influence the structure and function of the orbitofrontal region, it is important to examine these associations within the context of cognitive and brain aging generally. In this paper, we use data from the BLSA to highlight some aspects of cognition that show age-related declines and to characterize the age-associated orbitofrontal cortex (OFC) volume changes that motivated our studies of OFC function in non-BLSA samples. Next, we describe these studies targeted specifically to understanding age effects on behavioral performance and fMRI functional activation patterns using tasks that tap orbitofrontal functions.

REPRESENTATIVE BLSA STUDIES OF COGNITIVE FUNCTION

The BLSA is a volunteer cohort of community-dwelling adults followed by the National Institute on Aging to study prospectively the effects of normal aging.[13] The BLSA was initiated in 1958, with women enrolled since 1978, and is the longest running prospective study of aging in the United States. Since

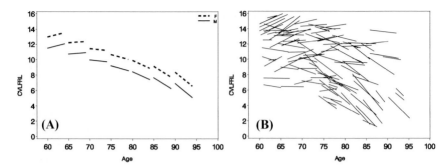

FIGURE 1. (**A** [*left*]) Mean predicted scores from mixed-effects regression for delayed free recall performance on the California Verbal Learning Test for the sample of 823 BLSA participants and (**B** [*right*]) individual trajectories for a random subset of 166 participants (modified from Lamar *et al.*[14]). CVLFRL is the long delay free recall score.

1986, a diagnostic battery of neuropsychological tests has been administered to older individuals in conjunction with other cognitive measures, and consensus conference–based diagnoses of dementia and cognitive impairment have been made. This clinical diagnostic information not only provides prospective information on dementia diagnoses, but also allows analysis of "normal aging," excluding individuals who subsequently receive diagnoses of dementia. Although some cognitively normal individuals will later develop dementia, these individuals are likely to be further from the onset of illness in comparison to studies dependent on cross-sectional evaluations.

BLSA studies have contributed to our understanding of age-related changes in specific aspects of cognitive function. Age differences and longitudinal age changes have been observed for verbal[14] and visual memory[1, 15] tasks in individuals without dementia. For example, on the California Verbal Learning Test[16] (CVLT), the ability to learn and remember a 16-item shopping list declines linearly with age. Interestingly, longitudinal studies of CVLT performance show that the nature of the longitudinal change observed is dependent on the age of the individual at base line, with greater practice effects in younger compared to older adults and greater apparent longitudinal decline in older individuals. Longitudinal trajectories for the BLSA sample as a whole and for a random subset of individuals are shown for CVLT delayed free recall in FIGURE 1A and B, respectively.[14]

Age differences and age changes over time also are apparent on a test of short-term visual memory and visuo-constructional ability, the Benton Visual Retention Test (BVRT).[17] As shown in FIGURE 2, numbers of errors increase with age,[1, 15] with accelerated increases in errors and decreases in performance after age 70. In addition, poor performance reflected in increased numbers of errors, predicts a subsequent diagnosis of Alzheimer's disease as long as 10–15 years prior to diagnosis.[18, 19]

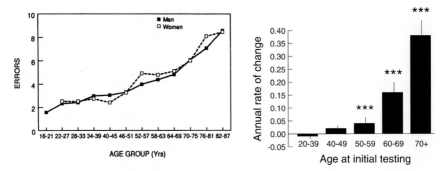

FIGURE 2. Cross-sectional age differences[1] and longitudinal increases[15] in errors on the Benton Visual Retention Test.

BLSA Studies of Structural Brain Aging

Age-Associated Changes in Brain Structure in Older Adults without Dementia

Age-related changes in cognitive performance described in the previous section indicate changes in average performance. However, as shown in FIGURE 1B, there are individual differences in the trajectories of cognitive performance over time. To better understand the possible neural underpinnings of these individual differences in cognitive aging, we began a longitudinal neuroimaging study of brain structure and function in 1994. A selected group of 158 BLSA participants with prior cognitive testing and between the ages of 55–85 years were enrolled in the BLSA neuroimaging study. At enrollment, participants were free of central nervous system disease (epilepsy, stroke, bipolar illness, prior diagnosis of dementia), severe cardiovascular disease (myocardial infarction, coronary artery disease requiring angioplasty or bypass surgery), severe pulmonary disease, and metastatic cancer. Neuroimaging participants had MRI studies of brain structure and positron emission tomography (PET) studies of regional cerebral blood flow during resting and memory task conditions, as well as neuropsychological assessments, annually through year 9 (8-year follow-up) and in conjunction with the BLSA visit schedule after the ninth evaluation. The primary reports of age-related changes in brain structure[7,20,21] and function[22,23] have been published. In the next section, we describe our findings showing structural brain changes in older adults without dementia to provide a context against which OFC tissue loss can be evaluated.

Our initial reports of the effects of age on brain structure focused on cross-sectional age differences and 1-year changes,[20] as well as on longitudinal changes over a 4-year follow-up.[7] Cross-sectional analysis of age differences in a subsample of 116 individuals (mean age at base line: 70.4 ± 7.5) completing two assessments showed modest negative associations between age

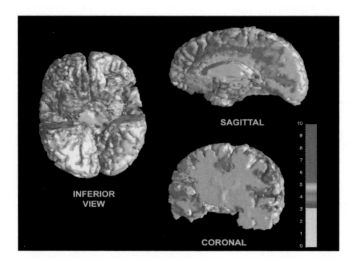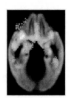

FIGURE 3. Three-dimensional view of specific gray-matter regions showing increased vulnerability to the effects of age.[7] Age-related tissue loss in the OFC is highlighted on a single gray-matter tissue density slice, with brighter areas reflecting greater tissue loss.

and total gray- ($r = -0.23$, $P < 0.05$) and white-matter ($r = -0.29$, $P < 0.05$) volumes.[20] Age effects were greater for frontal and parietal than temporal and occipital lobar volumes. Our studies of 4-year change in brain volume in 92 neuroimaging participants (mean age at base line: 70.4 ± 7.0) without dementia showed that brain volumes (gray and white matter) declined at a rate of 5.5 cm^3 per year, which reflects approximately 0.5% per year.[7] On average, gray-matter volumes declined 2.4 cm^3 per year, white-matter tissue loss was 3.1 cm^3 per year, and ventricular CSF, an indirect measure of central atrophy, increased 1.4 cm^3 per year. Rates of tissue loss in these global brain volumes and increased ventricular CSF remained significant in a subsample of 24 exceptionally healthy older adults without hypertension or other medical co-morbidities.

Against this background of more global tissue loss, we applied voxel-based analysis of stereotaxically normalized MRI images to identify local brain regions that showed the greatest sensitivity to age-related tissue loss. As shown in FIGURE 3, specific regions of vulnerability to age-related gray-matter loss included medial and lateral OFC, cingulate gyrus, insula, and medial temporal regions.

Accelerated Brain Changes in Cognitively Impaired Older Adults

We are continuing to follow our neuroimaging sample of older adults as they continue to age and pass through the risk period for cognitive impairment. To

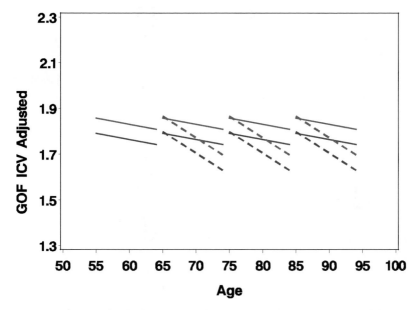

FIGURE 4. Longitudinal age changes in tissue loss, adjusted for intracranial volume, in OFC in men (blue) and women (red) with normal cognition (*solid line*) and MCI (*dashed line*). (In color in *Annals* online.)

date, 18 individuals have received diagnoses of mild cognitive impairment (MCI), defined as progressive memory impairment without evidence of functional loss in everyday activities.[24] Excluding all imaging data from evaluations coinciding with and subsequent to a diagnosis of dementia (5 of 18 with MCI had subsequent diagnosis of dementia), we compared the rates of global and regional brain changes in these 18 individuals with MCI to the rates of brain changes in 131 participants who remained cognitively healthy and did not develop MCI or dementia.[24] Mixed-effects regression analyses, adjusting for intracranial volume at baseline MRI, age at base line, sex, and diagnosis confirmed our prior findings of significant tissue loss over time in older adults without dementia for global brain structures and many individual brain regions. In addition, these studies demonstrated accelerated rates of brain-volume loss and ventricular CSF increase in individuals with MCI compared with cognitively unimpaired participants. Accelerated rates of tissue loss in association with MCI were observed in a number of specific regions, primarily in frontal and temporal cortex. Of note, the OFC (FIG. 4) was among those regions showing accelerated rates of tissue loss in individuals with MCI compared to those who remained cognitively normal (mean [SD] tissue loss per year: $0.17 \, \text{cm}^3$ in MCI; $0.09 \, \text{cm}^3$ in cognitively normal persons). In contrast, rates of tissue loss in the cingulate cortex as a whole were similar in MCI and cognitively healthy individuals.

Neuropathologic Changes in OFC

The accelerated rate of tissue loss in OFC in association with cognitive impairment in older adults is of particular interest in view of the delineation of the progression of plaque and neurofibrillary tangles reported by Braak and Braak.[25] While neurofibrillary tangles are first observed in mesial temporal lobe structures, particularly the hippocampus and entorhinal cortex, the OFC and more lateral aspects of the temporal cortex are among the first regions showing deposition of amyloid plaques. Thus, tissue loss in the OFC may reflect neurotoxic effects of plaque deposition, whereas tissue loss in the mesial temporal lobe structures may be due to tangle formation. Recently, methods for *in vivo* PET imaging of amyloid plaques have become available. Initial findings from studies of patients with early Alzheimer's disease and MCI have confirmed the early presence of amyloid plaques in OFC. Imaging findings also have revealed the presence of amyloid deposition in at least 10% of cognitively normal individuals,[26] a finding consistent with results from autopsy studies.[27,28] New PET imaging tracers for *in vivo* localization of Alzheimer's disease-type pathology will allow investigation of the impact of neuropathology in specific brain structures, including the OFC, on trajectories of cognitive change over time and the development of cognitive impairment.

The Effects of Age on Prefrontal Function

On the basis of our observations of the relative vulnerability of the OFC to MRI-assessed volume loss, we initiated a series of studies to further probe the effects of age on prefrontal function, focusing on the OFC. We recruited individuals from the larger community, as opposed to those in the BLSA, who were free of cognitive impairment and medical co-morbidities, including treated hypertension. In the first study,[29] we investigated behavioral performance differences in young compared to old individuals on a battery of tasks selected on the basis of lesion and/or neuroimaging studies demonstrating their differential reliance on the OFC versus dorsolateral prefrontal cortex (DLPFC). In the second study,[30] we probed OFC functional activation using functional fMRI and Delayed Match and Non-Match to Sample tasks previously shown to preferentially activate the medial versus lateral OFC, respectively.[31]

Age Differences in Task Performance

In the first study, we administered a battery of tasks considered to be sensitive to OFC and DLPFC function to groups of healthy younger ($n = 23$, 13 women; age $= 28.4 \pm 5.9$ years) and older ($n = 20$, 9 women; age $= 69.1 \pm 5.0$ years) participants; details of inclusion and exclusion criteria in this exceptionally

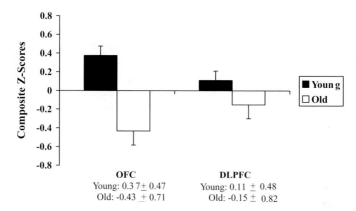

FIGURE 5. Mean composite z-scores for tasks preferentially assessing OFC ($P < 0.001$) and DLPFC by age group. (From Lamar and Resnick.[29] Reprinted by permission.)

healthy sample are in our original article.[29] Younger and older groups were comparable with respect to years of education and mental status, measured by the MMSE. Tasks considered to preferentially tap OFC function based on human neuroimaging and lesion studies (reviewed in Elliott *et al.*[32]) as well as rodent[33] and non-human primate[34] studies included the Delayed Match and Non-Match to Sample tasks and the Iowa Gambling Task. Tasks thought to preferentially involve DLPFC function based on human neuroimaging as well as animal lesion studies, outlined in detail elsewhere,[29] included Petrides' Self-Ordered Pointing Task, the WAIS-R Digit Span Backward, and Letter Fluency and Months Backward from the Boston Revision of the Wechsler Memory Scale (WMS) Mental Control Task.

Mean OFC and DLPFC composite performance scores were calculated from z-score transformations of the individual tests. A 2×2 repeated-measures analysis of variance showed the expected age effect ($P = 0.001$), with better overall performance in younger versus older participants. In addition, there was a significant interaction between age group and tasks differentially tapping OFC versus DLPFC functions, $P = 0.02$ (FIG. 5), with the young group significantly outperforming the old group only for the OFC composite score. Post-hoc analysis of the individual test scores for OFC function showed significant age effects for the Delayed Match and Non-Match to Sample tasks but not the Iowa Gambling Test. For the DLPFC tasks, only the Self-Ordered Pointing Task (effect size $= 0.78$) showed a significant age effect, and the magnitude of the effect size was reduced in comparison to the Delayed Match (effect size $= 1.48$) and Non-Match (effect size $= 1.53$) to Sample tasks. In summary, we found greater vulnerability of tasks emphasizing OFC compared to DLPFC function to age in these samples of young and old adults. These findings suggest that neuroanatomic data indicating differential effects of age within the OFC may have implications for behavioral performance.

Although it is unlikely that successful performance on any neuropsychological task is subserved exclusively by a single brain region, the specific tasks employed in this study were chosen to emphasize the relative contribution of OFC versus DLPFC function. For example, lesions of the DLPFC as well as other brain regions outside the prefrontal cortex, most notably the temporal lobe, have been shown to have a negative impact on delay task performance in monkeys. However, the relative degree of processing each task requires of OFC versus other regions is based on findings from prior fMRI studies.[31] Post-hoc analyses of data within the young and old groups in our behavioral sample did not show significant associations between performance on the delayed tasks and measures of learning and memory or working memory that are heavily reliant on temporal cortex and DLPFC, respectively. Furthermore, studies of these delay tasks and other measures of orbitofrontal functioning suggest that the 5-s delay incorporated into our match and non-match paradigms minimized the DLPFC burden[35] as well as the hippocampal contribution.[36] Additional studies, including functional imaging investigations, are needed to determine the relative contributions of OFC and other brain regions to these tasks. In addition, we are currently conducting testing with other measures of orbitofrontal functioning (e.g., object alternation) in younger and older adults to provide additional information on the differential aging of prefrontal functions served by the OFC and DLPFC.

Age Differences in fMRI Activation during Delayed Match and Non-Match to Sample Tasks

A subset of the participants in the behavioral studies of prefrontal function also participated in an event-related fMRI investigation, using BOLD imaging to assess functional activation during the Delayed Match and Non-Match to Sample tasks.[30] This exceptionally healthy sample included 16 young (8 female; mean age 26.7 ± 5.6 years) and 16 old (8 female; mean age 69.1 ± 5.6 years) individuals with similar levels of education and general cognitive functioning. To elicit OFC activation, we adopted the paradigm previously employed by Elliott *et al.* in young adults, which had shown greater medial OFC activation when contrasting the Match minus Non-Match tasks and greater lateral OFC activation for the Non-Match minus Match tasks.[31] Thus, participants chose the stimulus from a pair of stimuli matching a previously viewed target (*Match* to sample) or chose the non-target item (*Non-Match* to sample), depending upon a trial-specific instruction word. We adopted this paradigm because of its ability to discriminate medial from lateral OFC activation in young participants,[31] anticipating that other regions of brain both within and outside of the prefrontal cortex may be recruited for successful completion. We hypothesized that greater activations within medial and lateral OFC would

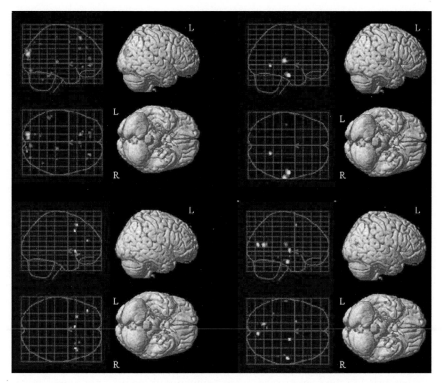

FIGURE 6. Comparisons of between-group analyses of Delayed Match to Sample minus Perceptual Control for young > old (*top left panel*) and old>young (*top right panel*) and Delayed Non-Match to Sample minus Perceptual Control for young > old (*bottom left panel*) and old > young (*bottom right panel*). (From Lamar et al.[30] Reprinted by permission.)

contribute to successful performance in young individuals for the match and non-match conditions, respectively, but that older individuals would show a different pattern of functional activation during successful performance based on the structural and behavioral vulnerability documented with regard to this region in our previous work.

Consistent with previous studies, voxel-based analyses of successful (correct responses) delay task performance revealed greater activation for medial OFC regions (BA 25) during the Match task compared to the Non-Match task and greater lateral OFC activation (BA 11) during the Non-Match task compared to the Match task for younger adults. In contrast, older adults showed superior prefrontal activation only during the Match relative to the Non-Match task and more posterior temporal and limbic involvement than anterior prefrontal involvement during the Non-Match relative to the Match task. Between-group analyses confirmed the within-group results, suggesting differential age-related recruitment of prefrontal regions when performing Match and Non-Match tasks (FIG. 6). For details of statistical analyses and

Talairach coordinates, readers are referred to the original article by Lamar and colleagues.[30] Our findings suggest that OFC recruitment during cognitive tasks differs as a function of age. Furthermore, they indicate that successful performance is dependent upon a different network of regional activation in old compared with young individuals. Such differences in functional activation patterns in older individuals are consistent with an emerging literature reporting functional compensation of the aging brain in association with maintenance of cognitive performance across a variety of tasks.[12,22,23] Additional studies are warranted to elucidate the nature and implications of the effects of age on OFC function, both in relation to other prefrontal regions and to more complex networks among frontal-temporal functioning.

SUMMARY AND CONCLUSIONS

In this paper, we highlight findings from the BLSA that provide information on cognitive and brain aging, emphasizing cross-sectional and longitudinal findings from studies of older adults. BLSA studies have contributed to our understanding of age-related changes in verbal and nonverbal memory, as well as other cognitive functions. Our initial structural MRI studies have helped define the magnitude and regional distribution of tissue loss in older adults free of dementia and have suggested that the OFC may be particularly vulnerable to age-associated tissue loss. These data from cognitively healthy aging individuals provide the background against which pathologic cognitive changes and accelerated tissue loss in association with cognitive impairment can be investigated.

In recent work, we compared rates of tissue loss and ventricular enlargement over 8 years in cognitively impaired and unimpaired BLSA neuroimaging study participants.[24] We identified a number of brain regions showing accelerated tissue loss in individuals with MCI. These brain regions predominately involved frontal and temporal structures, and included the OFC, consistent with neuropathologic evidence that the OFC is an early site of plaque and tangle deposition in the progression of Alzheimer's disease.[25]

Our observation that the OFC is among those brain structures particularly vulnerable to age-related tissue loss also motivated a series of studies to probe the effects of age on OFC function. These cross-sectional studies of differences between healthy young and old individuals provided behavioral and physiological evidence in support of age effects on OFC function. On a battery of tasks selected to preferentially assess OFC versus DLPFC function, better performance in young compared to old individuals was greater on the Delayed Match and Non-Match to Sample tasks (preferential OFC tasks) than DLPFC tasks.[29] An investigation of functional brain activation during performance of the Delayed Match and Non-Match to Sample tasks showed the predicted medial and lateral OFC activation, respectively, in young individuals. In contrast, old individuals showed activation of more–posterior brain regions in support of successful performance,[30] suggesting a compensatory response of neural networks in maintenance of cognitive function in older adults.

Together, these findings indicate a vulnerability of the OFC to age-related decline in brain structure and function, as well as early vulnerability to the pathologic processes characteristic of Alzheimer's disease. While there has been a wealth of emerging information on the role of the mesial temporal region in aging and dementia, OFC structure and function have been under-studied in normal and pathologic aging. Our data suggest that structural and functional OFC changes may contribute to age-associated changes in cognition and everyday function. A particularly fruitful area for future investigation may include investigation of the effects of age on OFC involvement in reward contingencies, given emerging evidence of the role of OFC in dissociating positive and negative valence of stimulus-reward values.[37,38] Age effects on reward contingencies, including monetary rewards, may have implications for decision making abilities and everyday functioning in older adults. Age differences in economic decision-making, also influenced by OFC functioning,[39,40] would be a particularly important area of investigation. Loss of the ability to make financial decisions is an early sign of functional impairment in dementia, often leading to the diagnosis in many individuals.

Future studies investigating the structure and function of the OFC across the life span will elucidate age-related changes in this region and how these changes affect cognition and everyday functioning. Furthermore, new *in vivo* imaging probes that allow prospective investigation of neuropathology will help determine the contribution of OFC pathology to these structural and functional changes in older adults.

ACKNOWLEDGMENT

This work was supported by the Intramural Research Program of the National Institute on Aging of the NIH.

REFERENCES

1. GIAMBRA, L.M. *et al.* 1995. Adult life span changes in immediate visual memory and verbal intelligence. Psychol. Aging **10:** 123–139.
2. PARK, D.C. & A.H. GUTCHESS. 2002. Aging, cognition, and culture: a neuroscientific perspective. Neurosci. Biobehav. Rev. **26:** 859–867.
3. BURKE, S.N. & C.A. BARNES. 2006. Neural plasticity in the ageing brain. Nat. Rev. Neurosci. **7:** 30–40.
4. BARENSE, M.D., M.T. FOX & M.G. BAXTER. 2002. Aged rats are impaired on an attentional set-shifting task sensitive to medial frontal cortex damage in young rats. Learn. Mem. **9:** 191–201.

5. ZYZAK, D.R. *et al*. 1995. Cognitive decline associated with normal aging in rats: a neuropsychological approach. Learn. Mem. **2:** 1–16.
6. PFEFFERBAUM, A. *et al*. 1994. A quantitative magnetic resonance imaging study of changes in brain morphology from infancy to late adulthood. Arch. Neurol. **51:** 874–887.
7. RESNICK, S.M. *et al*. 2003. Longitudinal magnetic resonance imaging studies of older adults: a shrinking brain. J. Neurosci. **23:** 3295–3301.
8. YUE, N.C. *et al*. 1997. Sulcal, ventricular, and white matter changes at MR imaging in the aging brain: data from the Cardiovascular Health Study. Radiology **202:** 33–39.
9. GUR, R.C. *et al*. 1991. Gender differences in age effect on brain atrophy measured by magnetic resonance imaging. Proc. Natl. Acad. Sci. USA **88:** 2845–2849.
10. RAZ, N. & K.M. RODRIGUE. 2006. Differential aging of the brain: patterns, cognitive correlates and modifiers. Neurosci. Biobehav. Rev. **30:** 730–748.
11. GRADY, C.L. *et al*. 1995. Age-related reductions in human recognition memory due to impaired encoding. Science **269:** 218–221.
12. CABEZA, R. 2002. Hemispheric asymmetry reduction in older adults: the HAROLD model. Psychol. Aging **17:** 85–100.
13. SHOCK, N.W. *et al*. 1984. Normal Human Aging: the Baltimore Longitudinal Study of Aging. U.S. Government Printing Office. Washington, DC.
14. LAMAR, M., S.M. RESNICK & A.B. ZONDERMAN. 2003. Longitudinal changes in verbal memory in older adults: distinguishing the effects of age from repeat testing. Neurology **60:** 82–86.
15. RESNICK, S.M. *et al*. 1995. Age-associated changes in specific errors on the Benton Visual Retention Test. J. Gerontol. Psychol. Sci. **50B:** P171–P178.
16. DELIS, D.C. *et al*. 1987. California Verbal Learning Test—Research Edition. The Psychological Corporation. New York.
17. BENTON, A.L., P.J. ESLINGER & A.R. DAMASIO. 1981. Normative observations on neuropsychological test performances in old age. J. Clin. Neuropsychol. **3:** 33–42.
18. KAWAS, C.H. *et al*. 2003. Visual memory predicts Alzheimer's disease more than a decade before diagnosis. Neurology **60:** 1089–1093.
19. ZONDERMAN, A.B. *et al*. 1995. Changes in immediate visual memory predict cognitive impairment. Arch. Clin. Neuropsychol. **10:** 111–123.
20. RESNICK, S.M. *et al*. 2000. One-year age changes in MRI brain volumes in older adults. Cereb. Cortex **10:** 464–472.
21. DAVATZIKOS, C. & S.M. RESNICK. 2002. Degenerative age changes in white matter connectivity visualized in vivo using magnetic resonance imaging. Cereb. Cortex **12:** 767–771.
22. BEASON-HELD, L.L., M.A. KRAUT & S.M. RESNICK. 2006. I. Longitudinal changes in aging brain function. Neurobiol. Aging. [Epuh ahead of print].
23. BEASON-HELD, L.L., M.A. KRAUT & S.M. RESNICK. 2006. II. Temporal patterns of longitudinal change in aging brain function. Neurobiol. Aging.
24. DRISCOLL, I. *et al*. 2007. Longitudinal brain changes in cognitively impaired and unimpaired older adults. Soc. Neurosci. Abstracts, San Diego.
25. BRAAK, H. & E. BRAAK. 1997. Frequency of stages of Alzheimer-related lesions in different age categories. Neurobiol. Aging **18:** 351–357.
26. MINTUN, M.A. *et al*. 2006. [11C]PIB in a nondemented population: potential antecedent marker of Alzheimer disease. Neurology **67:** 446–452.

27. GALVIN, J.E. *et al.* 2005. Predictors of preclinical Alzheimer disease and dementia: a clinicopathologic study. Arch. Neurol. **62:** 758–765.
28. DRISCOLL, I. *et al.* 2006. Impact of Alzheimer's pathology on cognitive trajectories in nondemented elderly. Ann. Neurol. **60:** 688–695.
29. LAMAR, M. & S.M. RESNICK. 2004. Aging and prefrontal functions: dissociating orbitofrontal and dorsolateral abilities. Neurobiol. Aging **25:** 553–538.
30. LAMAR, M., D.M. YOUSEM & S.M. RESNICK. 2004. Age differences in orbitofrontal activation: an fMRI investigation of delayed match and nonmatch to sample. Neuroimage **21:** 1368–1376.
31. ELLIOTT, R. & R.J. DOLAN. 1999. Differential neural responses during performance of matching and nonmatching to sample tasks at two delay intervals. J. Neurosci. **19:** 5066–5073.
32. ELLIOTT, R., R.J. DOLAN & C.D. FRITH. 2000. Dissociable functions in the medial and lateral orbitofrontal cortex: evidence from human neuroimaging studies. Cereb. Cortex **10:** 308–317.
33. RAMUS, S.J. & H. EICHENBAUM. 2000. Neural correlates of olfactory recognition memory in the rat orbitofrontal cortex. J. Neurosci. **20:** 8199–208.
34. BACHEVALIER, J. & M. MISHKIN. 1986. Visual recognition impairment follows ventromedial but not dorsolateral prefrontal lesions in monkeys. Behav. Brain Res. **20:** 249–261.
35. FUSTER, J. 1991. Role of prefrontal cortex in delay tasks: evidence from reversible lesion and unit recording in the monkey. *In* Frontal Lobe Function and Dysfunction. H. Levin, H. Eisenberg & A. Benton, Eds.: 59–71. Oxford University Press. New York.
36. CURTIS, C.E. *et al.* 2000. Object and spatial alternation tasks with minimal delays activate the right anterior hippocampus proper in humans. Neuroreport **11:** 2203–2207.
37. RAMNANI, N. *et al.* 2004. Prediction error for free monetary reward in the human prefrontal cortex. Neuroimage **23:** 777–786.
38. O'DOHERTY, J. *et al.* 2003. Dissociating valence of outcome from behavioral control in human orbital and ventral prefrontal cortices. J. Neurosci. **23:** 7931–7939.
39. DE MARTINO, B. *et al.* 2006. Frames, biases, and rational decision-making in the human brain. Science **313:** 684–687.
40. PADOA-SCHIOPPA, C. & J.A. ASSAD. 2006. Neurons in the orbitofrontal cortex encode economic value. Nature **441:** 223–226.

The Orbital Prefrontal Cortex and Drug Addiction in Laboratory Animals and Humans

BARRY J. EVERITT, DANIEL M. HUTCHESON, KAREN D. ERSCHE,
YANN PELLOUX, JEFFREY W. DALLEY, AND TREVOR W. ROBBINS

*Behavioural and Clinical Neuroscience Institute and Department
of Experimental Psychology, University of Cambridge, Cambridge, United
Kingdom*

ABSTRACT: In this chapter, we review evidence implicating the orbitofrontal cortex (OFC) in drug addiction. We show that the orbital
cortex is involved in conditioned reinforcement and is thereby important for the acquisition of cocaine-seeking behavior studied in a way
that provides an animal experimental homologue of orbital cortex activation and craving upon exposure of addicts to drug-associated stimuli.
We discuss the evidence indicating orbital prefrontal cortex dysfunction
in human drug addicts, reviewing both neuropsychological and neuroimaging studies. Finally, we consider animal experimental evidence
suggesting that addictive drugs may cause orbital cortex dysfunction
and thereby contribute to the transition to drug addiction. Reconciling
the observations that even brief periods of drug exposure can lead to
long-lasting functional and structural deficits associated with the OFC
together with those suggesting interactions between a vulnerable phenotype and chronic drug-self-administration will be an important topic of
future research.

KEYWORDS: drug seeking; compulsion; conditioned reinforcement

INTRODUCTION

The orbitofrontal cortex (OFC) has been implicated in drug addiction for
several reasons. First, functional imaging studies have demonstrated its activation, along with other limbic cortical areas, when addicts are exposed to
drug-associated stimuli that elicit craving.[1–5] Second, perhaps the greatest im-
petus for the growth in interest in the OFC and addiction is the evidence that
the compulsive drug-seeking behavior of addicts and its persistence despite
negative outcomes is similar to the behavior of individuals with damage to
or dysfunction of the OFC.[6–8] Third, persistent metabolic or neurochemical

Address for correspondence: Barry Everitt, Dept of Experimental Psychology, University if Cambridge, Downing Street, Cambridge CB2 3EB, UK. Voice: +44-1223-333583.
bje10@cam.ac.uk

Ann. N.Y. Acad. Sci. 1121: 576–597 (2007). © 2007 New York Academy of Sciences.
doi: 10.1196/annals.1401.022

changes have been demonstrated in the OFC of drug addicts, including those who have been abstinent for considerable periods of time, suggesting that long-term abuse of drugs may lead to functional changes that contribute to, or exacerbate, the development of drug addiction.[2,9,10] In addition, reduced dopamine D2-receptor binding in the striatum has been linked to the OFC hypometabolism seen in abstinent drug addicts,[11,12] and also to impulsive behavior and the tendency to escalate cocaine intake in rats.[13] The observations in humans have been made on a background of experimental data showing that the OFC plays a key role in encoding the value of outcomes, or goals, and in the flexible adjustment of both Pavlovian and instrumental responses when those values are altered.[14-18] Thus, the OFC may not only be involved in the fundamental mechanisms by which individuals learn to seek and take drugs, but its dysfunction may contribute to the emergence of the compulsive drug seeking characteristic of addiction.[19] We will discuss experimental studies in animals and humans that address some of these issues.

ROLE OF THE ORBITOFRONTAL CORTEX IN DRUG SEEKING IN ANIMALS

The OFC is activated not only by presentation of drug-associated stimuli in humans, but also in rats that have previously self-administered cocaine.[20,21] For example, in a cellular imaging study, the expression of *zif268*, a gene associated with activity and plasticity, measured using in situ hybridization histochemistry, was increased in the ventral and lateral OFC following the presentation of a discrete conditioned stimulus (CS) associated with self-administered cocaine.[21] Increased expression of *zif268* was also seen in the amygdala and anterior cingulate cortex, and these same areas are also reliably activated following presentation of drug-associated stimuli to cocaine and heroin addicts. These activations of the OFC, amygdala, and cingulate cortex are correlated with craving ratings in addicts,[1,4,5] suggesting a relationship between drug cue presentation and subjective states that may lead to drug use and relapse to drug seeking in addicts, sometimes long into a period of abstinence. Drug-associated CSs have a marked impact on drug seeking and relapse in animals, in particular when they act as conditioned reinforcers, i.e., are presented contingent on instrumental drug-seeking responses.[19,22] Thus, drug-associated conditioned reinforcers have a profound impact in rats responding for cocaine or heroin under a second-order schedule of reinforcement[23,24] and in models of relapse to drug seeking in animals having undergone,[25,26] or not,[27,28] prior extinction of the instrumental drug-seeking response. Conditioned reinforcers not only maintain behavior over prolonged periods of time, i.e., when reinforcement is delayed, but they can also act as goals for action, supporting the learning of new instrumental responses for CSs associated with both natural reinforcers (e.g., sucrose and water) and also drugs.[29-31]

Stimulant drugs greatly potentiate the control over behavior by conditioned reinforcers through their ability to increase dopamine release[32] in the nucleus accumbens shell.[33,34] Conditioned reinforcement assessed in acquisition of new instrumental response procedures[35] has been shown to depend upon the basolateral amygdala (BLA) and the nucleus accumbens core (AcbC) to which it projects.[33,36,37] More recently, it has been shown that selective lesions of the OFC, but not medial prefrontal cortex (mPFC), in a primate also impairs the acquisition of a new response with conditioned reinforcement.[38] A similar study in rats indicated the involvement of OFC mechanisms only when conditioned reinforcement was mediated by the representation of expected outcome, assessed in a blocking procedure and described in detail in this volume.[39] An impairment in the acquisition of a new instrumental response with conditioned reinforcement was also seen following OFC dopamine depletion in marmosets.[40]

In order to study the role of conditioned reinforcement in maintaining drug-seeking behavior and drug taking, we have utilized a second-order schedule of drug reinforcement in rats self-administering cocaine or heroin[24] adapted from those used in pioneering studies conducted using primates.[41,42] Drug seeking under a second-order schedule embodies several characteristics of addictive behavior in humans in that animals must forage (work instrumentally) for their intravenous drug over protracted periods of time, their seeking responses being reinforced in the interim by the contingent presentation of drug-associated stimuli acting, therefore, as conditioned reinforcers. We have demonstrated that, as predicted from our earlier findings on the neural basis of conditioned reinforcement, the acquisition of cocaine seeking was prevented by selective lesions of the BLA or AcbC.[34,43] Subsequent studies demonstrated the importance of a serial interaction between these structures using asymmetric, unilateral manipulations of dopamine and glutamate transmission in the BLA and AcbC, respectively.[44] On the background of the observations summarized above, showing that the OFC is activated by drug-associated stimuli in animals and humans and that the OFC is required for conditioned reinforcement measured under the theoretically rigorous requirements of an acquisition of a new response procedure, we have begun to investigate the effects of OFC lesions on cocaine self-administration and the acquisition of cocaine seeking under a second-order schedule of reinforcement.[45]

In this procedure, rats implanted with intravenous (i.v.) catheters attached to an infusion pump learn to lever press for cocaine under a continuous reinforcement schedule, designated Fixed Ratio (FR) 1. Each response delivers an i.v. bolus of cocaine preceded and overlapped by the illumination of a discrete light CS which, through Pavlovian conditioning, becomes associated with the effects of the drug. When responding has stabilized, the criteria for drug infusions increase, first by requiring rats to respond 10 times, earning 10 CS presentations, for an infusion of cocaine and then, in stages, increasing the response requirements for the CS to FR10, such that rats must make 10 responses for the CS and complete 10 such FR10 units to receive a single infusion of cocaine (in second-order terms, FR10(FR10:S)). In many studies, rats are at this point switched to an overall 15-min fixed interval (FI15(FR10:S)), but in the present experiments this stage was not included, for reasons that will become clear. Excitotoxic lesions of the OFC were made, sparing the rostral mPFC and similar to those used in other studies of OFC function.[46,47] In separate studies, OFC lesions were made either prior to the acquisition of cocaine self-administration (and, therefore, before the opportunity for cocaine-CS pairings), or afterwards, but before introduction of the increasingly demanding second-order schedule response requirements.

Lesions of the OFC had no significant effect on the acquisition of cocaine self-administration or its performance in those animals having received OFC lesions after acquisition. There was a non-significant tendency for rats with pre-training lesions to self-administer cocaine at a higher rate than controls, perhaps indicating reduced reinforcing efficacy of the drug, but this was not confirmed in a dose–response function analysis. The lack of effect of OFC lesions replicates other observations[48] and is consistent with a range of studies showing that similar OFC lesions do not impair the acquisition of responding for natural rewards.[18,49] The minor dysregulation of cocaine self-administration when lesions were made before any cocaine experience perhaps warrants more careful and systematic study, since it may indicate involvement in the interpretation of altered bodily states, such as autonomic responses, that undoubtedly accompany cocaine self-administration and contribute to the subjective states that are components of the drug's reinforcing effects.[19,50]

By contrast, OFC lesioned rats were markedly impaired in the acquisition of cocaine-seeking behavior, regardless of whether the lesions were made prior to or after the acquisition of cocaine self-administration and the formation of CS-cocaine Pavlovian associations. Thus, as the schedule requirements were increased from FR10(FR1:S) through FR10(FR7:S) to FR10(FR10:S), i.e., as the influence of the cocaine-associated conditioned reinforcer in controlling responding was increased, subjects with OFC lesions initially met the response criterion, but could not maintain it (FIG. 1). In the final analysis, only 30% or rats with pre-self-administration training lesions and 25% of those with lesions made afterwards maintained their drug seeking responding, as compared to 90% and 80% of controls, respectively. Therefore rats with OFC lesions could not sustain their drug seeking in a task that we have repeatedly shown depends upon the conditioned reinforcing properties of cocaine-associated cues.[22,23] But the effects of OFC lesions were quite different from those following selective lesions of the BLA, AcbC (or nucleus accumbens shell [AcbS]) and also mPFC areas. Lesions of the BLA or AcbC had similar effects, emphasizing their close functional interrelationship, such that rats with lesions failed at the earliest stages to acquire responding for the conditioned reinforcer, despite having readily acquired cocaine self-administration.[34]

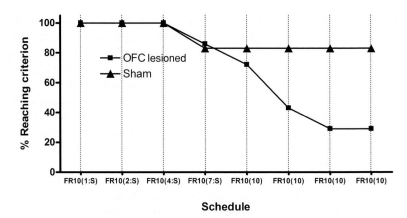

Schedule

FIGURE 1. The effects of OFC lesions on the acquisition of cocaine seeking in rats. The data show the percentage of animals reaching criterion at each stage of the second-order schedule as responding for conditioned reinforcement becomes increasingly important. All animals acquired cocaine self-administration under conditioned reinforcement, and the same proportions of sham and lesioned rats met the response requirements up to FR10(FR7:S)—i.e., when rats were responding seven times for each presentation of the cocaine-associated conditioned reinforcer, and completed 10 of these units of Fixed Ratio responding for each infusion of cocaine. However, although initially meeting the response requirements at FR10(FR10:S), rats with OFC lesions could not maintain their responding, which collapsed progressively over three additional sessions at this stage of the second-order schedule.

At no stage could they meet the response criteria and were therefore impaired in their acquisition of the drug-seeking task. Rats with mPFC lesions, by contrast, not only showed greatly enhanced acquisition of cocaine self-administration, but also readily responded at high rates as the second-order schedule requirements were introduced.[51] However, these animals were insensitive to CS omission and responded at high rates for delayed infusions of cocaine, their drug seeking therefore taking the form of perseverative or compulsive behavior that was not constrained by, or dependent upon, the control over performance exerted by conditioned reinforcers.

The interpretation of the effect of OFC lesions on responding under the second-order schedule of cocaine reinforcement requires further study. The effect is similar, but not identical, to that reported by Pears *et al.*[38] in marmosets with OFC lesions, which also readily acquired responding under a second-order schedule of food reinforcement, but were insensitive to CS omission. Thus, in both cases there was a loss of conditioned reinforcing efficacy of the CS, although it is difficult further to compare the studies because of the different histories of reinforcement. The increased responding seen in OFC-lesioned animals under second-order schedules may reflect the loss of general inhibitory control[38] and thus an inability to suppress, or alter, responding when task parameters change. The resultant perseveration in responding was perhaps more transient in OFC-lesioned rats than marmosets. Alternatively, since responding under second-order schedules is under the control of both secondary and primary reinforcers, OFC-lesioned subjects may have shown a compensatory enhancement of control by the primary reinforcer, cocaine in the present case, following impairment in the conditioned reinforcement process known to follow OFC lesions in tasks where no primary reinforcer is available.[38,39] There is also strong evidence that encoding of stimulus−reward associations in the BLA is impaired following lesions of OFC[49] and that cocaine treatment also affects this BLA encoding.[52] This perhaps suggests that in OFC-lesioned rats, the failure of contingent cocaine-associated conditioned reinforcer presentations to support vigorous cocaine seeking is a consequence of impaired or inflexible CS-cocaine encoding in the amygdala.

In studies with natural reinforcers, the OFC plays an important role in behavior emitted on the basis of active representations of the expected outcome, a process in which its interactions with the BLA are critically important.[17] Thus, OFC-lesioned subjects may be unable to utilize the representation of the value of the drug or food outcome held by the conditioned reinforcer, which is itself dependent upon encoding in the BLA. As we have speculated upon previously,[19] drug-seeking behavior may then be emitted with altered vigor because it has become both habitual and less dependent upon the value of the expected outcome (see also Ref. 12). Whatever the explanation, OFC lesions clearly impair the acquisition of cocaine seeking that depends greatly upon the conditioned reinforcing properties of a cocaine-associated CS. However, while lesions model to some extent the putative impairment in OFC function in addicts, they do not readily model the late-emerging deficits seen in addicts in imaging studies, or the enhanced metabolic response to presentations of drug cues on this hypometabolic background. Nor do they capture subtle changes in the structure and plasticity of OFC neurons seen upon exposure to self-administered and experimenter-administered amphetamine and cocaine.[53-55] The important issue of addictive drug-induced changes in OFC structure and function is considered further below.

ORBITOFRONTAL CORTEX DYSFUNCTION IN CHRONIC DRUG USERS

The behavior of chronic drug users has often been described as impulsive and maladaptive since their behavior becomes increasingly orientated toward further drug use despite consequent and progressively negative consequences, both social and personal.[56] Research in experimental animals has shown that drug seeking in the face of negative consequences can be modeled[57-61] and, moreover, it has been further suggested that the effects of cocaine pre-exposure on behavioral and neuronal responses to natural rewards may indicate OFC dysfunction[62] (also reviewed in this volume). Experiments on animals have in fact been led by data from neuropsychological research in human drug abusers and addicts, where there is evidence of functional impairments that may also vary with the specific drug of abuse.[6]

Poor behavioral adjustment may be due to lack of inhibitory control over the appropriate responses.[8,63] The ability to suppress a planned motor response in a laboratory setting is usually investigated using stop-signal or go/no-go paradigms.[64] For example, while participants are engaged in a primary choice reaction time task, they have to stop their prepared or ongoing response when an occasional stop-signal is presented. Stimulant users have repeatedly demonstrated poor performance on tasks requiring the inhibition of prepotent motor responses,[65,66] while the majority of studies could not identify response inhibition deficits in human opiate users.[67–69] The lateral OFC has been associated with response inhibition,[70] as has the inferior frontal gyrus.[64,71] The observation that inhibition failure on the stop-signal task was associated with the amount of methamphetamine previously consumed[66] has led to speculation that this might reflect dose-dependent neuroadaptive changes underlying poor behavioral inhibition in chronic methamphetamine abusers. Indeed, functional and structural abnormalities have been identified in the inferior frontal gyrus in methamphetamine users.[11,72]

Impairments in response reversal may account for the maladaptive behavior patterns in chronic drug users.[73] Probabilistic reversal learning requires participants to respond differentially to two stimuli under conditions of reward and punishment and to reverse their responses when reinforcement contingencies change. Thus, for example, an 80:20 discrimination means that subjects are rewarded 80% of the time for the correct response and that on 20% of trials they receive spurious negative feedback. In the reversal phase, the contingencies are reversed (20:80), rendering the task more difficult than the usual 100:0 to 0:100 paradigm. Although response reversal requires the inhibition of a prepotent response when stimulus–reward associations change, the cognitive demands during probabilistic reversal learning are somewhat different, namely the learning and reversal of stimulus–reward associations on the basis of degraded feedback. Cocaine addicts had major difficulties in adapting behavior to changes in reward contingencies, showing marked perseverative responding to the previously rewarded stimuli[73] (Ersche *et al.*, unpublished observations), while importantly, task performance in chronic users of amphetamine or of opiates and former drug users was not measurably impaired. The inability rapidly to modify an established response pattern in cocaine users may reflect dysfunction in the OFC and/or interconnected areas such as the ventrolateral part of the PFC (see also reviews by Refs. 74, 75). Supporting this contention, converging results from neuroimaging investigations suggest that chronic cocaine use is associated with OFC dysfunction (for reviews see Refs. 12, 76, 77) and reduced gray matter density in this area.[78] The divergent performance pattern in probabilistic reversal learning between amphetamine and cocaine users may lie in the distinct pharmacological profiles of these two substances on serotonergic neurotransmission. In contrast to amphetamine, cocaine has a strong affinity for the 5-HT transporter,[79] and chronic exposure has been associated with marked serotonergic dysregulation.[80] Amphetamine, by contrast, has a relatively low affinity for the 5-HT transporter,[79] which may explain why it is less potent than cocaine in increasing 5-HT levels in the PFC.[81] Since probabilistic reversal learning has been shown previously to be sensitive to modulation of serotonergic neurotransmission,[82,83] it seems likely that the different pharmacological profiles of cocaine and amphetamine may account for impaired response reversal and perseverative responding seen in chronic cocaine users but not in chronic amphetamine users.

Despite convincing evidence for performance impairments on tasks, such as response inhibition and response reversal, which are considered to be subserved by inferior frontal or orbitofrontal networks,[74,84] OFC dysfunction during more complex processes such as decision making may not always be reflected in behaviorally measurable impairment. Recruitment of additional OFC function may in some instances instead represent a compensatory response to pre-existing, or drug-induced, pathology. Whether or not this compensatory attempt is effective may depend upon the specific substance of abuse. Much evidence supports the important role of the OFC in reinforcement-guided decision making.[85–87] Decision making in patients with damage to the ventromedial PFC (i.e., in the medial OFC including areas on the medial wall) has been characterized as impulsive, irrational, and insensitive to its consequences.[88–91] Decision-making impairment in chronic amphetamine abusers on a computerized Gamble Task resembles in some respect the choices of patients with OFC lesions, as both groups chose the most favorable option less frequently than did controls.[6] However, it should be noted that this disadvantageous decision-making strategy in amphetamine abusers was not secondary to motor impulsivity; in fact the drug abusers deliberated longer on their decisional choices than controls. Furthermore, amphetamine abusers neither increased their gambles on the less favorable options nor did they choose significantly against the odds in the risky conditions, suggesting that their disadvantageous choice selection was due to difficulties in estimating outcome probabilities rather than a reflection of a reward-seeking strategy. Interestingly, neuroimaging research in chronic drug users has shown significant over-activation in the OFC during decision making, when behaviorally, decision-making performance was not measurably impaired,[92] as shown in FIGURE 2.[93] This may suggest that in chronic drug users, increased activation in the OFC during decision making reflects a compensation for an underlying pathology in the OFC or elsewhere, enabling drug users to meet the task demands. This proposal is consistent with findings from neuroimaging studies, showing a significant relationship between elevated OFC activation and improved cognitive controls in chronic cocaine users.[3,94]

Neurons in the OFC and striatum respond differentially to reward value and predictability of reward,[95–97] while information about the magnitude and the

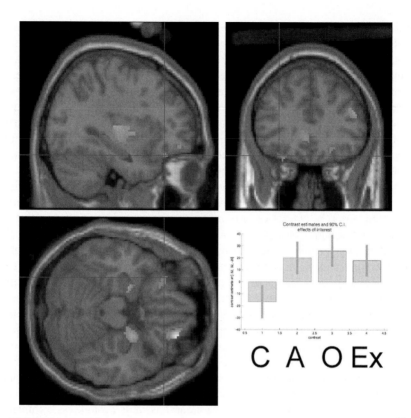

FIGURE 2. Decision making investigated using the Cambridge Risk Task during $H_2{}^{15}O$ positron emission tomography (PET) scans (Ersche *et al.* 2005). A specific feature of the Risk Task is the choice conflict between an unlikely large reward option and a likely small reward option. Four groups, each consisting of 15 participants, were compared: chronic amphetamine users, chronic opiate users, ex-drug users who had been long-term amphetamine/opiate users but were abstinent from all drugs of abuse for at least 1 year, and healthy matched controls without a drug-taking history. Although decision-making performance was not measurably impaired in drug users, there were significant differences in the pattern of brain activation in drug users compared to controls. Both current and former drug users showed relative over-activation in the OFC (as shown above) and under-activation in the dorsolateral PFC (data not shown). The plot in the lower right-hand corner shows the mean size of the significant task-related between-group effect in the OFC (x: −32, y: 32, z: −20) in the planned comparison (former drug abusers versus all three drug use groups). Abbreviations: C, cocaine abusers; A, amphetamine abusers; O, opiate abusers; Ex, former drug abusers. Reprinted with permission from. Ersche *et al.*[93]

likelihood of an upcoming event facilitates the selection of goal-directed responses by the OFC.[96] The processing of feedback information, on the basis of which outcome probabilities are estimated, has also been shown to be impaired in chronic drug users. For example, during a forced two-choice prediction task, Paulus *et al.*[98,99] found that although methamphetamine users demonstrated sensitivity to both positive and negative feedback, they were less able to use this feedback to guide their choices; an impairment that was reflected in reduced task-related OFC activation.[99] As a consequence, choice selection in methamphetamine users was quite stimulus bound and less influenced by outcome probabilities.[98] Opiate users, by contrast, showed a selective impairment in the processing of negative feedback, such as punishment[100] and errors.[67,101] During decision making, opiate users lacked the normal relationship between activation of the anterior cingulate cortex and adaptive responding to negative feedback,[102] but seemed to compensate for this impairment by significant task-related over-activation in the OFC compared to both controls and amphetamine users.[93,102] Both task-related under-activation in the OFC of methamphetamine users[98] and the over-activation in the OFC in opiate users[102] were significantly associated with the duration of methamphetamine and opiate use, respectively. This may suggest that the ability to compensate for abnormalities in feedback processing by the OFC is dependent on the drug of abuse. Alternatively, abnormal OFC activation may be influenced by the current state of drug use, e.g., the methamphetamine users in the Paulus *et al.*[98] study were drug abstinent, whereas the opiate users, studied by Ersche *et al.*,[102] had recently consumed opiates. At present, neuropathological changes associated with OFC dysfunction in chronic drug users are still relatively poorly defined. Evidence from studies in rats, however, suggests that different drugs may affect OFC morphology differentially; for example, chronic administration of amphetamine has been shown to decreases spine density in the OFC, while chronic opiate exposure appears to induce changes in the opposite direction.[53–55]

In summary, chronic drug abuse has clearly been associated with impairments in cognitive function and behavioral adjustment.[103,104] While deficits in cognitive function such as executive ability and memory are apparently abused-drug specific,[105,106] considerable evidence suggests that OFC-related processes involving decision making and impulsivity are differentially affected by different abused drugs. Future research will need to address substance-specific changes in the human OFC and their implications for behavior and cognition.

EFFECTS OF ADDICTIVE DRUGS ON OFC FUNCTION AND MODELS OF 'ADDICTION' IN ANIMALS

The data regarding alterations in behavior and cognition indicative of OFC dysfunction in chronic abusers of a variety of drugs strongly suggest that the drugs themselves may cause these deficits, contributing to the addictive state both directly and indirectly.[62,107] But even in situations where there is a relationship between the extent of drug use and specific deficits,[6,98,102] it remains possible that the alterations in OFC function pre-date, and may actually be causally related to, drug abuse and therefore represent a vulnerability factor.

These possibilities are not mutually exclusive. One way to investigate this further is to study the effects of addictive drugs on OFC-dependent processes in experimental animals and the consequences of chronic drug taking on behavior, including drug-seeking behavior. Such studies may provide insight into the mechanisms of drug addiction and, indeed, also address the issue of whether "addictive behavior," rather than simple drug self-administration, can be studied in animals.

Considerable evidence has accrued showing that even brief exposure to stimulant drugs, usually in a treatment regimen that induces behavioral (or rather locomotor) sensitization, is associated with changes in behavior and cognition measured subsequently. These changes may be compared with those seen in addicts, summarized above, and may contribute to the development of the compulsive drug seeking characteristic of addiction. Several studies are summarized in detail in this volume (Olavsson et al.; Schoenbaum et al.) and have been reviewed elsewhere.[62,107] Short-term, usually experimenter-administered rather than self-administered, cocaine or amphetamine enhances the development of impulsivity.[107,108] Cocaine-treated rats failed to adapt responding to a CS after food (not drug) reinforcer devaluation, also another characteristic effect of OFC lesions.[18] Perhaps especially impressive are consistent demonstrations of impaired reversal learning following cocaine treatment in monkeys[109] and in rats.[110] These demonstrations include the example of rats having self-administered and then been withdrawn from cocaine. These rats showed both increased extinction responding 1 and 30 days into withdrawal and a marked reversal deficit some 2 months into withdrawal, measured as persistent responding on the drug-seeking lever when an alternative response delivered a cocaine-associated conditioned reinforcer following introduction of the reversal contingency.[111] Schoenbaum and colleagues not only have emphasized the similarity between OFC lesions and these apparently long-lasting effects of relatively short-term treatment with cocaine, but have also shown that the deficit in reversal learning is reflected in a change in the properties of OFC neurons, such that they do not develop appropriate responses to cues predicting outcomes.[52] It remains to be seen in future studies whether the specific impairment in reversal learning in cocaine abusers, although not in those abusing amphetamine or opiates or in former drug users (Ersche et al., unpublished observations), is also observed in rats having self-administered cocaine, but not heroin or amphetamine.

It is clearly impressive that even brief periods of drug exposure, whether experimenter-administered or self-administered, can result in enduring changes in behavior indicative of OFC dysfunction. These changes are in many cases similar to the effects of OFC lesions, although, as discussed above, this may not be the best model of the OFC hypoactivity seen in addicts. Indeed, in the great majority of imaging and neuropsychological investigations of addicts, there has been an exceptionally long history of drug abuse, often poly-drug abuse. These drug-addicted individuals must represent, therefore, a relatively small proportion of the much larger number of individuals in a population who have abused drugs over varying periods of time, but who have not made the transition to an addicted state as characterized by compulsive drug seeking. Thus, it would seem unlikely that the experimental groups of rats receiving the fairly modest exposure to stimulant drugs in the experiments described above would in any sense fulfill the criteria for addiction, yet the changes in behavior indicative of OFC dysfunction are seen in the entire population of treated experimental animals. Clearly there is a need to understand whether more chronic exposure to self-administered drugs results in what might be regarded as an "addicted state" and whether this, too, involves the entire population of animals or a restricted sub-group that may more directly be compared with human addicts.

Dalley and co-workers have investigated the effects of a series of withdrawals from long access i.v. cocaine, amphetamine, heroin, and methylene-dioxymethamphetamine (MDMA) self-administration sessions over several weeks, using a five-choice serial reaction-time task (5CSRTT).[112–114] This task allows precise measurement of visual attentional function and impulsivity in rodents and depends upon the functional integrity of regions of the PFC and striatum as well of the dopaminergic, serotonergic, noradrenergic, and cholinergic innervation of these regions.[115] The results revealed marked changes in visual attentional accuracy and impulsivity following withdrawal from each drug, but generally these changes were relatively short-lived, recovering over 5 days of withdrawal. However, withdrawal from MDMA resulted in persistent deficits in accuracy and speed of responding under attentional challenge up to 6 weeks later, whereas withdrawal from heroin produced lasting and selective effects on the latency to collect food reward, reminiscent of anhedonic and related subjective states in human heroin addicts. The underlying neural basis of these changes can be speculated upon[112–114] and include adaptations in monoaminergic transmission, but a key finding was that enduring functional deficits were not observed, at least under the conditions of study. Indeed, the observations of Ersche *et al.*[102] also indicate that deficits in reversal learning seen specifically in cocaine addicts are not seen in long-abstinent individuals. However, it is important to note that while some deficits recover, some persist and these are most readily detected by taxing the cognitive functions mediated by the PFC.

A fundamentally important issue is whether the behavioral and cognitive changes caused by exposure to stimulant and other drugs that may reflect OFC dysfunction contribute to the development of compulsive drug seeking. According to the Diagnostic and Statistical Manual of Mental Disorders (DSM-IV), this is a key characteristic of "addictive behavior". There are few models of compulsive behavior in animals, but perhaps the perseverative responding, including drug seeking, in reversal learning tasks seen following cocaine exposure[109,111] provides one measure. However, in attempting to model drug addiction in animals, we and others have tried to capture the persistent, or compulsive, drug seeking despite negative outcomes. This meets a key DSM-IV diagnostic criterion which describes addicts (or substance-dependent individuals) as being unable to control their drug seeking despite aversive consequences, such as illness, impoverishment, social and family dysfunction, and the threat of actual punishment and incarceration. In developing such procedures, we and others have shown that compulsive drug seeking emerges following an extended, or chronic, history of cocaine taking.[59-61] In the study by Vanderschuren and Everitt,[59] rats were trained in what we have described as a "seeking–taking task" to learn to respond on one lever (the seeking lever) to gain access to a second, taking lever. Only responses on the taking lever result in an i.v. drug infusion and hence the seeking/taking distinction.[116,117] The rats then underwent fear conditioning (CS-mild foot shock pairings) and subsequently the ability of the fear CS to suppress seeking responses was assessed. Presentations of the CS readily suppressed drug seeking in rats with a limited history of self-administering cocaine, but in rats with an extended history of cocaine self-administration, including several long access sessions, no conditioned suppression of drug seeking was seen. In contrast, rats with a similarly long period of responding for sucrose on the same task readily suppressed their seeking responses in the presence of the fear CS, suggesting the change in behavior was specific for cocaine and not sucrose seeking. Thus, these data show that persistent or perseverative drug seeking despite negative consequences is an emergent phenomenon that is determined by chronic drug exposure. But even rats in the short cocaine history group, which showed no deficit in the conditioned suppression of drug seeking, had experienced more cocaine exposure than those in the studies summarized above showing impulsive responding and impaired reversal learning following relatively brief cocaine sensitization pre-treatments.

However, the results of the experiments by Vanderschuren and Everitt[59] still do not capture the fact that not all individuals self-administering drugs make the transition from regulated to "out-of-control" drug use, persisting despite aversive consequences, that we recognize as addiction. There is a vulnerable sub-group, often estimated to be less than 20% of the population that initially use drugs who progress to this addicted state.[118] Therefore, it is of interest that Deroche-Gamonet et al.[60] reported that while extended training increased the resistance to punishment of a nose-poking response for cocaine, this cocaine-exposure–dependent change in behavior was seen only in a sub-group of some 17% of individuals. Thus the vulnerability to develop compulsive drug seeking, as defined by its performance despite negative consequences (as well as two additional "addiction" criteria), is seen in only a sub-group of rats. In parallel studies we have confirmed the emergence of a similar pattern of compulsive behavior using a modified version of the drug "seeking–taking" task in which, in this case, 50% of the drug seeking periods in the chained schedule resulted in access to the cocaine-taking lever and the opportunity to self-administer cocaine, but 50% resulted instead in punishment of the seeking response, these

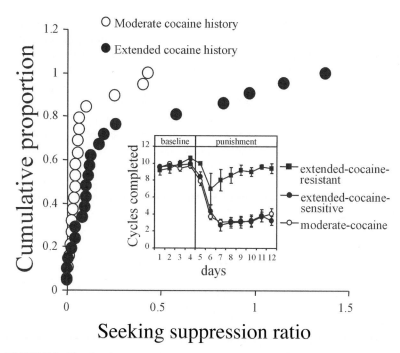

Seeking suppression ratio

FIGURE 3. The development of compulsive drug seeking in a subpopulation of outbred Lister-hooded rats. The graph shows the distribution of rats with a moderate (*open circles*) and extended (*filled circles*) cocaine self-administration history in terms of their suppression of drug-seeking responses when 50% of those responses resulted in punishment and 50% access to a cocaine-taking response (on an unpredictable basis). A subpopulation of rats failed to show any suppression of their drug-seeking behavior. The inset graph shows the suppression of cocaine seeking upon introduction of the shock contingency in rats with a moderate cocaine-taking history, rats with an extended cocaine history that were sensitive to punishment and suppressed their seeking, and the subpopulation of animals that showed resistance to punishment-induced suppression of cocaine seeking. Thus, persistent or "compulsive" drug seeking despite negative outcomes or consequences, which is a feature of "Substance Dependence" in DSM-IV, can be modeled in rats and occurs in a subpopulation of about 17% of individuals—similar to estimates of this propensity for compulsive drug use in humans.

outcomes occurring randomly.[61] After a limited history of cocaine taking, introduction of the punishment contingency readily suppressed drug seeking. But after an extended period of cocaine taking, some 17–20% of subjects were completely resistant to punishment, continuing to seek and take drugs despite the ongoing, daily experience of the negative outcome (FIG. 3). Thus, in both studies, a similarly sized subpopulation of rats with extended histories of cocaine self-administration showed the development of compulsive drug seeking. Such a vulnerable sub-group may bear more direct comparison with drug-addicted humans studied in neuropsychological and neuroimaging settings.

These individuals, rather than the entire population of drug users, are those who have progressed to drug "addiction" and the compulsive drug seeking, despite negative consequences, that this implies. These are the individuals who also display a range of behavioral deficits, some of which indicate impaired OFC function.

A challenge for future studies, then, is to understand how relatively long-lasting behavioral effects of acute drug exposure and the emergence of compulsive drug seeking, but only after chronic drug exposure, are related—especially their dependence upon drug-induced interactions with OFC-dependent processes. Additionally, it is becoming increasingly important to understand more about the predictive qualities of "vulnerable" endophenotypes[13] and how these relate to OFC function both prior to and following self-administered drug exposure.

ACKNOWLEDGMENTS

The research reported in this chapter was supported by the Medical Research Council and Wellcome Trust and was conducted within the Behavioural and Clinical Neuroscience Institute.

REFERENCES

1. CHILDRESS, A.R. *et al.* 1999. Limbic activation during cue-induced cocaine craving. American Journal of Psychiatry **156:** 11–18.
2. GOLDSTEIN, R.Z. & N.D. VOLKOW. 2002. Drug addiction and its underlying neurobiological basis: neuroimaging evidence for the involvement of the frontal cortex. American Journal of Psychiatry **159:** 1642–1652.
3. GOLDSTEIN, R.Z. *et al.* 2007. Role of the anterior cingulate and medial orbitofrontal cortex in processing drug cues in cocaine addiction. Neuroscience **144:** 1153–1159.
4. GARAVAN, H. *et al.* 2000. Cue-induced cocaine craving: neuroanatomical specificity for drug users and drug stimuli. Am. J. Psychiatry **157:** 1789–1798.
5. GRANT, S. *et al.* 1996. Activation of memory circuits during cue-elicited cocaine craving. Proceedings of the National Academy of Sciences, USA **93:** 12040–12045.
6. ROGERS, R.D. *et al.* 1999. Dissociable deficits in the decision-making cognition of chronic amphetamine abusers, opiate abusers, patients with focal damage to prefrontal cortex, and tryptophan-depleted normal volunteers: Evidence for monoaminergic mechanisms. Neuropsychopharmacology **20:** 322–339.
7. BECHARA, A. & M. VAN DER LINDEN. 2005. Decision-making and impulse control after frontal lobe injuries. Current Opinion in Neurology **18:** 734–739.
8. BECHARA, A. 2005. Decision making, impulse control and loss of willpower to resist drugs: a neurocognitive perspective. Nature Neuroscience **8:** 1458–1463.

9. VOLKOW, N.D., J.S. FOWLER & G.J. WANG. 2003. The addicted human brain: insights from imaging studies. Journal of Clinical Investigation **111:** 1444–1451.

10. VOLKOW, N.D., J.S. FOWLER & G.J. WANG. 2004. The addicted human brain viewed in the light of imaging studies: brain circuits and treatment strategies. Neuropharmacology **47:** 3–13.

11. VOLKOW, N.D. *et al.* 2001. Low level of brain dopamine D-2 receptors in methamphetamine abusers: Association with metabolism in the orbitofrontal cortex. American Journal of Psychiatry **158:** 2015–2021.

12. BALER, R.D. & N.D. VOLKOW. 2006. Drug addiction: the neurobiology of disrupted self-control. Trends in Molecular Medicine **12:** 559–566.

13. DALLEY, J.W. *et al.* 2007. Nucleus accumbens D2/3 receptors predict trait impulsivity and cocaine reinforcement. Science **315:** 1267–1270.

14. DALLEY, J.W., R.N. CARDINAL & T.W. ROBBINS. 2004. Prefrontal executive and cognitive functions in rodents: neural and neurochemical substrates. Neuroscience and Biobehavioral Reviews **28:** 771–784.

15. CARDINAL, R.N. *et al.* 2002. Emotion and motivation: the role of the amygdala, ventral striatum, and prefrontal cortex. Neuroscience and Biobehavioral Reviews **26:** 321–352.

16. SCHOENBAUM, G. & M. ROESCH. 2005. Orbitofrontal cortex, associative learning, and expectancies. Neuron. **47:** 633–636.

17. SCHOENBAUM, G. *et al.* 2003. Encoding predicted outcome and acquired value in orbitofrontal cortex during cue sampling depends upon input from basolateral amygdala. Neuron. **39:** 855–867.

18. GALLAGHER, M., R.W. MCMAHAN & G. SCHOENBAUM. 1999. Orbitofrontal cortex and representation of incentive value in associative learning. Journal of Neuroscience **19:** 6610–6614.

19. EVERITT, B.J. & T.W. ROBBINS. 2005. Neural systems of reinforcement for drug addiction: from actions to habits to compulsion. Nature Neuroscience **8:** 1481–1489.

20. THOMAS, K.L. & B.J. EVERITT. 2001. Limbic-cortical-ventral striatal activation during retrieval of a discrete cocaine-associated stimulus: a cellular imaging study with gamma protein kinase C expression. Journal of Neuroscience **21:** 2526–2535.

21. THOMAS, K.L., M. ARROYO & B.J. EVERITT. 2003. Induction of the learning and plasticity-associated gene Zif268 following exposure to a discrete cocaine-associated stimulus. European Journal of Neuroscience **17:** 1964–1972.

22. DI CIANO, P. & B.J. EVERITT. 2003. Differential control over drug-seeking behavior by drug-associated conditioned reinforcers and discriminative stimuli predictive of drug availability. Behav. Neurosci. **117:** 952–960.

23. ARROYO, M. *et al.* 1998. Acquisition, maintenance and reinstatement of intravenous cocaine self- administration under a second-order schedule of reinforcement in rats: effects of conditioned cues and continuous access to cocaine. Psychopharmacology **140:** 331–344.

24. EVERITT, B.J. & T.W. ROBBINS. 2000. Second-order schedules of drug reinforcement in rats and monkeys: measurement of reinforcing efficacy and drug-seeking behaviour. Psychopharmacology **153:** 17–30.

25. STEWART, J. & H. DE WIT. 1987. Reinstatement of drug-taking behavior as a method of Assessing Incentive Motivational Properties of Drugs. *In* Methods

of Assessing the Reinforcing Properties of Abused Drugs. M.A. Bozarth, Ed.: 211–227. Springer-Verlag. New York.

26. SHAHAM, Y. *et al.* 2003. The reinstatement model of drug relapse: history, methodology and major findings. Psychopharmacology **168:** 3–20.

27. LU, L. *et al.* 2004. Cocaine seeking over extended withdrawal periods in rats: different time courses of responding induced by cocaine cues versus cocaine priming over the first 6 months. Psychopharmacology **176:** 101–108.

28. LU, L. *et al.* 2005. Central amygdala ERK signaling pathway is critical to incubation of cocaine craving. Nature Neuroscience **8:** 212–219.

29. ROBBINS, T.W. *et al.* 1989. Limbic-striatal interactions in reward-related processes. Neuroscience and Biobehavioral Reviews **13:** 155–162.

30. CARDINAL, R.N. & B.J. EVERITT. 2004. Neural and psychological mechanisms underlying appetitive learning: links to drug addiction. Curr. Opin. Neurobiol. **14:** 156–162.

31. DI CIANO, P. & B.J. EVERITT. 2004. Conditioned reinforcing properties of stimuli paired with self-administered cocaine, heroin or sucrose: implications for the persistence of addictive behaviour. Neuropharmacology **47**(Suppl 1): 202–213.

32. TAYLOR, J.R. & T.W. ROBBINS. 1986. 6-hydroxydopamine lesions of the nucleus accumbens, but not of the caudate nucleus, attenuate enhanced responding with reward-related stimuli produced by intra-accumbens d-amphetamine. Psychopharmacology **90:** 390–397.

33. PARKINSON, J.A. *et al.* 1999. Dissociation in effects of lesions of the nucleus accumbens core and shell on appetitive Pavlovian approach behavior and the potentiation of conditioned reinforcement and locomotor activity by D-amphetamine. Journal of Neuroscience **19:** 2401–2411.

34. ITO, R., T.W. ROBBINS & B.J. EVERITT. 2004. Differential control over cocaine-seeking behavior by nucleus accumbens core and shell. Nature Neuroscience **7:** 389–397.

35. MACKINTOSH, N.J. 1983. Conditioning and Associative Learning. Oxford University Press. Oxford.

36. CADOR, M., T.W. ROBBINS & B.J. EVERITT. 1989. Involvement of the amygdala in stimulus-reward associations: interaction with the ventral striatum. Neuroscience **30:** 77–86.

37. BURNS, L.H., T.W. ROBBINS & B.J. EVERITT. 1993. Differential effects of excitotoxic lesions of the basolateral amygdala, ventral subiculum and medial prefrontal cortex on responding with conditioned reinforcement and locomotor activity potentiated by intraaccumbens infusions of D-amphetamine. Behavioural Brain Research **55:** 167–183.

38. PEARS, A. *et al.* 2003. Lesions of the orbitofrontal but not medial prefrontal cortex disrupt conditioned reinforcement in primates. J. Neurosci. **23:** 11189–11201.

39. BURKE, K.A. *et al.* 2007. Orbitofrontal lesions abolish conditioned reinforcement mediated by a representation of the expected outcome. Annals of the New York Academy of Sciences.

40. WALKER, S.C., T.W. ROBBINS & A.C. ROBERTS. 2007. Differential contributions of sertotonin and dopamine to reward processing within the orbitofrontal cortex. Annals of the New York Academy of Sciences. in press.

41. GOLDBERG, S.R. & A.H. TANG. 1977. Behavior maintained under second-order schedules of intravenous morphine injection in squirrel and rhesus monkeys. Psychopharmacology **51:** 235–242.

42. KATZ, J. 1979. A comparison of responding maintained under second-order schedules of intramuscular cocaine injection or food presentation in squirrel monkeys. J. Exp. Anal. Behav. **32:** 419–431.

43. WHITELAW, R.B. *et al.* 1996. Excitotoxic lesions of the basolateral amygdala impair the acquisition of cocaine-seeking behaviour under a second-order schedule of reinforcement. Psychopharmacology **127:** 213–224.

44. DI CIANO, P. & B.J. EVERITT. 2004. Direct interactions between the basolateral amygdala and nucleus accumbens core underlie cocaine-seeking behavior by rats. J. Neurosci. **24:** 7167–7173.

45. HUTCHESON, D.M. & B.J. EVERITT. 2003. The effects of selective orbitofrontal cortex lesions on the acquisition and performance of cue-controlled cocaine seeking in rats. Ann. N. Y. Acad. Sci. **1003:** 410–411.

46. PICKENS, C.L. *et al.* 2003. Different roles for orbitofrontal cortex and basolateral amygdala in a reinforcer devaluation task. Journal of Neuroscience **23:** 11078–11084.

47. WINSTANLEY, C.A. *et al.* 2004. Contrasting roles of basolateral amygdala and orbitofrontal cortex in impulsive choice. Journal of Neuroscience **24:** 4718–4722.

48. FUCHS, R.A. *et al.* 2004. Differential involvement of orbitofrontal cortex subregions in conditioned cue-induced and cocaine-primed reinstatement of cocaine seeking in rats. Journal of Neuroscience **24:** 6600–6610.

49. SCHOENBAUM, G. *et al.* 2003. Lesions of orbitofrontal cortex and basolateral amygdala complex disrupt acquisition of odor-guided discriminations and reversals. Learning & Memory **10:** 129–140.

50. NAQVI, N.H. *et al.* 2007. Damage to the insula disrupts addiction to cigarette smoking. Science **315:** 531–534.

51. WEISSENBORN, R., T.W. ROBBINS & B.J. EVERITT. 1997. Effects of medial prefrontal or anterior cingulate cortex lesions on responding for cocaine under fixed-ratio and second-order schedules of reinforcement in rats. Psychopharmacology **134:** 242–257.

52. STALNAKER, T.A. *et al.* 2006. Abnormal associative encoding in orbitofrontal neurons in cocaine-experienced rats during decision-making. European Journal of Neuroscience **24:** 2643–2653.

53. KOLB, B., S. PELLIS & T.E. ROBINSON. 2004. Plasticity and functions of the orbital frontal cortex. Brain and Cognition **55:** 104–115.

54. ROBINSON, T.E. & B. KOLB. 2004. Structural plasticity associated with exposure to drugs of abuse. Neuropharmacology **47:** 33–46.

55. CROMBAG, H.S. *et al.* 2005. Opposite effects of amphetamine self-administration experience on dendritic spines in the medial and orbital prefrontal cortex. Cerebral Cortex **15:** 341–348.

56. American Psychiatric Association. 1994. Diagnostic and Statistical Manual of Mental Disorders, 4th ed. American Psychiatric Association. Washington, DC.

57. SCHUSTER, C.R. 1986. Implications of laboratory research for the treatment of drug dependence. *In* Behavioral Analysis of Drug Dependence. S.R. Goldberg & I.P. Stolerman, Eds.: 357–386. Academic Press Inc. London.

58. WOLFFGRAMM, J. 1991. An ethopharmacological approach to the development of drug-addiction. Neuroscience and Biobehavioral Reviews **15:** 515–519.

59. VANDERSCHUREN, L.J.M.J. & B.J. EVERITT. 2004. Drug seeking becomes compulsive after prolonged cocaine self-administration. Science **305:** 1017–1019.
60. DEROCHE-GAMONET, V., D. BELIN & P.V. PIAZZA. 2004. Evidence for addiction-like behavior in the rat. Science **305:** 1014–1017.
61. PELLOUX, Y., B.J. EVERITT & A. DICKINSON. 2007. Compulsive drug seeking by rats under punishment: effects of drug taking history. Psychopharmacology **194:** 127–137.
62. SCHOENBAUM, G., M.R. ROESCH & T.A. STALNAKER. 2006. Orbitofrontal cortex, decision-making and drug addiction. Trends in Neurosciences **29:** 116–124.
63. FILLMORE, M.T., C.R. RUSH & C.A. MARCZINSKI. 2003. Effects of d-amphetamine on behavioral control in stimulant abusers: the role of prepotent response tendencies. Drug and Alcohol Dependence **71:** 143–152.
64. ARON, A.R. *et al.* 2004. Human midbrain sensitivity to cognitive feedback and uncertainty during classification learning. Journal of Neurophysiology **92:** 1144–1152.
65. FILLMORE, M.T. & C.R. RUSH. 2002. Impaired inhibitory control of behavior in chronic cocaine users. Drug and Alcohol Dependence **66:** 265–273.
66. MONTEROSSO, J.R. *et al.* 2005. Deficits in response inhibition associated with chronic methamphetamine abuse. Drug and Alcohol Dependence **79:** 273–277.
67. FORMAN, S.D. *et al.* 2004. Opiate addicts lack error-dependent activation of rostral anterior cingulate. Biological Psychiatry **55:** 531–537.
68. LEE, T.M.C. *et al.* 2005. Neural activity associated with cognitive regulation in heroin users: a fMRI study. Neuroscience Letters **382:** 211–216.
69. VERDEJO-GARCIA, A.J., J.C. PERALES & M. PEREZ-GARCIA. 2007. Cognitive impulsivity in cocaine and heroin polysubstance abusers. Addictive Behaviors **32:** 950–966.
70. ELLIOTT, R., R.J. DOLAN & C.D. FRITH. 2000. Dissociable functions in the medial and lateral orbitofrontal cortex: evidence from human neuroimaging studies. Cerebral Cortex **10:** 308–317.
71. ARON, A.R. *et al.* 2003. Stop-signal inhibition disrupted by damage to right inferior frontal gyrus in humans. Nature Neuroscience **6:** 115–116.
72. THOMPSON, P.M. *et al.* 2004. Structural abnormalities in the brains of human subjects who use methamphetamine. Journal of Neuroscience **24:** 6028–6036.
73. FILLMORE, M.T. & C.R. RUSH. 2006. Polydrug abusers display impaired discrimination-reversal learning in a model of behavioural control. Journal of Psychopharmacology **20:** 24–32.
74. ROLLS, E.T. 1999. The functions of the orbitofrontal cortex. Neurocase **5:** 301–312.
75. KRINGELBACH, M.L. & E.T. ROLLS. 2004. The functional neuroanatomy of the human orbitofrontal cortex: evidence from neuroimaging and neuropsychology. Progress in Neurobiology **72:** 341–372.
76. LONDON, E.D. *et al.* 2000. Orbitofrontal cortex and human drug abuse: functional imaging. Cerebral Cortex **10:** 334–342.
77. VOLKOW, N.D. & J.S. FOWLER. 2000. Addiction, a disease of compulsion and drive: involvement of the orbitofrontal cortex. Cerebral Cortex **10:** 318–325.
78. MATOCHIK, J.A. *et al.* 2003. Frontal cortical tissue composition in abstinent cocaine abusers: a magnetic resonance imaging study. Neuroimage **19:** 1095–1102.

79. WHITE, F.J. & P.W. KALIVAS. 1998. Neuroadaptations involved in amphetamine and cocaine addiction. Drug and Alcohol Dependence **51:** 141–153.

80. FILIP, M. *et al.* 2005. The serotonergic system and its role in cocaine addiction. Pharmacological Reports **57:** 685–700.

81. PUM, M. *et al.* 2007. Dissociating effects of cocaine and d-amphetamine on dopamine and serotonin in the perirhinal, entorhinal, and prefrontal cortex of freely moving rats. Psychopharmacology **193:** 375–390.

82. EVERS, E.A.T. *et al.* 2005. Serotonergic modulation of prefrontal cortex during negative feedback in probabilistic reversal learning. Neuropsychopharmacology **30:** 1138–1147.

83. CHAMBERLAIN, S.R. *et al.* 2006. Neurochemical modulation of response inhibition and probabilistic learning in humans. Science **311:** 861–863.

84. ARON, A.R., T.W. ROBBINS & R.A. POLDRAK. 2004. Inhibition and right inferior frontal cortex. Trends in Cognitive Sciences **8:** 170–177.

85. KRAWCZYK, D.C. 2002. Contributions of the prefrontal cortex to the neural basis of human decision making. Neuroscience and Biobehavioral Reviews **26:** 631–664.

86. WALLIS, J.D. 2007. Orbitofrontal cortex and its contribution to decision-making. Annual Review of Neuroscience **30:** 31–56.

87. RUSHWORTH, M.F.S. *et al.* 2007. Contrasting roles for cingulate and orbitofrontal cortex in decisions and social behaviour. Trends in Cognitive Sciences **11:** 168–176.

88. BECHARA, A. 2004. The role of emotion in decision-making: evidence from neurological patients with orbitofrontal damage. Brain and Cognition **55:** 30–40.

89. CLARK, L. *et al.* 2003. The contributions of lesion laterality and lesion volume to decision-making impairment following frontal lobe damage. Neuropsychologia **41:** 1474–1483.

90. MANES, F. *et al.* 2002. Decision-making processes following damage to the prefrontal cortex. Brain **125:** 624–639.

91. KOENIGS, M. & D. TRANEL. 2007. Irrational economic decision-making after ventromedial prefrontal damage: evidence from the ultimatum game. Journal of Neuroscience **27:** 951–956.

92. BOLLA, K.I. *et al.* 2003. Orbitofrontal cortex dysfunction in abstinent cocaine abusers performing a decision-making task. Neuroimage **19:** 1085–1094.

93. ERSCHE, K.D. *et al.* 2005. Abnormal frontal activations related to decision-making in current and former amphetamine and opiate dependent individuals. Psychopharmacology **180:** 612–623.

94. GOLDSTEIN, R.Z. *et al.* 2001. Addiction changes orbitofrontal gyrus function: involvement in response inhibition. Neuroreport **12:** 2595–2599.

95. ELLIOTT, R. *et al.* 2003. Differential response patterns in the striatum and orbitofrontal cortex to financial reward in humans: a parametric functional magnetic resonance imaging study. Journal of Neuroscience **23:** 303–307.

96. SCHULTZ, W., L. TREMBLAY & J.R. HOLLERMAN. 2000. Reward processing in primate orbitofrontal cortex and basal ganglia. Cerebral Cortex **10:** 272–283.

97. TOBLER, P.N. *et al.* 2007. Reward value coding distinct from risk attitude-related uncertainty coding in human reward systems. Journal of Neurophysiology **97:** 1621–1632.

98. PAULUS, M.P. *et al.* 2002. Behavioral and functional neuroimaging evidence for prefrontal dysfunction in methamphetamine-dependent subjects. Neuropsychopharmacology **26:** 53–63.
99. PAULUS, M.P. *et al.* 2003. Decision making by methamphetamine-dependent subjects is associated with error-rate-independent decrease in prefrontal and parietal activation. Biological Psychiatry **53:** 65–74.
100. ERSCHE, K.D. *et al.* 2005. Punishment induces risky decision-making in methadone-maintained opiate users but not in heroin users or healthy volunteers. Neuropsychopharmacology **30:** 2115–2124.
101. YUCEL, M. *et al.* 2007. A combined spectroscopic and functional MRI investigation of the dorsal anterior cingulate region in opiate addiction. Mol. Psychiatry. **12:** 691–702.
102. ERSCHE, K.D. *et al.* 2006. Differences in orbitofrontal activation during decision-making between methadone-maintained opiate users, heroin users and healthy volunteers. Psychopharmacology **188:** 364–373.
103. ROGERS, R.D. & T.W. ROBBINS. 2001. Investigating the neurocognitive deficits associated with chronic drug misuse. Current Opinion in Neurobiology **11:** 250–257.
104. ROGERS, R.D. *et al.* 2003. The neuropsychology of chronic drug abuse. *In* Disorders of Brain and Mind Vol. 2, Chapter 20. M.A. Ron & T.W. Robbins, Eds.: 447–467. Cambridge University Press. Cambridge.
105. ORNSTEIN, T.J. *et al.* 2000. Profiles of cognitive dysfunction in chronic amphetamine and heroin abusers. Neuropsychopharmacology **23:** 113–126.
106. ERSCHE, K.D. *et al.* 2006. Profile of executive and memory function associated with amphetamine and opiate dependence. Neuropsychopharmacology **31:** 1036–1047.
107. JENTSCH, J.D. & J.R. TAYLOR. 1999. Impulsivity resulting from frontostriatal dysfunction in drug abuse: implications for the control of behavior by reward-related stimuli. Psychopharmacology **146:** 373–390.
108. ROESCH, M.R. *et al.* 2007. Previous cocaine exposure makes rats hypersensitive to both delay and reward magnitude. Journal of Neuroscience **27:** 245–250.
109. JENTSCH, J.D. *et al.* 2002. Impairments of reversal learning and response perseveration after repeated, intermittent cocaine administrations to monkeys. Neuropsychopharmacology **26:** 183–190.
110. SCHOENBAUM, G. *et al.* 2004. Cocaine-experienced rats exhibit learning deficits in a task sensitive to orbitofrontal cortex lesions. European Journal of Neuroscience **19:** 1997–2002.
111. CALU, D.J. *et al.* 2007. Withdrawal from cocaine self-administration produces long-lasting deficits in orbitofrontal-dependent reversal learning in rats. Learning and Memory **14:** 325–328.
112. DALLEY, J.W. *et al.* 2005. Cognitive sequelae of intravenous amphetamine self-administration in rats: evidence for selective effects on attentional performance. Neuropsychopharmacology **30:** 525–537.
113. DALLEY, J.W. *et al.* 2005. Attentional and motivational deficits in rats withdrawn from intravenous self-administration of cocaine or heroin. Psychopharmacology **182:** 579–587.
114. DALLEY, J.W. *et al.* 2006. Enduring deficits in sustained visual attention during withdrawal of intravenous methylenedioxymethamphetamine self-administration in rats: results from a comparative study with d-amphetamine and methamphetamine. Neuropsychopharmacology **32:** 1195–1206.

115. ROBBINS, T.W. 2002. The 5-choice serial reaction time task: behavioural pharmacology and functional neurochemistry. Psychopharmacology **163:** 362–380.
116. OLMSTEAD, M.C. *et al.* 2000. Cocaine-seeking by rats: regulation, reinforcement and activation. Psychopharmacology **152:** 123–131.
117. HUTCHESON, D.M. *et al.* 2001. The role of withdrawal in heroin addiction: enhances reward or promotes avoidance? Nature Neuroscience **4:** 943–947.
118. WAGNER, F.A. & J.C. ANTHONY. 2002. From first drug use to drug dependence: Developmental periods of risk for dependence upon marijuana, cocaine, and alcohol. Neuropsychopharmacology **26:** 479–488.

Neural Correlates of Inflexible Behavior in the Orbitofrontal–Amygdalar Circuit after Cocaine Exposure

THOMAS A. STALNAKER,[a] MATTHEW R. ROESCH,[a] DONNA J. CALU,[b] KATHRYN A. BURKE,[b] TEGHPAL SINGH,[b] AND GEOFFREY SCHOENBAUM[a,c]

[a]*Departments of Anatomy and Neurobiology and Psychiatry, University of Maryland School of Medicine, Baltimore, Maryland 21201, USA*

[b]*Program in Neuroscience, University of Maryland School of Medicine, Baltimore, Maryland 21201, USA*

[c]*Department of Psychology, University of Maryland Baltimore County, Baltimore, Maryland 21228, USA*

ABSTRACT: Addiction is characterized by compulsive or inflexible behavior, observed both in the context of drug-seeking and in contexts unrelated to drugs. One possible contributor to these inflexible behaviors may be drug-induced dysfunction within circuits that support behavioral flexibility, including the basolateral amygdala (ABL) and the orbitofrontal cortex (OFC). Here we describe data demonstrating that chronic cocaine exposure causes long-lasting changes in encoding properties in the ABL and the OFC during learning and reversal in an odor-guided task. In particular, these data suggest that inflexible encoding in ABL neurons may be the proximal cause of cocaine-induced behavioral inflexibility, and that a loss of outcome-expectant encoding in OFC neurons could be a more distal contributor to this impairment. A similar mechanism of drug-induced orbitofrontal–amygdalar dysfunction may cause inflexible behavior when animals and addicts are exposed to drug-associated cues and contexts.

KEYWORDS: addiction; cocaine; orbitofrontal cortex; basolateral amygdala; reversal; associative learning

Addiction is characterized by poor decision making and a loss of control over drug-seeking. Memories for cues or contexts that occur in close proximity to drug-taking, such as syringes, crack pipes, people, or places, are often prominent features of these behaviors.[1–3] Activating these drug-associated memories elicits drug-seeking behavior and relapse in animal models and, it

Address for correspondence: Thomas A. Stalnaker, 20 Penn Street HSF-2, Rm S251, Baltimore, MD 21201. Voice: 410-706-8910; fax: 410-706-2512.
tstal002@umaryland.edu

Ann. N.Y. Acad. Sci. 1121: 598–609 (2007). © 2007 New York Academy of Sciences.
doi: 10.1196/annals.1401.014

is theorized, in human addicts.[4–9] The influence of drug-associated memories persists long into abstinence,[10,11] through extinction,[12] and, perhaps most strikingly, even in the face of adverse outcomes or cues that represent adverse outcomes.[13,14] These memories' persistence and apparent invulnerability to change have been argued to contribute to the lack of control that characterizes decision making in addiction.[8,15]

Addicts and drug-experienced animals also exhibit poor, inflexible decision making in experimental settings, far removed from drug-taking. For example, addicts exhibit an inability to shift or to reverse their response strategy in several gambling tasks.[16–18] Animal models, primarily of psychostimulant addiction, indicate that these deficits may be the result of drug exposure rather than a pre-existing condition. Thus, monkeys and rats exposed to chronic noncontingent cocaine show inflexible behavior in reversal-learning tasks up to a month after cocaine exposure.[19,20] As illustrated in FIGURE 1, we have recently found a similar reversal deficit in rats previously trained to self-administer cocaine.[21] The go, no-go odor discrimination task used in studies in our lab, illustrated in FIGURE 2, requires the rat to learn to associate one odor with a sucrose reward and a second odor with a bitter quinine punishment. Rats previously exposed to cocaine, either passively by 14 days of daily ip injections (30 mg/kg) or via 14 daily self-administration sessions (see FIG. 1 legend for details), learn these problems normally but require many more trials than controls to learn serial reversals of the final problem. Interestingly, drug-associated behavioral deficits, both in gambling tasks in humans and in reversal tasks, are similar to those caused by damage to the orbitofrontal cortex (OFC).[22–24]

Thus addiction involves inflexible behaviors both in drug-associated contexts and in normal learning contexts. What are the neural bases of these inflexible behaviors? One possibility is that addiction involves abnormalities in brain circuits that normally support flexible behavior. Below, we will describe evidence that chronic cocaine exposure causes long-lasting changes in information processing in a circuit including the OFC and the basolateral amygdala (ABL) that may contribute to the inflexibility of behavior in addiction.

INFLEXIBLE ASSOCIATIVE ENCODING IN BASOLATERAL AMYGDALA: A PROXIMAL CAUSE OF INFLEXIBLE DECISION MAKING IN ADDICTION

The ABL has been implicated in the persistent effects of drug-associated cues on drug-seeking, both in human cocaine addicts and in animal models of cocaine addiction.[25–29] For instance, imaging studies frequently reveal activations of the amygdala during exposure to cues that elicit craving in addicts,[25,27,28] and, in animal models, lesions or pharmacological manipulations of the ABL block cue-induced relapse.[9,30,31] Recently it has been shown that

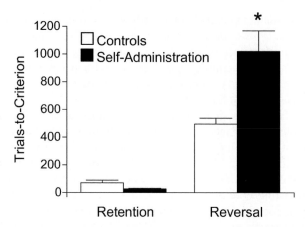

FIGURE 1. Effect of previous cocaine self-administration training on reversal learning. Training included 14 daily 3-hour sessions, with 0.75 mg/kg cocaine-HCl per infusion and an average of 24 infusions per day, and ended at least 1 month prior to behavioral testing on the go, no-go odor discrimination task described in the text. Rats first showed retention of a previously learned odor discrimination, and then acquired a reversal of that odor discrimination. Shown are average trials to criterion for two serial retention/reversals. Error bars indicate SEMs.*$P < 0.01$, compared to controls (data from Calu et al.[21]).

pharmacological manipulations of the ABL that block memory reconsolidation also impair cue-induced relapse, suggesting that memories stored in the amygdala may mediate this phenomenon.[32,33]

We have reported recently that the reversal-learning deficits that result from damage to the OFC are also mediated through the ABL. As reviewed elsewhere,[34] OFC lesions result in inflexible associative encoding in the ABL during reversal learning, and selective neurotoxic lesions of ABL, which eliminate these inflexible correlates, restore normal reversal learning in OFC-lesioned rats.[35,36] Based on these data, we have suggested that signals from the OFC normally facilitate changes in associative representations in other brain areas, particularly in the face of novel or unexpected outcomes[37]; damage to the OFC eliminates these signals, resulting in slower changes in encoding downstream in the ABL and slower reversal learning.

To ask whether a similar mechanism might mediate reversal-learning impairments caused by cocaine exposure, we recently compared neural correlates during reversal learning in the ABL in cocaine- and saline-treated rats.[38] Rats were again exposed to 14 daily ip injections of cocaine (30 mg/kg), and then beginning approximately 1 month later, neural activity was recorded in these rats as they learned and reversed a series of two-odor discrimination problems using the same go, no-go task described above (illustrated in FIG. 2). As we have reported previously for normal rats,[35,39] ABL neurons in both saline- and cocaine-treated rats rapidly developed differential firing to the odor cues as the

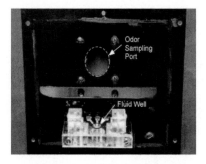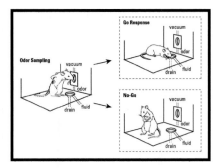

FIGURE 2. Schematic diagram demonstrating the odor-guided, go, no-go task described in the text. On the left is the panel used to train rats on this task. In each trial within a particular session, one of two odors was delivered to the odor port at the top of the panel. Odor 1 indicated that if the rat went to the fluid well below the odor port, sucrose solution would be available. Odor 2 indicated that if the rat went to the fluid well, unpalatable quinine solution would be available. Rats learned to go to the well (go response, shown on the right) after sampling odor 1, and to avoid going to the well (no-go response, shown on the right) after sampling odor 2. After rats had reached and maintained a behavioral criterion of 18 correct out of 20 trials, the odor-outcome contingencies were reversed until rats again reached criterion performance.

rats learned their meaning. In saline controls, these cue-selective populations reversed their cue-selectivity after reversal, such that they tracked the outcome predicted by the cue rather than the identity of the cue itself. In contrast, in cocaine-treated reversal-impaired rats, these populations failed to reverse their cue preference; instead they remained selective for the cue to which they fired before reversal. The contrast between the flexibility in cue-selectivity in controls and the inflexibility in cocaine-treated rats is illustrated by the population histograms and scatter plots shown in FIGURE 3.

To test whether the inflexibility of associative encoding in the ABL after reversal actually mediates the reversal-learning deficits in these rats, we exposed a second set of rats to cocaine or saline and then made bilateral neurotoxic or sham lesions of the ABL. After these rats recovered from surgery, we tested them in the same go, no-go odor discrimination task used earlier to assess reversal learning. As illustrated in FIGURE 4, we again found that cocaine exposure caused impaired reversal learning; however, this impairment was not observed in cocaine-exposed rats with ABL lesions. ABL lesions by themselves had no significant effect on reversal learning. Thus, in cocaine-exposed rats, encoding in the ABL seemed to be interfering with the ability to learn reversals quickly. These results are consistent with the hypothesis that rigid associative encoding in the ABL after reversal is the proximal cause of the cocaine-induced reversal impairment, just as it may be the proximal cause of cue-induced relapse to drug-seeking.

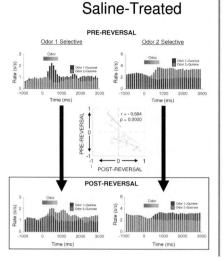
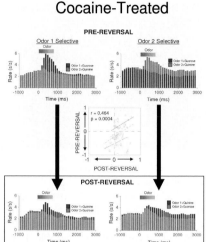

FIGURE 3. Population histograms before and after reversal for all neurons recorded in the ABL that were significantly selective for the sucrose-predictive cue (odor 1 selective) or the quinine-predictive cue (odor 2 selective) during the postcriterion prereversal-trial block. In saline-treated rats, neurons in both populations reversed their cue-selectivity across reversal. In contrast, in cocaine-treated rats, neurons that developed selectivity to the sucrose-predictive cue during learning remained selective for the same cue after reversal, even though it now predicted quinine. Neurons in cocaine-treated rats that developed selectivity to the quinine-predictive cue during learning failed to reverse their selectivity after reversal, instead showing a phasic response to both cues. Insets show a quantitative analysis of the flexibility of these populations across reversal. Neurons in saline-treated rats showed a negative correlation between their prereversal versus postreversal cue-selectivity indices; neurons in cocaine-treated rats showed a positive correlation between the two. Cue-selectivity index was defined as $(fr_{O1} - fr_{O2})/(fr_{O1} + fr_{O2})$, where $fr = $ firing rate during cue-sampling in the post-criterion trial block; $O1 = $ odor cue that predicted sucrose before reversal; $O2 = $ odor cue that predicted quinine before reversal (data adapted from Stalnaker *et al.*[38]). (In color in *Annals* online.)

A FAILURE TO SIGNAL EXPECTED OUTCOMES IN THE ORBITOFRONTAL CORTEX: A DISTAL CAUSE OF INFLEXIBLE DECISION MAKING IN ADDICTION

But why is associative encoding in the ABL resistant to change after drug exposure? An answer to this question may lie in the effects of addictive drugs on the OFC. Imaging studies in cocaine,[40] methamphetamine,[41] and heroin[42] users reveal altered metabolism in the OFC and abnormal neuronal activation in response to drug-associated cues.[42] Furthermore, as reviewed above, drug addicts and animals exposed to addictive drugs, such as patients and animals with OFC damage,[24,43,44] exhibit behavioral deficits on a variety of

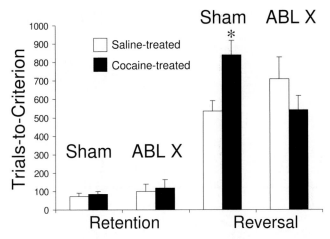

FIGURE 4. The effect of bilateral ABL lesions on retention and reversal learning in saline-treated rats (*white bars*) or cocaine treated rats (*black bars*). Previous cocaine treatment caused a severe reversal impairment that was abolished by ABL lesions. ABL lesions in the saline-treated rats had no significant effect. Shown is the average of three serial retention/reversals, in which rats first had to show retention of a previously learned odor discrimination, and then had to acquire a reversal of that odor discrimination. *$P < 0.05$ compared to the saline-treated sham-lesioned group and compared to the cocaine-treated ABL-lesioned group (data adapted from Stalnaker *et al.*[38]).

OFC-dependent tasks.[16,17,20,45–48] These observations have led to the proposal that addictive drugs cause long-lasting disruptions to OFC function.[49,50]

In the context of our reversal-learning task, we have proposed that the critical function of the OFC is to signal expected outcomes at the time a decision is made.[34] This signal is particularly evident in subpopulations of OFC neurons, like the one shown in FIGURE 5, that fire in anticipation of one of the outcomes early in learning and then, as learning progresses, become active in the presence of the odor cue that predicts that outcome. By this pattern of activity, these neurons appear to activate a representation of the expected outcome at the time of odor sampling, when a decision about whether to respond or not must be made. Signaling expected outcomes might facilitate changes in associative encoding in the ABL after reversal by contributing to the generation of teaching signals that occur when actual outcomes fail to match expectations. In other words, such teaching signals require there to be some record of what outcome was expected; the OFC may provide this signal, either in whole or in part. With the loss of this signal, as after OFC lesions, changes in the outcome predicted by the cues would result in less-robust teaching signals, thereby causing associative encoding in downstream regions—such as the ABL—to change more slowly.

To test whether cocaine exposure causes a disruption of this outcome-expectant signaling in the OFC, we compared neural correlates in the OFC

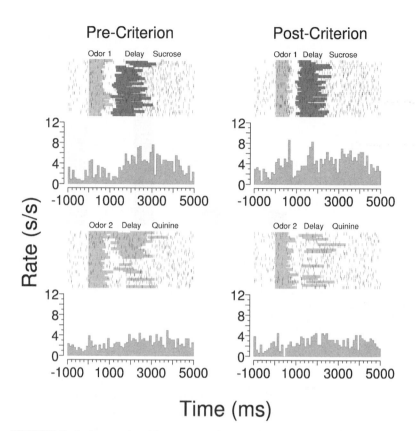

FIGURE 5. Peri-event time histograms and raster plots show activity of a single-unit recorded from the OFC of a control rat during learning of an odor discrimination. The gray shading on the raster plots represents the period of odor delivery on each trial, the subsequent blue shading on the upper rasters represents the delay after the response and immediately before sucrose delivery, and the subsequent red shading on the lower rasters represents the delay after the response and immediately before quinine delivery. In trials before the rat had reached behavioral criterion (precriterion, left histograms and raster plots) this neuron fired selectively during and immediately preceding the delivery of sucrose. In trials after the rat had reached criterion (postcriterion, right histograms and raster plots) this neuron fired selectively for the odor that predicted sucrose, while continuing to fire during and immediately preceding sucrose. Thus in the postcriterion phase, this neuron activated a representation of the expected outcome at the time of odor delivery (data adapted from Roesch et al.[54]). (In color in *Annals* online.)

in cocaine- and saline-treated rats during acquisition of a series of two-odor go, no-go discrimination problems, using the same procedures as in our ABL recording experiment described above.[51] Neural activity in saline-treated rats was similar to that reported previously,[4,52,53] with some neurons firing selectively in anticipation of one of the two outcomes (sucrose or quinine) early

Saline-treated   Cocaine-treated

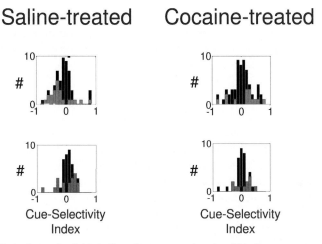

FIGURE 6. Cue-selectivity indices for neurons that developed outcome-expectant firing during the precriterion block, firing differentially after the rat's response in anticipation of either sucrose or quinine delivery. On the top row are shown the populations that developed quinine-expectant firing, and on the bottom row are shown the populations that developed sucrose-expectant firing. Red (top row) or blue (bottom row) bars represent neurons that were significantly selective for one or the other of the two odors. In both quinine-expectant and sucrose-expectant populations, neurons in control rats were more likely to develop cue-selectivity to the cue that predicted their preferred outcome. Thus, the distribution for quinine-expectant neurons is skewed to the left, and that in sucrose-expectant neurons is skewed to the right. In contrast, in both populations in cocaine-treated rats, neurons were equally likely to develop cue-selectivity to either cue. Thus, the distributions are symmetric around zero. Cue-selectivity indices were calculated from activity during odor sampling, using the same formula as in FIGURE 3 (data adapted from Stalnaker et al.[51]). (In color in *Annals* online.)

in learning and then becoming activated by the appropriate odor cue after learning (as in FIG. 5).[54] Rats that had been exposed to cocaine exhibited similar proportions of neurons that fired in anticipation of one or the other of the outcomes. However, these populations were not consistently activated by the appropriate odor cue after learning, and instead were equally likely to become activated by either odor cue. Thus, for example, quinine-expectant neurons were equally likely to become selective for the quinine-predictive odor cue or for the sucrose-predictive odor cue. This pattern of results is quantified in the distributions of cue-selectivity indices for the outcome-expectant populations, shown in FIGURE 6. These distributions are significantly skewed to the left for quinine-expectant neurons and to the right for sucrose-expectant neurons in saline-treated rats, but they are symmetrically distributed around zero for cocaine-treated rats. Thus, chronic cocaine exposure caused OFC neurons to fail to signal the expected outcome during odor sampling in this task. This failure may explain why these rats are unable to bias behavior to reflect the value of expected outcomes, both during odor discrimination learning[20] and possibly also after reinforcer devaluation.[47] In addition, such a loss of outcome-expectant encoding may be a distal cause of the long-lasting reversal deficit seen after chronic exposure to cocaine.

CONCLUSIONS

Here we have described data demonstrating that chronic cocaine exposure causes 1) inflexible encoding in the ABL across reversal of cue-outcome contingencies, 2) an ABL-dependent deficit in the ability to change behavior when cue-outcome contingencies change, and 3) long-lasting disruptions to outcome-expectant signaling in the OFC. These data support a model of cocaine-induced decision-making deficits in which cocaine exposure causes a critical loss of outcome-expectant encoding in the OFC, which leads to inflexible encoding of cue significance in the ABL. Such a model would be broadly consistent with data demonstrating that human addicts show abnormalities in the OFC and in OFC-dependent tasks, and with data from animal models of addiction suggesting that persistent ABL encoding underlies inflexible responding for drug-associated cues. Thus, while the changes in encoding properties described here were demonstrated during associative learning for nondrug outcomes, similar changes could also play a role in drug-seeking behavior itself. Future research should address whether the drug-induced changes to the encoding properties of the OFC–ABL circuit are similar in both drug and nondrug settings.

REFERENCES

1. EHRMAN, R.N., S.J. ROBBINS, A.R. CHILDRESS & C.P. O'BRIEN. 1992. Conditioned responses to cocaine-related stimuli in cocaine abuse patients. Psychopharmacology (Berl.) **107:** 523–529.
2. AVANTS, S.K., A. MARGOLIN, T.R. KOSTEN & N.L. COONEY. 1995. Differences between responders and nonresponders to cocaine cues in the laboratory. Addict. Behav. **20:** 215–224.
3. FOLTIN, R.W. & M. HANEY. 2000. Conditioned effects of environmental stimuli paired with smoked cocaine in humans. Psychopharmacology (Berl.) **149:** 24–33.
4. O'BRIEN, C.P., A.R. CHILDRESS, R. EHRMAN & S.J. ROBBINS. 1998. Conditioning factors in drug abuse: can they explain compulsion? J. Psychopharmacol. **12:** 15–22.
5. CROMBAG, H.S. & Y. SHAHAM. 2002. Renewal of drug seeking by contextual cues after prolonged extinction in rats. Behav. Neurosci. **116:** 169–173.
6. KALIVAS, P.W. & K. MCFARLAND. 2003. Brain circuitry and the reinstatement of cocaine-seeking behavior. Psychopharmacology (Berl.) **168:** 44–56.

7. SEE, R.E. 2005. Neural substrates of cocaine-cue associations that trigger relapse. Eur. J. Pharmacol. **526:** 140–146.
8. WEISS, F. 2005. Neurobiology of craving, conditioned reward and relapse. Curr. Opin. Pharmacol. **5:** 9–19.
9. FUCHS, R.A., M.W. FELTENSTEIN & R.E. SEE. 2006. The role of the basolateral amygdala in stimulus-reward memory and extinction memory consolidation and in subsequent conditioned cued reinstatement of cocaine seeking. Eur. J. Neurosci. **23:** 2809–2813.
10. CICCOCIOPPO, R., R. MARTIN-FARDON & F. WEISS. 2004. Stimuli associated with a single cocaine experience elicit long-lasting cocaine-seeking. Nat. Neurosci. **7:** 495–496.
11. LU, L., J.W. GRIMM, J. DEMPSEY & Y. SHAHAM. 2004. Cocaine seeking over extended withdrawal periods in rats: different time courses of responding induced by cocaine cues versus cocaine priming over the first 6 months. Psychopharmacology **176:** 101–108.
12. WEISS, F., R. MARTIN-FARDON, R. CICCOCIOPPO, *et al.* 2001. Enduring resistance to extinction of cocaine-seeking behavior induced by drug-related cues. Neuropsychopharmacology **25:** 361–372.
13. DEROCHE-GAMONET, V., D. BELIN & P.V. PIAZZA. 2004. Evidence for addiction-like behavior in the rat. Science **305:** 951–953.
14. VANDERSCHUREN, L.J.M.J. & B.J. EVERITT. 2004. Drug seeking becomes compulsive after prolonged cocaine self-administration. Science **305:** 1017–1019.
15. VANDERSCHUREN, L.J. & B.J. EVERITT. 2005. Behavioral and neural mechanisms of compulsive drug seeking. Eur. J. Pharmacol. **526:** 77–88.
16. ROGERS, R.D., B.J. EVERITT, A. BALDACCHINO, *et al.* 1999. Dissociable deficits in the decision-making cognition of chronic amphetamine abusers, opiate abusers, patients with focal damage to prefrontal cortex, and tryptophan-depleted normal volunteers: evidence for monoaminergic mechanisms. Neuropsychopharmacology **20:** 322–339.
17. GRANT, S., C. CONTOREGGI & E.D. LONDON. 2000. Drug abusers show impaired performance in a laboratory test of decision making. Neuropsychologia **38:** 1180–1187.
18. BECHARA, A., S. DOLAN & A. HINDES. 2002. Decision-making and addiction (part II): myopia for the future or hypersensitivity to reward? Neuropsychologia **40:** 1690–1705.
19. JENTSCH, J.D., P. OLAUSSON, R. DE LA GARZA & J.R. TAYLOR. 2002. Impairments of reversal learning and response perseveration after repeated, intermittent cocaine administrations to monkeys. Neuropsychopharmacology **26:** 183–190.
20. SCHOENBAUM, G., M.P. SADDORIS, S.J. RAMUS, *et al.* 2004. Cocaine-experienced rats exhibit learning deficits in a task sensitive to orbitofrontal cortex lesions. E. J. Neurosci. **19:** 1997–2002.
21. CALU, D.J., T.A. STALNAKER, T.M. FRANZ, *et al.* 2007. Withdrawal from cocaine self-administration produces long-lasting deficits in orbitofrontal-dependent reversal learning in rats. Learn. Mem. **14:** 325–328.
22. BECHARA, A., H. DAMASIO, D. TRANEL & A.R. DAMASIO. 1997. Deciding advantageously before knowing the advantageous strategy. Science **275:** 1293–1294.
23. SCHOENBAUM, G., B. SETLOW, S.L. NUGENT, *et al.* 2003. Lesions of orbitofrontal cortex and basolateral amygdala complex disrupt acquisition of odor-guided discriminations and reversals. Learn. Mem. **10:** 129–140.

24. IZQUIERDO, A.D., R.K. SUDA & E.A. MURRAY. 2004. Bilateral orbital prefrontal cortex lesions in rhesus monkeys disrupt choices guided by both reward value and reward contingency. J. Neurosci. **24:** 7540–7548.

25. CHILDRESS, A.R., P.D. MOZLEY, W. MCELGIN, *et al.* 1999. Limbic activation during cue-induced cocaine craving. Am. J. Psychiatry **156:** 11–18.

26. CICCOCIOPPO, R., P.P. SANNA & F. WEISS. 2001. Cocaine-predictive stimulus induces drug-seeking behavior and neural activation in limbic brain regions after multiple months of abstinence: reversal by D(1) antagonists. Proc. Natl. Acad. Sci. USA **98:** 1976–1981.

27. KILTS, C.D., J.B. SCHWEITZER, C.K. QUINN, *et al.* 2001. Neural activity related to drug craving in cocaine addiction. Arch. Gen. Psychiatry **58:** 334–341.

28. BONSON, K.R., S.J. GRANT, C.S. CONTOREGGI, *et al.* 2002. Neural systems and cue-induced cocaine craving. Neuropsychopharmacology **26:** 376–386.

29. CARELLI, R.M., J.G. WILLIAMS & J.A. HOLLANDER. 2003. Basolateral amygdala neurons encode cocaine self-administration and cocaine-associated cues. J. Neurosci. **23:** 8204–8211.

30. KRUZICH, P.J. & R.E. SEE. 2001. Differential contributions of the basolateral and central amygdala in the acquisition and expression of conditioned relapse to cocaine-seeking behavior. J. Neurosci. **21:** RC155.

31. SEE, R.E., J. MCLAUGHLIN & R.A. FUCHS. 2003. Muscarinic receptor antagonism in the basolateral amygdala blocks acquisition of cocaine-stimulus association in a model of relapse to cocaine-seeking behavior in rats. Neuroscience **117:** 477–483.

32. LEE, J.L., P. DI CIANO, K.L. THOMAS & B.J. EVERITT. 2005. Disrupting reconsolidation of drug memories reduces cocaine-seeking behavior. Neuron **47:** 795–801.

33. LEE, J.L., A.L. MILTON & B.J. EVERITT. 2006. Cue-induced cocaine seeking and relapse are reduced by disruption of drug memory reconsolidation. J. Neurosci. **26:** 5881–5887.

34. SCHOENBAUM, G., M.P. SADDORIS & T.A. STALNAKER. 2007. Reconciling the roles of orbitofrontal cortex in reversal learning and the encoding of outcome expectancies. Ann. N. Y. Acad. Sci. **1401:** xx–xx.

35. SADDORIS, M.P., M. GALLAGHER & G. SCHOENBAUM. 2005. Rapid associative encoding in basolateral amygdala depends on connections with orbitofrontal cortex. Neuron **46:** 321–331.

36. STALNAKER, T.A., T.M. FRANZ, T. SINGH & G. SCHOENBAUM. 2007. Basolateral amygdala lesions abolish orbitofrontal-dependent reversal impairments. Neuron **54:** 51–58.

37. SCHOENBAUM, G., M.R. ROESCH & T.A. STALNAKER. 2006. Orbitofrontal cortex, decision-making, and drug addiction. Trends. Neurosci. **29:** 116–124.

38. STALNAKER, T.A., M.R. ROESCH, T.M. FRANZ, *et al.* 2007. Cocaine-induced decision-making deficits are mediated by miscoding in basolateral amygdala. Nat. Neurosci. **10:** 949–951.

39. SCHOENBAUM, G., A.A. CHIBA & M. GALLAGHER. 1999. Neural encoding in orbitofrontal cortex and basolateral amygdala during olfactory discrimination learning. J. Neurosci. **19:** 1876–1884.

40. VOLKOW, N.D., J.S. FOWLER, A.P. WOLF, *et al.* 1991. Changes in brain glucose metabolism in cocaine dependence and withdrawal. Am. J. Psychiatry **148:** 621–626.

41. VOLKOW, N.D., L. CHANG, G.J. WANG, *et al.* 2001. Low level of brain dopamine D2 receptors in methamphetamine abusers: association with metabolism in the orbitofrontal cortex. Am. J. Psychiatry **158:** 2015–2021.

42. VOLKOW, N.D. & J.S. FOWLER. 2000. Addiction, a disease of compulsion and drive: involvement of the orbitofrontal cortex. Cerebral Cortex **10:** 318–325.

43. BECHARA, A., H. DAMASIO, A.R. DAMASIO & G.P. LEE. 1999. Different contributions of the human amygdala and ventromedial prefrontal cortex to decision-making. J. Neurosci. **19:** 5473–5481.

44. MOBINI, S., S. BODY, M.-Y. HO, *et al.* 2002. Effects of lesions of the orbitofrontal cortex on sensitivity to delayed and probabilistic reinforcement. Psychopharmacol **160:** 290–298.

45. BECHARA, A., S. DOLAN, N. DENBURG, *et al.* 2001. Decision-making deficits, linked to a dysfunctional ventromedial prefrontal cortex, revealed in alcohol and stimulant abusers. Neuropsychologia **39:** 376–389.

46. COFFEY, S.F., G.D. GUDLESKI, M.E. SALADIN & K.T. BRADY. 2003. Impulsivity and rapid discounting of delayed hypothetical rewards in cocaine-dependent individuals. Exp. Clin. Psychopharmacol. **11:** 18–25.

47. SCHOENBAUM, G. & B. SETLOW. 2005. Cocaine makes actions insensitive to outcomes but not extinction: implications for altered orbitofrontal-amygdalar function. Cerebral Cortex **15:** 1162–1169.

48. ROESCH, M.R., Y. TAKAHASHI, N. GUGSA, *et al.* 2007. Previous cocaine exposure makes rats hypersensitive to both delay and reward magnitude. J. Neurosci. **27:** 245–250.

49. JENTSCH, J.D. & J.R. TAYLOR. 1999. Impulsivity resulting from frontostriatal dysfunction in drug abuse: implications for the control of behavior by reward-related stimuli. Psychopharmacology **146:** 373–390.

50. VOLKOW, N.D. & J.S. FOWLER. 2000. Addiction, a disease of compulsion and drive: involvement of orbitofrontal cortex. Cerebral Cortex **10:** 318–325.

51. STALNAKER, T.A., M.R. ROESCH, T.M. FRANZ, *et al.* 2006. Abnormal associative encoding in orbitofrontal neurons in cocaine-experienced rats during decision-making. Eur. J. Neurosci. **24:** 2643–2653.

52. SCHOENBAUM, G., A.A. CHIBA & M. GALLAGHER. 1998. Orbitofrontal cortex and basolateral amygdala encode expected outcomes during learning. Nat. Neurosci. **1:** 155–159.

53. SCHOENBAUM, G., B. SETLOW, M.P. SADDORIS & M. GALLAGHER. 2003. Encoding predicted outcome and acquired value in orbitofrontal cortex during cue sampling depends upon input from basolateral amygdala. Neuron **39:** 855–867.

54. ROESCH, M.R., T.A. STALNAKER & G. SCHOENBAUM. 2007. Associative encoding in anterior piriform cortex versus orbitofrontal cortex during odor discrimination and reversal learning. Cerebral Cortex **17:** 643–652.

Orbitofrontal Cortex and Cognitive-Motivational Impairments in Psychostimulant Addiction

Evidence from Experiments in the Non-human Primate

PETER OLAUSSON,[a] J. DAVID JENTSCH,[b] DILJA D. KRUEGER,[a,c] NATALIE C. TRONSON,[a,d] ANGUS C. NAIRN,[a] AND JANE R. TAYLOR[a]

[a]Department of Psychiatry, Division of Molecular Psychiatry, Yale University, New Haven, Connecticut, USA

[b]Department of Psychology, UCLA, Los Angeles, California, USA

[c]The Picower Institute for Learning and Memory, Massachusetts Institute of Technology, Cambridge, Massachusetts, USA

[d]Department of Psychiatry & Behavioral Sciences, Feinberg School of Medicine, Northwestern University, Chicago, Illinois, USA

ABSTRACT: Addiction is characterized by compulsive drug use despite adverse consequences. The precise psychobiological changes that underlie the progression from casual use to loss of control over drug-seeking and drug-taking behavior are not well understood. Here we report that short-term cocaine exposure in monkeys is sufficient to produce both selective deficits in cognitive functions dependent on the orbitofrontal cortex (OFC) concurrent with enhancements in motivational processes involving limbic-striatal regions. Additional findings from behavioral studies and analyses of the synaptic proteome provide new behavioral and biochemical evidence that cocaine-induced neuroadaptations in cortical and subcortical brain regions result in dysfunctional decision-making abilities and loss of impulse control that in combination with enhancements of incentive motivation may contribute to the development of compulsive behavior in addiction.

KEYWORDS: reversal learning; prefrontal cortex; proteomics

Address for correspondence: Department of Psychiatry, Division of Molecular Psychiatry, Yale University, CMHC, 34 Park St, New Haven, CT 06508. Voice: (203) 974 7752; fax: (203) 974 7897. peter.olausson@yale.edu

Ann. N.Y. Acad. Sci. 1121: 610–638 (2007). © 2007 New York Academy of Sciences.
doi: 10.1196/annals.1401.016

INTRODUCTION

Behavior is the result of a variety of competing influences, including arousal, autonomic processes, and unconditioned responses. These processes allow for rapid and/or instinctual responses to environmental stimuli with primary reinforcing qualities (e.g., food, water, or a natural predator). The behavioral output can also be influenced by conditioned stimuli associated contingently with primary reinforcers. The acquisition and extinction of such learned responses typically require repeated experiences with the stimulus, the response, and the reward. Thus, the ability to rapidly modify behavior when conditions change is limited at this level of behavioral regulation. It is notably dysfunctional in addiction.

In more developed species, such as primates, this limitation is overcome by a cognitive level of behavioral regulation that provides the ability to suppress or override stimulus-controlled behavior. These neocortical functions include sophisticated processes monitoring the conditional associations between stimuli, responses, and reward and changes in the reinforcement contingencies, as well as mechanisms for planning for more distant goals that may be in conflict with immediate, but less desirable, outcomes. These functions, which are generally subsumed by the rubric of "cognitive control" or "executive functions," can enable the suppression of impulsive behaviors and underlie the capacity for altering responses with only a single or a few experiences with changes in the reinforcer contingency.

The frontal cortex is the neocortical region most expanded in primates, and a wealth of information suggests that it is this structure that mediates processes required for cognitive control, including decision making, attention, working memory, behavioral inhibition, and affective monitoring.[1–12] Importantly, the frontal cortex, in particular the orbitofrontal cortex (OFC) regions, may rapidly monitor and modulate behavior based upon changes in reinforcement contingency. Such OFC mechanisms may allow the individual to modulate behavior beyond the constraints of basic stimulus-driven behavior and are critical substrates of human cognitive and executive functions that may be especially impacted in addiction, a classic example of impulsive behavior.

The clinical manifestations of addictive disorders strongly suggest that the basic psychological functions that subserve cognitive control have eroded or become severely maladaptive. We have hypothesized that drug exposure modifies the function of neural circuits involved in cognitive control/behavioral regulation and results in a persistent state of enhanced drive to acquire and consume the drug, as well as a loss of voluntary control over drug-seeking and drug-taking behavior. Here, we will review the effects of psychostimulant exposure on the function of the cortico-limbic-striatal neural circuits that contribute to cognitive/behavioral control, focusing on the evidence that the OFC may be critically impacted even early on in the neuropathological processes that underlie addictive behavior. We will also discuss potential strategies to better understand the neurobiological substrate underlying these maladaptive effects of drug exposure on behavioral regulation and OFC function.

COGNITIVE-MOTIVATIONAL ALTERATIONS IN ADDICTION

Drug addiction is the consequence of complex interactions between genetic and environmental factors, including drug exposure, on the brain and behavior. Thus, the development of an addictive state is likely to result from drug-induced neurobiological changes in multiple brain circuits and networks that influence the complex psychological processes described above. The mechanisms by which drug exposure leads to the progression from voluntary use to the compulsive drug-seeking and drug-taking behavior that define addiction are, however, largely unknown. Preclinical studies have provided compelling evidence for persistent drug-induced neurochemical, molecular, and morphological changes within the cortico-limbic-striatal brain structures that regulate and coordinate cognitive and motivational functions.[13-17] Together, cognitive dysfunction and maladaptive motivational processes can have multiple adverse consequences for the individual and are likely to contribute to the transition from casual to compulsive drug use. Such inter-related drug-induced dysfunctions of amygdala, striatum, and frontal cortex are central to several developing hypotheses of neurocognitive deficits associated with the pathophysiology of addiction.[6,15,18,19] While both cognitive and motivational traits may be predisposing vulnerability factors that increase the susceptibility to addiction, the neurobiological consequences of drug exposure may be sufficient in themselves to facilitate this process. Here, we will provide evidence that, in the primate brain, short-term exposure to cocaine is sufficient to disrupt normal functioning of the OFC and regulated limbic-striatal circuits, resulting in deficits in inhibitory control of behavior while at the same time enhancing incentive motivational influences on behavior.

Clinical studies of cocaine addicts support the hypothesis that exposure to stimulants and other abused drugs is associated with cognitive-motivational abnormalities and altered brain activation patterns. Addicts display neurocognitive deficits involving behavioral disinhibition, poor decision making, and impaired cognitive control, and these phenomena are associated with abnormal task-induced brain activation patterns in frontal and limbic-striatal areas.[20-33] In additional studies, altered brain glucose metabolism and blood flow have also been found in OFC, anterior cingulate, and other related limbic and striatal regions.[34-39] Other experiments have demonstrated that these drug-induced neurobiological adaptations may contribute to the powerfully motivational effects (i.e., craving) of cocaine-associated cues.[40-44] Such cue-induced or imagery-induced cocaine craving is associated with limbic-striatal (amygdalar) and OFC activation.[27,41,42,44-47] Thus, available data from humans indicate multiple levels of drug-induced impairments; however, none of these studies has addressed whether, or the degree to which, such cognitive-motivational alterations are predisposing factors for substance abuse or represent the effect of repeated drug exposure.

ANIMAL STUDIES OF BEHAVIORAL REGULATION IN ADDICTION

Although animal models that mimic the negative personal and social consequences of addiction have not yet been created, there are compelling reasons to investigate neurocognitive deficits associated with repeated drug exposure in animals. Despite technical advances in imaging techniques, there are both methodological limitations and theoretical/ethical concerns with correlative studies of cognitive function in drug abusers. For example, brain-imaging studies cannot adequately attribute putative drug-induced behavioral deficits to alterations in documented cellular/molecular changes[48] or from those potentially produced by pre-existing conditions. Other issues include duration between last use, poly-drug abuse, concurrent medication for drug use and/or co-morbid psychiatric disorders, age, and/or duration of drug use.

Animal experiments have the potential to control for, and systematically investigate, these factors and to provide convincing evidence linking cognitive-motivational deficits with underlying neuronal changes. Our results, together with findings published by a number of groups, have provided important information about the nature of these links and suggest that addiction likely involves alterations within multiple circuits, including limbic-striatal circuits mediating motivational processes and cortico-limbic-striatal circuits mediating attentional, decision making, and inhibitory control mechanisms critical for executive function and cognitive control.[15,18,19,49] While the majority of research on the behavioral and biochemical consequences of chronic drug exposure has been performed in rodents, it is of great importance to conduct parallel studies in non-human primates because monkeys display close homology with humans in a number of relevant anatomical and functional domains. This is particularly true for the organization of the prefrontal cortex. For example, the prefrontal cortex is well developed in primates but less developed in rodents.[50] Thus, not surprisingly, there are both clear differences and similarities in the functional and organizational homologies between primate and rodent PFC, including both the medial and orbital sections.[50,51] Considerable research has begun to integrate these apparent inconsistencies and to clarify the contribution of specific brain structures and neurochemical systems to distinct cognitive domains. Studies in monkeys thus remain critically important for the progression of this research. In addition, such primate studies allow for investigation of behavioral and molecular alterations that are contributory to, and representative of, neurocognitive deficits in drug abuse.

DRUG-INDUCED DEFICITS IN COGNITIVE FUNCTION

To explore the consequences of drug-induced neuroadaptations on the processes supporting behavioral regulation and flexibility, we have conducted a number of experiments in non-human primates. Our focus has been to elucidate processes affected after short-term repeated cocaine exposure, as such exposure patterns have been demonstrated to produce drug-induced neuroadaptations and to increase cocaine self-administration in rodents (for a review, see Vezina[52]). We have hypothesized that these early changes will reduce cognitive control of behavior, facilitate drug consumption, and contribute to the transition to an addictive state.[19] However, the mechanisms by which the OFC is especially impacted or recruited in addiction are not known.

Using a task that measures response inhibition and that is sensitive to OFC lesions in the non-human primate, namely reversal learning (see below), we have demonstrated that cocaine, when administered daily for 14 days to juvenile vervet monkeys (*Cercopithecus aethiops sabaeus*), causes a striking and persistent deficit in the ability to stop or change behavior[53] (see FIG. 1). These deficits lasted for at least 1 month after the last injection. The impairment in reversal learning was associated with increased response perseveration such that cocaine-exposed monkeys continued to respond to the previously rewarded object even when the response-reward contingency changed and such responses were no longer reinforced. Cocaine exposure thus interfered with response flexibility. It did not, however, impact the ability to acquire a simple discrimination or to perform according to a set of well-learned rules. We recently confirmed these deficits in reversal learning in a new series of experiments where we also demonstrated that prior cocaine exposure did not influence behavior in a number of additional cognitive tests with little or no requirement for inhibitory control (Olausson *et al.*, unpublished observations). The ability of chronic experimenter-administered cocaine exposure to impair reversal learning has now also been confirmed both in rats[54] and mice (Krueger *et al.*, unpublished observations). These impairments have also been demonstrated after cocaine self-administration in rats[55] and in human addicts,[56] supporting our original findings in monkeys and demonstrating that the effects of chronic cocaine exposure on reversal learning do not require contingent administration.

Reversal learning requires the inhibition of innate response schemes or of previously established conditioned responses, and impairments in this task have been argued to reflect inhibitory control deficits (see Roberts[57] for a review of the associative structures involved in this task). Distinct regions of the prefrontal cortex appear to regulate inhibitory control processes within functionally specific cognitive domains. While lesions of the lateral prefrontal cortex in primates impair inhibitory control of attentional processing (i.e., extra-dimensional shifting), OFC lesions selectively impair inhibitory control of affective processes that modulate behavior in response to stimuli

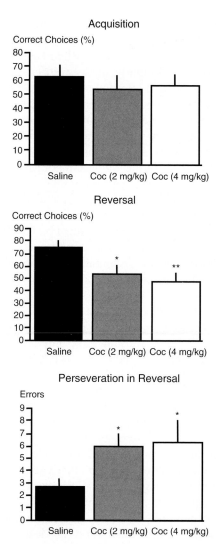

FIGURE 1. Chronic cocaine exposure produces persistent deficits in reversal learning in the non-human primate. Juvenile vervet monkeys were exposed to cocaine (2 or 4 mg/kg i.m.) or saline once daily for 14 days and tested on object discrimination acquisition and reversal after 9 or 30 days of withdrawal. A persistent deficit in reversal learning was observed in monkeys that had been exposed to cocaine, whereas this drug exposure schedule did not influence the acquisition of the task. The impairment in reversal learning was associated with increased perseverative responding. Cocaine thus appeared to interfere with cognitive flexibility required to shift responding when the reinforcement contingency changes. This pattern of result is reproduced by lesion of the OFC in humans, monkeys, or rodents, and cocaine may thus produce OFC-dependent cognitive defects *$P < 0.05$, **$P < 0.01$. Figure adapted by permission from Macmillan Publishers Ltd: Jentsch *et al.* *Neuropsychopharmacology 26:183–192,* copyright 2002.[53]

with motivational or emotional significance.[9] Moreover, in monkeys as well as in humans, lesions of the OFC produce response perseveration and impair the reversal of previously learned associations, while having little effect on discrimination acquisition.[58–66] Similarly, in rats, restricted lesions to the medial prefrontal cortex (prelimbic and infralimbic cortices), impair spatial reversal learning,[67,68] and recent experiments have confirmed deficits in reversal learning following lesion of the lateral OFC in rats.[69,70] Lesions of the OFC have also been reported to impair reversal of Pavlovian discriminations, a deficit that was associated with decreased response flexibility.[71] Recent behavioral and electrophysiological data further suggest that reversal of odor-based discriminations in rats is also dependent on the OFC.[72] Interestingly, a recent report has demonstrated that lesions of the basolateral amygdala ameliorated the reversal deficits caused by OFC lesions.[73] Thus, reversal learning and other cognitive functions appear to be dependent on inter-related cortical and subcortical structures,[59,64,74–79] and damage to dissociable subregions of the prefrontal cortex produces deficits in cognitive/executive functions associated with behavioral regulation, decision making, and impulsivity,[9,59,75,80,81] as well as working memory.[4,5,82]

While OFC lesions have selectively and repeatedly been demonstrated to impair reversal learning in a number of species, the normal neurobiological processes that mediate reversal learning have only recently begun to be determined. In a number of elegant studies, reversal learning has been assessed following neurochemically selective lesions of the prefrontal cortex in general, or the OFC specifically.[83–85] These studies demonstrate that OFC serotonin lesions produce reversal-learning deficits and increase response perseveration without affecting acquisition or performance of the discrimination task. These studies argue strongly that intact serotonin functioning is critical for reversal-learning on the non-human primate. However, while reduction in prefronto-cortical dopamine levels was not found to impact reversal learning,[85] recent data suggest that selective antagonism of dopamine D2/D3, but not D1/D5, receptors can produce powerful impairments in the ability to flexibly alter behavior in this task.[86] Importantly, one study revealed an additional mechanism that may contribute to the cocaine-induced reversal learning deficits, given the evidence for persistent down-regulation of dopamine D2 receptors in human cocaine addicts.[87]

Based upon our reversal learning data, indicating that short-term prior chronic cocaine exposure is sufficient to impair reversal learning in the non-human primate, we have recently sought to expand on these original findings by using an additional behavioral task that is sensitive to the functional integrity of the OFC. The object retrieval/detour task has been used to examine the inhibition of pre-potent responding.[88–96] Roberts and colleagues[94,95] have demonstrated that detour responses in this task were impaired by lesions of the OFC in non-human primates. In this task, monkeys that had been previously subjected to daily cocaine injections for 14 consecutive days, demonstrated

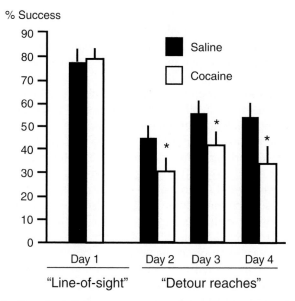

FIGURE 2. Chronic cocaine exposure impairs performance in the object retrieval/detour task. Vervet monkeys were treated daily with cocaine (2 mg/kg i.m.) for 14 days and tested on the object retrieval/detour task as previously described.[88,92,93] In this task, monkeys have to retrieve a fruit reward placed in a transparent box with an opening on only one side. The open side can be facing the monkey, such that it is simply required to reach along its "line-of sight." Here behavior is guided by previously conditioned or "prepotent" responses. In contrast, when the open side is directed to the side, the monkey needs to inhibit reaching directly at the transparent barrier for the reward and instead "negotiate" the barrier by making a detour reach in order to obtain the reward. Whereas both saline-treated and cocaine-treated monkeys performed identically in the "line-of-sight" trials on day 1, prior cocaine exposure resulted in impairments measured as reduced success on the subsequent days of testing (day 2–4) where hard trials, i.e., "detour reaches" that require response inhibition, were introduced. Prior cocaine exposure thus reduced the inhibition of pre-potent responding. This pattern of result is reproduced by lesion of the OFC in non-human primates, providing further support that repeated cocaine exposure produces OFC-dependent defects in cognitive behavioral control, rather than motivational or motoric impairments in this task. $*P < 0.05$.

a significant and selective deficit in detour responses when tested 2 weeks after the last injection (FIG. 2). Exposure to cocaine, however, had no effect on acquisition, showing that the impairments were not due to an inability of learning or performing the task. These data converge with similar studies in rodents to strongly support the idea that cocaine-induced neuroadaptations interfere with the cognitive processing involving the OFC.

Loss of cognitive control may underlie behavioral inflexibility, in which addicts are unable to shift or suppress thoughts and actions away from drugs and drug-related activities. As mentioned above, studies of human drug abusers suggest profound and complex cognitive deficits in several domains, involving behavioral inhibition, decision making, and cognitive flexibility. Although the cognitive impairment observed following prior cocaine exposure was restricted to functions thought to involve the OFC, more prolonged cocaine exposure may produce more widespread dysfunction of cortico-striatal circuits. For example, both additional cognitive deficits and abnormal brain activation patterns have been identified in other cortical areas, such as the anterior cingulate cortex and the dorsolateral prefrontal cortex, in human cocaine addicts (see below). Moreover, sensitization to amphetamine for 6 weeks in monkeys persistently impaired working memory performance.[97] However, this may be due to drug-specific effects, as short-term chronic amphetamine exposure impairs visuospatial attention and attentional set-shifting in rats.[98,99] Repeated cocaine exposure has also been found to produce impulsive responding in a go/no-go task in rats,[100] while such effects are not observed following cocaine exposure in mice (Krueger et al., unpublished observation). A modest impairment in working memory by prior cocaine exposure has, however, been observed (Krueger et al., unpublished observations). Moreover, withdrawal from either cocaine or amphetamine self-administration produces only a short-term deficit in attentional performance,[101,102] though animals with genetic vulnerability may have more profound disturbances.[103] Nevertheless, available data strongly suggest that OFC-mediated cognitive processes are particularly sensitive to drug exposure. We therefore hypothesize that psychostimulant-induced OFC dysfunction, even after relatively short-term use, underlies the initial losses of inhibitory control processes that are specifically involved in the transition from casual to compulsive drug use.

ALTERATIONS IN GOAL-DIRECTED BEHAVIORAL REGULATION

The development of cognitive deficits is, however, not likely to be solely responsible for the development of the compulsive drug-seeking and drug-taking behavior that characterizes the addictive state. Indeed, alterations in motivational processes are widely considered to be core features of this disorder. In particular, the increased impact of drug-associated cues on multiple components of addictive behavior has stimulated intense research. As part of our experimental analysis of the cognitive-motivational account of addiction, we have performed a series of experiments to examine the consequences of drug-exposure on motivational processes in rodents and primates.

A number of elegant studies have demonstrated increased motivation to self-administer drugs of abuse after prior drug exposure,[52,104] binge,[105-107] or extended self-administration experience.[108] Such increases in progressive ratio responding following experimenter-administered drugs have also been demonstrated for natural rewards.[109,110] Furthermore, repeated drug exposure consistently enhances the incentive influences on reward-motivated behavior. Such drug-induced changes in the control over behavior by cues can be assessed by investigating the conditioned reinforcing effects of reward-associated stimuli. Here, the ability of a conditioned stimulus to support new learning is a stringent measure of its reinforcing and motivational effects.[111–115] We have previously demonstrated augmented conditioned reinforcement following prior repeated exposure to cocaine or a number of other addictive drugs in rodents.[116–119] Other investigators have presented similar results in this[117] and other relevant rodent models.[120,121]

Notably, conditional cues that have been associated with cocaine in the operant self-administration procedures also gain the ability to reinstate drug-seeking behavior.[122,123] Consistent with this animal literature, drug-associated stimuli acquire conditioned reinforcing and incentive motivational properties and can evoke craving, drug seeking, and relapse in humans.[124–129] The motivational effects of drug-related cues increase over time following drug withdrawal, an effect that may contribute to high vulnerability to relapse after prolonged abstinence periods.[130–132] Whether repeated cocaine exposure also produces motivational alterations in primates has been an open question, particularly given that dopaminergic sensitization to the effects of psychostimulant drugs is less evident, or even absent, in monkeys.[133] We have therefore begun to characterize the effects of cocaine on conditioned motivational processes in monkeys. The acquisition of a second-order schedule of reinforcement has been used to examine aspects of conditioned reinforcement in primates.[134,135] In this study, monkeys were trained to associate a conditioned stimulus with fruit rewards and the ability of this cue to support instrumental responding was subsequently tested. Like rodents subjected to chronic cocaine exposure, monkeys that had been exposed to prior chronic cocaine injections also displayed increased responding to an object that was associated with contingent presentation of a conditioned stimulus, whereas other measures were not affected (FIG. 3). This observation suggests that chronic cocaine exposure produces lasting neuroadaptations that enhance the behavioral impact of reward-associated cues in the non-human primate. This experiment lends additional support to the conclusion that prior cocaine exposure augments conditioned reinforcement as measured by a variety of procedures.

Mesocorticolimbic dopaminergic innervation has long been implicated in mediating motivational state and the incentive value of established conditioned reinforcers. This work has primarily focused on the contributions of subcortical structures such as the nucleus accumbens and the amygdala.[111,114,115,134,136,137] However, in marmosets, lesions of the OFC also reduce responding with conditioned reinforcement and the ability of reward-associated conditioned stimuli to maintain responding under second-order schedules of reinforcement. In contrast, medial prefrontal cortex lesions do not affect these behaviors.[135] There is additional evidence suggesting that the OFC plays an important role in mediating the behavioral impact of reward-associated conditioned cues as

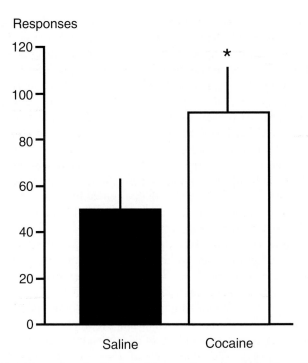

FIGURE 3. Enhanced motivational significance of reward-associated conditioned stimuli in cocaine-exposed monkeys. Vervet monkeys were treated daily with cocaine (2 mg/kg i.m.) for 14 days and tested on acquisition of a second-order schedule of reinforcement 19–21 days following the last injection. Animals were initially trained to associate the conditioned stimulus with food reinforcement and had previously been tested on additional behavioral tasks prior to the experiments detailed here. The ability of this conditioned stimulus to support responding was subsequently evaluated in the acquisition of a within-session, progressive, second-order schedule of reinforcement. In this test, monkeys had to make an increasing number of responses to elicit presentation of the conditioned stimulus and subsequently the food reinforcer. Cocaine-treated monkeys made more accurate responses than saline-treated controls, while there was no difference in inactive responses. These data suggest that prior chronic cocaine exposure enhanced the reinforcing or motivational effects of such stimuli, thus increasing the impact of such stimuli on behavioral regulation. *$P < 0.05$.

stimuli with incentive value, such as food or cues predictive of primary reinforcers, elicit physiological responses in the OFC.[138–141] Interestingly, dissociable parts of the human OFC are activated by processing of incentive value and goal selection.[142] Thus, in keeping with its role in the abovementioned processes, the OFC likely plays a role in representation of outcome value and response selection (for reviews see Refs. 7,10–12,57,143–145). Thus it has been argued that the primate OFC supports goal-directed behaviors that are maintained or elicited by the motivational effects of reward-associated stimuli by assessing the current incentive value of available reinforcers.[57]

The inability to generate accurate representations of the incentive value of reinforcers and thus to appropriately signal outcome value as a result of OFC damage or drug-induced dysfunction has been suggested to impair adaptive decision making and to underlie deficits in reversal learning.[145] Therefore, dysfunction produced by chronic cocaine exposure may interfere with this process and with the ability to generate and update the appropriate outcome representations during reversal learning when reward contingencies rapidly change. This view is supported by a recent report demonstrating that the OFC of cocaine-exposed rats fail to develop normal physiological responses during reversal learning.[146] Moreover, cocaine exposure renders Pavlovian behavior insensitive to the outcome,[147] supporting the idea that cocaine exposure disrupts the ability to guide behavior based on the current value of the outcome, a process dependent on the OFC.

Few studies have, however, examined the role of the OFC in drug self-administration. Rats with lesions of the OFC display a dysregulated response pattern and obtain cocaine infusions at a faster pace than control animals using an FR1 schedule of cocaine self-administration.[148] Fuchs *et al.* evaluated the effects of medial and lateral OFC lesions on cocaine self-administration and found no effect of these manipulations on cocaine self-administration at baseline.[149] In contrast, both studies report significant impairments in the ability of cocaine-associated cues to impact upon instrumental performance. First, the acquisition of a second-order schedule of reinforcement was impaired by OFC lesions.[148] Second, reversible inactivation of the lateral OFC also reduced the motivational effects of cocaine-associated cues in a cue-induced reinstatement procedure.[149] These findings converge upon the primate studies described above,[135] supporting the view that the OFC is required for the ability of reward-associated conditioned stimuli to support behavior. They also provide evidence that this process is of importance in the cocaine self-administration model. Finally, there is also evidence that the OFC, but not the medial prefrontal cortex, is necessary for stress-induced reinstatement of cocaine-seeking in rats.[150] Taken together, there is growing support for a role for the OFC in mediating the motivational effects of drug-associated stimuli and for the view that psychostimulant-induced neuroadaptations can enhance the incentive value of reward-associated stimuli. Whether this drug-induced enhancement is also dependent on the OFC remains, however, to be determined, but we hypothesize that these drug-induced alterations might be particularly important in the early phases of drug experimentation and may thus facilitate the transition to addiction.

Our new data, shown in FIGURE 3, strongly suggest that repeated exposure to cocaine increases conditioned reinforcement in monkeys, as has been previously shown for a number of addictive substances in rodents.[116–119] This new evidence may be consistent with enhanced motivational significance of reward-associated cues.[16] Our findings also provide support for theories that emphasize the development of habitual stimulus-response behavior in addiction.[15,18,151] This latter possibility is supported by observations that the acquisition of a new response with conditioned reinforcement is resistant to reinforcer devaluation.[152] Moreover, behavior maintained by stimulus-response relationships in a second-order schedule of reinforcement using cocaine-associated cues is associated with a shift in the activation of dopamine neurotransmission from the ventral to the dorsal striatum,[153,154] and antagonism of dopamine receptors in the dorsal striatum also blocks drug-seeking behavior in this model.[155] Together, these data suggest that drug-associated cues can increasingly come to maintain persistent drug-seeking behavior through processes involving habitual, rather than goal-directed, responses.

NEUROADAPTATIONS IN OFC: EVIDENCE FROM PRELIMINARY PROTEOMIC ANALYSES

Whereas the effects of chronic psychostimulant exposure in rodents have been the focus of numerous studies, very little is known about the neurobiological effects of such treatment on the OFC in rodents or in the non-human primate. Robinson and colleagues have demonstrated opposite effects of amphetamine self-administration on the density of dendritic spines in the medial prefrontal cortex and the OFC. Here, the spine density in the medial prefrontal cortex and the nucleus accumbens increased, whereas the OFC neurons had a reduced number of dendritic spines when measured one month after the last amphetamine self-administration session.[156] Additional evidence for psychostimulant-induced OFC alterations comes from Homayoun and Moghaddam. These investigators demonstrated that repeated amphetamine exposure alters the electrophysiological responses of the medial prefrontal cortex and OFC in rats engaged in a food-reinforced instrumental task, resulting in progressively more inhibitory responses of medial prefrontal cortex neurons and increasingly more excitatory responses of the OFC.[157] It seems highly plausible that these concurrent alterations in information processing of the prefrontal cortex may impact upon goal-directed behavior, consistent with our hypothesis.[19] While multiple studies on the effects of cocaine exposure on biochemical and molecular changes in cortical regions are available, a limited number of studies have directly examined cocaine-induced adaptations selectively within the OFC. For example, cocaine self-administration reduces glucose utilization in the primate OFC,[158,159] and presentation of a cocaine-associated conditioned stimulus increases the level of mRNA for the immediate early gene zif268 in a number of prefrontal cortical regions, including the ventral and lateral OFC.[160] Due to this relative paucity of data, we have recently begun to use large-scale proteomic screening techniques to identify target proteins and cellular functions that may be altered in the OFC and additional regions of the frontal cortex following repeated cocaine exposure (see further below).

As detailed above, our studies in the non-human primate provide strong evidence that prior drug exposure is sufficient to cause persistent dysfunction of OFC and related limbic-striatal circuits that contribute to neurocognitive and incentive motivational deficits associated with the pathophysiology of addiction. A remaining challenge is, however, to determine the neurobiological substrates associated with these cocaine-induced alterations. Given the idea that cocaine might induce aberrant synaptic plasticity in the mesolimbic dopamine system,[161–163] most studies have focused on investigating specific target proteins based on their previous link with other forms of plasticity, including those thought to underlie reward-related learning and memory.[164] While these studies have proven very valuable in characterizing certain aspects of drug-induced plasticity, they are by definition confined to previously known mechanisms. Therefore, drug-induced changes in cellular functions that are unrelated to classical mechanisms of experience-dependent plasticity are less likely to be uncovered. To overcome these limitations, unbiased approaches aimed toward identifying novel classes of molecules regulated by drugs of abuse are now being developed and used.

Until recently, the major strategy used for this purpose involved the large-scale assessment of mRNA levels by microarray analysis.[165–167] However, it is becoming increasingly clear that changes in mRNA abundance and protein levels often show limited correlation.[168,169] Since proteins represent the functional component of the cellular machinery and thus mediate the effects of drug exposure on the psychological and behavioral aspects of addiction, techniques that allow for unbiased analysis of the proteome directly offer great advantages.[170–172] One such technique that has recently gained popularity is DIGE, or differential 2D gel fluorescence electrophoresis.[173,174] DIGE allows for direct within-gel comparison of two separate protein samples (e.g., control and experimental) based on differential labeling of the two samples with unique fluorescent dyes. In this way, a ratio of the fluorescence emitted by the control- and experimental-labeled probes can be obtained for each protein individually, and this ratio corresponds to the relative levels of that protein in the control versus experimental samples. The identity of regulated proteins is then determined by mass spectrometry (MS). Another powerful technique is iTRAQ, or isobaric tagging for relative and absolute quantitation.[175,176] iTRAQ is an MS-based method in which control and experimental samples are labeled separately with isobaric tags prior to being pooled and subjected to liquid chromatography and tandem mass spectrometry (LC/MS/MS). These isobaric tags contain a reporter ion the abundance of which is directly correlated with the amount of the protein they are linked to in each sample. Thus, the reporter ions can be used to quantify the relative levels of each individual protein in the control versus experimental samples. Approaches, such as DIGE and iTRAQ, not only provide an unbiased assessment of the effects of chronic drug exposure, but by virtue of sampling hundreds of proteins simultaneously, they also have the potential to identify global patterns of changes in cellular processes and pathways that may be far more relevant to the neurobiology of addiction than any individual alteration alone.

To date, few reports have used neuroproteomics approaches in the study of drugs of abuse,[177–181] and only one of these relates to cocaine.[182] We thus took advantage of both DIGE and iTRAQ methodologies to begin to determine the cellular mechanisms underlying the persistent cocaine-induced alterations in cortico-limbic-striatal function observed in our behavioral studies. Using OFC tissue punches collected 3–4 weeks after the final cocaine injection, we previously reported alterations in metabolic proteins (e.g., ATP synthase, glyceraldehyde-3-phosphate dehydrogenase, and triosephosphate isomerase), protein folding and turnover (e.g., HSP-70), and cytoskeletal rearrangements (e.g., α-actin and β-tubulin).[183] Subsequently, we have repeated these experiments using synaptoneurosomes, a preparation in which the synaptic compartment in the OFC was specifically isolated. This approach reduces the sample complexity and thus facilitates the identification of changes with particular relevance to synaptic function. In a preliminary and ongoing study using a combined DIGE and iTRAQ approach, we have identified a number of cocaine-induced alterations in OFC synaptoneurosomes that confirm and expand our previous assessment (FIG. 4). To our knowledge, no previous studies have focused on the effects of psychostimulants specifically on protein expression in the synaptic compartment in non-human primates. These experiments have the potential to identify critical mediators of psychostimulant-induced alterations in synaptic plasticity.

One of the most striking observations arising from both sets of data from the OFC is the prominence of alterations in proteins related to metabolic function. Cocaine is well known to cause changes in brain metabolism, including in the OFC.[158,159,184,185] The concomitant regulation of a large number of these proteins may indicate that this is an important effect of chronic cocaine exposure, yet the functional significance of these alterations remains unknown. It is noteworthy that metabolic abnormalities in drug addicts occur in brain regions that are activated by set-shifting, reversal learning, and decision-making tasks in non-addicted humans (see above). One possibility is that these changes are reflective of an alteration in synapse number or function, possibly consistent with the structural changes observed in the OFC in abstinent cocaine users.[186,187] Indeed, synaptic transmission is a highly energy-intensive process, and there is increasing interest in the role of mitochondrial energy metabolism in both synaptic plasticity and psychiatric disorders.[188–190] Alternatively, the changes observed in our study may be a persistent response to the oxidative stress induced by elevated dopamine signaling, a possibility supported by the observation that the other main category of proteins identified as regulated by cocaine are those involved in the response to cell stress and protein degradation. It is thus tempting to speculate that long-lasting molecular alterations caused by oxidative stress in the OFC may result in functional consequences similar to those induced by lesions or pharmacological inactivation, and that

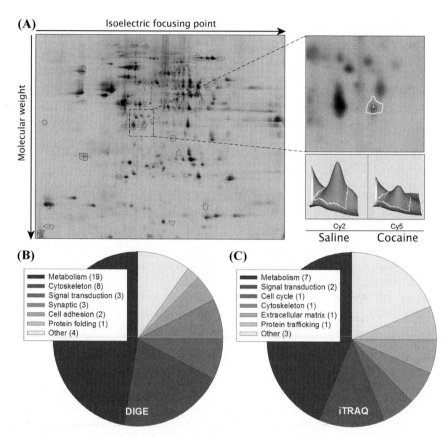

FIGURE 4. Proteomic analysis of the OFC of non-human primates following repeated exposure to cocaine. (**A**) DIGE gel comparing saline-exposed and cocaine-exposed synaptoneurosome tissue from vervet OFC area 11. Saline-exposed and cocaine-exposed samples were labeled with Cy2 and Cy5, respectively, and they were then pooled and run on a two-dimensional gel, separated first by isoelectric focusing point and then by molecular weight. Images were acquired using a Typhoon scanner (GE Healthcare Life Sciences, Piscataway, NJ), and Cy5/Cy2 ratios for each spot were analyzed using the Decyder software (GE Healthcare Life Sciences). *Left panel*: Cy5 image of the gel. Proteins up-regulated > 1.5x following cocaine exposure are marked in blue, those down-regulated > 1.5x are marked in red. *Right panels*: Magnified example of one of the spots changed following cocaine exposure. The peak on the left represents the Cy2 (saline) spot volume, while the peak on the right represents the Cy5 (cocaine) spot volume. (**B**) + (**C**) Classification of proteins identified as regulated > 1.5x by DIGE and iTRAQ approaches, respectively. (In color in *Annals* online.)

this may represent an important mechanism by which cocaine affects cortico-limbic-striatal function in addiction. Indeed, protracted cocaine abstinence is also associated with altered OFC metabolic activity in human cocaine addicts.[38,87] Interestingly, this change in metabolic activity was associated with reduced striatal D2 receptor availability,[87] possibly identifying a potential link between the neurobiological changes that occur in these regions and the neural substrate required for reversal learning as mentioned above.[86] However, while it is tempting to speculate about the consequences of these synaptic biochemical alterations observed after repeated cocaine exposures in the non-human primate, their significance remains to be clarified.

IMPLICATIONS FOR LOSS OF BEHAVIORAL CONTROL IN ADDICTION: DEVELOPMENT OF COMPULSIVE OR HABITUAL BEHAVIOR

We have argued that the cognitive and motivational sequelae of chronic drug exposure will result in reduced cognitive control of behavior, impulsivity, and poor response selection in the face of adverse consequences. The result is increased drug intake that may facilitate the development of habitual or compulsive drug-seeking behavior.[15,18] There is some experimental support for this hypothesis, as cocaine-seeking behavior rapidly becomes habitual[191] and repeated amphetamine exposure facilitates the development of instrumental habits.[192] Since prior chronic cocaine exposure also interferes with outcome devaluation,[147] a process that involves the OFC, it is possible that psychostimulant-induced dysfunction of this region contributes to this rapid development of habit. Moreover, insensitivity to aversive stimuli associated with drug or drug-related activities is a characteristic of addiction that could be argued to be habitual or compulsive in nature. The reduced impact of aversive consequences associated with drug self-administration was recently used to demonstrate the development of addictive behavior in animal models.[108,193] The role of the OFC in modulating responses to stimuli associated with aversive experiences or punishment may be particularly relevant in this respect.[10,11,141,146,194–197] In support of this notion, OFC neurons that fire in anticipation of aversive events fail to respond to cues predictive of this outcome following prior repeated cocaine exposure, reducing the ability of such stimuli to guide behavior.[146] While this circumstantial evidence may implicate the OFC in habitual or compulsive behavior, available data have focused on the contribution of the medial prefrontal cortex of rats in the expression of habit behavior.[198,199] Our recent studies have also implicated subregions of the prefrontal cortex in sensitivity to outcome value, where infusions of dopamine into the ventromedial prefrontal cortex can restore responding appropriate to the outcome value, i.e., reverse habit-like responding,[200] though the involvement of the OFC in these effects has yet to be determined.

Taken together, it seems possible that drug-induced dysfunction of the OFC will interfere with goal-directed behavior controlled by incentive stimuli as well as insensitivity to the influence of aversive or detrimental behavioral consequences. The drug-induced impairment of OFC-mediated processes may therefore be a critical and pervasive factor in the "loss of control," compulsive state of addiction. Our current studies are aimed at confirming directly the causal relationship between proteins identified in our monkey studies with the development of drug-seeking and drug-taking behaviors based on rodent models that include assessment of OFC-mediated cognitive-motivational function, and the development of habitual behavior patterns.

CONCLUSION

While the cognitive and motivational deficits observed in psychostimulant addicts could be related to predisposing factors increasing the vulnerability to addiction, the evidence presented here demonstrates that drug exposure is sufficient to produce both cognitive deficits (i.e., impairments in inhibitory control, especially when adaptive responding in the face of changing reward-associated events is required) and incentive motivational enhancements. We also provide evidence that the OFC may play a unique role in initial maladaptive responses to cocaine exposure in non-human primates and rodents. Such behavioral deficits, involving decision making, reward representation, and inhibitory control, can have several important maladaptive consequences for psychostimulant addicts. First, they may increase the incidence of drug-seeking and recidivism through deficits in impulse control and enhancements in incentive motivational processes. Second, such alterations may produce other forms of maladaptive behavior that may impact the normal functions of the individual and result in problems with social relationships, work, and the legal system. Third, they may enhance drug-taking behavior such that it is difficult to abstain from, or terminate, drug consumption. As such, the early impact of drug exposure on cognitive-motivational functions of the OFC and related circuits may facilitate the transition to addiction and/or the progression of substance abuse disorders by contributing to the development of the compulsive or habitual patterns of drug-seeking and drug-taking that characterize this disorder. Finally, these impairments in OFC function may interfere with rehabilitation programs involving cognitive therapy. It is thus imperative to investigate the biological and behavioral consequences of chronic drug exposure on cognitive and motivational functions and to identify why the OFC may be exceptionally sensitive to cocaine exposure in order to better understand the pathophysiology of addiction.

ACKNOWLEDGEMENTS

The authors like to thank Ms. Alexia Kedves and Mr. Drew Kiraly for valuable help on this project. The proteomic analyses were supported by the Yale/NIDA Neuroproteomics Center, and we are extremely grateful for contributions by Drs. Ken Williams, Christopher Colangelo, Kathy Stone, and Terence Wu. This research was supported by PHS grants DA11717 (JRT, PO), DA20598 (JDJ), DA22539 (JDJ), DA10044 (ACN).

REFERENCES

1. CHUDASAMA, Y. & T.W. ROBBINS. 2006. Functions of frontostriatal systems in cognition: comparative neuropsychopharmacological studies in rats, monkeys and humans. Biol. Psychol. **73:** 19–38.
2. CLARK, L., R. COOLS & T.W. ROBBINS. 2004. The neuropsychology of ventral prefrontal cortex: decision-making and reversal learning. Brain Cogn. **55:** 41–53.
3. DAMASIO, A.R. 1996. The somatic marker hypothesis and the possible functions of the prefrontal cortex. Phil. Trans. R. Soc. Lond. B. **351:** 1413–1420.
4. FUSTER, J.M. 1988. The Prefrontal Cortex. Raven Press. New York.
5. GOLDMAN-RAKIC, P.S. 1996. The prefrontal landscape: implications of functional architecture for understanding human mentation and the central executive. Philos. Trans. R. Soc. Lond. B. Biol. Sci. **351:** 1445–53.
6. JENTSCH, J.D., R.H. ROTH & J.R. TAYLOR. 2000. Role for dopamine in the behavioral functions of the prefrontal corticostriatal system: implications for mental disorders and psychotropic drug action. Prog. Brain Res. **126:** 433–453.
7. O'DOHERTY, J.P. 2004. Reward representations and reward-related learning in the human brain: insights from neuroimaging. Curr. Opin. Neurobiol. **14:** 769–776.
8. ROBBINS, T.W. 2000. From arousal to cognition: the integrative position of the prefrontal cortex. Prog. Brain Res. **126:** 469–483.
9. ROBERTS, A.C. & J.D. WALLIS. 2000. Inhibitory control and affective processing in the prefrontal cortex: neuropsychological studies in the common marmoset. Cereb. Cortex **10:** 252–262.
10. ROLLS, E.T. 2000. The orbitofrontal cortex and reward. Cereb. Cortex **10:** 284–294.
11. ROLLS, E.T. 2004. The functions of the orbitofrontal cortex. Brain Cogn. **55:** 11–29.
12. SCHOENBAUM, G. & M. ROESCH. 2005. Orbitofrontal cortex, associative learning, and expectancies. Neuron. **47:** 633–636.
13. EVERITT, B.J. & M.E. WOLF. 2002. Psychomotor stimulant addiction: a neural systems perspective. J. Neurosci. **22:** 3312–3320.
14. HYMAN, S.E. & R.C. MALENKA. 2001. Addiction and the brain: the neurobiology of compulsion and its persistence. Nat. Rev. Neurosci. **2:** 695–703.
15. ROBBINS, T.W. & B.J. EVERITT. 1999. Drug addiction: bad habits add up. Nature **398:** 567–570.
16. ROBINSON, T.E. & K.C. BERRIDGE. 1993. The neural basis of craving: an incentive-sensitization theory of addiction. Brain Res. Rev. **18:** 247–291.
17. VANDERSCHUREN, L.J. & P.W. KALIVAS. 2000. Alterations in dopaminergic and glutamatergic transmission in the induction and expression of behavioral sensitization: a critical review of preclinical studies. Psychopharmacology (Berl.) **151:** 99–120.
18. EVERITT, B.J. & T.W. ROBBINS. 2005. Neural systems of reinforcement for drug addiction: from actions to habits to compulsion. Nat. Neurosci. **8:** 1481–1489.

19. JENTSCH, J.D. & J.R. TAYLOR. 1999. Impulsivity resulting from frontostriatal dysfunction in drug abuse: implications for the control of behavior by reward-related stimuli. Psychopharmacology (Berl.) **146:** 373–390.
20. BEATTY, W.W. *et al.* 1995. Neuropsychological performance of recently abstinent alcoholics and cocaine abusers. Drug Alcohol Dep. **37:** 247–253.
21. BECHARA, A. *et al.* 2001. Decision-making deficits, linked to a dysfunctional ventromedial prefrontal cortex, revealed in alcohol and stimulant abusers. Neuropsychologia **39:** 376–389.
22. BOLLA, K. *et al.* 2004. Prefrontal cortical dysfunction in abstinent cocaine abusers. J. Neuropsychiatry Clin. Neurosci. **16:** 456–64.
23. BOLLA, K.I., J.L. CADET & E.D. LONDON. 1998. The neuropsychiatry of chronic cocaine abuse. J. Neuropsychiatry Clin. Neurosci. **10:** 280–289.
24. ERSCHE, K.D. *et al.* 2006. Profile of executive and memory function associated with amphetamine and opiate dependence. Neuropsychopharmacology **31:** 1036–1047.
25. ERSCHE, K.D. *et al.* 2005. Abnormal frontal activations related to decision-making in current and former amphetamine and opiate dependent individuals. Psychopharmacology (Berl.) **180:** 612–623.
26. GRANT, S., C. CONTOREGGI & E.D. LONDON. 2000. Drug abusers show impaired performance in a laboratory test of decision making. Neuropsychologia **38:** 1180–1187.
27. GRANT, S. *et al.* 1996. Activation of memory circuits during cue-elicited cocaine craving. Proc. Natl. Acad. Sci. USA **93:** 12040–12045.
28. HESTER, R. & H. GARAVAN. 2004. Executive dysfunction in cocaine addiction: evidence for discordant frontal, cingulate, and cerebellar activity. J. Neurosci. **24:** 11017–11022.
29. JOE, G.W. *et al.* 1991. Depression and decision-making among intravenous drug users. Psychol. Rep. **68:** 339–347.
30. KAUFMAN, J.N. *et al.* 2003. Cingulate hypoactivity in cocaine users during a GO-NOGO task as revealed by event-related functional magnetic resonance imaging. J. Neurosci. **23:** 7839–7843.
31. MCKETIN, R. & R.P. MATTICK. 1998. Attention and memory in illicit amphetamine users: comparison with non-drug-using controls. Drug Alcohol Dep. **50:** 181–184.
32. O'MALLEY, S. *et al.* 1992. Neuropsychological impairment in chronic cocaine abusers. Am. J. Drug Alcohol Abuse **18:** 131–144.
33. ORNSTEIN, T.J. *et al.* 2000. Profiles of cognitive dysfunction in chronic amphetamine and heroin abusers. Neuropsychopharmacology **23:** 113–126.
34. BREITER, H.C. *et al.* 1997. Acute effects of cocaine on human brain activity and emotion. Neuron **19:** 591–611.
35. HOLMAN, B.L. *et al.* 1991. Brain perfusion is abnormal in cocaine-dependent polydrug users: a study using technetium-99 m-HMPAO and ASPECT. J. Nucl. Med. **32:** 1206–1210.
36. LONDON, E.D. *et al.* 2000. Orbitofrontal cortex and human drug abuse: functional imaging. Cereb. Cortex **10:** 334–342.
37. VOLKOW, N.D. & J.S. FOWLER. 2000. Addiction, a disease of compulsion and drive: involvement of the orbitofrontal cortex. Cereb. Cortex **10:** 318–325.
38. VOLKOW, N.D. *et al.* 1991. Changes in brain glucose metabolism in cocaine dependence and withdrawal. Am. J. Psychiatry **148:** 621–626.

39. VOLKOW, N.D. *et al.* 1992. Long-term frontal brain metabolic changes in cocaine abusers. Synapse **11:** 184–190.
40. CHILDRESS, A.R. *et al.* 1988. Classically conditioned responses in opioid and cocaine dependence: a role in relapse? NIDA Res. Monogr. **84:** 25–43.
41. CHILDRESS, A.R. *et al.* 1999. Limbic activation during cue-induced cocaine craving. Am. J. Psychiatry **156:** 11–18.
42. KILTS, C.D. *et al.* 2001. Neural activity related to drug craving in cocaine addiction. Arch. Gen. Psychiatry **58:** 334–341.
43. NEGRETE, J.C. & S. EMIL. 1992. Cue-evoked arousal in cocaine users: a study of variance and predictive value. Drug Alcohol Depend. **30:** 187–192.
44. WANG, G.J. *et al.* 1999. Regional brain metabolic activation during craving elicited by recall of previous drug experiences. Life Sci. **64:** 775–784.
45. BONSON, K.R. *et al.* 2002. Neural systems and cue-induced cocaine craving. Neuropsychopharmacology **26:** 376–386.
46. GARAVAN, H. *et al.* 2000. Cue-induced cocaine craving: neuroanatomical specificity for drug users and drug stimuli. Am. J. Psychiatry **157:** 1789–1798.
47. MAAS, L.C. *et al.* 1998. Functional magnetic resonance imaging of human brain activation during cue-induced cocaine craving. Am. J. Psychiatry **155:** 124–126.
48. ROGERS, R.D. & T.W. ROBBINS. 2001. Investigating the neurocognitive deficits associated with chronic drug misuse. Curr. Opin. Neurobiol. **11:** 250–257.
49. VOLKOW, N.D. & T.K. LI. 2004. Drug addiction: the neurobiology of behaviour gone awry. Nat. Rev. Neurosci. **5:** 963–970.
50. UYLINGS, H.B., H.J. GROENEWEGEN & B. KOLB. 2003. Do rats have a prefrontal cortex? Behav. Brain Res. **146:** 3–17.
51. ONGUR, D. & J.L. PRICE. 2000. The organization of networks within the orbital and medial prefrontal cortex of rats, monkeys and humans. Cereb. Cortex **10:** 206–219.
52. VEZINA, P. 2004. Sensitization of midbrain dopamine neuron reactivity and the self-administration of psychomotor stimulant drugs. Neurosci. Biobehav. Rev. **27:** 827–839.
53. JENTSCH, J.D. *et al.* 2002. Impairments of reversal learning and response perseveration after repeated, intermittent cocaine administrations to monkeys. Neuropsychopharmacology **26:** 183–190.
54. SCHOENBAUM, G. *et al.* 2004. Cocaine-experienced rats exhibit learning deficits in a task sensitive to orbitofrontal cortex lesions. Eur. J. Neurosci. **19:** 1997–2002.
55. CALU, D.J. *et al.* 2007. Withdrawal from cocaine self-administration produces long-lasting deficits in orbitofrontal-dependent reversal learning in rats. Learn. Mem. **14:** 325–328.
56. FILLMORE, M.T. & C.R. RUSH. 2002. Impaired inhibitory control of behavior in chronic cocaine users. Drug Alcohol Depend. **66:** 265–273.
57. ROBERTS, A.C. 2006. Primate orbitofrontal cortex and adaptive behaviour. Trends Cogn. Sci. **10:** 83–90.
58. BUTTER, C.M. 1968. Perseveration in extinction and in discrimination reversal following selective frontal ablations in Macaca mulatta. Physiol. Behav. **4:** 163–171.
59. DIAS, R., T.W. ROBBINS & A.C. ROBERTS. 1996. Dissociation in prefrontal cortex of affective and attentional shifts. Nature **380:** 69–72.

60. DIAS, R., T.W. ROBBINS & A.C. ROBERTS. 1996. Primate analogue of the Wisconsin Card Sorting Test: effects of excitotoxic lesions of the prefrontal cortex in the marmoset. Behav. Neurosci. **110:** 872–886.
61. DIAS, R., T.W. ROBBINS & A.C. ROBERTS. 1997. Dissociable forms of inhibitory control within prefrontal cortex with an analog of the Wisconsin Card Sort test – restriction to novel situations and independence from on-line processing. J. Neurosci. **17:** 9285–9297.
62. GAFFAN, D., E.A. MURRAY & M. FABRE-THORPE. 1993. Interaction of the amygdala with the frontal lobe in reward memory. Eur. J. Neurosci. **5:** 968–975.
63. HORNAK, J. *et al.* 2004. Reward-related reversal learning after surgical excisions in orbito-frontal or dorsolateral prefrontal cortex in humans. J. Cogn. Neurosci. **16:** 463–478.
64. IZQUIERDO, A., R.K. SUDA & E.A. MURRAY. 2004. Bilateral orbital prefrontal cortex lesions in rhesus monkeys disrupt choices guided by both reward value and reward contingency. J. Neurosci. **24:** 7540–7548.
65. IVERSEN, S.D. & M. MISHKIN. 1970. Perseverative interference in monkeys following selective lesions of the inferior prefrontal convexity. Exp. Brain Res. **11:** 376–386.
66. ROLLS, E.T. *et al.* 1994. Emotion-related learning in patients with social and emotional changes associated with frontal lobe damage. J. Neurol. Neurosurg. Psychiatry **57:** 1518–1524.
67. LI, L. & J. SHAO. 1998. Restricted lesions to ventral prefrontal subareas block reversal learning but not visual discrimination learning in rats. Physiol. Behav. **65:** 371–379.
68. RAGOZZINO, M.E., S. DETRICK & R.P. KESNER. 1999. Involvement of the prelimbic-infralimbic areas of the rodent prefrontal cortex in behavioral flexibility for place and response learning. J. Neurosci. **19:** 4585–4594.
69. BOULOUGOURIS, V., J.W. DALLEY & T.W. ROBBINS. 2007. Effects of orbitofrontal, infralimbic and prelimbic cortical lesions on serial spatial reversal learning in the rat. Behav. Brain Res. **179:** 219–228.
70. MCALONAN, K. & V.J. BROWN. 2003. Orbital prefrontal cortex mediates reversal learning and not attentional set shifting in the rat. Behav. Brain Res. **146:** 97–103.
71. CHUDASAMA, Y. & T.W. ROBBINS. 2003. Dissociable contributions of the orbitofrontal and infralimbic cortex to pavlovian autoshaping and discrimination reversal learning: further evidence for the functional heterogeneity of the rodent frontal cortex. J. Neurosci. **23:** 8771–8780.
72. SCHOENBAUM, G., A.A. CHIBA & M. GALLAGHER. 2000. Changes in functional connectivity in orbitofrontal cortex and basolateral amygdala during learning and reversal training. J. Neurosci. **20:** 5179–5189.
73. STALNAKER, T.A. *et al.* 2007. Basolateral amygdala lesions abolish orbitofrontal-dependent reversal impairments. Neuron. **54:** 51–58.
74. BECHARA, A. 2005. Decision making, impulse control and loss of willpower to resist drugs: a neurocognitive perspective. Nat. Neurosci. **8:** 1458–1463.
75. BUSSEY, T.J. *et al.* 1997. Triple dissociation of anterior cingulate, posterior cingulate, and medial frontal cortices on visual discrimination tasks using a touch-screen testing procedure for the rat. Behav. Neurosci. **111:** 920–936.
76. HOLLAND, P.C., J.S. HAN & M. GALLAGHER. 2000. Lesions of the amygdala central nucleus alter performance on a selective attention task. J. Neurosci. **20:** 6701–6706.

77. KOLB, B. 1984. Functions of the frontal cortex of the rat: a comparative review. Brain Res. **320:** 65–98.
78. KOLB, B., S. PELLIS & T.E. ROBINSON. 2004. Plasticity and functions of the orbital frontal cortex. Brain Cogn. **55:** 104–115.
79. SWAINSON, R. *et al.* 2000. Probabilistic learning and reversal deficits in patients with Parkinson's disease or frontal or temporal lobe lesions: possible adverse effects of dopaminergic medication. Neuropsychologia **38:** 596–612.
80. DAMASIO, A.R. 1995. On some functions of the human prefrontal cortex. Ann. N. Y. Acad. Sci. **769:** 241–251.
81. SEAMANS, J.K., S.B. FLORESCO & A.G. PHILLIPS. 1995. Functional differences between the prelimbic and anterior cingulate regions of the rat prefrontal cortex. Behav. Neurosci. **109:** 1063–1073.
82. GOLDMAN-RAKIC, P.S. 1987. Circuitry of the frontal cortex and the regulation of behavior by representational knowledge. *In* Handbook in Physiology. The Nervous System, Vol. 5. F. Plum & V. Mountcastle, Eds.: 373–417. American Physiological Society. Bethesda.
83. CLARKE, H.F. *et al.* 2004. Cognitive inflexibility after prefrontal serotonin depletion. Science **304:** 878–880.
84. CLARKE, H.F. *et al.* 2005. Prefrontal serotonin depletion affects reversal learning but not attentional set shifting. J. Neurosci. **25:** 532–538.
85. CLARKE, H.F. *et al.* 2007. Cognitive inflexibility after prefrontal serotonin depletion is behaviorally and neurochemically specific. Cereb. Cortex **17:** 18–27.
86. LEE, B. *et al.* 2007. Dopamine D(2)/D(3) Receptors Play a Specific Role in the Reversal of a Learned Visual Discrimination in Monkeys. Neuropsychopharmacology **32:** 2125–2134.
87. VOLKOW, N.D. *et al.* 1993. Decreased dopamine D2 receptor availability is associated with reduced frontal metabolism in cocaine abusers. Synapse **14:** 169–177.
88. JENTSCH, J.D. *et al.* 1997. Enduring cognitive deficits and cortical dopamine dysfunction in monkeys after long-term administration of phencyclidine. Science **277:** 953–955.
89. JENTSCH, J.D., R.H. ROTH & J.R. TAYLOR. 2000. Object retrieval/detour deficits in monkeys produced by prior subchronic phencyclidine administration: evidence for cognitive impulsivity. Biol. Psychiatry **48:** 415–424.
90. JENTSCH, J.D. *et al.* 1999. Altered frontal cortical dopaminergic transmission in monkeys after subchronic phencyclidine exposure: involvement in frontostriatal cognitive deficits. Neuroscience **90:** 823–832.
91. JENTSCH, J.D. *et al.* 1999. Dopamine D4 receptor antagonist reversal of subchronic phencyclidine-induced object retrieval/detour deficits in monkeys. Psychopharmacology (Berl.) **142:** 78–84.
92. TAYLOR, J.R. *et al.* 1990. Cognitive and motor deficits in the acquisition of an object retrieval/detour task in MPTP-treated monkeys. Brain **113:** 617–637.
93. TAYLOR, J.R. *et al.* 1990. Cognitive and motor deficits in the performance of an object retrieval/detour task with barrier in monkeys treated with MPTP: Long-term performance and effect of transparency of the barrier. Behav. Neurosci. **104:** 564–576.
94. WALKER, S.C. *et al.* 2006. Selective prefrontal serotonin depletion impairs acquisition of a detour-reaching task. Eur. J. Neurosci. **23:** 3119–3123.

95. WALLIS, J.D. *et al.* 2001. Dissociable contributions of the orbitofrontal and lateral prefrontal cortex of the marmoset to performance on a detour reaching task. Eur. J. Neurosci. **13:** 1797–1808.

96. WILKINSON, L.S. *et al.* 1997. Contrasting effects of excitotoxic lesions of the prefrontal cortex on the behavioural response to D-amphetamine and presynaptic and postsynaptic measures of striatal dopamine function in monkeys. Neuroscience **80:** 717–730.

97. CASTNER, S.A., P.S. VOSLER & P.S. GOLDMAN-RAKIC. 2005. Amphetamine sensitization impairs cognition and reduces dopamine turnover in primate prefrontal cortex. Biol. Psychiatry **57:** 743–751.

98. FLETCHER, P.J. *et al.* 2005. Sensitization to amphetamine, but not PCP, impairs attentional set shifting: reversal by a D1 receptor agonist injected into the medial prefrontal cortex. Psychopharmacology (Berl.) **183:** 190–200.

99. FLETCHER, P.J. *et al.* 2007. A sensitizing regimen of amphetamine impairs visual attention in the 5-choice serial reaction time test: reversal by a D1 receptor agonist injected into the medial prefrontal cortex. Neuropsychopharmacology **32:** 1122–1132.

100. PAINE, T.A. & M.C. OLMSTEAD. 2004. Cocaine disrupts both behavioural inhibition and conditional discrimination in rats. Psychopharmacology (Berl.) **175:** 443–450.

101. DALLEY, J.W. *et al.* 2005. Attentional and motivational deficits in rats withdrawn from intravenous self-administration of cocaine or heroin. Psychopharmacology (Berl.) **182:** 579–587.

102. DALLEY, J.W. *et al.* 2005. Cognitive sequelae of intravenous amphetamine self-administration in rats: evidence for selective effects on attentional performance. Neuropsychopharmacology **30:** 525–537.

103. DALLEY, J.W. *et al.* 2007. Nucleus accumbens D2/3 receptors predict trait impulsivity and cocaine reinforcement. Science **315:** 1267–1270.

104. LORRAIN, D.S., G.M. ARNOLD & P. VEZINA. 2000. Previous exposure to amphetamine increases incentive to obtain the drug: long-lasting effects revealed by the progressive ratio schedule. Behav. Brain Res. **107:** 9–19.

105. MORGAN, D., Y. LIU & D.C. ROBERTS. 2006. Rapid and persistent sensitization to the reinforcing effects of cocaine. Neuropsychopharmacology **31:** 121–128.

106. MORGAN, D. & D.C. ROBERTS. 2004. Sensitization to the reinforcing effects of cocaine following binge-abstinent self-administration. Neurosci. Biobehav. Rev. **27:** 803–812.

107. MORGAN, D., M.A. SMITH & D.C. ROBERTS. 2005. Binge self-administration and deprivation produces sensitization to the reinforcing effects of cocaine in rats. Psychopharmacology (Berl.) **178:** 309–316.

108. DEROCHE-GAMONET, V., D. BELIN & P.V. PIAZZA. 2004. Evidence for addiction-like behavior in the rat. Science **305:** 1014–1017.

109. BRUNZELL, D.H. *et al.* 2006. beta2-Subunit-containing nicotinic acetylcholine receptors are involved in nicotine-induced increases in conditioned reinforcement but not progressive ratio responding for food in C57BL/6 mice. Psychopharmacology (Berl.) **184** (3–4): 328–338.

110. OLAUSSON, P. *et al.* 2006. DeltaFosB in the nucleus accumbens regulates food-reinforced instrumental behavior and motivation. J. Neurosci. **26:** 9196–9204.

111. EVERITT, B.J. *et al.* 2003. Appetitive behavior: impact of amygdala-dependent mechanisms of emotional learning. Ann. N. Y. Acad. Sci. **985:** 233–250.

112. MACKINTOSH, N.J. 1974. The Psychology of Animal Learning. Academic Press. New York.
113. ROBBINS, T.W. 1978. The acquisition of responding with conditioned reinforcement: effects of pipradrol, methylphenidate, d-amphetamine, and nomifensine. Psychopharmacology (Berl.) **58:** 79–87.
114. TAYLOR, J.R. & T.W. ROBBINS. 1984. Enhanced behavioral control by conditioned reinforcers following microinjections of d-amphetamine into the nucleus accumbens. Psychopharmacology **84:** 405–412.
115. TAYLOR, J.R. & T.W. ROBBINS. 1986. 6-Hydroxydopamine lesions of the nucleus accumbens, but not of the caudate nucleus, attenuate enhanced responding with reward-related stimuli produced by intra-accumbens d-amphetamine. Psychopharmacology **90:** 390–397.
116. JENTSCH, J.D. & J.R. TAYLOR. 2001. Impaired inhibition of conditioned responses produced by subchronic administration of phencyclidine to rats. Neuropsychopharmacology **24:** 66–74.
117. MEAD, A.N., H.S. CROMBAG & B.A. ROCHA. 2004. Sensitization of psychomotor stimulation and conditioned reward in mice: differential modulation by contextual learning. Neuropsychopharmacology **29:** 249–258.
118. OLAUSSON, P., J.D. JENTSCH & J.R. TAYLOR. 2004. Repeated nicotine exposure enhances responding with conditioned reinforcement. Psychopharmacology (Berl.) **173:** 98–104.
119. TAYLOR, J.R. & B.A. HORGER. 1999. Enhanced responding for conditioned reward produced by intra-accumbens amphetamine is potentiated after cocaine sensitization. Psychopharmacology (Berl.) **142:** 31–40.
120. MILES, F.J. *et al.* 2004. Conditioned activity and instrumental reinforcement following long-term oral consumption of cocaine by rats. Behav. Neurosci. **118:** 1331–1339.
121. WYVELL, C.L. & K.C. BERRIDGE. 2001. Incentive sensitization by previous amphetamine exposure: increased cue-triggered "wanting" for sucrose reward. J. Neurosci. **21:** 7831–7840.
122. BOSSERT, J.M. *et al.* 2005. Neurobiology of relapse to heroin and cocaine seeking: an update and clinical implications. Eur. J. Pharmacol. **526:** 36–50.
123. SHAHAM, Y. *et al.* 2003. The reinstatement model of drug relapse: history, methodology and major findings. Psychopharmacology (Berl.) **168:** 3–20.
124. CHILDRESS, A.R. *et al.* 1993. Cue reactivity and cue reactivity interventions in drug dependence. NIDA Res. Monogr. **137:** 73–95.
125. CHILDRESS, A.R., A.T. MCLELLAN & C.P. O'BRIEN. 1986. Role of conditioning factors in the development of drug dependence. Psychiatr. Clin. North Am. **9:** 413–425.
126. EHRMAN, R.N. *et al.* 1992. Conditioned responses to cocaine-related stimuli in cocaine abuse patients. Psychopharmacology **107:** 523–529.
127. O'BRIEN, C.P. *et al.* 1998. Conditioning factors in drug abuse: can they explain compulsion? J. Psychopharmacol. **12:** 15–22.
128. O'BRIEN, C.P. *et al.* 1993. Developing treatments that address classical conditioning. NIDA Res. Monogr. **135:** 71–91.
129. TIFFANY, S.T. & B.L. CARTER. 1998. Is craving the source of compulsive drug use? J. Psychopharmacol. **12:** 23–30.
130. GRIMM, J.W. *et al.* 2001. Neuroadaptation. Incubation of cocaine craving after withdrawal. Nature **412:** 141–142.

131. Lu, L. *et al.* 2004. Cocaine seeking over extended withdrawal periods in rats: different time courses of responding induced by cocaine cues versus cocaine priming over the first 6 months. Psychopharmacology (Berl.) **176**: 101–108.

132. Lu, L. *et al.* 2004. Incubation of cocaine craving after withdrawal: a review of preclinical data. Neuropharmacology **47**(Suppl 1): 214–226.

133. BRADBERRY, C.W. & S.R. RUBINO. 2006. Dopaminergic responses to self-administered cocaine in Rhesus monkeys do not sensitize following high cumulative intake. Eur. J. Neurosci. **23**: 2773–2778.

134. PARKINSON, J.A. *et al.* 2001. The role of the primate amygdala in conditioned reinforcement. J. Neurosci. **21**: 7770–7780.

135. PEARS, A. *et al.* 2003. Lesions of the orbitofrontal but not medial prefrontal cortex disrupt conditioned reinforcement in primates. J. Neurosci. **23**: 11189–11201.

136. PARKINSON, J.A. *et al.* 1999. Dissociation in effects of lesions of the nucleus accumbens core and shell on appetitive pavlovian approach behavior and the potentiation of conditioned reinforcement and locomotor activity by D-amphetamine. J. Neurosci. **19**: 2401–2411.

137. WYVELL, C.L. & K.C. BERRIDGE. 2000. Intra-accumbens amphetamine increases the conditioned incentive salience of sucrose reward: enhancement of reward "wanting" without enhanced "liking" or response reinforcement. J. Neurosci. **20**: 8122–8130.

138. COX, S.M., A. ANDRADE & I.S. JOHNSRUDE. 2005. Learning to like: a role for human orbitofrontal cortex in conditioned reward. J. Neurosci. **25**: 2733–2740.

139. O'DOHERTY, J. *et al.* 2003. Dissociating valence of outcome from behavioral control in human orbital and ventral prefrontal cortices. J. Neurosci. **23**: 7931–7939.

140. ROESCH, M.R. & C.R. OLSON. 2004. Neuronal activity related to reward value and motivation in primate frontal cortex. Science **304**: 307–310.

141. SCHOENBAUM, G., A.A. CHIBA & M. GALLAGHER. 1998. Orbitofrontal cortex and basolateral amygdala encode expected outcomes during learning. Nat. Neurosci. **1**: 155–159.

142. ARANA, F.S. *et al.* 2003. Dissociable contributions of the human amygdala and orbitofrontal cortex to incentive motivation and goal selection. J. Neurosci. **23**: 9632–9638.

143. ELLIOTT, R. & B. DEAKIN. 2005. Role of the orbitofrontal cortex in reinforcement processing and inhibitory control: evidence from functional magnetic resonance imaging studies in healthy human subjects. Int. Rev. Neurobiol. **65**: 89–116.

144. KRINGELBACH, M.L. 2005. The human orbitofrontal cortex: linking reward to hedonic experience. Nat. Rev. Neurosci. **6**: 691–702.

145. SCHOENBAUM, G., M.R. ROESCH & T.A. STALNAKER. 2006. Orbitofrontal cortex, decision-making and drug addiction. Trends Neurosci. **29**: 116–124.

146. STALNAKER, T.A. *et al.* 2006. Abnormal associative encoding in orbitofrontal neurons in cocaine-experienced rats during decision-making. Eur. J. Neurosci. **24**: 2643–2653.

147. SCHOENBAUM, G. & B. SETLOW. 2005. Cocaine makes actions insensitive to outcomes but not extinction: implications for altered orbitofrontal-amygdalar function. Cereb. Cortex **15**: 1162–1169.

148. HUTCHESON, D.M. & B.J. EVERITT. 2003. The effects of selective orbitofrontal cortex lesions on the acquisition and performance of cue-controlled cocaine seeking in rats. Ann. N. Y. Acad. Sci. **1003**: 410–411.

149. FUCHS, R.A. *et al.* 2004. Differential involvement of orbitofrontal cortex subregions in conditioned cue-induced and cocaine-primed reinstatement of cocaine seeking in rats. J. Neurosci. **24:** 6600–6610.
150. CAPRILES, N. *et al.* 2003. A role for the prefrontal cortex in stress- and cocaine-induced reinstatement of cocaine seeking in rats. Psychopharmacology (Berl.) **168:** 66–74.
151. EVERITT, B.J., A. DICKINSON & T.W. ROBBINS. 2001. The neuropsychological basis of addictive behaviour. Brain Res. Brain Res. Rev. **36:** 129–138.
152. PARKINSON, J.A. *et al.* 2005. Acquisition of instrumental conditioned reinforcement is resistant to the devaluation of the unconditioned stimulus. Q. J. Exp. Psychol. B. **58:** 19–30.
153. ITO, R. *et al.* 2000. Dissociation in conditioned dopamine release in the nucleus accumbens core and shell in response to cocaine cues and during cocaine-seeking behavior in rats. J. Neurosci. **20:** 7489–7495.
154. ITO, R. *et al.* 2002. Dopamine release in the dorsal striatum during cocaine-seeking behavior under the control of a drug-associated cue. J. Neurosci. **22:** 6247–6253.
155. VANDERSCHUREN, L.J., P. DI CIANO & B.J. EVERITT. 2005. Involvement of the dorsal striatum in cue-controlled cocaine seeking. J. Neurosci. **25:** 8665–8670.
156. CROMBAG, H.S. *et al.* 2005. Opposite effects of amphetamine self-administration experience on dendritic spines in the medial and orbital prefrontal cortex. Cereb. Cortex **15:** 341–348.
157. HOMAYOUN, H. & B. MOGHADDAM. 2006. Progression of cellular adaptations in medial prefrontal and orbitofrontal cortex in response to repeated amphetamine. J. Neurosci. **26:** 8025–8039.
158. BEVERIDGE, T.J. *et al.* 2006. Chronic cocaine self-administration is associated with altered functional activity in the temporal lobes of non human primates. Eur. J. Neurosci. **23:** 3109–3118.
159. LYONS, D. *et al.* 1996. Cocaine alters cerebral metabolism within the ventral striatum and limbic cortex of monkeys. J. Neurosci. **16:** 1230–1238.
160. THOMAS, K.L., M. ARROYO & B.J. EVERITT. 2003. Induction of the learning and plasticity-associated gene Zif268 following exposure to a discrete cocaine-associated stimulus. Eur. J. Neurosci. **17:** 1964–1972.
161. HYMAN, S.E., R.C. MALENKA & E.J. NESTLER. 2006. Neural mechanisms of addiction: the role of reward-related learning and memory. Annu. Rev. Neurosci. **29:** 565–598.
162. KELLEY, A.E. 2004. Memory and addiction: shared neural circuitry and molecular mechanisms. Neuron **44:** 161–179.
163. ROBINSON, T.E. & B. KOLB. 2004. Structural plasticity associated with exposure to drugs of abuse. Neuropharmacology **47**(Suppl 1): 33–46.
164. NESTLER, E.J. 2004. Molecular mechanisms of drug addiction. Neuropharmacology **47:** 24–32.
165. NESTLER, E.J. 2001. Psychogenomics: opportunities for understanding addiction. J. Neurosci. **21:** 8324–8327.
166. NESTLER, E.J. & D. LANDSMAN. 2001. Learning about addiction from the genome. Nature **409:** 834–835.
167. POLLOCK, J.D. 2002. Gene expression profiling: methodological challenges, results, and prospects for addiction research. Chem. Phys. Lipids **121:** 241–256.
168. GREENBAUM, D. *et al.* 2003. Comparing protein abundance and mRNA expression levels on a genomic scale. Genome Biol. **4:**117.

169. GYGI, S.P. *et al.* 1999. Correlation between Protein and mRNA abundance in yeast. Mol. Cell. Biol. **19:** 1720–1730.

170. ABUL-HUSN, N.S. & L.A. DEVI. 2006. Neuroproteomics of the synapse and drug addiction. J. Pharmacol. Exp. Ther. **318** (2): 461–468.

171. TANNU, N.S. & S.E. HEMBY. 2006. Methods for proteomics in neuroscience. Prog. Brain Res. **158:** 41–82.

172. WILLIAMS, K. *et al.* 2004. Recent advances in neuroproteomics and potential application to studies of drug addiction. Neuropharmacology **47:** 148–166.

173. UNLU, M., M.E. MORGAN & J.S. MINDEN. 1997. Difference gel electrophoresis: a single gel method for detecting changes in protein extracts. Electrophoresis **18:** 2071–2077.

174. VAN DEN BERGH, G. & L. ARCKENS. 2004. Fluorescent two-dimensional difference gel electrophoresis unveils the potential of gel-based proteomics. Curr. Opin. Biotechnol. **15:** 38–43.

175. AGGARWAL, K., L.H. CHOE & K.H. LEE. 2006. Shotgun proteomics using the iTRAQ isobaric tags. Brief. Funct. Genomic. Proteomic **5:** 112–120.

176. ROSS, P.L. *et al.* 2004. Multiplexed protein quantitation in saccharomyces cerevisiae using amine-reactive isobaric tagging reagents. Mol. Cell. Proteomics **3:** 1154–1169.

177. BIERCZYNSKA-KRZYSIK, A. *et al.* 2006. Proteomic analysis of rat cerebral cortex, hippocampus and striatum after exposure to morphine. Int. J. Mol. Med. **18:** 775–784.

178. FREEMAN, W.M. *et al.* 2005. Distinct proteomic profiles of amphetamine self-administration transitional states. Pharmacogenomics J. **5:** 203–214.

179. IWAZAKI, T., I.S. MCGREGOR & I. MATSUMOTO. 2006. Protein expression profile in the striatum of acute methamphetamine-treated rats. Brain Res. **1097:** 19–25.

180. LI, K.W. *et al.* 2006. Intermittent administration of morphine alters protein expression in rat nucleus accumbens. Proteomics **6:** 2003–2008.

181. YEOM, M. *et al.* 2005. Proteomic analysis of nicotine-associated protein expression in the striatum of repeated nicotine-treated rats. Biochem. Biophys. Res. Commun. **326:** 321–328.

182. TANNU, N., D.C. MASH & S.E. HEMBY. 2007. Cytosolic proteomic alterations in the nucleus accumbens of cocaine overdose victims. Mol. Psychiatry **12:** 55–73.

183. KRUEGER, D.D. *et al.* 2005. Proteomic analysis of persistent cortico-limbic-striatal neuroadaptations following repeated cocaine exposure in Vervet monkeys. Program # 1030.6, 2005 Abstract Viewer/Itinerary Planner. Society for Neuroscience. Washington, DC, Online.

184. CLOW, D.W. & R.P. HAMMER, JR. 1991. Cocaine abstinence following chronic treatment alters cerebral metabolism in dopaminergic reward regions. Bromocriptine enhances recovery. Neuropsychopharmacology **4:** 71–75.

185. PORRINO, L.J. & D. LYONS. 2000. Orbital and medial prefrontal cortex and psychostimulant abuse: studies in animal models. Cereb. Cortex **10:** 326–333.

186. FRANKLIN, T.R. *et al.* 2002. Decreased gray matter concentration in the insular, orbitofrontal, cingulate, and temporal cortices of cocaine patients. Biol. Psychiatry **51:** 134–142.

187. MATOCHIK, J.A. *et al.* 2003. Frontal cortical tissue composition in abstinent cocaine abusers: a magnetic resonance imaging study. Neuroimage **19:** 1095–1102.

188. LI, Z. *et al.* 2004. The importance of dendritic mitochondria in the morphogenesis and plasticity of spines and synapses. Cell **119:** 873–887.
189. LY, C.V. & P. VERSTREKEN. 2006. Mitochondria at the synapse. Neuroscientist **12:** 291–299.
190. MATTSON, M.P. 2007. Mitochondrial regulation of neuronal plasticity. Neurochem. Res. **32:** 707–715.
191. MILES, F.J., B.J. EVERITT & A. DICKINSON. 2003. Oral cocaine seeking by rats: action or habit? Behav. Neurosci. **117:** 927–938.
192. NELSON, A. & S. KILLCROSS. 2006. Amphetamine exposure enhances habit formation. J. Neurosci. **26:** 3805–3812.
193. VANDERSCHUREN, L.J. & B.J. EVERITT. 2004. Drug seeking becomes compulsive after prolonged cocaine self-administration. Science **305:** 1017–1019.
194. BUTTER, C.M., J.A. MCDONALD & D.R. SNYDER. 1969. Orality, preference behavior, and reinforcement value of non-food objects in monkeys with orbital frontal lesions. Science **164:** 1306–1307.
195. BUTTER, C.M., D.R. SNYDER & J.A. MCDONALD. 1970. Effects of orbital frontal lesions on aversive and aggressive behaviors in rhesus monkeys. J. Comp. Physiol. Psychol. **72:** 132–144.
196. O'DOHERTY, J. *et al.* 2001. Abstract reward and punishment representations in the human orbitofrontal cortex. Nat. Neurosci. **4:** 95–102.
197. THORPE, S.J., E.T. ROLLS & S. MADDISON. 1983. The orbitofrontal cortex: neuronal activity in the behaving monkey. Exp. Brain Res. **49:** 93–115.
198. COUTUREAU, E. & S. KILLCROSS. 2003. Inactivation of the infralimbic prefrontal cortex reinstates goal-directed responding in overtrained rats. Behav. Brain Res. **146:** 167–174.
199. KILLCROSS, S. & E. COUTUREAU. 2003. Coordination of actions and habits in the medial prefrontal cortex of rats. Cereb. Cortex **13:** 400–408.
200. HITCHCOTT, P.K., J.J. QUINN & J.R. TAYLOR. 2007. Bidirectional Modulation of Goal-Directed Actions by Prefrontal Cortical Dopamine. Cereb. Cortex. Feb. 24 [E pub ahead of print].

The Orbitofrontal Cortex, Impulsivity, and Addiction

Probing Orbitofrontal Dysfunction at the Neural, Neurochemical, and Molecular Level

CATHARINE A. WINSTANLEY

University of British Columbia, Department of Psychology, Vancouver, BC, Canada

ABSTRACT: The association between impulsivity and addiction is currently a topic of intense research interest. Investigations into the neurobiological basis of aspects of impulse control have revealed some striking parallels between the brain circuitry and neurochemical systems implicated in drug dependence and impulsive behavior. Both processes are heavily regulated by limbic corticostriatal circuits including the orbitofrontal cortex (OFC) and nucleus accumbens (NAC), and are modulated by dopamine (DA) and serotonin (5-HT). Hypoactivity within the OFC has been observed in recently abstinent cocaine users, and this is thought to contribute to the cognitive deficits associated with drug abuse, including impairments in impulse control. However, the neurobiological mechanisms underlying these functional and behavioral deficits are unclear. In parallel to observations made in the NAC, recent data indicate that chronic cocaine use also induces the transcription factor ΔFosB in the OFC and that this plays a role in the cognitive sequelae of chronic cocaine administration. In particular, ΔFosB appears to be involved in the development of tolerance to the disruptive effects of acute cocaine on impulsivity and motivation observed after repeated cocaine administration. Increased ΔFosB also contributes to increased impulsivity during withdrawal from the drug. Both effects could be attributed to the upregulation of local inhibitory processes in the OFC after over-expression of ΔFosB and chronic cocaine treatment. Through integrating what is known of the interaction between addictive drugs and impulsivity at the neural, neurochemical, and molecular level, novel insight may be obtained into the multi-faceted regulation of the addicted state.

KEYWORDS: cocaine; five-choice serial reaction time task; delay-discounting; ΔFosB; dopamine; serotonin

Address for correspondence: Catharine A. Winstanley, Ph.D., University of British Columbia, Department of Psychology, 2136 West Mall, Vancouver BC, V6T 1Z4, Canada. Voice: (604) 822 3128; fax: (604) 822 6923.

cwinstanley@psych.ubc.ca

Ann. N.Y. Acad. Sci. 1121: 639–655 (2007). © 2007 New York Academy of Sciences.
doi: 10.1196/annals.1401.024

INTRODUCTION

Broadly defined as action without sufficient foresight, high levels of impulsivity are associated with a range of psychiatric disorders, most notably bipolar depression and attention-deficit hyperactivity disorder (ADHD). However, contemporary studies have identified deficits in impulse control as a contributing factor to drug addiction. Although research to date has largely focused on understanding the reinforcing effects of addictive drugs,[1] recent evidence indicates that cognitive changes caused by cocaine and other drugs of abuse are also important in the generation and maintenance of addiction and may determine whether therapy is successful.[2,3] Research into the biological basis of impulse control indicates that some of the same brain structures and neurotransmitter systems are implicated in both addiction and impulsivity. In particular, the orbitofrontal cortex (OFC) and nucleus accumbens (NAC) have been identified as important loci of impulse control. In terms of its role in addiction, it has been firmly established that drug-induced changes in dopamine (DA) within the NAC signal the rewarding properties of addictive drugs and the stimuli associated with them.[4] However, the role played by the OFC in the development of addiction and how hypoactivity in this region may relate to the maladaptive decision making and impulsive behavior seen in substance abusers, have not been sufficiently clarified. Following a brief discussion of the definition and measurement of impulsivity, the relationship between impulsivity and addiction will be reviewed with a focus on the OFC. Current information regarding the extent to which manipulations of the OFC at the neural, neurochemical, and molecular level alter impulsivity and addiction will be presented and future directions for research outlined.

DEFINING IMPULSIVITY

Understanding exactly what we mean by the term "impulsivity" has proven more problematic than superficial discussion would suggest. Clinical psychologists have designed self-report questionnaires to measure impulsive behavior, such as the Barratt Impulsiveness scale[5] and the I7.[6] Factor analysis of data from such questionnaires largely suggests that impulsive behavior consists of several independent dimensions, although there is considerable variation as to the precise definition of these constituent parts (see Ref. 7 for review). However, common themes include decreased inhibitory control (or behavioral disinhibition), intolerance of delay to rewards, and quick decision making due to lack of consideration. Aspects of impulsivity are also thought to relate to poor attentional ability and hyperactivity. Bearing in mind this diversity of processes, one definition of impulsivity which still seems particularly appropriate is that "impulsivity encompasses a range of actions which are poorly conceived, prematurely expressed, unduly risky or inappropriate to the situation and that often result in undesirable consequences" (p. 23).[8]

Given the apparent multifaceted nature of the phenomena collectively described as impulsive, it has been suggested that impulsivity is not a unitary construct, but rather incorporates multiple distinct psychological processes, which may have independent underlying biological mechanisms.[7,9] This has led some to question the utility of the concept of impulsivity in and of itself. However, in exploring the neural bases of aspects of impulsivity, it becomes clear that similar, interconnecting networks of neural structures are employed in regulating different forms of impulse control, although the relative importance of different structures or neurotransmitter systems may vary with the exact process under examination.[10] Furthermore, the combined use of two independent measures of impulsivity is able to accurately diagnose ADHD far more effectively than the use of either measure in isolation, suggesting that the impulsivity construct is still of significant clinical import despite its apparent complexity.[11]

Measuring Impulsivity

Through focusing on different aspects of impulsive behavior, it has proved possible to devise a variety of behavioral paradigms to measure impulsivity in both human and non-human subjects. These can be broadly divided into two categories: those measuring impulsive choice or impulsive decision making and those measuring impulsive action or motoric impulsivity.

Impulsive action can be broadly defined as the inability to withhold from making a response. One of the most ubiquitous and well-characterized tasks designed for rats is the five-choice serial reaction time task (5CSRT).[12] This task was developed as a test of sustained and divided attention for rodents based on the continuous performance task (CPT) used to monitor attentional function in humans.[13] During the 5CSRT, the animal is required to make a nosepoke response in one of five apertures upon brief illumination of a stimulus light located therein. Subsequent to beginning a trial and prior to illumination of a stimulus light, there is a 5 s inter-trial interval during which the animal must withhold from responding at the five-hole array. Any responses made during this time are described as premature responses, and are punished. These premature responses provide an index of motoric impulsivity and are potentially analogous to "false alarm" errors made in the CPT.

In order to model impulsive decision making, an alternative task must be used. One of the most widely used measurements of impulsive decision making in laboratory animals is the delay-discounting or delay-to-gratification model of impulsive choice. Here, the subject chooses between a small reward delivered immediately and a larger reward delivered after a delay. Although the concept appears simple, many variants of the task have been developed.

One of the most prevalent is that first published by Evenden and Ryan in which animals choose to respond on two levers, one of which provides a small reward of one pellet, the other a large reward of four pellets.[14] Each session is divided into blocks of 12 trials, the first two of which are forced choice. In each successive block, the delay to the large reward increases from 0 s in the first block, to 10, 20, 40, and finally 60 s in the last block. In order to ensure that choice of the large reward option would always maximize the amount of reward earned, the length of each trial is kept constant so that the animal cannot accrue more pellets or increase the rate of reinforcement by repeatedly choosing the small reward. Using this paradigm, a within-session delay-discounting curve can be obtained. Animals typically show a strong preference for the larger reward early in the session when the delay to its delivery is short or absent, but shift their preference to the smaller reward as delay to the larger reward increases. This shift indicates an increase in impulsive choice. There is no measure of motoric impulsivity in this paradigm.

Together, these behavioral paradigms have been used in numerous studies to probe the neural and neurochemical mechanisms that regulate impulsivity. For example, manipulations of the NAC and medial prefrontal cortex (mPFC) have been found to affect performance of these tasks, e.g.[15,16] However, the same brain regions are not always involved in all measures of impulse control, and damage to the same region can sometimes have discordant and even opposing effects on impulse control depending on how impulsivity is defined. For example, lesions to the anterior cingulate cortex have been shown to increase premature responding on the 5CSRT,[16] but lesions to this region do not alter impulsive choice.[15] Damage to the NAC increases impulsive choice dramatically,[15] but the effects on 5CSRT performance are subtle.[17] More specifically, when the data are averaged over the whole session, there is no clear effect of NAC lesions on the level of premature responding. However, on closer analysis, it becomes apparent that NAC-lesioned rats were generally more likely to make a premature response after they had made an incorrect choice, an effect which was also observed after disconnection lesions of the NAC and mPFC. Such effects highlight the importance of frontostriatal circuitry in integrating information about task contingencies and response selection, and may also relate to the putative relationship between the assessment of negative feedback and the propensity to be impulsive.[18]

It would therefore appear that, although common regions within the affective frontostriatal loop are implicated in multiple forms of impulse control, the precise role that an individual area plays in a specific aspect of impulsivity varies according to the task demands and likely reflects the roles these regions play in other aspects of goal-directed behavior. Furthermore, the behavioral effects of modulating neurotransmitter levels in these different regions may also be an important consideration (see Ref. 10 for further discussion). In light of these observations, the following paragraphs will focus on data pertaining to the OFC.

COMMON NEURAL CIRCUITRY IN IMPULSIVITY
AND ADDICTION: FOCUS ON THE OFC

In humans, damage to the OFC results in a pattern of maladaptive decision making and aberrant social behavior that is often described as impulsive, despite relatively normal IQ, language ability, and general measurements of cognitive ability. The impairment noted in OFC patients is often exemplified by their poor performance on laboratory-based gambling tasks, such as that devised by Bechara, Damasio, and colleagues (the Iowa gambling task).[19] On each trial, subjects choose cards from four decks to accumulate points. The optimal strategy is to choose cards from the two decks associated with small immediate gains but also low and infrequent losses, an approach which healthy volunteers learn during the course of the session. Persistent selection from the two disadvantageous decks leads to large immediate gain but heavy losses in the long term. This pattern of risky decision making is observed in pathological gamblers,[20] substance abusers,[21] and patients with damage to the OFC or basolateral amygdala.[22]

Imaging studies have revealed that the OFC is hypoactive in recently abstinent cocaine abusers,[23–25] and it has been suggested that this reduced cortical activity may contribute to the elevated levels of impulsivity seen in addicts. In addition to their poor performance on gambling tasks, people with a history of drug addiction make more premature-like responses on a version of the CPT known as the immediate and delayed memory task.[26] Data from such behavioral experiments complement results obtained from self-report questionnaires, such as those measuring delay-discounting performance, which indicate that addicts are less tolerant to delay of reward.[27,28] Collectively, these data suggest that addicts show deficits in a variety of different types of impulse control.

In terms of animal models of addiction and impulsivity, lesions to the OFC increase premature and perseverative responding on the 5CSRT. Furthermore, animals that were innately more impulsive on the 5CSRT also self-administered significantly more cocaine.[29] PET scans of more impulsive animals that were drug naive also revealed decreases in DA D_2 receptor binding within the NAC. Interestingly, a similar pattern of data has been observed in human drug addicts.[30] These data suggest that changes in dopaminergic function within the NAC may be a trait marker for impulsivity, which impacts upon the development of addiction. Whether these animals also show alterations in OFC function is yet to be established. However, using the delay-discounting paradigm developed by Evenden and Ryan, damage to the OFC has been reported to increase choice of the larger, delayed reward,[31] i.e., decrease impulsive choice. Although seemingly paradoxical, this persistent choice of the large reward despite its associated aversive consequences (i.e., the delay) could reflect a "myopia for the future" comparable to that reported on laboratory-based gambling tasks in human patients with OFC damage.[19] As such, damage to the OFC may prevent the adequate integration of information about the consequences of responding for a reward with the subjective value of that rewarding outcome,[32] such that delay fails to sufficiently devalue the larger reward.

In summary, there appears to be considerable overlap between the effects of damage or reduced activity within the OFC and the effects of long-term exposure to addictive drugs on measures of impulse control. Although other brain regions such as the NAC are almost certainly involved in the generation of the addicted state, drug-induced changes within the OFC may also be important in mediating the cognitive sequelae of addiction.

NEUROCHEMICAL REGULATION OF IMPULSIVITY: FOCUS ON THE OFC

Amphetamine and cocaine acutely increase measures of impulsive action in rats.[33,34] However, stimulant drugs are also used to treat the increased impulsivity evident in ADHD, an apparent paradox that may reflect the fact that the effects of dopaminergic drugs may depend on the basal level of dopaminergic activity.[35] In parallel to the effects of OFC lesions, psychostimulants have also been shown to increase choice of the larger, delayed reward in delay-discounting paradigms.[36–40] It would therefore appear that cocaine and amphetamine acutely increase behavioral disinhibition and promote the selection of larger rewards regardless of the aversive consequences. Such a pattern of behavior is strikingly similar to the effects of OFC lesions and has been interpreted as reflecting an increase in incentive motivation for reward.[41] The ability of addictive drugs to hijack the reward system has been largely attributed to their enhancement of dopaminergic activity, and it is clear that the dopaminergic system also has an important role to play in the regulation of impulsivity. The ability of amphetamine to increase premature responding on the 5CSRT can be blocked by lesions to the dopaminergic terminals within the NAC and can be attenuated by systemic administration of the DA D_2 receptor antagonist eticlopride.[34,42] However, global reductions in serotonin (5-HT) levels also impair the ability of amphetamine to increase impulsivity on the 5CSRT,[43] and levels of 5-HT rather than DA within the mPFC correlate with the number of premature responses made by individual animals.[44] Thus, although both 5-HT and DA are implicated in the regulation of this form of impulsivity, there may be some redundancy within these signaling pathways. The effects of dopaminergic or serotonergic manipulations targeting the OFC on 5CSRT performance have yet to be determined.

In parallel to impulsive action, the ability of amphetamine to modulate delay-discounting performance can also be affected by both dopaminergic and serotonergic manipulations,[37,39] although the dopaminergic input to the NAC appears less important for amphetamine's effects in this paradigm.[40] However, selective lesions to the dopaminergic terminals within the OFC produced effects similar to the amphetamine and OFC lesions in that choice of the larger but delayed reward was increased.[45] It would therefore seem that too much or too little DA in the OFC may limit the ability of this region to update the representation of the value of a reward when that value changes, i.e. to decrease the subjective value of the larger reward as it becomes increasingly delayed.

Exactly what DA is signaling within the OFC therefore remains an intriguing question. Data using *in vivo* microdialysis reveal that increases in dopaminergic activity are observed when animals are engaged in performing delay-discounting judgments, but not in animals that were yoked to those making the choice between the large and small rewards.[46] Levels of the dopaminergic metabolite DOPAC were also higher at the beginning of the session, when delay to the large reward was short, compared to the end of the session, when delay to the large reward was longer. These findings suggest that DA in this region does more than signal the occurrence or expectation of reward delivery, and it is tempting to speculate that dopaminergic innervation to the OFC is indeed involved in signaling the changing value of the larger reward as it becomes progressively more delayed. However, further work is needed to determine the validity of this hypothesis. Likewise, whether DA in this region is also involved in mediating 5CSRT performance remains to be investigated either through *in vivo* microdialysis or direct drug infusions. Given the parallels between psychostimulant medication and OFC damage observed in the delay-discounting paradigm, it is possible to speculate that too much or too little DA in the OFC would likewise increase premature responding.

EXPLORING THE COGNITIVE SEQUELAE OF ADDICTIVE DRUGS ON TEST OF IMPULSIVITY

While it is clear that drugs which act on the dopaminergic and serotonergic systems can acutely alter impulsive responding, less is known about the effects of repeated administration of drugs of abuse, and how such administration may affect the cognitive response to a subsequent drug challenge. Exploring these issues may provide insight into the cognitive changes which accompany the development of addiction, as well as the neurobiological mechanisms which lead to under-activity of the OFC in cocaine addicts.

Acute administration of cocaine (0–20 mg/kg intraperitoneally [IP]) produces a range of cognitive impairments on the 5CSRT, increasing premature responding and the number of omissions, as well as decreasing the accuracy of target detection and the number of trials completed at higher doses.[34,47] In comparison to the effects of amphetamine, cocaine also increases choice of the larger delayed reward in the delay-discounting paradigm (0–15 mg/kg IP).[47] However, if animals are treated chronically with cocaine (2 × 15 mg/kg

IP for 21 days) and then challenged again with an acute injection of cocaine on-task, many of these cognitive changes are no longer evident.[47] A similar reduction in the ability of amphetamine to increase premature responding in animals with a history of cocaine self-administration has also been reported.[48] Surprisingly, it would therefore appear that repeated exposure to an addictive substance produces tolerance to its disruptive effects on motivation and impulsivity. These effects are particularly unexpected given that chronic exposure to cocaine increases the hyperactivity caused by an acute injection of the drug, a phenomenon known as locomotor sensitization.

However, tolerance to the effects of addictive drugs is hardly a new concept in the addiction literature. The rewarding or euphoric effects of cocaine certainly diminish with repeated use, and one of the major criticisms of the use of locomotor sensitization to model addiction is that sensitization to the arousing effects of cocaine are not reported clinically.[49] Furthermore, tolerance to the effects of cocaine may be one factor which contributes to escalating drug use and increased drug dependency.[50] Hence, repeated drug use leads to compensatory processes in the brain which combat the drugs' enjoyable effects, and these compensatory processes may lead to increased drug intake. In parallel, compensatory processes may limit the impact on cognition of an acute dose of cocaine, but could also have disadvantageous consequences. For example, given that cocaine is a stimulant drug and increases excitatory activity in the OFC, it is probable that any compensatory process designed to reduce the impact of cocaine on OFC function would be inhibitory in nature. Upregulating inhibitory processes in the OFC is unlikely to be without consequences (see previous discussion) and may lay the groundwork for cognitive deficits during withdrawal. The following theoretical framework therefore emerges: during chronic cocaine use, stimulation of the OFC is higher than normal and inhibitory processes are engaged to reduce OFC activation level to the optimal status quo. However, if cocaine intake ceases, as in withdrawal, drug-induced stimulation of the OFC stops. The compensatory inhibitory processes which developed to preserve OFC function now act to reduce OFC activation below the level of optimal functioning, and cognitive impairment may result.

Consistent with this hypothesis are the findings from imaging studies indicating that the OFC is under-active in recently abstinent cocaine addicts (see above) and that this under-activity can be reversed by administration of the cocaine analogue procaine.[51] If the cortex really does adapt to drug-induced stimulation such that the threshold for activation is higher, and if this does contribute to cognitive dysfunction during withdrawal, then controlled administration of the abused drug or a pharmacological analogue may be beneficial in the treatment of addiction. Certainly maintenance therapy of this kind is available for opiate dependence,[52] but its efficacy is thought to stem from reduced craving or a decrease in the pleasant sensations induced by the abused drug; the effects of maintenance therapy on cognitive function has not been determined. Interestingly, the stimulant drug modafinil has recently been used in clinical trials to reduce cocaine dependence and relapse.[53] Whether modafinil improves cognitive dysfunction in abstinent cocaine users has not been determined, though it has been shown to have pro-cognitive effects in and of itself.[54]

Another question concerns the mechanism underlying the induction of these putative compensatory changes. In addition to their effects on monoaminergic neurotransmitter systems, the impact of addictive drugs on brain function can also be determined at the level of intracellular signaling pathways and gene transcription. Some observations made within this domain may reveal how repeated exposure to addictive drugs causes such long-term changes in brain function and behavior[55–57] and may provide insight into drug-induced dysfunction within the OFC.

MOLECULAR CHANGES ASSOCIATED WITH ADDICTION WITHIN THE OFC: ROLE IN IMPULSIVITY

One line of investigation has focused on transcription factors, nuclear proteins which bind to the regulatory regions of certain genes and change the rate at which they are transcribed. It has been observed that a truncated splice variant of FosB known as ΔFosB is only expressed at high levels after chronic rather than acute administration of a variety of abused substances, including cocaine, morphine, and nicotine.[58] Once expressed, it is relatively stable and can persist in the brain for weeks after the last drug exposure. Furthermore, downstream targets of ΔFosB include proteins involved in synaptic plasticity, such as cyclin-dependent kinase 5, induction of which could lead to relatively permanent changes in neuronal connectivity.[59] As such, induction of ΔFosB may contribute to the regulation of gene transcription in a manner relevant to the development of addiction. The majority of work undertaken to investigate this hypothesis has focused on the NAC and striatum, where induction of ΔFosB by addictive drugs depends on their ability to modulate the dopaminergic system.[60] Interestingly, dopaminergic lesions of the striatum also lead to an increase in ΔFosB expression, suggesting that chronic perturbations of the DA system may induce the protein.[61] Transgenic mice engineered to over-express ΔFosB within striatal regions showed enhanced locomotor sensitization to cocaine and increased conditioned place preference for both cocaine and morphine.[62,63] These mice also show a greater level of incentive motivation for cocaine in self-administration studies, as indicated by more rapid acquisition of self-administration behavior and higher breakpoints in progressive ratio responding for drug.[64]

In addition to its effects in the striatum, it has recently been observed that repeated administration of cocaine also increases expression of ΔFosB within the OFC of the rat.[47] Given the role that the OFC is thought to play in mediating 5CSRT and delay-discounting performance, it is therefore plausible that increased ΔFosB in this region may influence drug-induced changes in task performance. In order to address this question, viral-mediated gene transfer was used to over-express ΔFosB (or the dominant negative protein ΔJunD, which binds to ΔFosB and prevents it from activating gene transcription) within the OFC of animals trained to perform the 5CSRT or delay-discounting task.

Although induction of these proteins did not by itself alter task performance, it did alter the response of these animals to cocaine. In parallel to the effects of repeated administration of cocaine, over-expression of ΔFosB in the OFC significantly attenuated the effects of cocaine on both the 5CSRT and delay-discounting paradigms. Chronic treatment with cocaine further reduced the impact on task performance of an acute cocaine challenge. In contrast, over-expression of ΔJunD within the OFC prevented repeated cocaine treatment from inducing tolerance to the acute effects of cocaine on these tasks. In keeping with the hypothesis suggested above, one interpretation of these findings is that cocaine-induced increases in the expression of ΔFosB within the OFC could reflect part of an adaptive response by the brain to repeated stimulation by cocaine. To reiterate, given that cocaine increases neuronal activity within the OFC,[65] such a compensatory response could involve upregulation of local inhibitory networks to dampen the excitatory effects of the drug. This would theoretically limit the impact of an acute cocaine challenge on OFC function. In support of this general hypothesis, DNA microarray analysis of tissue taken from the OFC following chronic cocaine treatment revealed an upregulation of GABA$_A$ receptor subunits, substance P, and the mGluR5 receptor, each of which has been shown to dampen cortical activity.[66–68] Furthermore, these changes were also observed in the OFC following over-expression of ΔFosB, and cocaine's regulation of these genes is blocked by over-expression of ΔJunD.[47]

As postulated above, although adaptations of this kind may preserve cortical function to some extent when drug is on-board, it may also contribute to the cognitive impairments observed after cessation of drug use, potentially by reducing the sensitivity of the OFC to normal levels of stimulation. Preliminary support for this hypothesis has been observed by using the 5CSRT to track the evolution of cognitive changes resulting from daily cocaine self-administration.[70] 5CSRT testing was carried out Monday–Friday morning, and animals were trained to self-administer cocaine (0.5 mg/kg/infusion) Sunday–Friday afternoons for 2 hours. Initially, animals became more impulsive when learning to self-administer cocaine, but this effect was no longer evident after 4 weeks of training, i.e., the animals grew tolerant to the dyscognitive effects of cocaine. However, when withdrawn from the drug (i.e., rats remained in their homecages and did not self-administer cocaine), animals became significantly more impulsive. Over-expression of ΔFosB within the OFC led to increased premature responding during withdrawal from a period of prolonged cocaine access (6 hours versus 2 hours). These animals

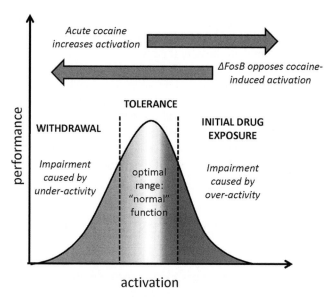

FIGURE 1. Theoretical schematic of how induction of ΔFosB by repeated cocaine administration may alter neuronal activation and cognitive performance within the OFC. Acute cocaine over-stimulates the OFC leading to a decrease in cognitive performance and changes in impulsive behavior. Repeated cocaine exposure leads to adaptive processes within the OFC, potentially including the induction of ΔFosB. This dampens cortical activity in order to counter the excitatory effect of cocaine, leading to tolerance to the cognitive disruption caused by an acute cocaine challenge. However, activation of these inhibitory processes may also lead to under-activation of the OFC during withdrawal, i.e., when cocaine is no longer stimulating cortical activity, leading to a decline in cognitive performance and impairments in impulse control.

also tended to take more of the drug during these longer sessions. Although the dose–response curves were similar in shape to those of control animals, animals over-expressing ΔFosB took more infusions of the highest dose of drug. Interestingly, lesions to the OFC impair rats' ability to regulate their cocaine intake during self-administration sessions, as indicated by an irregular pattern of responding on the drug-paired lever.[70] Although the temporal profile of responding for cocaine within each session was comparable in both control animals and those over-expressing ΔFosB, the latter appeared less able to regulate their drug intake when the amount of cocaine available was increased.

When these data are integrated together with what is already known about the effects of cocaine on OFC function and activation, the following hypothesis emerges, which is summarized in FIGURE 1. Acute administration of cocaine increases neuronal activity within the OFC. Repeated administration induces expression of ΔFosB, which may reflect or engage an attempt to compensate for this over-stimulation through activation of local inhibitory processes. A role for ΔFosB in compensating for excessive cortical activation has been suggested previously.[71] If true, increasing ΔFosB expression would essentially adjust the dynamic range of the neural networks in the OFC to account for the acute effects of cocaine treatment. This mechanism would lead to recovery of normal behavioral functioning in OFC-dependent tasks with ongoing drug exposure, as we observed, while also causing a deficit to be unmasked upon sudden cessation of drug exposure. Although the precise effects of increasing ΔFosB on neuronal excitability within the OFC remain to be tested, this model provides a theoretical mechanistic explanation of how repeated activation of the OFC leads to long-term inhibition of this region, and how both processes are inherent in the development of addiction.[51]

SUMMARY AND FUTURE DIRECTIONS

Understanding how functioning within the OFC is altered by addictive drugs and the extent to which such changes contribute to cognitive impairments, craving, and relapse is increasingly recognized as a research priority.[72] Progress on this issue is being made at a number of levels of brain function, including identification of important neural circuits, understanding how different neurotransmitters are involved in regulating relevant behavioral changes, and how these drugs alter processing at the molecular level. Through integrating what is known about the process of addiction at all these levels, it will be possible to obtain a deeper understanding of how addictive drugs alter brain function. Such information may also illuminate questions of how behavior is regulated, both under normal conditions and in other related psychopathologies, such as impulse control disorders.

Reviewing the data presented here from this perspective, it still remains to be determined whether induction of ΔFosB within the OFC is modulated by dopaminergic neurotransmission, in comparison to its expression in the striatum. There are certainly parallels to be observed between the effects of systemic administration of DA D_2 antagonists and the over-expression of ΔFosB within the OFC in that both attenuate the ability of psychostimulant drugs to modulate levels of impulsivity. Little is known regarding the role of 5-HT within the OFC, both in terms of its precise role in regulating impulsivity or drug intake, or in the downstream regulation of cellular processes. Bearing in mind the overlap between the effects of more global dopaminergic and serotonergic manipulations at the behavioral level, it would be interesting if common molecular endpoints could be identified that may explain their redundancy in the regulation of impulse control.

It is becoming clearer that high levels of impulsivity are associated with use of addictive drugs, but whether those who are innately more impulsive are more likely to become addicts, or whether repeated intake of addictive drugs increases impulsivity, is difficult to determine from clinical data. These two alternatives need not be mutually exclusive. Indeed, bearing in mind that similar areas of the brain are involved in both the regulation of impulsivity and the development of addiction and that both processes are heavily influenced by dopaminergic and serotonergic innervation, it may not be surprising to find that not only can high levels of impulsivity predict use of addictive drugs, but increasing drug intake can also increase levels of impulsivity. Preclinical investigations are starting to reveal that both situations can arise. Improving our understanding of the interaction between impulsivity and addiction could provide the basis for novel avenues of research and therapeutic strategies to target the development of drug dependence.

REFERENCES

1. EVERITT, B.J. & T.W. ROBBINS. 2005. Neural systems of reinforcement for drug addiction: from actions to habits to compulsion. Nat. Neurosci. **8:** 1481–1489.
2. JENTSCH, J.D. & J.R. TAYLOR. 1999. Impulsivity resulting from frontostriatal dysfunction in drug abuse: implications for the control of behavior by reward-related stimuli. Psychopharmacology **146:** 373–390.
3. ROGERS, R.D. & T.W. ROBBINS. 2001. Investigating the neurocognitive deficits associated with chronic drug misuse. Curr. Opin. Neurobiol. **11:** 250–257.
4. WISE, R.A. 1996. Neurobiology of addiction. Curr. Opin. Neurobiol. **6:** 243–251.
5. BARRATT, E.S. 1994. Impulsiveness and aggression. In Violence and Mental Disorder. J. Monahan & H.J. Steadman, Eds.: 61–79. University of Chicago Press. Chicago.
6. EYSENCK, S.B.G. 1993. The I7: development of a measure of impulsivity and its relationship to the superfactors of personality. In The Impulsive Client: Theory, Research and Treatment. W.G. McCown, J.L. Johnson & M.B. Shure, Eds.: 141–149. American Psychological Association. Washington, DC.
7. EVENDEN, J.L. 1999. Varieties of impulsivity. Psychopharmacology **146:** 348–361.
8. DARUNA, J.H. & P.A. BARNES. 1993. A neurodevelopmental view of impulsivity. In The Impulsive Client: Theory, Research and Treatment. W.G. McCown, J.L. Johnson & M.B. Shure, Eds.: 23. American Psychological Association. Washington, DC.
9. MOELLER, F.G. et al. 2001. Psychiatric aspects of impulsivity. Am. J. Psychiatry **158:** 1783–1793.
10. WINSTANLEY, C.A., D.M. EAGLE & T.W. ROBBINS. 2006. Behavioral models of impulsivity in relation to ADHD: translation between clinical and preclinical studies. Clin. Psychol. Rev. **26:** 379–395.
11. SOLANTO, M.V. et al. 2001. The ecological validity of delay aversion and response inhibition as measures of impulsivity in AD/HD: a supplement to the NIMH multi-modal treatment study of AD/HD. J. Abnorm. Child Psychol. **29:** 215–228.
12. CARLI, M. et al. 1983. Effects of lesions to ascending noradrenergic neurons on performance of a 5-choice serial reaction time task in rats—implications for theories of dorsal noradrenergic bundle function based on selective attention and arousal. Behav. Brain Res. **9:** 361–380.

13. ROSVOLD, H.E. *et al.* 1956. A continuous performance test of brain damage. J. Consult. Psychol. **20:** 343–350.
14. EVENDEN, J.L. & C.N. RYAN. 1996. The pharmacology of impulsive behaviour in rats: the effects of drugs on response choice with varying delays of reinforcement. Psychopharmacology **128:** 161–170.
15. CARDINAL, R.N. *et al.* 2001. Impulsive choice induced in rats by lesions of the nucleus accumbens core. Science **292:** 2499–2501.
16. MUIR, J.L., B.J. EVERITT & T.W. ROBBINS. 1996. The cerebral cortex of the rat and visual attentional function: dissociable effects of mediofrontal, cingulate, anterior dorsolateral, and parietal cortex lesions on a five-choice serial reaction time task. Cereb. Cortex **6:** 470–481.
17. CHRISTAKOU, A., T.W. ROBBINS & B.J. EVERITT. 2004. Prefrontal-ventral striatal systems involved in affective modulation of attentional performance: implications for corticostriatal circuitry function. J. Neurosci. **24:** 773–780.
18. GOMEZ, R. 2003. Underlying processes in the poor response inhibition of children with Attention-Deficit/Hyperactivity Disorder. J. Atten. Disord. **6:** 111–122.
19. BECHARA, A. *et al.* 1994. Insensitivity to future consequences following damage to human prefrontal cortex. Cognition **50:** 7–15.
20. CAVEDINI, P. *et al.* 2002. Frontal lobe dysfunction in pathological gambling patients. Biol. Psychiatry **51:** 334–341.
21. BECHARA, A. *et al.* 2001. Decision-making deficits, linked to a dysfunctional ventromedial prefrontal cortex, revealed in alcohol and stimulant abusers. Neuropsychologia **39:** 376–389.
22. BECHARA, A. *et al.* 1999. Different contributions of the human amygdala and ventromedial prefrontal cortex to decision-making. J. Neurosci. **19:** 5473–5481.
23. VOLKOW, N.D. & J.S. FOWLER. 2000. Addiction, a disease of compulsion and drive: involvement of the orbitofrontal cortex. Cereb. Cortex **10:** 318–325.
24. VOLKOW, N.D., J.S. FOWLER & G.-J. WANG. 2004. The addicted human brain viewed in the light of imaging studies: brain circuits and treatment strategies. Neuropharmacology **47:** 3–13.
25. VOLKOW, N.D. *et al.* 2002. Role of dopamine, the frontal cortex and memory circuits in drug addiction: insight from imaging studies. Neurobiol. Learn. Mem. **78:** 610–624.
26. MOELLER, F.G. *et al.* 2004. P300 event-related potential amplitude and impulsivity in cocaine-dependent subjects. Neuropsychobiology **50:** 167–173.
27. PETRY, N.M. 2002. Discounting of delayed rewards in substance abusers: relationship to antisocial personality disorder. Psychopharmacology **162:** 425–432.
28. KIRBY, K.N. & N.M. PETRY. 2004. Heroin and cocaine abusers have higher discount rates for delayed rewards than alcoholics or non-drug-using controls. Addiction **99:** 461–471.
29. DALLEY, J.W. *et al.* 2007. Nucleus accumbens D2/3 receptors predict trait impulsivity and cocaine reinforcement. Science **315:** 1267–1270.
30. VOLKOW, N.D. *et al.* 1996. Cocaine addiction: hypothesis derived from imaging studies with PET. J. Addict. Dis. **15:** 55–71.
31. WINSTANLEY, C.A. *et al.* 2004. Contrasting roles for basolateral amygdala and orbitofrontal cortex in impulsive choice. J. Neurosci. **24:** 4718–4722.
32. SCHOENBAUM, G., A.A. CHIBA & M. GALLAGHER. 1999. Neural encoding in orbitofrontal cortex and basolateral amygdala during olfactory discrimination learning. J. Neurosci. **19:** 1876–1884.

33. COLE, B.J. & T.W. ROBBINS. 1987. Amphetamine impairs the discriminative performance of rats with dorsal noradrenergic bundle lesions on a 5-choice serial reaction time task: new evidence for central dopaminergic-noradrenergic interactions. Psychopharmacology 91: 458–466.

34. VAN GAALEN, M.M. et al. 2006. Behavioral disinhibition requires dopamine receptor activation. Psychopharmacology (Berl.) 187: 73–85.

35. ROBBINS, T.W. & B.J. SAHAKIAN. 1979. "Paradoxical" effects of psychomotor stimulant drugs in hyperactive children from the standpoint of behavioural pharmacology. Neuropharmacology 18: 931–950.

36. CARDINAL, R.N., T.W. ROBBINS & B.J. EVERITT. 2000. The effects of d-amphetamine, chlordiazepoxide, alpha- flupenthixol and behavioural manipulations on choice of signalled and unsignalled delayed reinforcement in rats. Psychopharmacology 152: 362–375.

37. VAN GAALEN, M.M. et al. 2006. Critical involvement of dopaminergic neurotransmission in impulsive decision making. Biol. Psychiatry 60: 66–73.

38. WADE, T.R., H. DE WIT & J.B. RICHARDS. 2000. Effects of dopaminergic drugs on delayed reward as a measure of impulsive behavior in rats. Psychopharmacology 150: 90–101.

39. WINSTANLEY, C.A. et al. 2003. Global 5-HT depletion attenuates the ability of amphetamine to decrease impulsive choice in rats. Psychopharmacology 170: 320–331.

40. WINSTANLEY, C.A. et al. 2005. Interactions between serotonin and dopamine in the control of impulsive choice in rats: therapeutic implications for impulse control disorders. Neuropsychopharmacology 30: 669–682.

41. USLANER, J.M. & T.E. ROBINSON. 2006. Subthalamic nucleus lesions increase impulsive action and decrease impulsive choice—mediation by enhanced incentive motivation? Eur. J. Neurosci. 24: 2345–2354.

42. COLE, B.J. & T.W. ROBBINS. 1989. Effects of 6-Hydroxydopamine lesions of the nucleus accumbens septi on performance of a 5-choice serial reaction time task in rats—Implications for theories of selective attention and arousal. Behav. Brain Res. 33: 165–179.

43. HARRISON, A.A., B.J. EVERITT & T.W. ROBBINS. 1997. Central 5-HT depletion enhances impulsive responding without affecting the accuracy of attentional performance: interactions with dopaminergic mechanisms. Psychopharmacology 133: 329–342.

44. DALLEY, J.W. et al. 2002. Deficits in impulse control associated with tonically-elevated serotonergic function in rat prefrontal cortex. Neuropsychopharmacology 26: 716–728.

45. KHERAMIN, S. et al. 2004. Effects of orbital prefrontal cortex dopamine depletion on inter-temporal choice: a quantitative analysis. Psychopharmacology 175: 206–214.

46. WINSTANLEY, C.A. et al. 2006. Double dissociation between serotonergic and dopaminergic modulation of medial prefrontal and orbitofrontal cortex during a test of impulsive choice. Cereb. Cortex 16: 106–114.

47. WINSTANLEY, C.A. et al. 2007. ΔFosB induction in orbitofrontal cortex regulates tolerance to cocaine-induced cognitive dysfunction. J. Neurosci. 27: 10497–10507.

48. DALLEY, J.W. et al. 2005. Attentional and motivational deficits in rats withdrawn from intravenous self-administration of cocaine or heroin. Psychopharmacology (Berl.) 182: 579–587.

49. ROBINSON, T.E. & B. KOLB. 2004. Structural plasticity associated with exposure to drugs of abuse. Neuropharmacology **47**(Suppl 1): 33–46.
50. KOOB, G.F. 1996. Drug addiction: the yin and yang of hedonic homeostasis. Neuron. **16**: 893–896.
51. ADINOFF, B. *et al.* 2001. Limbic responsiveness to procaine in cocaine-addicted subjects. Am. J. Psychiatry **158**: 390–398.
52. KREEK, M.J. *et al.* 2004. Evolving perspectives on neurobiological research on the addictions: celebration of the 30th anniversary of NIDA. Neuropharmacology **47**(Suppl 1): 324–344.
53. DACKIS, C.A. *et al.* 2005. A double-blind, placebo-controlled trial of modafinil for cocaine dependence. Neuropsychopharmacology **30**: 205–211.
54. TURNER, D.C. *et al.* 2003. Cognitive enhancing effects of modafinil in healthy volunteers. Psychopharmacology (Berl.) **165**: 260–269.
55. HYMAN, S.E. & R.C. MALENKA. 2001. Addiction and the brain: the neurobiology of compulsion and its persistence. Nat. Rev. Neurosci. **2**: 695–703.
56. KALIVAS, P.W. 2004. Glutamate systems in cocaine addiction. Curr. Opin. Pharmacol. **4**: 23–29.
57. NESTLER, E.J. 2004. Molecular mechanisms of drug addiction. Neuropharmacology **47**(Suppl 1): 24–32.
58. NESTLER, E.J., M. BARROT & D.W. SELF. 2001. DeltaFosB: a sustained molecular switch for addiction. Proc. Natl. Acad. Sci. USA **98**: 11042–11046.
59. BIBB, J.A. *et al.* 2001. Effects of chronic exposure to cocaine are regulated by the neuronal protein Cdk5. Nature **410**: 376–380.
60. MULLER, D.L. & E.M. UNTERWALD. 2005. D1 dopamine receptors modulate deltaFosB induction in rat striatum after intermittent morphine administration. J. Pharmacol. Exp. Ther. **314**: 148–154.
61. DOUCET, J.P. *et al.* 1996. Chronic alterations in dopaminergic neurotransmission produce a persistent elevation in deltaFosB-like protein(s) in both the rodent and primate striatum. Eur. J. Neurosci. **8**: 365–381.
62. KELZ, M.B. *et al.* 1999. Expression of the transcription factor deltaFosB in the brain controls sensitivity to cocaine. Nature **401**: 272–276.
63. ZACHARIOU, V. *et al.* 2006. An essential role for DeltaFosB in the nucleus accumbens in morphine action. Nat. Neurosci. **9**: 205–211.
64. COLBY, C.R. *et al.* 2003. Striatal cell type-specific overexpression of DeltaFosB enhances incentive for cocaine. J. Neurosci. **23**: 2488–2493.
65. HOMAYOUN, H. & B. MOGHADDAM. 2006. Progression of cellular adaptations in medial prefrontal and orbitofrontal cortex in response to repeated amphetamine. J. Neurosci. **26**: 8025–8039.
66. CHU, Z. & J.J. HABLITZ. 1998. Activation of group I mGluRs increases spontaneous IPSC frequency in rat frontal cortex. J. Neurophysiol. **80**: 621–627.
67. DUNN, E. *et al.* 1996. Differential distribution of gamma-aminobutyric acidA receptor subunit (alpha 1, alpha 2, alpha 3, alpha 5 and beta 2 + 3) immunoreactivity in the medial prefrontal cortex of the rat. Neurosci. Lett. **210**: 213–217.
68. MAUBACH, K.A., C. CODY & R.S. JONES. 1998. Tachykinins may modify spontaneous epileptiform activity in the rat entorhinal cortex in vitro by activating GABAergic inhibition. Neuroscience **83**: 1047–1062.
69. WINSTANLEY, C.A. *et al.* 2006. Withdrawal from cocaine self-administration increases impulsivity in rats: role for DeltaFosB in the orbitofrontal cortex. Program No. 482.22, 2006 Neuroscience Meeting Planner. Atlanta, GA: Society for Neuroscience, 2006. Online.

70. HUTCHESON, D.M. & B.J. EVERITT. 2003. The effects of selective orbitofrontal
    cortex lesions on the acquisition and performance of cue-controlled cocaine
    seeking in rats. Ann. N.Y. Acad Sci. **1003:** 410–411.
71. POWELL, K.J. *et al.* 2006. Neonatal ventral hippocampal lesions produce an eleva-
    tion of DeltaFosB-like protein(s) in the rodent neocortex. Neuropsychopharma-
    cology **31:** 700–711.
72. KALIVAS, P.W. 2001. Drug addiction: to the cortex and beyond! Am. J. Psychiatry
    158: 349–350.

Abstracts of Poster Presentations

1

COCAINE EFFECTS ON BRAIN AREAS RELATED TO EMOTION PROCESSING

Samuel Asensio, B.Sc.,[1] María J. Romero, M.D., Ph.D.,[1,3] Francisco Bosch-Morell, Ph.D.,[1] Maria Miranda, Ph.D.,[1] César Ávila, Ph.D.,[2] Francisco J. Romero, M.D., Ph.D.

[1]*Instituto de Drogas y Conductas Adictivas (IDYCA), Universidad CEU Cardenal Herrera, Valencia, Spain;* [2]*Department Psychobiology, Universitat Jaume I, Castellón, Spain;* [3]*MR Unit, Arnau de Vilanova Hospital (ERESA), Valencia, Spain*

We have used a block functional magnetic resonance imaging (fMRI) design to investigate the capacity of positive emotional pictures to study the brain areas related to the appetitive system (*i.e.*, nucleus accumbens, prefrontal cortex), in order to apply this approach to subjects with cocaine addiction. This includes emotional pictures as background while participants performed a vowel-consonant discrimination task. Importantly, participants of the control and study groups were heterosexual males and all positive pictures were related to erotic couples, opposite sex erotica, or romantic scenes. Negative pictures were similar to those used in previous studies. All pictures were taken from IAPS. Results in control subjects were consistent with previous studies using event-related designs showing activation of amygdala, lateral prefrontal cortex, and occipito-temporal areas, but positive pictures showed a significant activation in the left nucleus accumbens in controls. The results confirm that addicts show alterations of brain areas related to the emotional processing of stimuli not related to drug addiction: hypoactivation of n. accumbens, amygdala, anterior cingulate, and orbitofrontal cortex with positive pictures, and hypoactivation of anterior cingulate with negative pictures, in both cases when compared with the control group.

2

THE ORBITOFRONTAL CORTEX, IMPULSIVITY, AND BORDERLINE PERSONALITY DISORDER

Heather A. Berlin, Ph.D., MPH,[1,2] Edmund T. Rolls, D.Sc.,[1] Susan D. Iversen, Ph.D., Sc.D.[1]

Ann. N.Y. Acad. Sci. 1121: 656–689 (2007). © 2007 New York Academy of Sciences.
doi: 10.1196/annals.1401.039

[1] *University of Oxford, Department of Experimental Psychology, Oxford, England;* [2] *Mount Sinai School of Medicine, Department of Psychiatry, New York, NY*

Objective: Orbitofrontal cortex (OFC) lesions produce disinhibited or socially inappropriate behavior and emotional irregularities. Characteristics of Borderline Personality Disorder (BPD) include impulsivity and affective instability. We investigated whether aspects of BPD, in particular impulsivity, are associated with OFC dysfunction.

Methods: Measures of personality, emotion, impulsivity, time perception, sensitivity to reinforcers, and spatial working memory (SWM), were administered to BPD, OFC lesion, non-OFC prefrontal cortex lesion control, and normal control participants.

Results: OFC and BPD patients performed similarly in that they were more impulsive, reported more inappropriate behaviors, BPD characteristics, anger, and less happiness than both control groups. They were less open to experience and had a faster perception of time (underproduced time) than normal controls. They performed differently on other tasks: BPD patients were less extraverted and conscientious and more neurotic and emotional than all other groups. OFC patients had deficits in reversing stimulus-reinforcer associations and a faster perception of time (overestimated time) than normal controls.

Conclusions: OFC dysfunction may contribute to some of the core characteristics of BPD, in particular impulsivity. Other characteristics of BPD, such as high emotionality and personality irregularities, do not appear to be related to the type of dysfunction produced by OFC damage. The similarities and dissociations found between BPD and OFC patients may lead to a better understanding of the aetiology of BPD and the functions of the OFC. These findings could have significant implications for treatment.

3

DOUBLE DISSOCIATIONS IN THE EFFECTS OF PREFRONTAL CORTEX LESIONS IN MACAQUE MONKEYS ON A WISCONSIN CARD SORTING TASK ANALOGUE

Mark J. Buckley, D.Phil.,[1] Keiji Tanaka, Ph.D.,[2] Majid Mahboubi, B.Sc.,[2] Farshad A. Mansouri, Ph.D.[2]

[1] *Department Experimental Psychology, Oxford University, United Kingdom;* [2] *Cognitive Brain Mapping Lab., RIKEN Brain Science Institute, Wako, Japan*

Macaque monkeys were trained on an analogue of the human clinical Wisconsin Card Sorting Task (WCST). This task had two dimensions (color and shape) and in each trial animals had to choose (on a touchscreen) one of three stimuli surrounding a central sample stimulus that matched the sample according to the currently reinforced matching dimension (one stimulus matched only in color, one matched only in shape, and one did not match in either dimension). No cues were given as to the currently correct matching rule so the animals had to base their decisions on their memory of reinforcement history of previous responses. Whenever performance criterion was attained in a session (85% correct in 20 consecutive trials) the rule was switched unannounced and we observed how long it took the animals to switch their performance to the new rule. Animals became highly proficient in the task, switching between rules on average 12 times per daily session and typically made only a few 'perseverative' errors prior to recovering to a high performance level after each rule switch.

Macaques with bilateral lesions of the orbitofrontal cortex (OFC) were unimpaired on control tasks that demanded color and shape matching even in the presence of response conflicts. However, the OFC group was considerably worse on the WCST task post-operatively, achieving significantly fewer rule-shifts per daily session than they had done pre-operatively. The effects of OFC lesions are dissociable from the effects of bilateral lesions to the medial portion of the dorsolateral prefrontal cortex (mdlPFC) as this latter group was not impaired at all upon the WCST. However, when we compared the effects of OFC lesions to the deleterious effects of bilateral principal sulcus lesions (PS) on the WCST, we observed double-dissociations between the effects of OFC and PS lesions upon different post-operative performance measures. Only the PS group had impaired rule memory and impaired error correction whereas only the OFC group had impaired reaction times and impaired sensitivity to positive feedback. This strongly supports the notion that these regions of prefrontal cortex are functionally distinct.

4

ORBITOFRONTAL CORTEX LESIONS ABOLISH CONDITIONED REINFORCEMENT MEDIATED BY A REPRESENTATION OF THE EXPECTED OUTCOME

Kathryn A. Burke, B.S.,[1,2] Danielle N. Miller,[1] Theresa M. Franz,[1] Geoffrey Schoenbaum, M.D., Ph.D.[1,2]
[1]Department of Anatomy and Neurobiology and [2]Program in Neuroscience, University of Maryland, Baltimore, MD

Neurophysiological and behavioral data suggest that orbitofrontal cortex (OFC) is critical for using representations of expected outcomes to guide Pavlovian responding. Here we show a similar role for OFC in responding for conditioned reinforcers in an instrumental setting. Using the transreinforcer blocking task (Rescorla, 1999), rats were initially trained to associate two different light cues (A and B) with two different flavored pellets (A-O1, B-O2). Next, in compound conditioning, cues A and B were paired with two new auditory cues, X and Y respectively, leading to either the same outcome (AX-O1) or a new outcome (BY-O1). This procedure resulted in creation of a partially blocked cue (Y), biased to evoke outcome representations, a fully blocked cue (X), as well as two fully conditioned cues (A/B). Subsequently, rats were given the opportunity to respond on levers to obtain one second presentations of these cues in a standard conditioned reinforcement procedure. We found that rats with OFC lesions learned to respond for the fully conditioned cues, like controls, but failed to acquire any instrumental conditioned responding for the partially blocked cue. Instrumental responding for this cue in controls was completely abolished by devaluation of the predicted outcome. These results show that OFC is critical for instrumental responding for conditioned reinforcement when that responding is mediated by a representation of the outcome predicted by the conditioned reinforcer.

5

A COMPARISON OF REWARD-RELATED ACTIVITY DURING LEARNING IN VTA AND OFC

Donna J. Calu, B.S., M. R. Roesch, G. Schoenbaum
Department of Anatomy & Neurobiology, University of Maryland, Baltimore, MD

Learning and decision making depend on the ability to form expectations for rewards and to detect when those expectations are violated. Evidence from recording studies suggests that orbitofrontal cortex (OFC) is responsible for the former function, whereas the latter function is mediated by midbrain dopamine neurons (DA). However recordings have not been made in comparable tasks in the two areas. To address this, we recorded DA neurons from rat VTA in a choice task we have previously used to characterize neural activity in OFC. Rats were trained to respond for rewards at two fluid wells. Across trial blocks in each recording session, we manipulated the relative value of the rewards by changing the size of or time to reward at one well. In both studies rats biased behavior toward more valued rewards, i.e., short delays and large rewards. Consistent with the proposal that DA neurons signal prediction errors, we found that reward-related activity of putative DA neurons increased significantly whenever the value of the reward available at the well increased, and then declined as the rat learned to expect that reward. Signaling of prediction errors in individual neurons was not modulated by response direction and co-varied with delay and reward size manipulations. This pattern of signaling clearly differed from reward-related activity in OFC, which tended to develop as the rats learned to expect reward. This was particularly evident when the timing of the reward changed; delay-selective OFC neurons showed anticipatory and reward-related activity that strengthened during the block as the rats learned when to expect the delayed reward. Additionally, encoding of delayed reward in OFC was modulated by response direction and did not co-vary with encoding of reward size. These data are consistent with the proposal that OFC maintains detailed information about the current value of expected outcomes, whereas VTA signals when those expectations have been violated.

6

REVERSAL LEARNING WITHIN ORBITOFRONTAL-SUBCORTICAL NETWORKS: THE ROLES OF THE VENTROMEDIAL STRIATUM AND THE AMYGDALA

Hannah F. Clarke, Ph.D., T. W. Robbins, A. C. Roberts*
*Departments of Experimental Psychology and *Physiology, Development and Neuroscience, and the Behavioural and Clinical Neurosciences Institute, University of Cambridge, Cambridge, United Kingdom*

The ability to switch responding between two visual stimuli, due to their changing relationship with reward, is dependent upon the orbitofrontal cortex (OFC). OFC lesions in monkeys, humans and rats disrupt performance on a commonly used test of this ability, the visual serial discrimination reversal (SDR) task. This finding is of particular significance to our understanding of psychiatric disorders such as obsessive–compulsive disorder (OCD) and schizophrenia, in which behavioural inflexibility is a prominent symptom. Although OFC dysfunction can occur in these disorders, there is considerable evidence for more widespread dysfunction within OFC-subcortical networks including the ventromedial striatum (VMS) and amygdala. Since the contribution of these subcortical structures to behavioural flexibility is poorly understood, the present study compared the effects of excitotoxic lesions of the OFC, amygdala and VMS in the marmoset monkey on performance of the SDR task.

All monkeys were able to learn a novel stimulus–reward association but, compared to both control and amygdala-lesioned monkeys, those with VMS or OFC lesions were impaired in their ability to reverse this association. In both cases, the deficit was due specifically to perseverative responding to the previously rewarded stimulus, although differences in the pattern of perseveration across reversals may suggest differences in the contribution of VMS and OFC to behavioural inflexibility. These findings suggest that both the OFC and the VMS support behavioural flexibility during changes in reward contingencies, and are consistent with the hypothesis that OFC and striatal dysfunction can contribute to pathological perseveration.

7

INVESTIGATIONS OF ORBITOFRONTAL CORTEX FUNCTION IN OPERANT EXTINCTION AND RESPONSE REVERSAL LEARNING APPLIED TO PSYCHOPATHY

Elizabeth C. Finger, M.D.,[1] Abigail A. Marsh, Ph.D.,[1] Derek G. V. Mitchell, Ph.D.,[2] Maggie Reid,[1] Courtney Sims,[1] Matthew Jones,[1] Daniel Pine, M.D.,[1] James R. Blair, Ph.D.[1]

[1]National Institute of Mental Health, Bethesda, MD; [2]University of Western Ontario, London, Ontario

Patients with psychopathy, a disorder featuring antisocial behaviors and a poverty of emotional responding featuring callousness and lack of guilt or remorse, demonstrate behavioral impairments in response reversal and extinction of operant responses. Studies of patients with prefrontal cortex lesions have found a positive correlation between inappropriate social behaviors and deficits in response reversal and extinction learning. Based on these findings, we investigated whether abnormalities in regions of orbitofrontal cortex (OFC) underlie the dual deficits in response reversal and operant extinction observed in psychopathy. To investigate whether (OFC) dysfunction contributes to aberrant decision making and emotional responding in psychopathy, we conducted fMRI studies of operant extinction and response reversal learning. Using a modified passive avoidance task requiring learned approach to stimuli associated with reward and avoidance of stimuli associated with punishment, we conducted an event related fMRI study to identify the neural regions recruited for extinction of instrumentally learned responses. Our results demonstrate that neural responses during operant extinction learning exhibit shared and unique features when compared with Pavlovian extinction and response reversal learning. While the role of ventrolateral and dorsomedial PFC likely differs in response reversal and operant extinction, both types of learning exhibit similar activation patterns in medial OFC. Results from our imaging studies of response reversal in children with psychopathic traits suggest marked dysfunction within medial OFC consistent with this hypothesis.

8

OFC LESIONS AFFECT MONKEYS' NEURAL RESPONSES TO A HUMAN INTRUDER

Andrew S. Fox, B.A.,[1,3] Steven E. Shelton,[2] Terrence R. Oakes,[3] Alexander K. Converse,[3] Richard J. Davidson,[1,2,3] Ned H. Kalin[2,3]

Departments of [1]Psychology, [2]Psychiatry and [3]Waisman Laboratory of Brain Imaging and Behavior at the University of Wisconsin-Madison, Madison, WI

Background: In primates, disruption of the OFC decreases fear related responding (Izquierdo *et al.*, 2005; Rudebeck *et al.*, 2006). In a recent study, Kalin and colleagues (In Preparation) demonstrated that OFC lesions decrease freezing behavior in response to the anxiety inducing presentation of a human intruder making no eye contact (NEC) with the monkey. Interestingly, an imaging study found individual differences in freezing behavior to be associated with activation of a region that included the Bed Nucleus of the Stria Terminalis and Nucleus Accumbens (BNST/NAcc) (Kalin *et al.*, 2005). Since the OFC projects to the BNST/NAcc and has been hypothesized to be involved with emotion regulation, it may be possible that regions of the OFC function to regulate BNST/NAcc activation during anxiety provoking situations.

Methods: Five monkeys that received aspiration lesions of the OFC were compared to matched controls. Each animal underwent pre- and post-lesion 18FDG microPET imaging to observe the brain activation associated with the NEC condition. We examined regions that showed a significant Group (Lesion vs. Control) by Time (Pre- vs. Post-Surgery) interaction ($P < 0.05$) and a significant post-lesion main effect of Group ($P < 0.005$).

Results: FDG-PET analyses revealed OFC-lesioned animals had decreased activity in regions that included the BNST/NAcc, medial dorsal thalamus, and the OFC. Increased metabolic activity occurred in regions that included middle cingulate and motor cortex. Individual differences in BNST/NAcc activity significantly predicted freezing.

Summary: These findings have implications for adaptive and maladaptive anxiety responses in that the OFC plays a role in modulating anxiety by affecting BNST/NAcc activity.

9

THE RODENT ORBITOFRONTAL CORTEX SIMULTANEOUSLY REPRESENTS EXPECTED OUTCOMES AND SPACE-RELATED INFORMATION ASSOCIATED WITH ONGOING BEHAVIORAL EVENTS

Tomoyuki Furuyashiki, M.D., Ph.D., Peter C. Holland, Ph.D., Michela Gallagher, Ph.D.

Department of Psychological and Brain Sciences, Johns Hopkins University, Baltimore, MD

The orbitofrontal cortex (OFC) has been implicated in behavioral guidance based on expected outcomes. OFC neurons were shown to encode the incentive value of expected outcomes. However, how the value of expected outcomes is used to guide behavior is not understood. Here we recorded single units from the rodent OFC, while rats performed a four-odor discrimination task in which the contingencies between odor cues, correct behavioral actions and rewarding outcomes were specifically manipulated. A significant number of OFC neurons encoded either spatial information tied with behavioral choices ("space selectivity") or the expectancy of either sucrose or water outcome ("outcome selectivity") or both during odor sampling, response and reward-waiting periods. Outcome selectivity was relatively stable across multiple behavioral phases: The selectivity that emerged during odor sampling was significantly maintained until the reward delivery. In contrast, space selectivity was mostly transient and confined within single behavioral phases. Furthermore, the comparison between space selectivity in correct and error trials revealed that space selectivity during and after odor sampling was correlated with locations of correct and actual behavioral choices, respectively. Taken together, the rodent OFC simultaneously represents expected outcomes and space-related information associated with ongoing behavioral events. Thus the rodent OFC may provide the mechanism by which the outcome expectancy influences behavioral actions.

10

HIGH-FREQUENCY ELECTRICAL BRAIN STIMULATION IN SEVERE, TREATMENT-REFRACTORY OBSESSIVE-COMPULSIVE DISORDER: A NEW TREATMENT OPTION

Loes Gabriëls, M.D., M.Sc.Eng.,[1] Bart Nuttin, M.D.,[2] Paul Cosyns, M.D.[1,3]
[1] Collaborative Antwerp Psychiatric Research Institute (CAPRI), University of Antwerpen, Belgium; [2] Department of Neurosurgery, University Hospital Gasthuisberg, Leuven, Belgium; [3] Department of Psychiatry, University Hospital Antwerpen, Belgium

Obsessive-compulsive disorder (OCD) is an anxiety disorder hallmarked by intrusive obsessive thoughts and compulsive repetitive actions, which often runs a chronic course. Dysfunctional corticostriatothalamocortical (CSTC) circuitry is implicated in OCD, with a relative hyperactivity of the orbitofrontal cortex and anterior cingulate cortex, impacting both affect and action. A minority of patients does not improve by any available psychopharmacological and/or psychotherapeutic treatment. About 50% of these treatment-refractory OCD patients improve by neurosurgical lesioning of the anterior limbs of the internal capsules. We hypothesized that reversible high-frequency stimulation in this target could improve symptoms of OCD.

In 10 carefully selected patients with severe, longstanding, treatment-refractory OCD quadripolar electrodes were stereotactically implanted in both anterior limbs of the internal capsules electrodes and the grey matter of the fundus of the striatum. Severity of OCD was measured with the Yale-Brown Obsessive Compulsive Scale (YBOCS). The mean YBOCS at base line was 33.8 (SD = 3.1). Patients served as their own control in a two-branched double blind randomized crossover design with a 3-month episode with stimulation on (crossover-ON) or off (crossover-OFF), followed by an episode of the opposite condition. YBOCS decreased by 54% from a mean of 29.5 (SD = 9.5) during crossover-OFF to 14.0 (SD = 9.3) during crossover-ON.

These results support the hypothesis that electrical stimulation may cause a reversible functional disruption of the dysfunctional CSTC circuit implicated in OCD, passing through the internal capsule and the grey matter below.

11

PROTRACTED DEVELOPMENT OF THE ORBITAL FRONTAL CORTEX RELATIVE TO THE NUCLEUS ACCUMBENS MIGHT UNDERLIE RISK-TAKING BEHAVIOR DURING ADOLESCENCE

Adriana Galvan, Ph.D.,[1] Todd A. Hare,[1] Henning Voss,[1] Gary Glover,[2] B. J. Casey[1]

[1] The Sackler Institute for Developmental Psychobiology, Weill Medical College of Cornell University, New York, NY; [2] Department of Radiology and Neurosciences Program, Stanford University, Palo Alto, CA

Adolescence has been characterized by risk taking behaviors that can lead to fatal outcomes. This study examined the neurobiological development of subcortical and cortical (e.g., nucleus accumbens and orbital frontal cortex, respectively) neural systems implicated in reward seeking behaviors Thirty-seven participants, 7–29 years, were scanned using event-related fMRI and a paradigm that parametrically manipulated reward values. The results show exaggerated accumbens activity, relative to orbital frontal cortex activity in adolescents, compared to children and adults, which appeared to be driven by different time courses of development for these regions. Accumbens activity in adolescents looked like adults in both extent of activity and sensitivity to reward values, although the magnitude of activity was exaggerated. In contrast, the extent of orbital frontal cortex activity in adolescents looked more like children, than adults, with less focal patterns of activity. These findings suggest that maturing subcortical systems become disproportionately activated relative to later maturing top-down control systems, biasing the adolescent's action toward immediate over long-term gains.

12

AFTER 9/11/01: GREY MATTER DENSITY IN RIGHT VENTROMEDIAL PREFRONTAL CORTEX (vmPFC) PREDICTS SALIVARY CORTISOL LEVELS IN HEALTHY TRAUMA-EXPOSED ADULTS

Barbara L. Ganzel, Ph.D.,[1,2] Pilyoung Kim, M.S.,[2] Margaret Altemus, Ph.D.,[3] Henning U. Voss, Ph.D.,[4] Elise Temple, Ph.D.[2]

[1] Sackler Institute for Developmental Psychobiology, Weill Medical College of Cornell University; [2] Department of Human Development, Cornell University; [3] Department of Psychiatry, Weill Medical College of Cornell University; [4] CitiGroup Biomedical Imaging Center, New York, NY

We previously found higher levels of amygdala activation to fearful versus calm faces in healthy adults who had closer proximity to the World Trade Center (WTC) on 9/11/01 (Ganzel et al., in press). The present study uses salivary cortisol and voxel-based morphometry (VBM) to examine the relationship between trauma exposure, grey matter density, and hypothalamic-pituitary-adrenal (HPA) axis function in 36 healthy adults: 17 (6 female) were near the WTC on 9/11/01 and 17 (9 female) who lived more than 200 miles away. Following the work of Wang et al. (2005), we hypothesized that grey matter density in the right vmPFC would better predict group differences in cortisol than grey matter density in the amygdala.

Although grey matter density in the amygdala represented the most significant regional density difference between groups ($[-23, -9, -13]$, $Z = 3.47$, $P < 0.001$), it was not related to salivary cortisol. Conversely, grey matter density in the right vmPFC OFC ($[30, 45, -6]$, $Z = 2.79$, $P = 0.003$) predicted group differences in morning salivary cortisol levels ($beta = -0.48$, $P = 0.03$). Our results provide evidence that both the amygdala and OFC experience stress-related plasticity, with OFC playing a more central role in the HPA response to trauma.

13

ORBITO-FRONTAL CORTEX SENSITIVITY TO REVERSAL OF PRE-POTENT RESPONDING

Dara G. Ghahremani, Ph.D.,[1] John Monterosso,[2] J. David Jentsch,[1] Robert M. Bilder,[2] Russell A. Poldrack[1]
[1] Department of Psychology, [2] Semel Institute for Neuroscience, University of California, Los Angeles, CA

The orbito-frontal cortex (OFC) is implicated in supporting behavioral flexibility: the ability to adaptively control behavioral responding. In humans and non-human animals, lesions to the OFC lead to perseveration on tasks that require flexibly inhibiting or altering well-established responses for optimal performance. Reversal learning is one such task that tests the ability of participants to inhibit conditioned responding to permit re-learning stimulus-response contingencies when an established set of associations are reversed. We conducted a functional MRI study during acquisition and reversal of a set of visual discriminations. Our aim was to examine the role of OFC in the ability to inhibit a prepotent response in favor of a more optimal one. Participants performed a deterministic feedback-driven discrimination task. On each trial, they were presented with an abstract visual pattern and had to deliver either a left or right key response, receiving immediate performance feedback. Monetary reward or no reward was given for correct and incorrect responses, respectively. To manipulate pre-potency of stimulus-response association, we varied the number of stimulus presentations prior to reversal, assuming that participants would show more perseverative behavior when required to reverse more practiced responses. Our results indicate that, although striatal and ventrolateral prefrontal areas showed strong activation during reversal, only the dorso-medial OFC showed a prepotency effect—a larger response when reversing stronger versus weaker stimulus-response associations. Moreover, greater activation of OFC was associated with faster behavioral responses, suggesting greater recruitment of OFC with more pre-potent responding. Combined with findings from previous lesion studies, our results suggest that the OFC may provide an important control signal for redirecting previously learned behavior in service of optimal performance.

14

INCREASED GRAY MATTER VOLUME IN THE LATERAL ORBITOFRONTAL CORTEX OF CURRENT COCAINE USERS

Ali S. Gonul, M.D.,[1,2] P. A. Woicik,[1] D. Tomasi,[1] N. Alia-Klein,[1] T. Maloney,[1] C. Wong,[1] G.-J. Wang,[1] M. Sedler,[2] N. D. Volkow,[3] R. Z. Goldstein[1]

[1]*Brookhaven National Laboratory;* [2]*University of Stony Brook Department of Psychiatry and Behavioral Sciences;* [3]*National Institute on Drug Abuse/NIH*

Functional deficits in the striato-thalamic-OFC circuit are common in drug-addicted individuals. The current study was designed to examine whether structural changes in this circuit can similarly differentiate cocaine-addicted individuals from healthy controls. The T1 weighted MRI images of 25 individuals with current cocaine use disorders and 25 age, sex, and race-matched controls were processed by an optimized voxel-based morphometry algorithm. Gray matter was compared via SPM2 in nine a priori selected regions (statistical threshold was $P < 0.05$ family-wise corrected). Consistent with previous results, the cocaine subjects in the current study demonstrated reduced volumes of the bilateral mid cingulate cortex (BA 24, 18% within the cluster) and larger volumes of the subcortical basal ganglia (bilateral putamen, 18%; left caudate, 16%). Unexpectedly, larger gray matter volumes were also detected in the right lateral OFC (BA 11, 22.5%); the larger the volume, the longer was the self-reported lifetime abstinence from drugs (r = 0.56, $P = 0.003$). Although there were no group differences in thalamic volume, the bilateral thalamus was similarly correlated with length of abstinence (r > 0.66, $P < 0.001$); they further correlated with the amount of recent cocaine use (r > -0.4, $P < 0.03$).

Consistent with previously documented functional abnormalities, the current results implicate structural changes in the striato-thalamic-OFC circuit in individuals with current cocaine use disorders. In particular, the enlarged lateral OFC may reflect mechanisms that compensate for the decreased inhibitory control characterizing drug addiction. Indeed, the individuals with the largest OFC volumes were also the ones who reported greater ability to maintain longer abstinence periods.

15

IMPAIRMENTS IN REVERSAL RESPONDING, DECREASED BDNF, AND INCREASED GluR1 PHOSPHORYLATION IN ORBITOFRONTAL CORTEX IN A CHRONIC DEPRESSION MODEL

Shannon L. Gourley, M.S.,[1,2] Alexia T. Kedves, B.S.,[2] Jane R. Taylor, Ph.D.[1,2,3]
[1]Interdepartmental Neuroscience Program, [2]Department Psychiatry, [3]Department Psychology, Yale Univ., New Haven, CT

The orbitofrontal cortex (OFC) regulates flexible responding and aspects of decision making in appetitive tasks, e.g., lesions impair performance in reversal-learning tasks. A rodent depression model that induces perseverative responding (characteristic of OFC damage) may aid in understanding the neurochemical mechanisms of perseverative behavior in depressive illness. Using a novel model of depression (chronic administration of corticosterone [CORT] and wash-out), we observed increased perseveration in a spatial reversal task. Initially, mice were trained to perform an operant response (nose poke) for a food reinforcer. After CORT exposure, the response requirement was reversed, such that the previously inactive responding was reinforced. Mice were tested using either a variable ratio (VR) 2 schedule of reinforcement—in which the response:reinforcement ratio varies minimally—or a VR8 schedule—in which the ratio varies widely, and the animal receives few reinforcers and less feedback regarding the efficacy of its response. CORT-exposed VR8 mice performed more perseverative responses and fewer accurate responses compared to CORT-exposed VR2 mice, while control mice did not differ. To independently dissect cortical sub-regions for biochemical analyses, rats in a parallel study were exposed to CORT and sacrificed. Western blot analyses revealed decreased NMDA and AMPA receptor subunit expression in the medial prefrontal cortex (mPFC), with increased phosphorylation of the AMPA receptor subunit, GluR1, in the OFC, coincident with decreased Brain-derived Neurotrophic Factor (BDNF), as analyzed by RT-PCR. Elevated cortisol may thus exert persistent deleterious effects on both the mPFC and OFC that confer risk for cognitive deficit in depression. Abhorrent glutamatergic activity and decreased neurotrophic support in the OFC might contribute to inhibitory control deficits in depression. Support: PHS MH25642.

16

RULES OF OPERATION OF THE PRIMATE INCLUDING HUMAN ORBITOFRONTAL CORTEX

Fabian Grabenhorst, M.Sc., Edmund T. Rolls, Ciara McCabe, Amy Bilderbeck

University of Oxford, Department of Experimental Psychology, Oxford, England

The reward values of sensory stimuli that are primary reinforcers, such as taste, touch and oral temperature, are represented in the OFC. (2) The OFC implements visual and olfactory stimulus-reward association learning. (3) The OFC implements one-trial visual stimulus-reward reversal which is so fast that it must be non-associative and rule-based. (4) The OFC contains error neurons that may help to implement one-trial reversal. (5) Neuronal activity in the OFC is largely sensory and reward/punishment-related, and not response related, so that the OFC can influence actions by specifying the reward value of goals, but does not link these to actions in action-outcome learning. In human fMRI studies: (6) The OFC represents the subjective hedonic value of oral temperature stimuli, with activity in the medial OFC correlated with pleasantness and the lateral with unpleasantness. (7) The interaction between the taste of glutamate and a consonant vegetable odor elicits supralinear activation in the medial OFC to produce the pleasant flavour of umami. (8) Top-down cognitive effects from the word level modulate reward and emotion-related representations of odor and touch in the OFC. (9) Paying attention to the hedonic value versus intensity of olfactory stimuli also has a top-down influence on OFC activations. (10) OFC activations reflect individual differences and decision making, in that responses to chocolate in the human OFC are greater in chocolate cravers than non-cravers. The OFC is by these computations involved in processing the goal values that produce emotional states; and projects to regions such as the anterior cingulate cortex that may link actions to these OFC predicted and signaled goals. Rolls, E.T. (2005) Emotion Explained. Oxford University Press: Oxford.

17

FINANCIAL DECISIONS IN NORMAL AGING

Michael Hernandez, B.S.,[1] Catherine A. Cole, Ph.D.,[2] Allison R. Kaup, B.S.,[1] Daniel Tranel, Ph.D.,[1] Antoine Bechara, Ph.D.,[1,3] Natalie L. Denburg, Ph.D.[1]

[1]*Department of Neurology, University of Iowa College of Medicine, Iowa City, IA;* [2]*Department of Marketing, University of Iowa, Iowa City, IA;* [3]*Department of Psychology, University of Southern California, Los Angeles, CA*

Financial responsibilities accumulate throughout the life span, yet little research has addressed our ability to handle this increasing burden in our later years. The research that does exist suggests that people may have difficulty making advantageous decisions late in life. A wealth of multidisciplinary research exists documenting preferential aging of the frontal lobes. The age-associated morphological changes in this region may have a detrimental effect on complex cognitive processes such as decision making. Ongoing research in our lab has yielded a subset of older adults who demonstrate poor performance on the Iowa Gambling Task (IGT), a laboratory test of decision making that factors in reward, punishment, risk, and ambiguity. We have developed a battery of financial scenarios to determine the ability of older adults to make advantageous financial decisions. Participants are required to make three investment decisions, each increasing in the size of the investment and the potential loss. Our preliminary results indicate that there are age-related differences in investment strategies. Among the older adults, IGT performance interacts with investment strategy. Those who perform poorly on the IGT tend to select more aggressive investment strategies. The IGT has repeatedly been shown to be sensitive to brain damage within the orbitofrontal cortex (OFC), suggesting that the aggressive investment behavior may be associated with OFC dysfunction.

18

NEURAL ANTICIPATION OF MONETARY LOSS CORRELATES WITH SUBSEQUENT REINFORCEMENT LEARNING IN YOUNGER AND OLDER ADULTS

Nick Garber Hollon, B.A., Gregory R. Samanez Larkin, Brian Knutson
Stanford University, Stanford, CA

Recent converging evidence has highlighted the contribution of affective responding in the ventral prefrontal cortex for behavioral action. Studies have suggested that attenuated incentive anticipation (as assessed by skin conductance) in patients with ventral prefrontal lesions and healthy non-lesioned older adults may be associated with suboptimal decision making (Denburg *et al.*, 2006). However, no previous studies have used functional imaging to link anticipatory neural activation with subsequent learning or decision-making behavior in healthy older adults. The present study found that relative to younger adults, older adults show reduced activation of the anterior insula and ventrolateral prefrontal cortex while anticipating monetary losses (Samanez Larkin *et al.*, under review) and that anticipatory activation in these regions correlates with subsequent loss avoidance learning. The results highlight the importance of assessing anticipatory neural responses to incentives and suggest that sensitivity to potential losses may decline with age. Further, the present findings may facilitate the identification of neural markers of decisional impairment in old age.

19

GENETIC MODULATION OF COGNITIVE AND SOCIOEMOTIONAL BEHAVIOR IN RHESUS MONKEYS

Alicia Izquierdo, Ph.D.,[1] Timothy K. Newman,[2,3] J. Dee Higley,[3] Elisabeth A. Murray[1]

[1] Laboratory of Neuropsychology, National Institute of Mental Health, NIH, Bethesda MD; [2] Laboratory of Neurogenetics, National Institute on Alcohol Abuse and Alcoholism, NIH, Rockville MD; [3] Laboratory of Clinical & Translational Studies, National Institute on Alcohol Abuse and Alcoholism, NIH, Poolesville, MD

Structural variants of the gene encoding the serotonin transporter (5-HTT) differentially affect extracellular clearance of serotonin as well as the function of the amygdala and ventromedial prefrontal cortex, regions critical for regulation and expression of emotion. Relatively little is known about the impact of the 5-HTT allelic variants (S, short; L, long) on cognition. To address this question, we tested rhesus monkeys (Macaca mulatta) carrying different structural variants of the 5-HTT gene on a battery of tasks assessing cognition and socioemotional behavior. In comparison to L-allele carriers, monkeys carrying two copies of the short allele (SS) show significantly reduced cognitive flexibility as measured by two tasks in the battery: object discrimination reversal learning and instrumental extinction. Monkeys with the SS genotype also displayed increased aggression in response to a human intruder relative to L-allele carriers. Although emotional alterations associated with 5-HTT gene variation have been described as the primary phenotype, the present results suggest that cognitive flexibility is also affected. In addition, the behaviors modulated by 5-HTT gene variation appear to be a subset of those dependent on the orbital prefrontal cortex (PFo). An analysis of structural and functional correlates of gene variation in this region may inform the nature of the genetic modulation of both cognitive flexibility and socioemotional behavior.

20

RISK, INCENTIVE SALIENCE, AND AMBIGUITY: EFFECTS ON DECISION MAKING IN ADHD

A. M. Clare Kelly, Ph.D.,[1] Lucina Q. Uddin, Ph.D.,[1] Manely Gaffari, M.D.,[1] Lenard A. Adler, M.D.,[2,3] John Rotrosen, M.D.,[2,3] F. Xavier Castellanos, M.D.,[1] Michael P. Milham, M.D., Ph.D.[1]

[1]The Phyllis Green and Randolph Cowen Institute for Pediatric Neuroscience, NYU Child Study Center, New York, NY; [2]Department of Psychiatry, NYU Medical Center, New York, NY; [3]New York Veterans Affairs Medical Center, New York, NY

The orbitofrontal cortex (OFC), ventral striatum (VS), and anterior cingulate cortex (ACC) are core nodes in the brain's decision making (DM) and reward processing networks. Abnormalities in these areas in Attention Deficit/Hyperactivity Disorder (ADHD) may be related to the impulsive behavior that is characteristic of the disorder. We constructed a "Wheel of Fortune" task in order to examine DM in ADHD. Participants "gambled" by betting on one of two sections of a wheel that was divided up according to three levels of ambiguity; 6:1 (low ambiguity), 2:5 (medium), and 3:4 (high). The sections were worth either the same (no risk) or different (risky) amounts, which were either large (high incentive salience-IS) or small (low IS). After making their decision, the wheel was "spun" and the participant was informed of the outcome. Real prize money was awarded. Sixteen adults with ADHD (mean age 35 years) and 16 healthy controls (32 years) played the task while fMRI images were acquired (3T; TR = 2 s; $3 \times 3 \times 4$ mm resolution). Standard image preprocessing was carried out using FSL. Data were analyzed at the group level in a GLM which examined activity related to each variable and their interactions. Behavioral data were entered into a 2(group) × 2(risk) × 2(IS) × 3(ambiguity) ANOVA. This analysis revealed that participants chose the less likely outcome (i.e., they gambled) more often on risky and high ambiguity trials. This effect was greater for the ADHD group, who gambled more often than controls. ADHD individuals also responded more rapidly at higher levels of ambiguity, particularly at high levels of risk and IS. There were no main effects of group, indicating that these effects are the result of differential responses to the DM parameters by the ADHD group. Initial analyses of the fMRI data indicate that ACC is activated by risk while IS activates VS, OFC, and the default mode network. Further analyses will focus on interactions between these areas in DM and group differences. Results will be discussed in terms of our understanding of risky and impulsive behavior in ADHD.

21

NEURAL CORRELATES OF EMOTION DYSREGULATION IN BORDERLINE PERSONALITY DISORDER

Harold W. Koenigsberg, M.D.,[1,2] Jin Fan, Ph.D.,[1] Kevin Ochsner, Ph.D.,[3] Scott Pizzarello,[1] Antonia New, M.D.,[1] Marianne Goodman, M.D.,[1,2] Larry J. Siever, M.D.[1,2]

[1]Mount Sinai School of Medicine, New York, NY; [2]James J. Peters VA Medical Center, Bronx. NY; [3]Columbia University, New York, NY

Affective instability, a hallmark feature of borderline personality disorder (BPD), is associated with many of its most disabling symptoms such as suicidality, inappropriate anger, and stormy relationships, yet the mechanism of emotional dysregulation in BPD is poorly understood. One possible explanation is that BPD patients cannot modulate their emotional reactions as effectively as healthy individuals. The present study employs fMRI to compare regional activation in BPD patients and healthy volunteers as they employ cognitive reappraisal strategies to down-regulate their emotional responses. We hypothesized that BPD patients would be less able to activate brain regions involved in emotional control. Method: BOLD fMRI images were acquired at 3.0 T while 8 BPD patients and 8 healthy volunteers (HC's) maintained or attempted to suppress their emotional reaction while viewing emotionally negative images. Activation data were analyzed with SPM2. Results: The HCs showed greater activation in the suppress relative to maintain condition, compared to the BPDs, in the anterior cingulate cortex, the pregenual anterior cingulate cortex, and the intraparietal sulci (IPS) bilaterally and a trend for increased activation in the tempero-parietal junction. The BPDs demonstrated greater activation in the striatum bilaterally than the HCs. Conclusions: These pilot findings suggest that BPD patients activate brain regions implicated in control of emotion (dorsal and pregenual ACC) and in attentional disengagement (IPS) to a lesser degree than healthy volunteers when trying to suppress their emotional reactions to negative stimuli.

22

GREATER ACTIVATION OF FRONTAL AND STRIATAL REGIONS FOR MONETARY OUTCOMES IN OLDER ADULTS: COUNTERFACTUAL LOSS AND LOSS AVOIDANCE

Gregory R. Samanez Larkin, B.A., Kabir Khanna, Laura L. Carstensen, Brian Knutson

Stanford University, Stanford, CA

A vast literature on reward has implicated the role of mesolimbic brain regions (ventral striatum, prefrontal/orbitofrontal cortex) in the processing of monetary incentives. However, very little is presently known about age-related changes in these regions during incentive processing. Recent evidence using both neural activation and self-reported affect suggests that although younger and older adults do not differ in anticipatory responding to potential monetary gain, older adults do show an attenuated discriminatory response while anticipating potential losses (Samanez Larkin *et al.*, under review). However, at outcomes older adults more strongly activate (greater negative signal change) the medial prefrontal cortex and ventral striatum for both missing the opportunity to win (counterfactual loss) and actual monetary loss than younger adults. Further, for older adults counterfactual losses elicit greater negative activation than actual monetary loss. The present study highlights the importance of investigating the differential contributions of activation in mesolimbic regions over time (anticipation and outcome), especially when making comparisons between groups. Further, age differences in the processing of monetary incentives may have implications for reward-related decision making and risk taking.

23

A SHOCK TO THE SENSES: OLFACTORY AVERSIVE LEARNING IN HUMAN ORBITOFRONTAL CORTEX

Wen Li, Ph.D., James D. Howard, B.S., Mark Benton, B.S., Jay A. Gottfried, M.D., Ph.D.
Cognitive Neurology and Alzheimer's Disease Center, Feinberg School of Medicine, Northwestern University, Chicago, IL

It is widely presumed that odor quality is a direct outcome of odorant molecular structure, but increasing evidence suggests that learning, experience, and context play an equally important role in human olfactory perception (Schoenbaum & Eichenbaum, 1995; Shepherd, 2004). To explore the perceptual and neural correlates of olfactory aversive learning, we focused on odor enantiomers, mirror-symmetric (chiral) molecules that are often perceptually indistinguishable. Subjects ($n = 12$) smelled two pairs of enantiomers in an fMRI paradigm of classical conditioning. During the conditioning phase, a target odorant (tgCS+) was repeatedly paired with electric shock, while the other three odorants were delivered without shock. A triangle test was administered at the beginning and end of the experiment; discrimination between tgCS+ and its chiral counterpart (chCS+) improved significantly from pre- to post-conditioning (0.25 to 0.56, $P < 0.05$; chance performance, 0.33), but was unchanged for the non-conditioned enantiomers (0.33 to 0.31). Group-level fMRI analysis showed increased activation in bilateral posterior OFC ($-14, 24, -24$; and $26, 18, -24, P < 0.001$) for tgCS+ at post- versus pre-conditioning relative to the non-conditioned pair of enantiomers. Also, activation enhancement in anterior OFC correlated strongly with the magnitude of discrimination improvement (r $= 0.87, P < 0.001$; coordinates: 8, 54, -14). These findings not only provide the first evidence concerning updated odor coding in human olfactory OFC via aversive learning, but also suggest that OFC plasticity may underlie modified odor representation such that odorants initially smelling the same can be made perceptually distinct.

24

NEURAL DYNAMICS OF OFC IN RESPONSE TO FACIAL THREAT PROCESSING AS REVEALED BY GAMMA BAN SYNCHRONIZATION USING MEG

Qian Luo, Ph.D.,[1] Tom Holroyd, Ph.D.,[2] Matthew Jones, B.Sc.,[1] Talma Hendler, M.D.,[3] James Blair, Ph.D.[1]
[1]*Mood and Anxiety Disorders Program, NIMH/NIH;* [2]*NIMH MEG Core Facility, NIMH/NIH;* [3]*Laboratory of Brain and Cognition, NIMH/NIH*

Facial threat conveys important information about imminent environmental danger and the rapid detection of it is critical for survival and social interaction. So far the spatiotemporal profile for facial threat processing is unknown. By using MEG, Synthetic Aperture Magnetometry and sliding window analysis, we identified the spatiotemporal development of facial threat processing in the gamma band. In particular, we were interested in determining the temporal response of OFC to emotional expression information. OFC is thought to be involved in emotional processing, in particular, at a later stage of higher-level emotional evaluation and emotional/cognitive control. However, due to lack of temporal information, direct evidence has been lacking. By using MEG, we attempted to reveal the dynamic response profile of OFC in processing emotional expressions in the gamma band.

We found significant event-related synchronizations (ERS) in the left OFC (BA 10) in response to angry faces. Significant ERS onset at around 170–180 ms, peaked at around 200–210 ms and offset at around 230–240 ms. Compared with ERS onset in the visual cortex (20–30 ms) and the amygdala (150–160 ms), the ERS in OFC was later. These data will be discussed with reference to models of expression processing.

25

THE ROLE OF THE ORBITOFRONTAL CORTEX AND VENTROMEDIAL STRIATUM IN THE REGULATION OF PREPOTENT RESPONSES TO FOOD REWARD

Mei-See Man, Ph.D.,[1,3] Hannah Clarke, Ph.D.,[2,3] Angela C. Roberts, Ph.D.[1,3]
[1]*Depts. of Physiology,* [2]*Development and Neuroscience & Experimental Psychology,* [3]*Institute of Behavioural and Clinical Neurosciences, University of Cambridge, Cambridge, United Kingdom*

The orbitofrontal cortex (OFC) has been implicated in the regulation of prepotent responses toward food and stimuli associated with food. Recently however, Chudasama *et al.* (Cereb.Cortex, 2006, doi:10.1093/cercor /bh1025) reported that rhesus monkeys with bilateral OFC ablations could learn, as well as controls, to inhibit a prepotent tendency to select the larger of two food rewards, using the reversed reward contingency task (RRCT). This result contrasts with previous findings that OFC-lesioned marmosets are impaired on the detour reaching task (DRT), which also requires inhibition of a prepotent tendency to reach for food reward (Wallis *et al.* Eur. J Neurosci. 13, 1797, 2001). Since the overall cognitive demands of the RRCT are considerably greater than those of the DRT and even control performance on the RRCT is very poor, the present study used a simplified version of the RRCT to determine whether OFC involvement in the latter could be unmasked. In addition, performance of OFC-lesioned marmosets was compared to marmosets with either a lesion of the ventromedial striatum (vmS) or amygdala, in order to define the OFC-subcortical circuitry involved in such regulation. Compared to controls and amygdala-lesioned marmosets, OFC and vmS-lesioned marmosets showed significantly greater difficulty in inhibiting a prepotent tendency to select the preferred of two food rewards, despite being rewarded for selecting the less preferred. These findings highlight the importance of both the OFC and vmS in the regulation of prepotent responses and will be discussed in relation to the specific control processes governing performance of such tasks.

26

EFFECTS OF PRIOR COCAINE EXPOSURE AND ORBITOFRONTAL CORTEX LESIONS ON INSTRUMENTAL RESPONDING

Ian A. Mendez, M.A., Nicholas W. Simon, M.S., Barry Setlow, Ph.D.
Department of Psychology, Texas A&M University, College Station, TX

Addiction to drugs of abuse (particularly psychostimulants) is associated with deficits in the ability to use delayed outcomes to guide appropriate behavior. This "myopia for the future" is manifest as a preference for short-term over long-term rewards, and is similar to deficits observed in patients with damage to orbitofrontal cortex (OFC). Exposure to psychostimulants can also result in sensitization of reward-directed behavior, such that subjects display enhancements in behavior directed by reward-related cues. To examine how a psychostimulant drug of abuse, cocaine, would affect free-operant instrumental responding, rats given prior exposure to cocaine (30 mg/kg/day $\times$ 14 days, i.p.) or saline vehicle were trained 2 months later in a lever-pressing task under a progressive ratio schedule of responding. Cocaine-exposed rats had lower "break-points" than controls on the progressive ratio schedule, suggestive of deficits in either general motivation, "effort," or response-outcome integration across delays. Rats were then tested at 6 months post injection using fixed ratio schedules. Cocaine-exposed rats showed significantly less lever pressing under high fixed ratio schedules, but performed normally under low fixed ratios, arguing against a general motivational deficit. These cocaine-induced deficits were mimicked by OFC lesions in drug-naïve rats, suggesting that cocaine-induced alterations to this structure may mediate the observed behavioral deficits.

A follow-up experiment examined the influence of pre-training in the progressive ratio task on subsequent effects of cocaine exposure on progressive ratio performance. This pre-training prevented the appearance of cocaine-induced deficits in progressive ratio responding. The results of these experiments provide no evidence for cocaine exposure-induced increases in instrumental reward-directed behavior (at least at the doses tested). However, they do suggest that prior cocaine exposure impairs learning (but not performance) of relationships between effortful responding and outcomes and/or responses and delayed outcomes, possibly through alterations in orbitofrontal cortex.

27

THE IMPORTANCE OF NATURAL OLFACTORY STIMULATION ON THE PERCEPTION OF WELL-BEING AND HAPPINESS

Gayil Nalls, Ph.D.
SMARTlab, University of East London, United Kingdom

This study surveyed the officials of 230 countries to identify dominant natural aromas retained through odor memory by a majority of people of each country. The study established that there are highly associative natural scents that work as olfactory imprints and memory triggers for large numbers of people of cultures in every region of the world. The results of this empirical analysis suggest that early ambient chemosensory stimulation of environmental flora is encoded, stored in the long-term memory and influences of the orbitofrontal cortex. Certain flora is attributed symbolic meaning. When aromatic cues trigger those memory influences, people can experience potent emotion, feelings, and memories, and this can often restore positive feelings and perceptions of well-being. Group identity is sometimes linked to collective response to natural odors relating to geographic location and cultural practices.

The results of the study show that early stimulation of the olfactory brain by aromatic volatile oils of regional flora may have a positive effect on well-being and on the cognitive processing and storage of olfactory information. The results of the study may also show that the use of olfactory therapy with oils of plants attributed symbolic cultural meaning may have applications in the treatment of problems associated with aging, addiction, and psychiatric disorders.

28

CHILDREN EXHIBITING HIGHER LEVELS OF EXTERNALIZING PSYCHIATRIC SYMPTOMS IN CHILDHOOD DEMONSTRATE STRONGER ORBITOFRONTAL—AMYGDALA FUNCTIONAL CONNECTIVITY IN ADOLESCENCE

Jonathan A. Oler, Ph.D.,[1] T. Johnstone,[1] J. Z. Kirkland,[1] E. C. Mazzulla,[1] J. M. Armstrong,[1] P. J. Whalen,[2] N. H. Kalin,[1] M. J. Essex,[1] R. J. Davidson[1]
[1]University of Wisconsin-Madison; [2]Dartmouth College, Hanover, NH

Functional MRI data were collected from 61 adolescent subjects (29 male, mean age: 14.7 years) during a volitional emotion-regulation task. Participants were recruited from the Wisconsin Study of Family and Work, a prospective longitudinal study of child and adolescent development. Subjects were shown photographs from the International Affective Picture System containing scenes selected to induce negative affect, and were instructed to alter their emotional response through cognitive reappraisal of the image. Psychiatric symptom data obtained earlier from the subjects at ages 7, 9, 11, and 13, were compiled and individual overall levels of externalizing symptoms were computed. The externalizing scores included subscales for oppositional-defiant and conduct problems, aggression, hyperactivity, and inattention. The orbitofrontal cortex (OFC) and the amygdala are reciprocally connected structures, and both have been implicated in processing the affective and motivational value of environmental stimuli. Importantly, both have also been associated with externalizing behaviors, including aggression, impulsivity and addiction. Functional connectivity was assessed by extracting amygdala time-series and running whole-brain temporal correlation analyses for each subject. This produced a 3D statistical brain map representing the correlation of all brain regions with amygdala signal over time. Each subject's temporal correlation was then entered into a whole-brain regression analysis with the averaged psychiatric symptom data. The analysis revealed that tighter temporal coupling between bilateral amygdala and the right OFC was related to higher overall levels of externalizing symptoms. Results of the current investigation may offer important information about the role of OFC/amygdala interactions in the development of a broad range of externalizing behaviors.

29

INSTRUMENTAL PERFORMANCE REMAINS SENSITIVE TO REWARD VALUE AFTER EXTENSIVE ORBITOFRONTAL DAMAGE

Sean B. Ostlund, Ph.D., Bernard W. Balleine, Ph.D.
Department of Psychology and the Brain Research Institute, University of California, Los Angeles, CA

In an earlier study, we found evidence that the orbitofrontal cortex (OFC) plays a role in Pavlovian, but not instrumental, outcome encoding. Specifically, lesions of the OFC made after initial training left intact the sensitivity of instrumental performance to a reduction in reward value (i.e., outcome devaluation performance; a test of action-outcome learning), but abolished its sensitivity to presentations of a cue that signaled reward (i.e., Pavlovian-instrumental transfer; a test of stimulus-outcome learning). Interestingly, lesions made before training were found to have no effect on either task. In this study, however, damage was restricted primarily to lateral and ventrolateral regions of the OFC, leaving open the possibility that larger lesions would have disrupted the influence of reward value over instrumental performance.

We are currently investigating this issue by examining the impact of large pretraining OFC lesions (extending into the medial OFC and agranular insular cortex) on outcome devaluation performance and Pavlovian-instrumental transfer. The initial results are consistent with our previous findings; OFC lesions had no effect on control by outcome value but disrupted transfer. These findings provide further evidence that the OFC is selectively involved in encoding stimulus-outcome relations.

30

DISTINCT GABAERGIC NETWORKS WITHIN THE ORBITOFRONTAL CORTEX OF NORMALLY BEHAVING AND PHARMACOLOGICALLY IMPAIRED RATS

Michael C. Quirk, Ph.D.,* D. L. Sosulski, C. E. Feierstein, N. Uchida, Z. F. Mainen

  *Cold Spring Harbor Laboratory, NY; *Present address: AstraZeneca Pharmaceuticals, Wilmington, DE*

Neocortical neurons have diverse cellular and circuit properties but little is known about how firing patterns observed in the intact brain relate to these features. Here, we used multi-electrode recordings to study the activity of fast-spiking interneurons in the orbitofrontal cortex of behaving rats. Extracellular waveforms and firing patterns were used to classify narrow spiking units into subclasses. We identified one distinct group, termed NS1 neurons, that show high firing rates, prominent spike after-hyperpolarization and little activity-dependent spike broadening—properties consistent with those of basket and chandelier interneurons. Cross-correlation analysis indicated a high incidence of coupling from wide-spiking units to nearby NS1 neurons and robust synchrony between NS1 neurons. Examination of event-triggered firing rate histograms showed that NS1 cells have relatively homogeneous behavioral correlates, suggesting that these neurons form a coherent functional ensemble with a potentially large impact on the dynamics of local cortical activity. Under acute ketamine administration—a pharmacological model of schizophrenia—firing of NS neurons was inhibited and this reduction was significantly greater for NS1 neurons compared to other cell types. Given that NS1 neurons show strong coupling to neighboring pyramidal cells, these data suggest that local feed-back inhibition is selectively vulnerable within these animals—a finding consistent with models positing that disinhibition of prefrontal cortex contributes to the cognitive deficits seen in schizophrenia. Together, these results provide novel insight into the functions of cortical networks during behavior and suggest strategies whereby large-scale in vivo recordings can be used as a tool for discovering novel therapeutic pathways for a host of psychiatric conditions involving disruptions to normal GABAergic processing.

31

THE NEURAL BASIS FOR THE COMPUTATION OF DECISION VALUES IN SIMPLE ECONOMIC CHOICE

Hilke Plassman, John O'Doherty, Antonio Rangel, Ph.D.
California Institute of Technology, Pasadena, CA

Almost all models of decision making assume that choices are made in two stages: first a decision value (DV) is computed for each alternative, then the DVs are compared to generate a choice. We study the neural mechanisms underlying the first set of computations in simple choice situations. These types of choices are defined by the following characteristics: individuals choose between two highly familiar items, the chosen object is consumed immediately, there is no uncertainty about the costs and benefits generated by the items, and the individual faces no self-control problem regarding their consumption.

We present results from a series of fMRI experiments that combine tools from experimental economics and cognitive neuroscience to identify brain areas associated with the computation of DVs. There are two difficulties in finding the neural basis for the computation of DVs. First, a trial-by-trial measure of DVs is necessary. Second, it is important to dissociate anticipatory reward and DV signals. We propose a novel experimental design that solves both problems. A key innovation is the use of incentive compatible Becker-DeGroot auctions to reliably measure DVs on each trial.

We find that areas of the orbitofrontal and anterior cingulate cortex are associated with the computation of DVs in simple choices. Our results are consistent with recent primate electrophysiology studies by Padoa-Schioppa (Nature, 2006).

32

THE ROLE OF THE ORBITOFRONTAL CORTEX IN THE REGULATION OF POSITIVE EMOTION

M. S. Yvonna Reekie, K. Braesicke, M. Man, R. Cummings, A. C. Roberts

Department of Physiology, Development and Neuroscience, University of Cambridge, Cambridge, United Kingdom

An important, as well as advantageous, element of adaptive behavior is the ability to regulate appropriately our emotional responses to stimuli within an ever-changing environment. This regulation may be relatively automatic, as in the case of the decline in an emotional response once the emotion-eliciting stimulus has been withdrawn, or may involve higher-order cognitive control, as when required to actively suppress an emotional response upon presentation of an emotion-eliciting stimulus. A number of recent studies in rats and humans have highlighted the importance of the medial and lateral prefrontal cortex (PFC) in certain aspects of emotional regulation such as extinction of fear responses, active suppression and re-appraisal. In contrast, the role of the orbital PFC (OFC) in emotion regulation remains poorly understood. Thus, the aim of the present study was to explore the specific involvement of the OFC in regulating autonomic and behavioral arousal that accompanies the presentation of conditioned stimuli that predict food reward.

The results revealed that the rapid suppression of autonomic arousal that accompanies reward omission in the control group was significantly slowed in the OFC-lesioned group. In addition, compared to controls, OFC-lesioned animals took longer to adapt to the reversal of reward contingencies, both in terms of their autonomic responses as well as in terms of their behavior. Together these findings demonstrate the importance of the OFC in the regulation of autonomic and behavioral responses in positive affect.

33

ORBITOFRONTAL CORTEX INACTIVATION AFFECTS REVERSAL LEARNING IN MALE RATS DURING A SEXUALLY MOTIVATED TASK

Francisco Robles-Aguirre, Ph.D.,[1] Marisela Hernandez-González, Ph.D.,[1] G. L. Quirarte, Ph.D.,[2] Paulina Haro, B.Sc.,[1] M. A. Guevara, Ph.D.[1]

[1] *Institute of Neuroscience, University of Guadalajara,* [2] *Institute of Neurobiology, Campus UNAM-UAQ, México*

This study was designed to analyze if inactivation of the orbitofrontal cortex (OFC) with tetrodotoxin (TTX) modifies the performance of male rats in a T maze during two learning sessions, of discrimination and reversal, using sexual interaction as reward.

The OFC of male rats was bilaterally infused with a 0.9% saline solution (0.5 μL) or tetrodotoxin, at lower (2.5 ng/0.5 μL), or higher (5 ng/0.5 μL) doses. Thirty minutes later, rats were allowed an intromission with a receptive female to induce a sexually motivated state and immediately after proceed with the experiment in the T maze. A receptive female was placed at one goal-box of the T maze and a non-receptive female at the other, with the male reinforced when it reached the goal-box of the receptive female and returned to the start box when it reached the non-receptive female box. During reversal learning, the receptive female was changed to the opposite goal box of the T maze. Each learning session, both of discrimination and reversal, consisted of seven trials, with an intertrial interval of 1–2 min and with an intersession interval of 30 min. Rats with inactivated OFC did not present a significant deficit in discrimination. Rats infused with the higher doses of TTX showed a significant deficit in the number of correct responses during the reversal-learning session with respect to the discrimination session in the same group. These data agree with other studies which suggest that a functionally intact OFC appears to be essential for adequate learning behavior.

34

A GENERAL DISPOSITION "DISINTEGRATION OF REGULATIVE FUNCTION" AS A BASIS OF MALADAPTATION

Goran Knezevic, Ph.D.,[1,2] Danka Savic, Ph.D.,[1,3] Vesna Kutlesic, Ph.D.,[4] Vlada Jovic, MD, Ph.D.,[1] Goran Opacic, Ph.D.[1,2]
[1]International Aid Network, Belgrade, Serbia; [2]University of Belgrade, School of Psychology, Belgrade, Serbia; [3]Institute of Nuclear Sciences "Vinca," Belgrade, Serbia; [4]National Institutes of Health, Bethesda, MD

Various aspects of schizotypal and dissociative behavior strongly converge on a general dimension assessed by 23 self-report measures on a sample of 2193 high school students (age mean 17.78 years, $SD = 0.56$). School psychologists were trained in the administration of the self-report measures. The assessment lasted about two months. Factor analysis based on 205 subscales (composed of smaller groups of items derived from 23 self-report scales) yielded nine symptom groups converging to this general dimension (working title "Disintegration of regulative function"): general prefrontal dysfunction, schizotypy-dissociation, paranoia, depression, flattened affect, magical thinking, absorption, hypomania, and somatoform dissociation.

This dimension should be understood as a basic personality trait (behavioral disposition), mainly responsible for various types of maladaption. Taking into account our previous findings that this dimension is strongly correlated with criminal behavior, we expect that it is substantially related to orbitofrontal functioning, especially through the 'flattened affect' facet.

35

LATERAL AND MEDIAL ORBITOFRONTAL CORTEX MEDIATE REVERSAL OF FEAR LEARNING IN HUMANS

Daniela Schiller, Ph.D.,[1,2] Yael Niv, M.A.,[3] Joseph E. LeDoux, Ph.D.,[1] Elizabeth A. Phelps, Ph.D.[1,2]

[1]Center for Neural Science, [2]Psychology Department, New York University, New York, NY; [3]Gatsby Computational Neuroscience Unit, University College London, London, United Kingdom

Fear learning is typically rapid and resistant to modification. This prevents the need for relearning about danger and is adaptive in promoting avoidance. However, the ability to flexibly readjust behavior is also advantageous, and might be impaired in fear disorders. One way of studying fear modification involves reversal of reinforcement contingencies. Investigations of the neural circuitry of reversal learning strongly implicated the orbitofrontal cortex (OFC) across species. However, these studies typically used appetitive reinforcement while the mechanisms underlying fear reversal in humans are largely unknown. To investigate these mechanisms we used whole brain fMRI during a Pavlovian fear acquisition and reversal paradigm. During Acquisition, one stimulus co-terminated with a shock on some trials while another stimulus was never paired with the shock, and vice verse during Reversal. Galvanic skin responses (GSR) served as an index of fear.

BOLD responses in the amygdala and the striatum were correlated with GSR responding and more selectively with the pattern predicted by the temporal difference model, suggesting that these areas promote fear learning and reversal by updating the aversive value of the conditioned stimuli based on prediction errors. The OFC subareas showed dissociable effects during reversal: the lateral OFC was the first to detect a change in reinforcement contingencies by quickly reversing its differential responding to the predictive and non-predictive stimuli in early reversal. The medial OFC represented this change in the late phase of reversal by increased responding to the no longer reinforced stimuli. These results point to a specific role of the OFC subareas in change detection, inhibition of fear and possibly in providing a "reward" signal when cues cease to predict aversive outcomes.

36

A NOVEL DECISION-MAKING TASK TO MEASURE SUBJECTIVE VALUING

Alison Simioni, Ph.D. Candidate, Lesley K. Fellows, M.D., Ph.D.
Montreal Neurological Institute, McGill University, Montreal, Quebec, Canada

Converging evidence from animal models suggests that orbitofrontal cortex (OFC) represents the relative 'economic' value of potential choices. OFC is also thought to play a critical role in human decision making, but the precise nature of that role remains ill-defined. The bulk of the human literature to date has focused on relatively complex decision tasks involving learning, uncertainty, punishment, and reward. Here, we aimed to develop a simple behavioral measure of subjective value suitable for use in humans. Drawing on parallels between perceptual and preference judgments first noted in the 1930s, and on tasks used in monkeys, we developed a novel task requiring pairwise preference judgments across several categories of stimuli: foods, landscapes, colors, and puppies. Such preference judgments have no objectively correct response; instead, we measured how consistent subjects were in their choices across all possible stimulus pairs. We also examined reaction times for each decision. Twelve healthy participants (mean age 55 years), and 12 patients with OFC damage were tested. The control group made few inconsistent choices, and performance was comparable across categories. There was an inverse relationship between RT and the 'value distance' between choices: that is, subjects were slowest to choose between pairs that were closest in the individualized rank order of value inferred from their overall pattern of choices. A subset of patients with OFC damage were impaired on this task, with an increase in the number of erratic preference choices, and a loss of the orderly relationship between RT and value order. These results indicate that subjective value can be isolated from other aspects of decision making and measured in the laboratory. Further, the preliminary findings suggest that OFC damage can sometimes disrupt the ability to reliably establish the subjective value of stimuli.

37

PRIOR AMPHETAMINE EXPOSURE ALTERS APPROACH STRATEGY DURING PAVLOVIAN CONDITIONING

Nicholas W. Simon, M.S., Ian A. Mendez, Barry Setlow
Department of Psychology, Texas A&M University, College Station, TX
Exposure to drugs of abuse can cause long-term alterations in attentional processes and reward approach behavior. When a discrete visual cue is as-

sociated with a reward and not located at the specific reward site, subjects tend to prefer one of two strategies: maintaining attention to the site of reward delivery, or orienting directly to the cue itself, which is termed *autoshaping*. Normal autoshaping behavior depends upon the orbitofrontal cortex (OFC), the structure and function of which are altered by stimulant drugs. We tested the effects of prolonged exposure to amphetamine on attentional strategy in Long-Evans rats.

Rats received daily intraperitoneal injections of 2.0 mg/kg d-amphetamine or saline for 5 consecutive days ($n = 10$/group). Following treatment, rats were given seven days of withdrawal, then tested in a discriminative Pavlovian autoshaping task. On each trial in this task, rats were presented with a 10 s visual cue (consisting of simultaneous illumination of a small light bulb and extension of a retractable lever) located either to the left or right of a centrally located food receptacle. One cue (CS+) was always followed by food delivery, whereas the other (CS−) was not. Both autoshaped behavior (responses on the lever cue) and entries into the food receptacle were assessed throughout training.

Amphetamine-exposed rats were impaired in their ability to discriminate between the CS+ and CS− in terms of autoshaping behavior, but not in their ability to enter the food trough at the appropriate time (during the CS+ as opposed to the CS−). Rats exposed to amphetamine also demonstrated less autoshaping to the CS+ than saline-exposed rats overall. Conversely, amphetamine-exposed rats spent more time than saline-exposed rats entering the food receptacle during the CS+ period. As an additional control, a second group of amphetamine- and saline-exposed rats were tested in a non-discriminative (CS+ only) version of the autoshaping task. Amphetamine-exposed rats demonstrated less autoshaping to the CS+ than saline-exposed rats in this condition as well, implying that the observed impairment in discriminative learning was not responsible for the amphetamine-induced shift in attentional strategy.

These experiments demonstrate that amphetamine can cause impairments in discriminative learning, and also appear to support a hypothesis of increased attention to rewards rather than reward-predictive cues following drug exposure. This could provide insight into the overall reward motivation and attentional processes related to rewards (such as drugs themselves) in addicts. Additionally, the observed decrease in autoshaping behavior is similar to that observed in OFC-lesioned rats, suggesting that amphetamine-induced changes in OFC metabolism or structure may play a role in shifts in attention to rewards.

38

MAPPING FUNCTIONAL CONNECTIVITY OF ORBITOFRONTAL CORTEX

Gregory Z. Tau, M.D. Ph.D., Amy L. Krain, Ph.D., Daniel S. Margulies, B.A., Lucina Uddin, Ph.D., A. M. Clare Kelly, Ph.D., F. Xavier Castellanos, M.D., Michael P. Milham, M.D., Ph.D.

The Phyllis Green and Randolph Cowen Institute for Pediatric Neuroscience, NYU Child Study Center, New York, NY

As a processing center for social cues and affective information, the orbitofrontal cortex (OFC) is critical for sensory integration, regulation of emotion and for motivated behavior. Reflecting this key role, a body of research in non-human primates demonstrates that OFC is functionally and structurally heterogeneous. Human data is largely derived from structural analyses, lesion studies, and more recently fMRI studies. In contrast to task-based approaches, the application of correlation analyses to resting state fMRI data enables the characterization of task-independent patterns of functional connectivity. Previous studies using this analytic approach showed have demonstrated that functionally relevant pattern of activity commonly observed during task performance are intrinsically represented in spontaneous brain activity.

In the present study we explore functional differentiation within OFC using a seed-based regression analyses of resting state data from 24 healthy adults. We examined patterns of functional connectivity for 15 seed ROIs systematically placed throughout the right OFC. This novel method has been successfully used to map functional segregation within the anterior cingulate cortex and basal ganglia uncovering more subtle regional differentiation than traditional approaches (submitted). We show anterior/posterior and medial/lateral distinctions in connectivity within OFC. We expect that completed analysis will provide novel evidence of regional OFC differentiation and can have potential application to the study of brain development and clinical populations.

39

ALPHA 7 NICOTINIC ACETYLCHOLINE RECEPTORS ACTIVATE IMMEDIATE EARLY GENES IN THE MEDIAL PREFRONTAL AND ORBITOFRONTAL CORTICES: A LINK TO ATTENTION?

Morten S. Thomsen, M.Sc.,[1,2] Henrik H. Hansen,[1] Søren E. Kristensen,[1,2] Daniel B. Timmerman,[1] Anders Hay-Schmidt[2] Jens D. Mikkelsen[1]
[1]*Department of Translational Neurobiology, NeuroSearch A/S, Denmark*
[2]*University of Copenhagen, Denmark*

Activation of $\alpha 7$ nicotinic acetylcholine receptors ($\alpha 7$ nAChRs) is considered to enhance attentional function and perhaps aspects of memory function in experimental models and in man, but it remains to be shown that these actions are in fact mediated by $\alpha 7$ nAChRs using selective pharmacological tools. Furthermore, it is unclear which neurons in the brain are activated and may translate immediate receptor activation into cognitive behavioral consequences. Recently, novel and selective $\alpha 7$ nAChR agonists have been developed. We have examined the expression of the immediate early genes (IEGs) arc/arg3.1 and c-fos in various parts of the rat brain after acute administration of the α7 nAChR agonists SSR180711 and A-582941 to determine which neurons are affected by these molecules. The protein encoded by the effector IEG arc/arg3.1 has been shown to be strongly implicated in long-term memory and c-fos encodes the transcriptional factor Fos, which has been used extensively in detecting cellular activity in the brain. We analyzed the expression of the arg3.1/arc gene in various brain regions using quantitative *in situ* hybridization and detected the activation of both arc/arg3.1 and c-fos at the cellular level using immunocytochemistry. Administration of the novel and selective α7 nAChR agonist, SSR180711 (1, 3, and 10 mg/kg) to adolescent rats, produced a dose- and time-dependent increase in the expression of arc/arg3.1 mRNA in the medial prefrontal cortex and the lateral orbitofrontal cortex. By contrast, no change in arc/arg3.1 mRNA levels was detected in the parietal cortex and the CA1 of the hippocampus. Similarly, acute administration A-582941 (10 mg/kg) to adult male rats produced an induction of Fos protein in the medial prefrontal cortex and the orbitofrontal cortices. In addition, induction of Fos was observed in the limbic striatum. These data are consistent with the hypothesis that α7 nAChRs activate a subset of neurons in the rat orbitofrontal cortex and medial frontal cortex, and this activation is likely to be important for the attentional effects of this new class of drugs.

40

PREFRONTAL CONTRIBUTIONS TO THE RECOGNITION OF SUBTLE EMOTIONAL EXPRESSIONS IN HUMANS

Ami Tsuchida, M.Sc.,[1,2] Lesley K. Fellows, M.D., Ph.D.[1,2]
[1]*McGill University,* [2]*Montreal Neurological Institute, Montreal, Quebec*

Recent evidence from neuroimaging and lesion studies implicates the prefrontal cortex (PFC) in emotion processing. In particular, several studies suggest the critical involvement of orbitofrontal regions in emotion recognition from facial expression. However, there is little consensus regarding the precise roles of prefrontal regions in the processing of different emotions. We administered a sensitive facial emotion recognition task to 18 human subjects with focal frontal lobe damage, and 23 demographically matched healthy controls. Subjects with frontal lobe damage were grouped according to the main site of damage: orbitofrontal ($n = 5$), lateral ($n = 5$), and medial PFC ($n = 8$). Replicating previous work using the same experimental paradigm, we found an overall impairment in recognizing emotional expressions in individuals with orbitofrontal damage. Patients with OFC damage were particularly impaired at differentiating negative emotional expressions from neutral expressions, with a relatively preserved ability to recognize happiness. In addition, although patients with lateral PFC damage successfully distinguished subtle negative emotions from neutral expressions, they had difficulty distinguishing between specific emotions such as anger, sadness, and disgust. The results confirm the importance of orbitofrontal cortex in recognition of facial emotion expression, and suggested that this effect might be specific to negatively-valenced emotions. These findings also suggest a distinct role of more lateral prefrontal regions in making finer discriminations between subtle emotional expressions.

41

ORBITOFRONTAL DYSFUNCTION IN BORDERLINE PERSONALITY DISORDER: AN fMRI-STUDY

Oliver Tüscher, M.D., Ph.D.,[1,8] J. Clarkin,[2] M. Goldstein,[1] O. Kernberg,[2] H. Pan,[1] K. Levy,[1,3] G. Brendel,[1] M. Beutel,[4] M. Pavoni,[1] J. Epstein,[1] M. Lenzenweger,[5] K. Thomas,[6] M. Posner,[7] E. Stern,[1] D. Silbersweig[1]

[1]Functional Neuroimaging Laboratory and [2]Borderline Personality Disorder Institute, Department of Psychiatry, Weill Medical College of Cornell University; [3]Pennsylvania State University; [4]Johannes Gutenberg University, Mainz, Germany; [5]State University of New York at Binghamton; [6]University of Minnesota; [7]University of Oregon; [8]Albert-Ludwigs-University, Freiburg, Germany

Affective dysregulation plays a large role in individuals with Borderline Personality Disorder (BPD) and manifests itself as emotional instability, with a propensity toward intense negative emotional states (anger, anxiety, dysphoria). Impulsive behaviors (impulsivity/impulsive aggression), particularly in the setting of negative affective states, are considered to be another underlying dimension in BPD, and best predict the persistence of borderline psychopathology across time. A specifically designed emotional linguistic fMRI Go/NoGo paradigm was used to tested hypotheses concerning decreased prefrontal inhibitory function in the context of negative emotion in BPD. Statistical Parametric Mapping analyses revealed decreased orbitofrontal (including medial orbitofrontal and subgenual anterior cingulate) activation for the interaction contrast of behavioral inhibition and negative emotion (NegvsNeu × NoGovsGo), compared to healthy subjects. Behavioral inhibition compared to no inhibition in the context of negative emotion (NegNoGovsNegGo) showed decreased orbitofrontal and increased amygdalar-ventral striatal activity. Under conditions of behavioral inhibition in the context of negative compared to neutral emotion, ventromedial prefrontal activity correlated highly with measures of decreased constraint, reflecting the inability to inhibit and restrain impulse expression, and left amygdala/ventral striatal activity correlated with measures of increased negative emotion, in BPD patients. These findings suggest specific fronto-limbic neural substrates associated with core clinical features of BPD.

42

DIFFERENTIAL CONTRIBUTIONS OF SEROTONIN & DOPAMINE TO REWARD PROCESSING WITHIN THE ORBITOFRONTAL CORTEX

Susannah C. Walker, Ph.D.,[1,3] Trevor W. Robbins[1,3] Angela C. Roberts[2,3]

[1]Departments of Experimental Psychology, Physiology, [2]Development and Neuroscience and [3]Institute of Behavioral and Clinical Neurosciences, University of Cambridge, Cambridge, United Kingdom

Recent neurochemical work from our laboratory has highlighted the selective contribution of serotonin (5-HT) to the inhibitory control functions of the orbitofrontal cortex (OFC). Specifically, 5-HT lesions, but not dopamine (DA) lesions of the OFC in marmosets induced perseverative responding on a discrimination reversal task (Clarke et al., 2006). However, since both monoamines are present within the OFC, the aim of the present study was to determine the contribution of the DA innervations to orbitofrontal functioning and to further characterize the specific role of 5-HT. Thus, marmosets received either 6-hydroxydopamine-induced DA lesions or 5,7,dihydroxytryptamine-induced 5-HT lesions of the OFC and were tested on their ability to learn a novel visual discrimination based upon the conditioned reinforcing properties of an auditory stimulus, an ability dependent upon the OFC (Pears et al., 2003). Animals were presented with two visual stimuli, a response to one resulting in the presentation of a sound previously paired with reward (CS+), a response to the other resulting in a sound not previously associated with reward. While control animals biased their responding to the stimulus paired with the CS+, preliminary findings show that DA-lesioned monkeys respond equally to both stimuli and 5-HT-lesioned monkeys display stimulus-bound responding. These findings will be discussed in relation to the differential roles of DA and 5-HT in the reinforcement and inhibitory control functions of the OFC.

43

ORBITOFRONTAL CORTEX AND SEROTONIN: EFFECTS OF CITALOPRAM PHARMACOTHERAPY ON ORBITO-FRONTO-AMYGDALA FUNCTION

James M. Warwick, B.Sc., MBChB, FCNP(SA), P. D. Carey, D. J. Stein

MRC Unit for Stress and Anxiety Disorders, Stellenbosch University, Cape Town, South Africa

Introduction: There is rich innervation of orbitofrontal cortex (OFC), and closely connected regions such as the amygdala, by serotonergic neurons. Previous work has established that anxiety disorders are mediated by amygdala hyperactivation, and that selective serotonin reuptake inhibitor (SSRI) treatment of anxiety disorders results in OFC deactivation. However, the effect of SSRIs on OFC-amygdala connectivity is not been established.

Materials & Methods: Seventeen patients meeting DSM-IV criteria for generalized Social Anxiety Disorder (SAD) underwent resting brain SPECT using [Tc-99m]-HMPAO before and following 8 weeks of citalopram pharmacotherapy. Data were analyzed in a voxel-wise manner using SPM2, with a focus on detecting changes in resting OFC function, and in OCF connectivity with the amygdala, after treatment with this SSRI.

Results: A 22 voxel ($1.3\,\text{cm}^3$) cluster of significantly decreased resting perfusion was found in orbito-frontal cortex, just to the left of the midline ($P < 0.001$). A functional connectivity analysis of the scans revealed a positive correlation between the OFC and the right amygdala on citalopram ($P < 0.05$) that was not present prior to therapy.

Conclusion: These data confirm previous data that SSRI treatment of an anxiety disorder results in reduced activity in OFC. Further, there was evidence for enhanced connectivity between the OFC and right amygdala following SSRI therapy. Optimization of OCF-amygdala interaction by SSRIs may facilitate processes such as reversal learning, and so decrease anxiety symptoms.

Index of Contributors

691